Huszar's
BASIC DYSRHYTHMIAS
and Acute Coronary Syndromes

Interpretation and
Management

Fourth Edition

Huszar's BASIC DYSRHYTHMIAS and Acute Coronary Syndromes

Interpretation and Management

Keith Wesley, MD
Medical Director
HealthEast Medical Transportation
St. Paul, Minnesota

Medical Director
United EMS
Wisconsin Rapids, Wisconsin

Medical Director
Chippewa Fire District
Chippewa Falls, Wisconsin

ELSEVIER
MOSBY JEMS

3251 Riverport Lane
St. Louis, Missouri 63043

HUSZAR'S BASIC DYSRHYTHMIAS: INTERPRETATION
AND MANAGEMENT, FOURTH EDITION

ISBN: 978-0-323-03974-1

Copyright © 2011, 2007, 2002, 1998 by Mosby, Inc., an affiliate of Elsevier Inc.

Notices

Knowledge and best practice in this field are constantly changing. As new research and experience broaden our understanding, changes in research methods, professional practices, or medical treatment may become necessary.

Practitioners and researchers must always rely on their own experience and knowledge in evaluating and using any information, methods, compounds, or experiments described herein. In using such information or methods they should be mindful of their own safety and the safety of others, including parties for whom they have a professional responsibility.

With respect to any drug or pharmaceutical products identified, readers are advised to check the most current information provided (i) on procedures featured or (ii) by the manufacturer of each product to be administered, to verify the recommended dose or formula, the method and duration of administration, and contraindications. It is the responsibility of practitioners, relying on their own experience and knowledge of their patients, to make diagnoses, to determine dosages and the best treatment for each individual patient, and to take all appropriate safety precautions.

To the fullest extent of the law, neither the Publisher nor the authors, contributors, or editors, assume any liability for any injury and/or damage to persons or property as a matter of products liability, negligence or otherwise, or from any use or operation of any methods, products, instructions, or ideas contained in the material herein.

ISBN: 978-0-323-03974-1

Vice President and Publisher: Andrew Allen
Executive Editor: Linda Honeycutt Dickison
Senior Developmental Editor: Laura Bayless
Publishing Services Manager: Julie Eddy
Senior Project Manager: Andrea Campbell
Design Direction: Jessica Williams

Printed in China

Last digit is the print number: 9 8 7 6 5 4 3 2 1

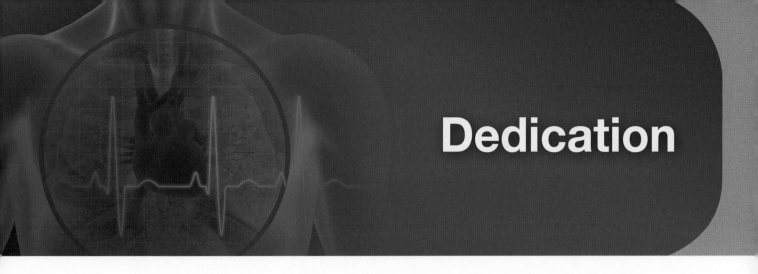

Dedication

This book is dedicated to my wife Karen and three sons JT, Austin, and Camden.

Without your love, confidence, and patience, I could not have pursued my dream.

I love you.

It is with great gratitude and humility that I continue Dr. Huszar's legacy of this wonderful text.

Keith Wesley, MD

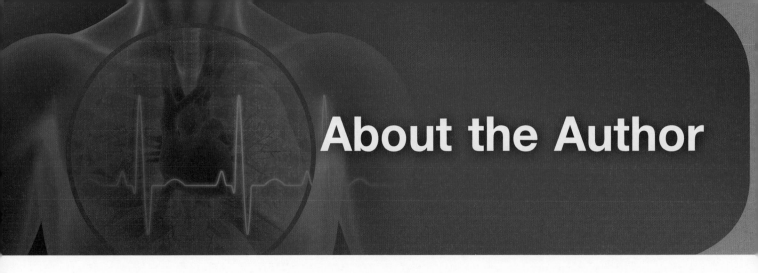

About the Author

Keith Wesley is a board-certified emergency medicine physician living in Wisconsin. Originally from Tyler, Texas, he graduated from Brigham Young University in 1982 and Baylor College of Medicine in Houston, Texas in 1986. He completed an Emergency Medicine Residency at Methodist Hospital in Indianapolis, Indiana, where he gained his first exposure to EMS flying air medical missions.

Dr. Wesley has been involved in EMS since 1989, working with many services in Wisconsin. In 1992, he was selected by the Governor as a founding member of the Wisconsin State Physician Advisory Committee and served for 12 years, the last 4 years as Chair. In 2006, Dr. Wesley was selected as the Wisconsin State EMS Medical Director and continues to provide medical oversight to several services throughout Wisconsin.

From 1992 to 2004, Dr. Wesley was a Clinical Assistant Professor, University of Wisconsin Family Practice Residency, Eau Claire, Wisconsin responsible for the training and education of family practice residents rotating through the emergency department. During the same period, Dr. Wesley was an ACLS instructor overseeing the courses throughout south central Wisconsin.

In 2008, Dr. Wesley moved his practice to Minnesota when he accepted the position as the Minnesota State EMS Medical Director. He currently works for HealthEast Care Systems in St. Paul, where he is the EMS Medical Director for HealthEast Medical Transportation.

Dr. Wesley is a former chair of the National Council of State EMS Medical Directors and is active in the National Association of EMS Physicians. Dr. Wesley has co-authored four textbooks and numerous articles and papers and is a frequent speaker at state and national conferences. He is currently on the editorial board for JEMS magazine.

An active member of the American College of Emergency Physicians and the National Association of EMS Physicians, Dr. Wesley has been actively involved in the creation of educational programs for medical and nursing students, EMTs, and physicians.

When not engaged in EMS duties, Dr. Wesley enjoys sailing on Lake Superior with his wife Karen and spending time with his three sons.

Acknowledgments

First, I would like to thank the dedicated men and women of my EMS services who provided me encouragement, criticism, and reams of rhythms strips and 12 leads. They include HealthEast Medical Transportation, Chippewa Fire District, Higgins Ambulance, and the EMT-Basic services of Ashland and Bayfield Counties.

Next, I must acknowledge the successful foundation upon which this book is based. Dr. Huszar expertly crafted this text in three previous editions. To be given the opportunity to carry on where this great man left off is an honor.

Finally, no author can accomplish anything without an editor. I have been most fortunate to have not one but two excellent editors with Laura Bayless and Andrea Campbell. Thank you both for the encouragement to make this project a success. Also, I'd like to thank Linda Honeycutt for giving me this opportunity and her tireless support.

Keith Wesley, MD

Publisher Acknowledgments

The editors wish to acknowledge the reviewers of the fourth edition of this book for their invaluable assistance in developing and fine-tuning this manuscript.

Janet Fitts, RN, BSN, CEN, TNS, EMT-P
Owner/Educational Consultant
Prehospital Emergency Medical Education
Pacific, Missouri
Paramedic/Training Officer
New Haven Ambulance District
New Haven, Missouri

Mark Goldstein, RN, MSN, EMT-P I/C
Emergency Services Operations Manager
Memorial Health System–Emergency & Trauma Center
Colorado Springs, Colorado

Kevin T. Collopy, BA, CCEMT-P, NREMT-P, WEMT
Lead Instructor
Wilderness Medical Associates
Flight Paramedic
Spirit MTS, St. Joseph's Hospital
Marshfield, Wisconsin

Robert L. Jackson, Jr., BA, MAPS, MAR, NREMT-P, CCEMT-P
Paramedic
University of Missouri Healthcare
Columbia, Missouri

Ronald N. Roth, MD, FACEP
Professor of Emergency Medicine
University of Pittsburgh, School of Medicine
Medical Director, City of Pittsburgh
Department of Public Safety
Pittsburgh, Pennsylvania

Lynn Pierzchalski-Goldstein, PharmD
Clinical Coordinator
Penrose St Francis Health System
Colorado Springs, Colorado

David L. Sullivan, PhD, NREMT-P
Program Director
Emergency Medical Services–Continuing Medical Education
St. Petersburg College–Health Education Center
Pinellas Park, Florida

Gilbert N. Taylor FF/NREMT-P,I/C
Fire Investigator
Bourne Fire and Rescue
Bourne, Massachusetts

Our continued thanks also go out to the previous edition reviewers, whose hard work continues to contribute to the ongoing success of this book: Robert Carter, Robert Cook, Robert Elling, Timothy Frank, Glen A. Hoffman, Kevin B. Kraus, Mikel Rothenburg, Judith Ruple, Ronald D. Taylor, Glen Treankler, and Andrew W. Stern.

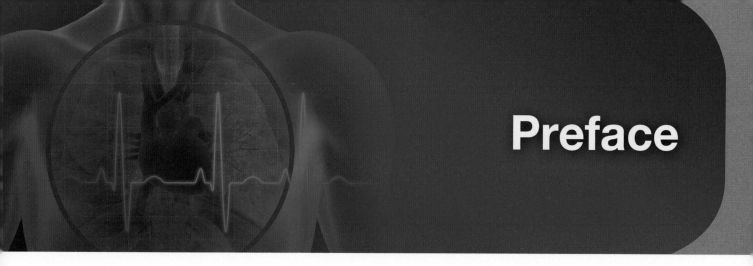

Preface

This text was written to teach medical, nursing, and EMS providers the basic skills in cardiac dysrhythmia interpretation. Once this is accomplished, the student discovers advanced instruction in the clinical signs, symptoms, and management of patients presenting with cardiac dysrhythmias.

With the advent of ECG monitoring has come readily accessible 12-lead electrocardiography, an essential tool in the detection and management of acute coronary syndromes. It is for that reason that this edition has added several chapters dedicated to 12-lead ECG interpretation. Following these, the student is provided an in-depth review of the pathophysiology, clinical signs and symptoms, and management of acute coronary syndromes.

The amount of anatomy, physiology, and pathophysiology has been significantly increased from previous versions to better enable the student to develop a more comprehensive understanding of the cause of particular dysrhythmias and coronary syndromes. This knowledge provides the student additional tools to accurately interpret and manage the presented dysrhythmias and conditions.

Each dysrhythmia is presented in its "classic," form with an associated table listing its unique characteristics. These tables can be used as a quick reference. The accompanying text contains a more detailed and extensive discussion of these characteristics.

The majority of rhythm strips are from real patients and will not always include all of the "classic" characteristics described in the text. This is the challenge of ECG dysrhythmia interpretation, and the student should take this into consideration when examining any rhythm strip.

The treatment algorithms are based on the latest information from the American Heart Association and the American College of Cardiology recommendations. However, because the science continues to evolve and local policy and protocol may vary, the student should remain abreast of new treatments and consult local medical experts to ensure that their treatment remains current.

Throughout the text, the student will encounter text contained in boxes that provides particularly important information. They include:

Key Point

These contain a summary of the most important information presented on the associated text.

Author Notes

These contain information related to how the information is being presented and how it may differ from other text. This information is provided to ensure that the student clearly understands the conventions used by the author.

Clinical Notes

These contain information related specifically to the medical diagnosis and management of a particular condition.

Key Definition

These contain an extensive definition of a particular term discussed in the text. A full glossary is enclosed in the back of the text; however, these Key Definitions will elaborate on the relevant term

Chapter summary questions covering the major points are presented and, in combination with the self-assessment questions in Appendix C, provide the student additional practice in ECG interpretation intended to increase competency. For those particularly interested in ECG axis interpretation, Appendix A provides an extensive review of the subject.

Each chapter builds on the points and interpretation skills previously presented, and by moving sequentially through them, each the student will have all the information they need to intelligently interpret ECG dysrhythmias and 12-lead ECGs, and develop a clinically sound management plan.

Welcome to this exciting, critical, and sometimes challenging subject.

Keith Wesley, MD

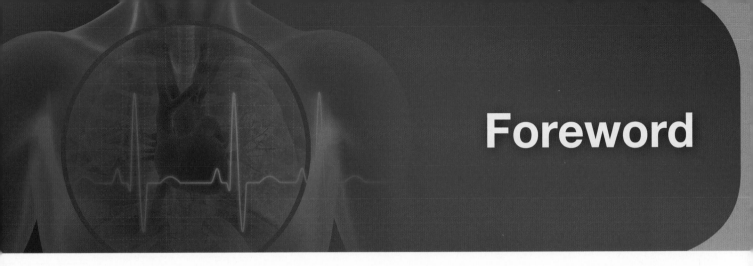

Foreword

This 2010 edition of Drs. Wesley and Huszar's *Basic Dysrhythmias and Acute Coronary Syndromes: Interpretation and Management* marks the 109th year since the technique known as electrocardiography was first reported by the eminent Dutch physiologist William Einthoven. With this fundamental discovery came a new methodology that has forever changed the face of medicine and guided the care of patients with heart disease, especially those with acute cardiac pathology. Given that the correct interpretation of an electrocardiogram provides a non-invasive legend to diagnosing and treating heart rhythm disorders and acute coronary syndromes, it is critical that all clinicians who care for patients with the potential for cardiac disease feel comfortable knowing how to understand and use this vital tool.

In the span of a little over a century since the ECG was introduced, the squiggly lines of print on a piece of paper have become a clinical guide and call to action. Knowing how to interpret this code and what to do with the correct interpretation requires knowledge and practice. This new edition provides this comprehensive information in a concise and straightforward manner. Each chapter is user-friendly and provides state-of-the art information. Dr. Wesley is an emergency department physician, EMS Medical Director with decades of clinical experience, *and* a skilled writer and educator. He has supplemented the previous edition with up-to-date information, especially in the area of the treatment of acute coronary syndromes and cardiac arrest. The text is easy to read, the figures are refreshing and easy to understand, and each section contains a self-assessment test to help reinforce the key messages.

This book builds on the adage that knowledge is power: this book provides knowledge that can be life-saving. Rooted upon the foundation of vector cardiography and electrophysiology that forms the geometric and physiological underpinnings of ECG analysis and understanding, the chapters on ECG interpretation, pacemakers and defibrillators, and treatment algorithms are a translational toolkit for emergency medical technicians, paramedics, nursing student and nurses, medical students, and physicians. They provide a means to learn at one's own pace and then deliver care based on a solid understanding of the essentials of cardiac pathophysiology, especially in the acute care setting. This book is particularly helpful for the new clinician: it helps take the fear out of treating patients with life-threatening cardiac abnormalities and empowers them by providing the tools for action.

Finally it is important to re-emphasize that, although *Basic Dysrhythmias and Acute Coronary Syndromes* is encyclopedic in size and content, it is organized in a way such that it can be used on the job in the emergency department, on the telemetry wards, in an intensive care unit, or on the street in the back of an ambulance. When taking care of a patient with a dysrhythmia or acute infarction, the clinician can see this text as a blueprint and will not need to look beyond it for complete guidance.

As you turn the pages of this book as a reference or use it to learn the essentials of cardiac care, I hope you enjoy this learning process. We are living in an extraordinary age in medicine and the teaching messages in this text reflect the incredible progress over the past century. From the first ECG tracings reported at the beginning of the 20th century, we now have the clinical tools to transform the information from an ECG into definitive and life-saving care. That translational process is dynamic: this text provides the key up-to-date pathways to successfully treat patients and save lives based on the widespread use of cardiac electrogram. I encourage you to use it as a vital resource.

Keith Lurie, MD
Cardiac electrophysiologist
Professor of Emergency and Internal Medicine
University of Minnesota
Minneapolis, Minnesota

Publisher's Note

The author and publisher have made every attempt to check dosages and advanced life support content for accuracy. The care procedures presented here represent accepted practices in the United States. They are not offered as a standard of care. Advanced life support–level emergency care is performed under the authority of a licensed physician. It is the student's responsibility to know and follow local care protocols as provided by his or her medical advisors. It is also the student's responsibility to stay informed of emergency care procedure changes, including the most recent guidelines set forth by the American Heart Association and printed in their textbooks.

Contents

1

Anatomy and Physiology of the Heart

OBJECTIVES *Upon completion of this chapter, you should be able to:*

1. Name and identify the following anatomical features of the heart:
   - The right atria, right ventricle, left atria, and left ventricle of the heart
   - The three layers of the ventricular walls
   - The base and apex of the heart
   - The layers of the pericardium and its associated spaces
2. Define the right heart and left heart and the primary function of each with respect to the pulmonary and systemic circulations.
3. Name and locate on an anatomical drawing the following major structures of the circulatory system:
   - The aorta
   - The pulmonary artery
   - The superior and inferior vena cavae
   - The coronary sinus
   - The pulmonary veins
   - The four heart valves
4. Define the following:
   - Atrial systole and diastole
   - Ventricular systole and diastole
5. Name and identify the components of the electrical conduction system of the heart.
6. Name the two basic types of cardiac cells and describe their function.
7. List and define the three major types of accessory conduction pathways, including their location, conduction capabilities, and potential for disrupting normal cardiac function.
8. Name and define the four properties of cardiac cells.
9. Describe the difference between a resting, a polarized, and a depolarized cardiac cell.
10. Define the following:
    - Depolarization process
    - Repolarization process
    - Threshold potential
11. Name and locate on a schematic of a cardiac action potential the five phases of a cardiac potential.

12. Define and locate on an ECG the following:
    - Absolute refractory period
    - Relative refractory period
13. Explain the property of automaticity (spontaneous depolarization) and how the slope of phase-4 depolarization relates to the rate of impulse formation.
14. On a chart of the heart, trace the normal conduction pathway of the heart.
15. Define the following:
    - Dominant and escape pacemaker cells
    - Nonpacemaker cells
16. Define and locate the primary, escape, and ectopic pacemakers of the heart.
17. Define inherent firing rate and give the inherent firing rates of the following:
    - SA node
    - AV junction
    - Ventricles
18. Give three conditions under which an escape pacemaker may assume the role of pacemaker of the heart.
19. List and define the three basic mechanisms that are responsible for ectopic beats and rhythms.
20. Describe the components of the nervous system controlling the heart.
21. List the effects on the heart produced by the stimulation of the sympathetic and parasympathetic nervous system.

ANATOMY AND PHYSIOLOGY OF THE HEART

Anatomy of the Heart

The heart, whose sole purpose is to circulate blood through the circulatory system (the blood vessels of the body), consists of four hollow chambers (Figure 1-1). The upper two chambers, the *right and left atria*, are thin-walled; the lower two chambers, the *right and left ventricles*, are thick-walled and muscular. Because the heart is anchored to the vascular system at the atria, the two atria are referred to as the base of the heart while the ventricles are called the apex of the heart.

The walls of the atria and ventricles are composed of three layers of tissue: the innermost thin layer is called the *endocardium* and is smooth to promote low friction movement of blood; the middle layer is the *myocardium* and contains the muscle cells. The outermost layer, the *epicardium,* is a thin layer of smooth connective tissue.

In the ventricles the myocardium is divided into the *subendocardial area,* which is the inner half of the myocardium, and the *subepicardial area*, the outer half of the myocardium. Compared to the right ventricles, the walls of the left ventricle are more muscular and therefore approximately three times thicker. The atrial walls are also composed of three layers of tissue, like those of the ventricles, but the middle muscular layer is much thinner.

The heart is enclosed in the *pericardium*, which consists of an outer tough layer the *fibrous pericardium* (Figure 1-2), which comes into direct contact with the lung. The inner layer of the pericardium is called the *serous pericardium*. The *visceral pericardium*, or, as it is more commonly known, the *epicardium*, covers the heart itself. Between the visceral pericardium and the pericardial sac is the *pericardial space or cavity*. It normally contains up to 50 mL of *pericardial fluid*, which helps to lubricate the movements of the heart within the pericardium.

Inferiorly, the pericardium is attached to the center of the diaphragm. Anteriorly, it is attached to the sternum; posteriorly, to the esophagus, trachea, and main bronchi; and at the base of the heart, to the aorta, vena cava, and pulmonary veins. In this way, the pericardium anchors the heart to the chest and limits its movement within the mediastinum.

The *interatrial septum* (a thin membranous wall) separates the two atria, and a thicker, more muscular wall, the *interventricular septum*, separates the two ventricles. The two septa, in effect, divide the heart into two pumping systems, the *right heart* and *left heart*, each one consisting of an atrium and a ventricle.

Circulation of the Blood Through the Heart

The right heart pumps blood into the pulmonary circulation. The left heart pumps blood into the systemic circulation. The systemic circulation includes the coronary circulation, which supplies the heart through the coronary arteries.

The right atrium receives deoxygenated blood from the body via two of the body's largest veins (the superior vena cava and inferior vena cava) and from the heart itself by way of the coronary sinus (see Figure 1-1). The blood is delivered to the right ventricle through the tricuspid valve. The right ventricle then pumps the deoxygenated blood through the pulmonic valve and into the lungs via the pulmonary artery. In the lungs, the blood picks up oxygen and releases carbon dioxide.

The left atrium receives the newly oxygenated blood from the lungs via the pulmonary veins and delivers it to the left ventricle through the mitral valve. The left ventricle then pumps the oxygenated blood out through the aortic valve and into the aorta, the largest artery in the body. From the aorta, the blood is distributed throughout the body, including the heart, where the blood releases oxygen to the cells.

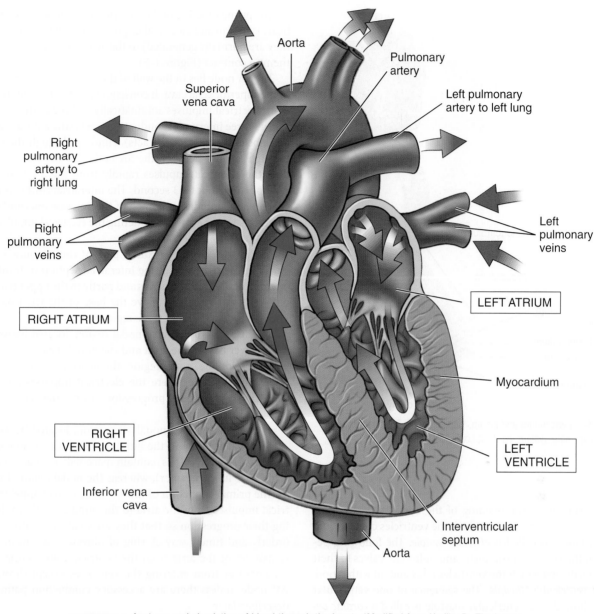

FIGURE 1-1 Anatomy and circulation of blood through the heart. (Modified from Herlihy B: *The human body in health and illness*, ed 3, St Louis, 2007, Saunders.)

Atrial and Ventricular Diastole and Systole

The heart performs its pumping action over and over in a rhythmic sequence as follows (Figure 1-3):

1. First, the atria relax (atrial diastole), allowing the blood to pour in from the vena cavae and lungs.
2. As the atria fill with blood, the atrial pressure rises above that in the ventricles, forcing the tricuspid and mitral valves *(atrioventricular valves)* to open and allowing the blood to empty rapidly into the relaxed ventricles.
3. Then, the atria contract (atrial systole), filling the ventricles to capacity. After the contraction of the atria, the pressures in the atria and ventricles equalize and the tricuspid and mitral valves begin to close.
4. Then, the ventricles contract vigorously (ventricular systole), causing the ventricular pressure to rise sharply. As the tri-

cuspid and mitral valves close completely, the aortic and pulmonic valves snap open, allowing the blood to be ejected forcefully into the pulmonary and systemic circulations.

5. Meanwhile, the atria are again relaxing and filling with blood. As soon as the ventricles empty of blood and begin to relax (ventricular diastole), the ventricular pressure falls, the aortic and pulmonic valves shut tightly, the tricuspid and mitral valves open, and the rhythmic cardiac sequence begins anew.

> It is during ventricular diastole when the aortic valve is closed that coronary perfusion occurs.

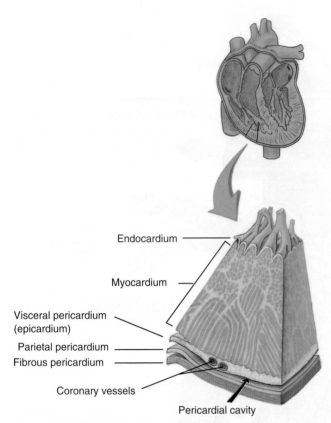

Endocardium

Myocardium

Visceral pericardium (epicardium)

Parietal pericardium

Fibrous pericardium

Coronary vessels

Pericardial cavity

FIGURE 1-2 Pericardium and pleura. (Applegate E: *The anatomy and physiology learning system*, ed 3, St Louis, 2006, Saunders.)

The period from the opening of the aortic and pulmonic valves to their closing, during which the ventricles contract and empty of blood, is called *ventricular systole*. The following period from the closure of the aortic and pulmonic valves to their reopening, during which the ventricles relax and fill with blood, is called *ventricular diastole*. The sequence of one ventricular systole followed by a ventricular diastole is called a *cardiac cycle*, commonly defined as the period from the beginning of one heart beat to the beginning of the next.

ELECTRICAL CONDUCTION SYSTEM OF THE HEART

The electrical conduction system of the heart (Figure 1-4) is composed of the following structures:
- The sinoatrial (SA) node
- The internodal conduction tracts and the interatrial conduction tract (Bachmann bundle)
- The atrioventricular (AV) junction, consisting of the AV node and bundle of His
- The right bundle branch and left bundle branch and its left anterior and posterior fascicles
- The Purkinje network

The prime function of the electrical conduction system of the heart is to transmit electrical impulses from the SA node (where they are normally generated) to the atria and ventricles, causing them to contract (Figure 1-5).

The SA node lies in the wall of the right atrium near the inlet of the superior vena cava. It consists of pacemaker cells that generate electrical impulses automatically and regularly.

The three internodal conduction tracts (the anterior, middle, and posterior internodal tracts), running through the walls of the right atrium between the SA node and the AV node, conduct the electrical impulses rapidly from the SA node to the AV node in about 0.03 second. The interatrial conduction tract (Bachmann's bundle), a branch of the anterior internodal tract, extends across the atria, conducting the electrical impulses from the SA node to the left atrium.

The AV node, the proximal part of the AV junction, lies partly in the right side of the interatrial septum in front of the opening of the coronary sinus and partly in the upper part of the interventricular septum above the base of the tricuspid valve. The AV node consists of three regions:
- The small, upper atrionodal region, located between the lower part of the atria and the nodal region
- The middle, nodal region, the major large central area of the AV node where the electrical impulses are slowed down in their progression from the atria to the ventricles
- The small, lower nodal-His region, located between the nodal region and the bundle of His. The atrionodal and nodal-His regions contain pacemaker cells (described later in the chapter), whereas the nodal region does not.

The primary function of the AV node is to channel the electrical impulses from the atria to the bundle of His while slowing their progression so that they arrive at the ventricles in an orderly and timely way. A ring of fibrous tissue insulates the remainder of the atria from the ventricles, preventing electrical impulses from entering the ventricles except through the AV node, unless there are accessory conduction pathways as described later.

The electrical impulses slow as they travel through the AV node, taking about 0.06 to 0.12 second to reach the bundle of His. The delay is such that the atria can contract and empty, and the ventricles can fill before they (the ventricles) are stimulated to contract.

The bundle of His, the distal part of the AV junction, lies in the upper part of the interventricular septum, connecting the AV node with the two bundle branches. Once the electrical impulses enter the bundle of His, they travel more rapidly on their way to the bundle branches, taking 0.03 to 0.05 second.

The right bundle branch and the left common bundle branch arise from the bundle of His, straddle the interventricular septum, and continue down both sides of the septum. The left common bundle branch further divides into two major divisions: the left anterior fascicle and the left posterior fascicle.

The bundle branches and their fascicles subdivide into smaller and smaller branches, the smallest ones connecting with the Purkinje network, an intricate web of tiny Purkinje fibers spread

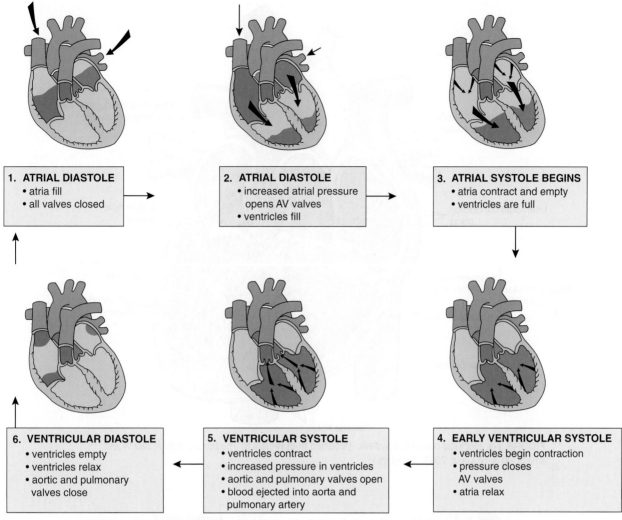

FIGURE 1-3 Ventricular diastole and systole. (Gould BE: *Pathophysiology for the health professions*, ed 3, St Louis, 2006, Saunders.)

widely throughout the ventricles beneath the endocardium. The ends of the Purkinje fibers finally terminate at the myocardial cells. The bundle of His, the right and left bundle branches, and the Purkinje network are also known as the *His-Purkinje system* of the ventricles. Pacemaker cells are located throughout the His-Purkinje system.

The electrical impulses travel very rapidly to the Purkinje network through the bundle branches in less than 0.01 second. All in all, it normally takes the electrical impulses less than 0.2 second on the average to travel from the SA node to the Purkinje network in the ventricles.

Accessory Conduction Pathways

Several distinct electrical conduction pathways have been found in the heart that conduct electrical impulses from the atria to the ventricles more directly, bypassing the AV node, the bundle of His, or both. These accessory conduction pathways (Figure 1-6) activate the ventricles earlier than they would be if the electrical impulses traveled down the electrical conduction

system normally. These pathways exists in all hearts but under certain conditions can lead to premature depolarization of the ventricles, resulting in *ventricular preexcitation* and *preexcitation syndrome.*

The most common of these accessory conduction pathways are the accessory AV pathways (or connections), which conduct the electrical impulses from the atria directly to the ventricles. Less commonly, other accessory conduction pathways conduct the electrical impulses from the atria to the bundle of His (the atrio-His fibers or tracts) and from the AV node and bundle of His to the ventricles (the nodoventricular and fasciculoventricular fibers, respectively). These pathways cannot only conduct electrical impulses forward (anterograde), but most of them can conduct the impulses backward (retrograde) as well, setting up the mechanism for reentry tachydysrhythmias.

Accessory Atrioventricular Pathways

Accessory AV pathways (also known as the *bundles of Kent*) consist of bundles of conductive myocardial fibers bridging the

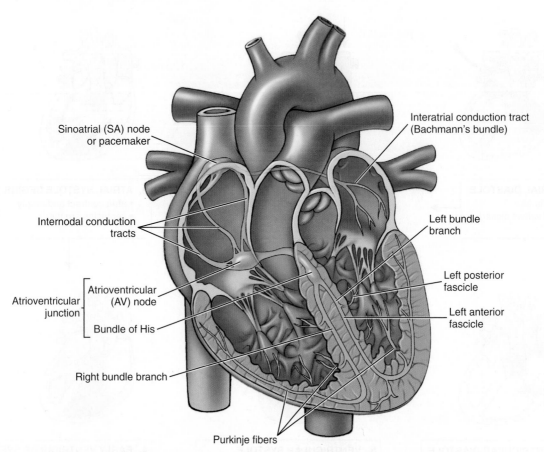

FIGURE 1-4 Electrical conduction system. (Modified from Herlihy B: *The human body in health and illness*, ed 3, St Louis, 2007, Saunders.)

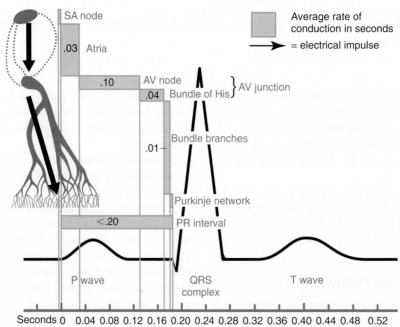

FIGURE 1-5 The average rate of conduction of the electrical impulse through various parts of the electrical conduction system.

fibrous layer insulating the atria from the ventricles. The accessory AV pathways have been found in the following locations:

- Between the posterior free wall of the left atrium and that of the left ventricle (type A Wolff-Parkinson-White [WPW] conduction pathway)
- Between the posterior atrial and ventricular walls in the septal region (posteroseptal WPW conduction pathway)
- Between the anterior free wall of the right atrium and that of the right ventricle (type B WPW conduction pathway)

These accessory AV pathways are responsible for accessory AV pathway conduction, also known as the *Wolff-Parkinson-White conduction*, resulting in abnormally wide QRS complexes, the classic form of ventricular preexcitation. When this type of AV conduction is associated with a paroxysmal supraventricular tachycardia with normal QRS complexes, it is known as the *Wolff-Parkinson-White syndrome*.

Atrio-His Fibers

The atrio-His fibers, an accessory conduction pathway also known as the *James fibers*, connect the atria with the lowermost part of the AV node near the origin of the bundle of His, bypassing the AV node. This form of anomalous AV conduction is classified as *atrio-His preexcitation*.

Nodoventricular/Fasciculoventricular Fibers

The nodoventricular and fasciculoventricular fibers (also known as the *Mahaim fibers*) are accessory conduction pathways that provide bypass channels between the AV junction and the ventricles in the following locations:

- Between the lower part of the AV node and the right ventricle (the nodoventricular fibers)
- Between the bundle of His and the ventricles (the fasciculoventricular fibers)

Such anomalous AV conduction is called nodoventricular/fasciculoventricular preexcitation.

CARDIAC CELLS

The heart is composed of cylindrical cardiac cells (Figure 1-7, Table 1-1) that partially divide at their ends into two or more branches. These connect with the branches of adjacent cells, forming a branching and anastomosing network of cells called a *syncytium*. At the junctions where the branches join together are specialized cellular membranes not found in any other cells—the *intercalated disks*. These membranes contain areas of low electrical resistance called "gap junctions" that permit very rapid conduction of electrical impulses from one cell to another. The ability of cardiac cells to conduct electrical impulses is called the *property of conductivity*.

Cardiac cells are enclosed in a semipermeable cell membrane that allows certain charged chemical particles (ions), such as sodium, potassium, and calcium ions, to flow in and out of the

TABLE 1-1 Myocardial Cells

Kinds of Cardiac Cells	Primary Function
Myocardial cells	Contraction and relaxation
Specialized cells of the electrical conduction system	Generation and conduction of electrical impulses

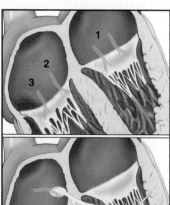
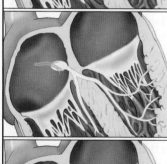
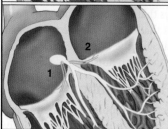

A. Accessory AV pathways (Bundles of Kent)
1. Type A
2. Posteroseptal
3. Type B

B. Atrio-His fibers (James fibers)

C. Mahaim fibers
1. Nodoventricular fibers
2. Fasciculoventricular fibers

FIGURE 1-6 Accessory conduction pathways.

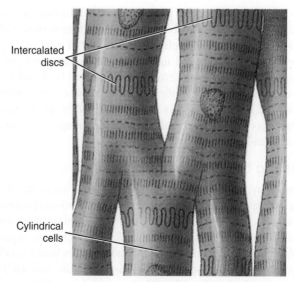

Intercalated discs

Cylindrical cells

Cardiac muscle cells

FIGURE 1-7 Cardiac cells. (McCance KL, Huether SE: *Pathophysiology: The biologic basis for disease in adults and children*, ed 5, St Louis, 2006, Mosby.)

cells, making the contraction and relaxation of the heart and the generation and conduction of electrical impulses possible.

There are two basic kinds of cardiac cells in the heart—the myocardial (or "working") cells and the specialized cells of the electrical conduction system of the heart. The myocardial cells form the thin muscular layer of the atrial wall and the much thicker muscular layer of the ventricular wall—the myocardium. These cells contain numerous thin myofibrils that consist of contractile protein filaments called *actin* and *myosin*. The myofibrils give the myocardial cells the *property of contractility* (i.e., the ability to shorten and return to their original length when stimulated by an electrical impulse).

The force of myocardial contractility increases in response to certain drugs (e.g., digitalis, sympathomimetics) and physiologic conditions (e.g., increased venous return to the heart, exercise, emotion, hypovolemia, anemia). In contrast, other drugs (e.g., procainamide, quinidine, beta-blockers, potassium) and pathophysiologic conditions (e.g., shock, hypocalcemia, hypothyroidism) decrease the force of myocardial contractility.

The specialized cells of the electrical conduction system do not contain myofibrils and therefore cannot contract. They do, however, contain more gap junctions than do myocardial cells, permitting them to conduct electrical impulses very rapidly (at least six times faster than myocardial cells). Specialized cells of the electrical conduction system—the pacemaker cells—are also capable of generating electrical impulses spontaneously, unlike myocardial cells, which cannot do so normally. This capability, the *property of automaticity*, will be discussed in greater detail later in this chapter.

ELECTROPHYSIOLOGY OF THE HEART

Cardiac cells are capable of generating and conducting electrical impulses that are responsible for the contraction of myocardial cells. These electrical impulses are the result of brief but rapid flow of positively charged ions (primarily sodium and potassium ions and, to a lesser extent, calcium ions) back and forth across the cardiac cell membrane. The difference in the concentration of these ions across the cell membrane at any given instant produces an electrical potential (or voltage) and is measured in millivolts (mV).

Resting State of the Cardiac Cell

When a myocardial cell is in the resting state, a high concentration of positively charged sodium ions (Na^+) (cations) is present outside the cell. At the same time, a high concentration of negatively charged ions (especially organic phosphate ions, organic sulfate ions, and protein ions) (anions) mixed in with a smaller concentration of positively charged potassium ions (K^+) is present inside the cell, making the interior of the cell electrically negative with reference to its exterior.

Under these conditions, a negative electrical potential exists across the cell membrane. This is made possible by the cell

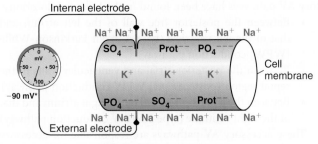

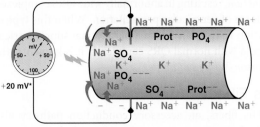

*Resting membrane potential 〰️ = Electrical impulse

Na^+	sodium ion
K^+	potassium ion
PO_4^{---}	phosphate ion
SO_4^{--}	sulfate ion
$Prot^{--}$	protein ion

FIGURE 1-8 Membrane potentials of polarized and depolarized cardiac cells.

membrane being impermeable to (1) positively charged sodium ions outside the cell membrane during the resting state and (2) negatively charged phosphate, sulfate, and protein ions inside the cell during the resting state (Figure 1-8). When a cell membrane is impermeable to an ion, it does not permit the free flow of that ion across it.

The resting cardiac cell can be depicted as having a layer of positive ions surrounding the cell membrane and an equal number of negative ions lining the inside of the cell membrane directly opposite each positive ion. When the ions are so aligned, the resting cell is called *polarized*.

The electrical potential across the membrane of a resting cardiac cell is called the *resting membrane potential*. The resting membrane potential in atrial and ventricular myocardial cells and the specialized cells of the electrical conduction system is normally −90 mV except in the SA and AV nodal cells, where it is slightly less negative at −70 mV. In summary, a negative (−) membrane potential indicates that the concentration of positive ions outside the cell is greater than that inside the cell; a positive (+) membrane potential indicates the opposite, that there are more positive ions inside the cell than outside.

Depolarization and Repolarization

When stimulated by an electrical impulse, the membrane of a polarized myocardial cell becomes permeable to positively charged sodium ions, allowing sodium to flow into the cell. This causes the interior of the cell to become less negative with respect to its exterior.

When the membrane potential drops to about −65 mV (−60 to −70 mV) from its resting potential of −90 mV, large pores in the membrane (the fast sodium channels) momentarily open. These channels facilitate the rapid, free flow of sodium across the cell membrane, resulting in a sudden large influx of positively charged sodium ions into the cell. This causes the interior of the cell to become rapidly positive. The moment the concentration of positively charged ions within the cell reaches that outside the cell, the membrane potential becomes 0 mV and the myocardial cell is "depolarized." The influx of positively charged sodium ions continues, resulting in a transient rise in the membrane potential to about 20 to 30 mV (the so-called "overshoot"). The process by which the cell's resting, polarized state is reversed is called *depolarization* (Figure 1-9).

The fast sodium channels are typically found in the myocardial cells and the specialized cells of the electrical conduction system other than those of the SA and AV nodes. The cells of the SA and AV nodes, on the other hand, have slow calcium-sodium channels that open when the membrane potential drops to about −50 mV. They permit the entry of positively charged calcium and sodium ions into the cells during depolarization at a slow and gradual rate. The result is a slower rate of depolarization as compared with the depolarization of cardiac cells with fast sodium channels.

As soon as a cardiac cell depolarizes, positively charged potassium ions flow out of the cell, initiating a process by which the cell returns to its resting, polarized state. This process, called *repolarization* (see Figure 1-9), involves a complex exchange of sodium, calcium, and potassium ions across the cell membrane. It must be noted here that the electrical potential external to a resting cardiac cell is more positive than that external to a depolarized cardiac cell. This difference in electrical potential between the resting, polarized cardiac cells and the depolarized cells is the basis of the electric current generated during depolarization and repolarization and detected and displayed as the electrocardiogram (ECG).

Depolarization of one cardiac cell acts as an electrical impulse (or stimulus) on adjacent cells and causes them to depolarize. The propagation of the electrical impulse from cell to cell produces a wave of depolarization that can be measured as an electric current flowing in the direction of depolarization. As the cells repolarize, another electric current is produced that is similar to, but opposite in direction to the first one. The direction of flow and magnitude of the electric currents generated by depolarization and repolarization of the myocardial cells of the atria and ventricles can be detected by surface electrodes and recorded as the ECG. Depolarization of the myocardial cells produces the P waves and QRS complexes (which include the Q, R, and S waves), and repolarization of the cells results in the T waves in the ECG.

Threshold Potential

A cardiac cell need not be repolarized completely to its resting, polarized state (−90 mV) before it can be stimulated to

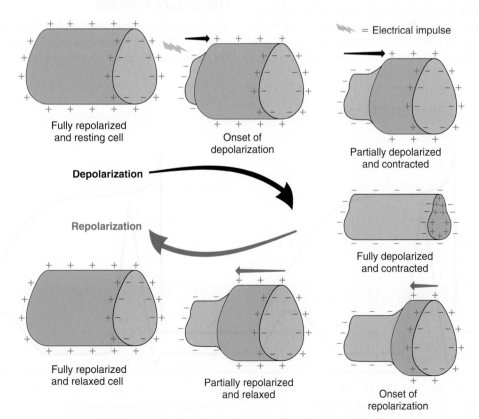

FIGURE 1-9 Depolarization and repolarization of a myocardial cell.

depolarize again. The cells of the SA and AV nodes can be depolarized when they have been repolarized to about −30 to −40 mV. The rest of the cells of the electrical conduction system of the heart and the myocardial cells can be depolarized when they have been repolarized to about −60 to −70 mV. The level to which a cell must be repolarized before it can be depolarized again is called the *threshold potential.*

It is important to note that a cardiac cell cannot generate or conduct an electrical impulse or be stimulated to contract until it has been repolarized to its threshold potential.

Cardiac Action Potential

A cardiac action potential is a schematic representation of the changes in the membrane potential of a cardiac cell during depolarization and repolarization (Figure 1-10). The cardiac action potential is divided into five phases: phase 0 to phase 4. The following are the five phases of the cardiac action potential of a typical myocardial cell.

- **Phase 0.** Phase 0 (depolarization phase) is the sharp, tall upstroke of the action potential during which the cell membrane reaches the threshold potential, triggering the fast sodium channels to open momentarily and permit the rapid entry of sodium into the cell. As the positively charged ions flow into the cell, the interior of the cell becomes electrically positive to about 20 mV to 30 mV with respect to its exterior. During the upstroke, the cell depolarizes and begins to contract.
- **Phase 1.** During phase 1 (early rapid repolarization phase), the fast sodium channels close, terminating the rapid flow of sodium into the cell, followed by a loss of potassium from the cell. The net result is a decrease in the number of positive electrical charges within the cell and a drop in the membrane potential to about 0 mV.

- **Phase 2.** Phase 2 is the prolonged phase of slow repolarization (plateau phase) of the action potential of the myocardial cell, allowing it to finish contracting and begin relaxing. During phase 2, the membrane potential remains about 0 mV because of a very slow rate of repolarization. In a complicated exchange of ions across the cell membrane, calcium slowly enters the cell through the slow calcium channels as potassium continues to leave the cell and sodium enters it slowly.
- **Phase 3.** Phase 3 is the terminal phase of rapid repolarization, during which the inside of the cell becomes markedly negative and the membrane potential once again returns to about −90 mV, its resting level. This is caused primarily by the flow of potassium from the cell. Repolarization is complete by the end of phase 3.
- **Phase 4.** At the onset of phase 4 (the period between action potentials), the membrane has returned to its resting potential and the inside of the cell is once again negative (−90 mV) with respect to the outside. But there is still an excess of sodium in the cell and an excess of potassium outside. At this point, a mechanism known as the *sodium-potassium pump* is activated, transporting the excess sodium out of the cell and potassium back in. Because of this mechanism and the impermeability of the cell membrane to sodium during phase 4, the myocardial cell normally maintains a stable membrane potential between action potentials.

Refractory Periods

The time between the onset of depolarization and the end of repolarization is customarily divided into periods during which the cardiac cells can or cannot be stimulated to depolarize.

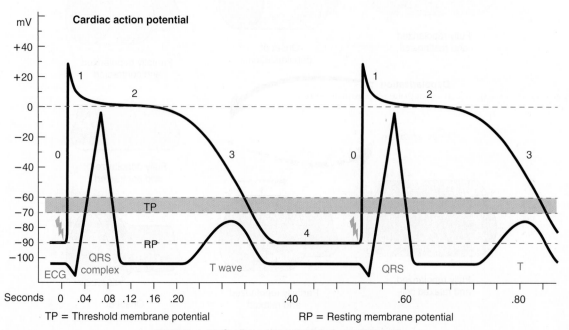

FIGURE 1-10 Cardiac action potential of myocardial cells.

Refractory and Supernormal Periods

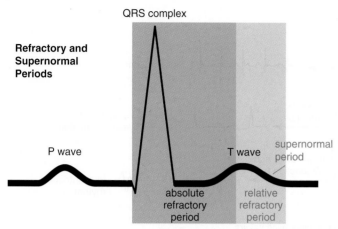

FIGURE 1-11 Refractory periods.

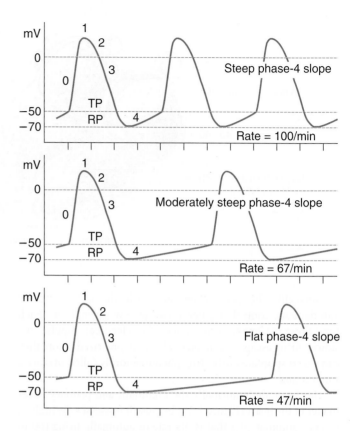

FIGURE 1-12 Cardiac action potential of pacemaker cells. Rate of spontaneous depolarization is dependent on the slope of phase-4 depolarization. TP = Threshold potential; RP = Resting membrane potential.

These are the *refractory periods* (absolute and relative) (Figure 1-11).

The refractory period of cardiac cells (e.g., those of the ventricles) begins with the onset of phase 0 of the cardiac action potential and ends just before the end of phase 3. On the ECG, it extends from the onset of the QRS complex to about the end of the T wave.

The refractory period is further divided into the absolute and relative refractory periods. The absolute refractory period (ARP) begins with the onset of phase 0 and ends midway through phase 3 at about the peak of the T wave, occupying over two thirds of the refractory period. During this period, the cardiac cells—having completely depolarized—are in the process of repolarizing. Because they have not repolarized to their threshold potential, the cardiac cells cannot be stimulated to depolarize. In other words, myocardial cells cannot contract, and the cells of the electrical conduction system cannot conduct an electrical impulse during the absolute refractory period.

The relative refractory period (RRP) extends through most of the second half of phase 3, corresponding to the downslope of the T wave. During this period, the cardiac cells, having repolarized to their threshold potential, can be stimulated to depolarize if the stimulus is strong enough. This period is also called the *vulnerable period of repolarization.*

The capability of a cardiac cell to depolarize spontaneously during phase 4—to reach threshold potential and to depolarize completely without being externally stimulated—is called the *property of automaticity.*

Spontaneous depolarization depends on the ability of the cell membrane to become permeable to sodium during phase 4, thus allowing a steady leakage of sodium ions into the cell. This causes the resting membrane potential to become progressively less negative. As soon as the threshold potential is reached, rapid depolarization of the cell (phase 0) occurs.

The rate of spontaneous depolarization is dependent on the slope of phase 4 depolarization (Figure 1-12). The steeper the slope of phase 4 depolarization, the faster is the rate of spontaneous depolarization and the rate of impulse formation (the firing rate). The flatter the slope is, the slower the firing rate.

Increase in sympathetic activity and administration of catecholamines increase the slope of phase 4 depolarization, resulting in an increase in the automaticity of the pacemaker cells and their firing rate. On the other hand, an increase in parasympathetic activity and administration of such drugs as lidocaine, procainamide, and quinidine decrease the slope of phase 4 depolarization, causing a decrease in the automaticity and firing rate of the pacemaker cells.

Dominant and Escape Pacemakers of the Heart

The specialized cells in the electrical conduction system that normally have the property of automaticity are called the pacemaker cells. These cells are located in the SA node, in some areas of the internodal atrial conduction tracts and AV node, and throughout the bundle of His, bundle branches, and Purkinje network. The pacemaker cells of the SA node, having the fastest firing rate, are normally the dominant (or primary) pacemaker cells of the heart. The pacemaker cells in the rest of the electrical conduction system hold the property of automaticity in reserve should the SA node fail to function properly or electrical impulses fail to reach them for any reason, such as a disruption in the electrical conduction system. For this reason, these pacemaker cells are called *escape pacemaker cells.*

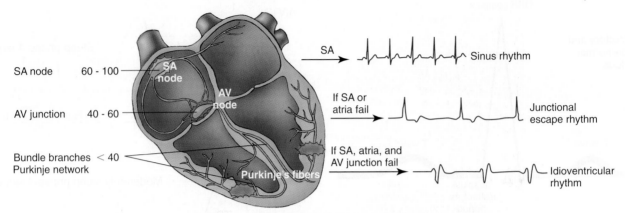

FIGURE 1-13 Dominant and escape pacemakers.

Normally, the pacemaker cells with the fastest rate of automaticity control the heart rate at any given time. Each time these pacemaker cells generate an electrical impulse, the slower-firing escape pacemaker cells are depolarized before they can do so spontaneously. This phenomenon is called *overdrive suppression.*

The SA node is normally the dominant and primary pacemaker of the heart (Figure 1-13) because it possesses the highest level of automaticity; that is, its rate of automatic firing (60 to 100 times per minute) is normally greater than that of the other pacemaker cells.

If the SA node fails to generate electrical impulses at its normal rate or stops functioning entirely, or if the conduction of the electrical impulse is blocked for any reason (e.g., in the AV node), escape pacemaker cells in the AV junction will usually assume the role of pacemaker of the heart but at a slower rate (40 to 60 times per minute). If the AV junction is unable to take over as the pacemaker because of disease, an escape pacemaker in the electrical conduction system below the AV junction in the ventricles (i.e., in the bundle branches or Purkinje network) may take over at a still slower rate (less than 40 times per minute). In general, the farther the escape pacemaker is from the SA node, the slower it generates electrical impulses.

The rate at which the SA node or an escape pacemaker normally generates electrical impulses is called the *pacemaker's inherent firing rate.* A beat or a series of beats arising from an escape pacemaker is called an *escape beat* or *rhythm* and is identified according to its origin (e.g., junctional, ventricular).

Mechanisms of Abnormal Electrical Impulse Formation

Under certain circumstances, cardiac cells in any part of the heart, whether they are escape pacemaker cells or nonpacemaker, myocardial cells, start generating extraneous electrical impulses. Such activity is referred to as ectopy because it originates outside the normal conduction pathway. The result can be abnormal ectopic beats and rhythms, such as premature con-

tractions, tachycardias, flutters, and fibrillations. These dysrhythmias are identified according to the location of the ectopic pacemaker (e.g., atrial, junctional, ventricular). The three basic mechanisms that are responsible for ectopic beats and rhythms (ectopy) are (1) enhanced automaticity, (2) reentry, and (3) triggered activity.

Enhanced Automaticity

Enhanced automaticity is an abnormal condition of ectopy in which their firing rate is increased beyond their inherent rate. This occurs when the cell membrane becomes abnormally permeable to sodium during phase 4. The result is an abnormally high leakage of sodium ions into the cells and, consequently, a sharp rise in the phase-4 slope of spontaneous depolarization. Even myocardial cells that do not ordinarily possess automaticity (nonpacemaker cells) may acquire this property under certain conditions and depolarize spontaneously. Enhanced automaticity can cause atrial, junctional, and ventricular ectopic beats and rhythms.

Common causes of enhanced automaticity are an increase in catecholamines, digitalis toxicity, and administration of atropine. In addition, hypoxia, hypercapnia, myocardial ischemia or infarction, stretching of the heart, hypokalemia, hypocalcemia, and heating or cooling of the heart may also cause enhanced automaticity.

Reentry

Reentry is a condition in which the progression of an electrical impulse is delayed or blocked (or both) (Figure 1-14, *A-B*) in one or more segments of the electrical conduction system while being conducted normally through the rest of the conduction system. This results in delayed antegrade or retrograde conduction of electrical impulses into adjacent cardiac cells that have just been depolarized by the normally conducted electrical impulse. If these cardiac cells have repolarized sufficiently, the delayed electrical impulse depolarizes them prematurely, producing ectopic beats and rhythms. Myocardial ischemia and hyperkalemia are the two most common causes of delay or block in the conduction of an electrical impulse through

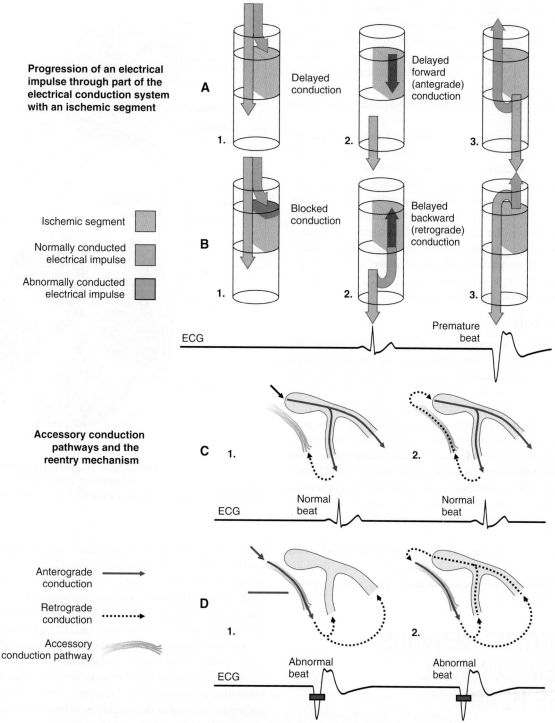

FIGURE 1-14 Examples of reentry mechanism. **A**, Delayed conduction. **B**, Blocked and delayed conduction. **C**, Anterograde conduction through the electrical conduction system. **D**, Retrograde conduction through the electrical conduction system.

the electrical conduction system responsible for the reentry mechanism.

Another cause of the reentry mechanism is the presence of an accessory conduction pathway (Figure 1-14, *C* and *D*), such as the accessory AV pathways located between the atria and ventricles described earlier in this chapter. After normal

antegrade progression of an electrical impulse through the electrical conduction system and depolarization of the cardiac cells, the electrical impulse enters the accessory conduction pathway and progresses in a *retrograde* fashion to reenter the proximal end of the electrical conduction system much sooner than the next expected normal electrical impulse. The electrical impulse is then conducted anterogradely as before, causing depolarization of the cardiac cells prematurely. Thus a reentry circuit is set up that can result in the conduction of a rapid series of electrical impulses through the electrical conduction system and a tachydysrhythmia. The electrical impulse can also progress anterogradely through the accessory conduction pathway and retrogradely through the electrical conduction system.

The reentry mechanism can result in the abnormal generation of single or repetitive electrical impulses in the atria, AV junction, bundle branches, and Purkinje network. This produces atrial, junctional, or ventricular ectopic beats and rhythms, such as atrial, junctional, and ventricular tachycardias. Such reentry tachycardias typically start and stop abruptly. If the delay in the conduction of the electrical impulse through the reentry circuit responsible for ectopic beats is constant for each conduction cycle, the abnormal beat will always follow the normal one at exactly the same interval of time. This is called *fixed coupling and bigeminal rhythm*, or simply *bigeminy*.

Triggered Activity

Triggered activity is an abnormal condition of myocardial cells (nonpacemaker cells) in which the cells may depolarize more than once after stimulation by a single electrical impulse. The level of membrane action potential spontaneously increases after the first depolarization until it reaches threshold potential, causing the cells to depolarize, once or repeatedly. This phenomenon, called *afterdepolarization*, can occur almost immediately after depolarization in phase 3 (early afterdepolarization [EAD]) or later in phase 4 (delayed afterdepolarization [DAD]).

Triggered activity can result in atrial or ventricular ectopic beats occurring singly, in groups of two (paired or coupled beats), or in bursts of three or more beats (paroxysms of beats or tachycardia).

Common causes of triggered activity, like those of enhanced automaticity, include an increase in catecholamines, digitalis toxicity, hypoxia, myocardial ischemia or injury, and stretching or cooling of the heart.

AUTONOMIC NERVOUS SYSTEM CONTROL OF THE HEART

The heart is under constant control of the autonomic nervous system, which includes the sympathetic (adrenergic) and parasympathetic (cholinergic) nervous systems (Figure 1-15), each producing opposite effects when stimulated. These two systems work together to cause changes in cardiac output (by regulating the heart rate and stroke volume) and blood pressure.

Nervous control of the heart originates in two separate nerve centers located in the medulla oblongata, a part of the brainstem. One is the cardioaccelerator center, a part of the sympathetic nervous system; the other is the cardioinhibitor center, a

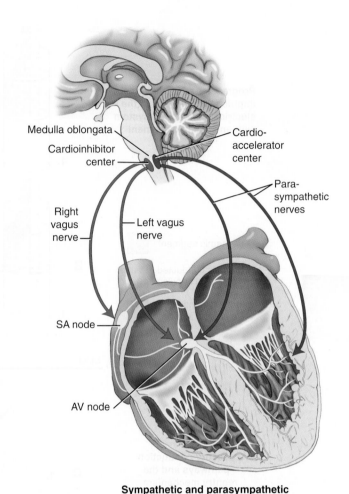

Sympathetic and parasympathetic innervation of the heart

FIGURE 1-15 Sympathetic and parasympathetic innervation of the heart.

part of the parasympathetic nervous system. Impulses from the cardioaccelerator center reach the electrical conduction system of the heart and the atria and ventricles by way of the sympathetic nerves. Impulses from the cardioinhibitor center innervate the SA node, atria, and AV junction and to a small extent the ventricles by way of the right and left vagus nerves.

Another important cardioinhibitor (parasympathetic) nerve center is the carotid sinus, a slight dilatation of the common carotid artery, located at the point where it branches into the internal and external carotid arteries. It contains sensory nerve endings important in the regulation of blood pressure and heart rate.

As the blood requirements of the body change, multiple sensors in the body relay impulses to the cardioinhibitor and cardioaccelerator centers for analysis. From here, the sympathetic and parasympathetic nerves transmit the appropriate impulses to the electrical conduction system of the heart and the atrial and ventricular myocardium, where they influence the automaticity, excitability conductivity, and contractility of the heart's cardiac cells.

Stimulation of the sympathetic nervous system produces the following adrenergic effects on the cardiovascular system:

- An increase in the firing rate of the SA node and escape and ectopic pacemakers throughout the heart by increasing their automaticity and excitability
- An increase in the conductivity of electrical impulses through the atria and ventricles, especially through the AV node
- An increase in the force of atrial and ventricular contractions

The result is an increase in heart rate, cardiac output, and blood pressure. This is accomplished by direct stimulation of the cardiac cells and indirectly by the secretion of catecholamines, such as epinephrine (adrenaline), and their effect on the cardiac cells

Stimulation of the parasympathetic nervous system produces the following cholinergic (vagal) effects on the cardiovascular system:

- A decrease in the firing rate of the SA node and escape and ectopic pacemakers in the atria and AV junction by decreasing their automaticity and excitability
- A slowing of conduction of electrical impulses through the AV node
- The result is a decrease in heart rate, cardiac output, and blood pressure and, sometimes, an AV block.

The following maneuvers and bodily functions stimulate the parasympathetic nervous system:

- Pressure on the carotid sinus
- The Valsalva maneuver (the action of straining against a closed glottis)
- Straining to move the bowels
- Distention of the urinary bladder

Nausea, vomiting, bronchial spasm, sweating, faintness, and hypersalivation are examples of excessive parasympathetic activity. The drug atropine, a parasympathetic blocking agent, effectively blocks parasympathetic activity.

CHAPTER SUMMARY

- The heart lies in the center of the chest with its base at the atria and its apex at the ventricles. It is surrounded by the pericardium and is lined on the outside by the epicardium and on the inside by the endocardium.
- The heart muscle is called the myocardium.
- Blood from the vena cava and lungs enters the atria and empties into the ventricles and is then pumped to the lungs and body during the cardiac cycle.
- The specific properties of excitability, conductivity, automaticity, and contractility allow the cardiac muscles to perform their unique duties to ensure a coordinated contraction of the heart to generate blood flow through the body.
- The properties of excitability, conductivity, and automaticity allow the cardiac cells involved in the conduction system to propagate an electrical impulse through pathways in the heart resulting in myocardial contraction.
- The electrophysiology of the heart is regulated by the movement of positive and negative ions across cell membranes, which change their permeability based on their own unique properties.
- The process of depolarization and repolarization results in the movement of electrical impulses down the conduction pathways and can be influenced by the autonomic nervous system and other environmental stimuli and pathological conditions.
- The presence of dominant and escape pacemakers ensures that the heart has back-up mechanisms in place to generate a pulse in the event that normal nervous system stimulation to the heart is interrupted.

CHAPTER REVIEW

1. The inner layer of the pericardium, which covers the heart itself, is more commonly called the:
   A. endocardium
   B. epicardium
   C. myocardium
   D. pericardium

2. The the_____ side of the heart pumps blood into the the_____ circulation, while the the_____ side of the heart pumps blood into the the_____ circulation.
   A. left, pulmonary: right, systemic
   B. left, ventricular: right, atrial
   C. right, pulmonary: left, systemic
   D. right, systemic: left, pulmonic

3. The right ventricle pumps deoxygenated blood through the the_____ valve and into the lungs through the the_____ artery
   A. aortic: mitral
   B. mitral: tricuspid
   C. pulmonic: pulmonary
   D. tricuspid: pulmonary

4. The period of relaxation and filling of the ventricles with blood is called:
   A. atrial diastole
   B. atrial systole
   C. ventricular diastole
   D. ventricular systole

5. Which structure is a normal component of the heart's electrical conduction system?
   A. atrial septa
   B. coronary sinus
   C. right bundle branch
   D. vagus nerve

6. The property of cardiac cells to spontaneously depolarize is:
   A. automaticity
   B. conductivity
   C. contractility
   D. self-excitation

7. In the resting state, a myocardial cell has a high concentration of the_____ charged the_____ ions present outside the cell.
   A. negatively: potassium
   B. negatively: sodium
   C. positively: potassium
   D. positively: sodium

8. Cardiac cells cannot be stimulated to depolarize during the:
   A. absolute refractory period
   B. ectopic period
   C. relative refractory period
   D. resting state

9. The normal and dominant pacemaker of the heart is the_____.
   A. AV node
   B. bundle of His
   C. Purkinje fibers
   D. SA node

10. The vagus nerve is part of the parasympathetic nervous system. Slowing of the heart by the vagus nerve occurs when
    A. the nerve fires more rapidly
    B. the nerve is blocked by atropine
    C. the nerve is severed
    D. the patient is given a stimulant

11. Label the figure.

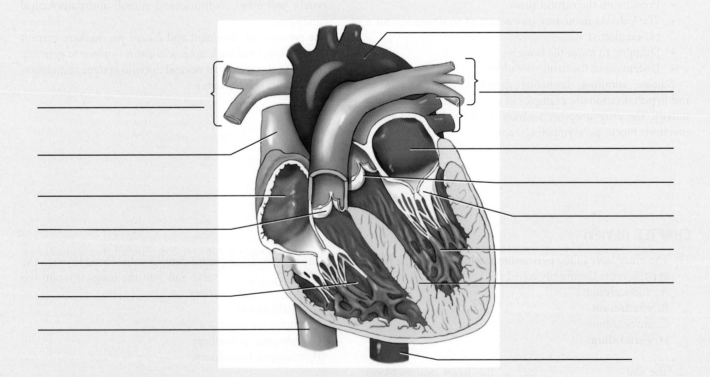

The Electrocardiogram: Basic Concepts and Lead Monitoring

2

OBJECTIVES *Upon completion of this chapter, you should be able to:*

1. Explain what the electrocardiogram (ECG) represents.
2. Identify the measurements of time and amplitude as represented by the dark and light vertical and horizontal lines on an ECG grid.
3. Name and identify the components of the ECG, including the waves, complexes, segments, and intervals.
4. List at least four causes of artifacts in the ECG.
5. Define an ECG lead and differentiate between a bipolar lead, and a unipolar lead.
6. Describe how monitoring leads I, II, and III are obtained.
7. Describe the sequence and direction of normal ventricular depolarization and its depiction of the QRS complex in lead II.
8. Explain what monitoring leads MCL$_1$ and MCL$_6$ are, and under what circumstances they are useful, and how they are obtained.

BASIC ECG CONCEPTS

AUTHOR'S NOTE Throughout this text the term "ECG" will be used. Some texts use the abbreviation "EKG," which is derived from the German word "Elektrokardiogramm." Also, "EKG" is often the abbreviation used verbally because "ECG" can be confused with "EEG," which refers to "electroencephalogram."

Electrical Basis of the ECG

The *electrocardiogram* (ECG) is a graphic record of the changes in magnitude and direction of the electrical activity (Figure 2-1), or more specifically, the electric current generated by the wave of depolarization that progresses through the atria and ventricles followed by the wave of repolarization of the atria and ventricles in the opposite direction. This electrical activity is readily detected by electrodes attached to the skin. More specifically, the ECG detects the depolarization and repolarization of the atrial and ventricular myocardial cells. The electrical activity that generates and transmits impulses responsible for triggering the depolarization are too weak to be detected by skin electrodes.

ECG Paper

The paper used in recording ECGs has a grid to permit the measurement of time in seconds (sec) along the horizontal axis and voltage (amplitude) in millimeters (mm) along the vertical axis (Figure 2-2).

The grid consists of intersecting dark and light vertical and horizontal lines that form large and small squares. The distance between the vertical lines depends on the paper speed at the time of the ECG recording (i.e., 25 mm or 50 mm per second). The standard recording speed is 25 mm/sec. Other speeds are used only for specialized purposes to attempt to capture uncommon electrical signals.

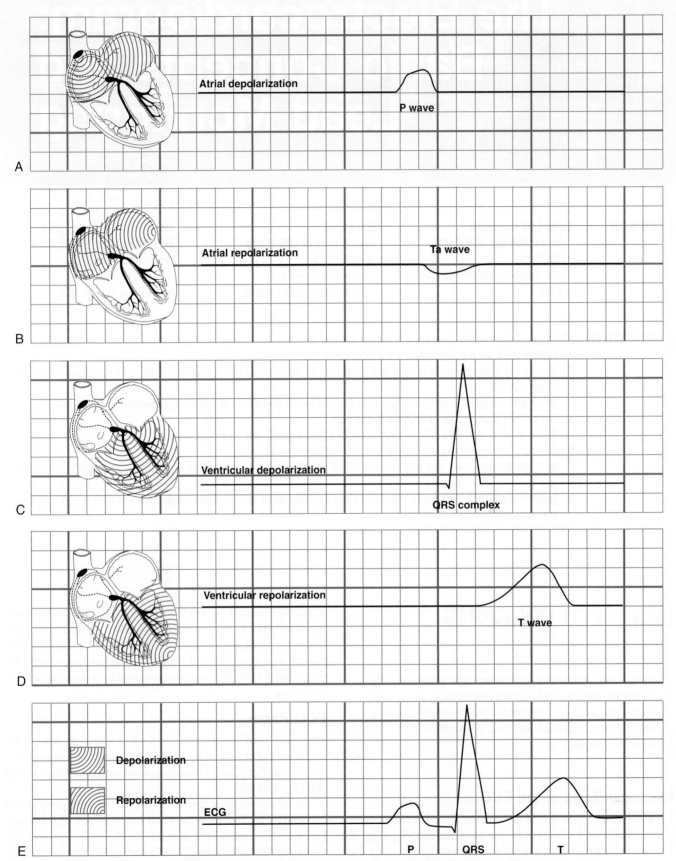

FIGURE 2-1 Electrical basis of the ECG. **A,** Atrial depolarization. **B,** Atrial repolarization. **C,** Ventricular depolarization. **D,** Ventricular repolarization. **E,** ECG.

When the ECG is recorded at the standard speed of 25 mm/sec, the measurements between the vertical lines are as follows:

- The dark vertical lines are 5 mm apart
- If 1 second = 25 mm, then 5 mm = $^1/_5$ of second or 0.20 seconds
- The light vertical lines are 1 mm apart
- If 5 mm = $^1/_5$ of second, then 1 mm = $^1/_{25}$ of second or 0.04 seconds

Regardless of the speed of the recording, the measurements between the horizontal lines are as follows:

- The dark horizontal lines are 5 mm apart.
- The light horizontal lines are 1 mm apart.

Therefore at the standard paper speed of 25 mm/sec, the large and small squares have the following characteristics.

- One large square is 5 mm tall × 0.2 second long.
- One small square is 1 mm tall × 0.04 second long.

Conventionally, the sensitivity of the ECG machine is adjusted (i.e., calibrated or standardized) so that a 1-millivolt (mV) electrical signal produces a 10-mm deflection (two large squares or 10 small squares) on the ECG.

Printed along one edge of the ECG paper, either the top or the bottom, are regularly spaced short, vertical lines (or small arrowheads) denoting intervals of time (time lines). Time lines are spaced 15 large squares apart (75 mm, or about 3 inches apart). When the ECG is recorded at the standard paper speed of 25 mm/sec, the vertical lines are 3 seconds apart, and every third vertical line is 6 seconds apart. Some ECG papers have the time lines spaced every five large squares apart (25 mm, or about 1 inch apart) so they are 1 second apart at the standard paper speed.

BASIC COMPONENTS OF THE NORMAL ECG

It is vital to understand the relationship between the various components of the ECG and the electrical activity occurring in the heart. The current generated by depolarization and repolarization of the atria and ventricles is detected by electrodes. It is then amplified and displayed on an oscilloscope, and recorded on ECG paper as waves and complexes. The combination of the waves and complexes is referred to as the ECG waveform (Figure 2-3). The next chapter will discuss each component in greater detail but the basics are as follows.

The electric current generated by atrial depolarization is recorded as the *P wave*, and that generated by ventricular depolarization is recorded as the *Q, R,* and *S waves*—which together are referred to as the *QRS complex*. Ventricular repolarization is manifested by the *T wave*. Because atrial repolarization

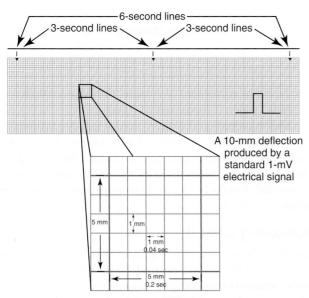

FIGURE 2-2 ECG paper.

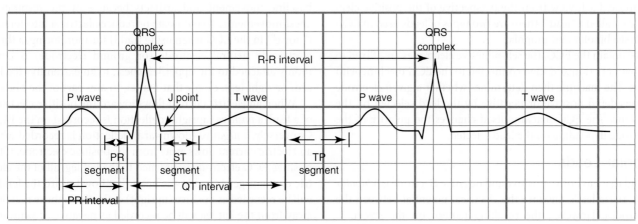

FIGURE 2-3 Components of the ECG.

normally occurs during ventricular depolarization, it is hidden in the QRS complex.

In a normal ECG waveform, the P wave occurs first, followed by the QRS complex and then the T wave. The sections of the ECG between waves and complexes are called segments and intervals, and their shape and length provide information related to the speed of the electrical conduction through the heart. The PR-segment occupies the period of time from the end of the P wave to the beginning for the QRS complex. The ST segment is that portion of the ECG from the end of the QRS complex until the beginning of the T wave. This start of the ST segment, where the QRS complex ends, is referred to as the "J point." The final segment to mention is the TP segment, which begins at the end of the T wave and terminates at the beginning of the next P wave.

The P-R interval is defined as starting at the beginning of the P wave and ending at the QRS complex. The Q-T interval starts at the QRS complex and terminates at the end of the T wave. And finally, the R-R "R to R" interval is measured from two consecutive R waves.

Following each wave and complex the ECG waveform (see Figure 2-3) returns to a near flat line, which is called the "baseline" or "isoelectric line." During this period there is no electrical activity occurring. Generally speaking when examining the ECG waveform we will be evaluating the waves and complexes based on their shape and timing, intervals based on their length, and segments based on their relationship with the baseline.

ECG LEADS

The Basics of ECG Leads

An ECG is obtained by using electrodes (usually designated as either negative or positive) attached to the skin that detect the electric current generated by the depolarization and repolarization of the heart. The placement of the positive electrodes on specified areas of the body (the right or left arm, the left leg, or one of several locations on the anterior chest wall) determines what view of the heart's electrical activity is obtained. This view occurs because the energy of the electrical impulse is the movement of negatively charged electrons toward or away from the electrode. Each view from the perspective of the positive electrode is called a "lead." There are two types of leads used in ECG analysis: bipolar and unipolar.

To obtain the ECG, the self-adhesive electrodes are affixed to the patient's skin and then connected to the ECG machine with wires. The machine then determines whether a given electrode is considered positive or negative by the lead selected on the machine. The ECG machine itself changes the polarity of the electrode depending on the lead selected.

Bipolar Leads

A lead that has both a positive and negative electrode is a *bipolar lead*. These leads measure the electrical potential between the electrodes. However, the resulting pattern on the screen is "viewed" from the positive electrode's perspective. Bipolar leads

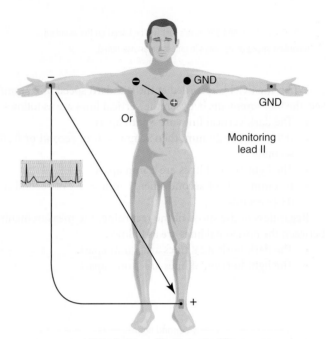

FIGURE 2-4 Monitoring lead II.

are referred to as *standard limb leads*. The standard limb leads are Leads I (one), II (two), and III (three).

When monitoring the heart solely for dysrhythmias, a single bipolar ECG lead, such as lead II (Figure 2-4), is commonly used. Another commonly used bipolar monitoring lead is lead MCL_1, particularly in the monitoring of dysrhythmias in the hospital. Bipolar leads less frequently used for monitoring include leads III, and MCL_6.

Monitoring Lead II

Lead II is obtained by attaching the negative electrode to the right arm and the positive electrode to the left leg. Lead II can also be obtained by attaching the negative electrode to the upper right anterior chest wall below the right clavicle and the positive electrode to the lower left anterior chest wall over the apex of the heart (usually in the fifth left intercostal space in the midclavicular line). However, such electrode placement may cause baseline movement and artifacts because of the respiratory chest movements. To eliminate or reduce electrical interference ("noise") in the ECG when using lead II for monitoring, a third, electrically neutral electrode (or ground electrode) is commonly attached to the upper left chest, to an extremity (the left arm or right leg), or, for that matter, to any part of the body.

When an electric current flows toward the positive electrode of a lead, a *positive* (upright) deflection is recorded on the ECG. Conversely, a *negative* (downward) deflection is recorded when an electric current flows away from the positive electrode. If the positive ECG electrode is attached to the left leg, all of the electric currents generated in the heart that flow toward the left leg will be recorded as positive (upright) deflections; those that flow away from the left leg will be recorded as negative (downward) deflections (Figure 2-5).

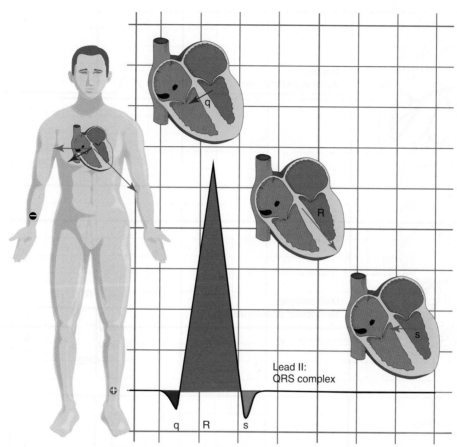

FIGURE 2-5 Sequence and direction of normal depolarization.

It should be noted here that because normal depolarization of the atria and ventricles generally progresses from the right upper chest downward toward the left leg, the electric currents generated during normal depolarization of the heart will, for the most part, flow toward the left leg and be recorded as two positive (upright) deflections—a positive P wave (atrial depolarization) and a large positive R wave (ventricular depolarization)—in lead II.

The relationship between the depolarization and repolarization of the atria and ventricles and the P wave, QRS complex, and the T wave (Figure 2-6) is as follows:

- **P wave.** Depolarization of the atria normally begins near the SA node and then proceeds downward and to the left, producing a positive P wave.
- **QRS complex.** Depolarization of the ventricles usually starts with the depolarization of the relatively thin interventricular septum from left to right, resulting in a small negative (inverted) deflection—the Q wave. This is immediately followed by the depolarization of the large left ventricle from right to left, which overshadows the almost simultaneous left-to-right depolarization of the smaller right ventricle, resulting in a large R wave. In addition, depending on the position of the heart in the chest, the size of the ventricles, and the rotation of the heart, depolarization of the base of the left ventricle from left to right

produces a small negative (inverted) deflection after the R wave—the S wave.
- **T wave.** Finally, as the ventricles repolarize from left to right, the T wave is produced.

> **AUTHOR'S NOTE** The ECG components and strips shown in this book are depicted as they would appear in lead II unless otherwise noted.

Monitoring Leads I and III

The two other bipolar leads, leads I and III, are also used for ECG monitoring (Figure 2-7). The placement of the electrodes for these leads is as follows:

- **Lead I.** Lead I is obtained by attaching the negative electrode to the right arm, the positive electrode to the left arm, and the ground electrode to the right leg. Lead I can also be obtained by attaching the negative electrode to the upper right anterior chest wall below the right clavicle and the positive electrode to the upper left anterior chest wall below the left clavicle. The ground electrode is attached to the right or left lower chest wall.
- **Lead III.** Lead III is obtained by attaching the negative electrode to the left arm, the positive electrode to the left

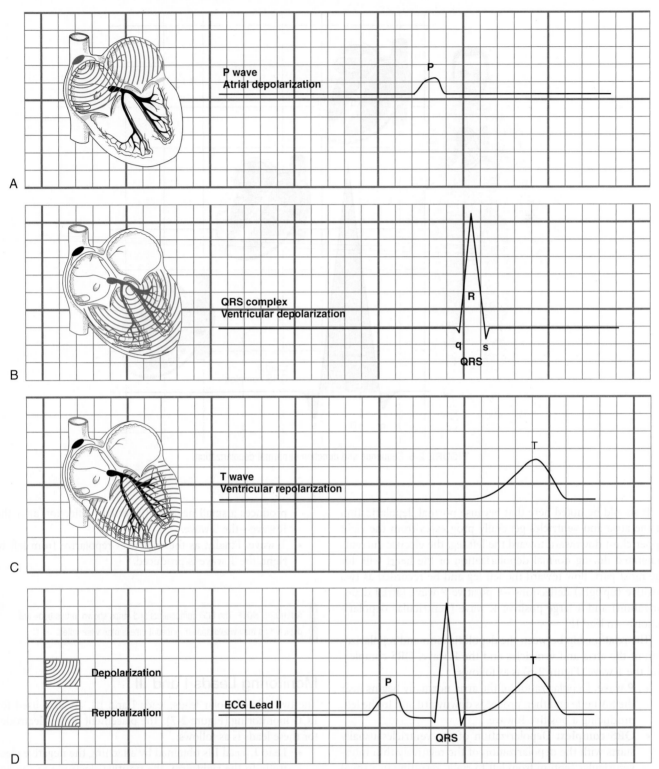

FIGURE 2-6 Depolarization and repolarization of the atria and ventricles and the ECG. **A,** P wave. **B,** QRS complex. **C,** T wave. **D,** ECG lead II.

leg, and the ground electrode to the right leg. Lead III can also be obtained by attaching the negative electrode to the upper left anterior chest wall below the left clavicle and the positive electrode to the lower left anterior chest wall at the intersection of the fifth intercostal space and the middavicular line. The ground electrode is attached to the right lower chest wall.

Leads I and III in normal hearts may or may not resemble lead II because of the normal variations in the mean QRS axis (the average direction of ventricular depolarization), which

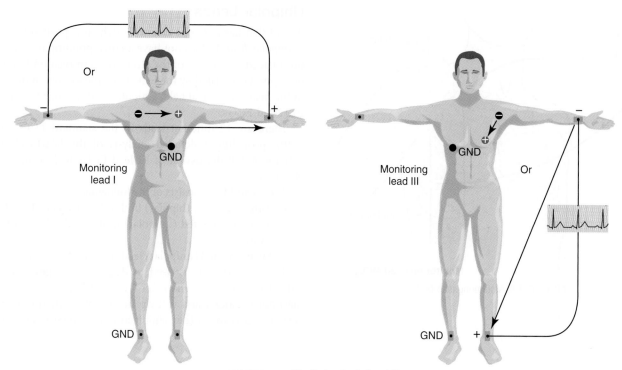

FIGURE 2-7 Monitoring leads I and III.

affects the direction of the QRS deflection in these three leads. This is discussed in Chapters 12 and 13.

Modified Chest Leads (MCL)

Modified chest leads (MCL) are similar to the unipolar chest leads used in 12 lead ECGs but have less sensitivity. They can, however, be used for monitoring of certain rhythms.

Monitoring Lead MCL₁

Lead MCL_1 is a bipolar lead similar to lead V_1 of the 12-lead ECG (Figure 2-8). It is obtained by attaching the positive electrode from lead III to the right side of the anterior chest in the fourth intercostal space just right of the sternum and the negative electrode to the left chest in the midclavicular line below the clavicle. Lead MCL_1 is helpful in identifying the origin of certain dysrhythmias with wide QRS complexes. This will be discussed later in the book.

Unlike lead II in which has a predominantly positive QRS complex with a large R wave is normally present, the electric current generated during normal ventricular depolarization will flow away from the positive electrode on the right chest toward the left leg, producing a predominantly negative QRS complex with a large negative S wave in lead MCL_1. The small electric current that flows toward the right shoulder, producing the Q and S waves in lead II, will produce small R waves in lead MCL_1. The P wave in lead MCL_1 may be positive, negative, or biphasic (partly positive and partly negative).

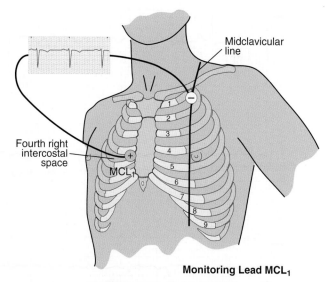

Monitoring Lead MCL₁

FIGURE 2-8 Monitoring lead MCL_1.

Monitoring Lead MCL₆

Lead MCL_6, a bipolar lead that resembles V_6 of the 12-lead ECG, is obtained by attaching the positive electrode of lead III to the left chest in the sixth intercostal space in the midaxillary line and the negative electrode in the midclavicular line below the clavicle on the same side (Figure 2-9). The P waves, QRS complexes, and T waves are similar to those in lead II when the ECG is normal, but in certain heart conditions (e.g., ACS, including acute MI, bundle branch block) the QRS complexes and T waves are usually dissimilar.

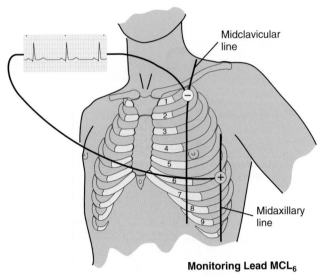

Monitoring Lead MCL₆

FIGURE 2-9 Monitoring lead MCL₆.

Unipolar Leads

A lead that has only one electrode (which is positive) is called a *unipolar lead*. It does not have a corresponding negative lead but instead the "view" of the electrode is in relation to a reference point calculated by the ECG machine located in the center of the heart's electrical field. Unipolar leads are used extensively in 12-led ECGs.

There are 12 different leads in the standard ECG (Figure 2-10), providing a detailed analysis of the heart's electrical activity. A full discussion of 12-lead ECGs will occur in later chapters.

A 12-lead ECG consists of the following:

- Three standard (bipolar) limb leads (leads I, II, and III)
- Three augmented (unipolar) leads (leads aVR, aVL, and aVF)
- Six precordial (unipolar) leads (V_1, V_2, V_3, V_4, V_5, and V_6)

The 12-lead ECG is used to diagnose changes associated with *acute coronary syndromes* (ACS) or "heart attacks," bundle branch blocks, and to help in the differentiation between certain tachycardias (i.e., supraventricular versus ventricular).

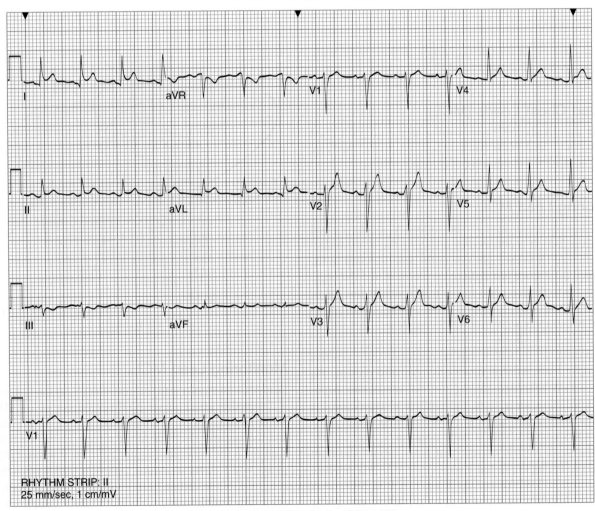

FIGURE 2-10 Sample of a 12-lead ECG.

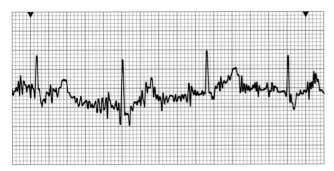

FIGURE 2-11 Muscle tremor.

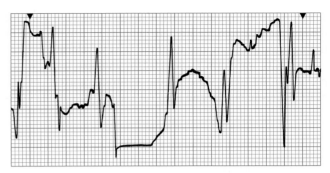

FIGURE 2-13 Loose electrodes.

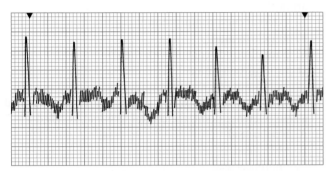

FIGURE 2-12 AC interference.

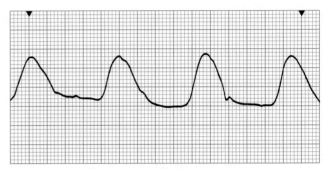

FIGURE 2-14 External chest compression.

The 12-lead ECG is used commonly in the hospital setting; its use is rapidly becoming the standard of care in prehospital medicine to more effectively identify patients with acute coronary syndromes and deliver them efficiently to the closest, most appropriate facility.

Acquiring A Quality ECG

Artifacts

Abnormal waves and spikes in an ECG that result from sources other than the electrical activity of the heart and interfere with or distort the components of the ECG are called *artifacts*. The causes of artifacts include muscle tremor, alternating current (AC) interference, poor electrode contact with the skin, and external chest compression.

Muscle tremor (Figure 2-11) can occur in tense or nervous patients or those shivering from the cold, and it can give the ECG a fine or coarsely jagged appearance.

AC interference (Figure 2-12) can occur when an improperly grounded, AC-operated ECG machine is used, or when an ECG is obtained near high tension wires, transformers, or electric appliances. This results in a thick baseline composed of 60-cycle waves.

Loose electrodes, or electrodes that are in poor electrical contact with the skin (Figure 2-13) because of insufficient or dried electrode paste or jelly, can cause multiple, sharp spikes and waves in the ECG and are the most common cause of artifacts. Loose connecting wires can also cause similar artifacts. In addition, any extraneous matter on the skin, such as blood, vomit, sweat, and hair can result in poor electrode contact and the appearance of artifacts.

External chest compressions (Figure 2-14) during cardiopulmonary resuscitation (CPR) cause regularly spaced, wide, upright waves synchronous with the downward compressions of the chest. It must be emphasized that such waves do not indicate that the chest compressions are producing adequate cardiac output and circulation.

QRS Size and Wandering Baseline

The ECG machine has the capability to amplify the signal it receives and display it on the monitor. If the signal strength is low, most machines have a control that allows you to increase the amplitude. The control is called the "gain." Increasing the gain will not affect the depiction of the ECG waveform printed on the ECG graph paper but can be very helpful when using only the monitor to interpret the rhythm. Other causes of low amplitude waveforms that will result in low amplitude ECG when printed include patients with large barrel chests and obesity (due to increased resistance of the signal passing through the chest). Another problem can arise when the ECG waveform does not maintain a steady baseline. This can make measuring portions of the waveform difficult. This occurs when the patient moves, breathes heavily, or when the electrodes are attached too close to the torso.

CHAPTER SUMMARY

An electrocardiogram is a graphical representation of the current generated during the depolarization and repolarization of the atria and ventricles. This current is detected by electrodes attached to the body and the resulting ECG waveform is displayed on the monitor and printed on ECG graph paper for analysis. The ECG graph paper is designed to allow accurate measurement of both the strength (amplitude) and duration or timing of various components of the ECG waveform.

The ECG waveform is detected by multiple leads, which provide a different view of the electrical current of the heart. There are bipolar and unipolar leads. Dysrhythmia inter-pretation generally relies on the use of bipolar leads, while unipolar leads are used in the assessment of acute coronary syndromes.

Acquiring a quality ECG if vital to enables accurate measurement of the various components of the ECG waveform required in dysrhythmia interpretation.

CHAPTER REVIEW

1. The electrocardiogram (ECG) is a record of the electrical activity generated by:
   A. the depolarization and repolarization of the atria and ventricles
   B. the flow of blood through the heart
   C. the mechanical contraction and relaxation of the atria and ventricles
   D. the transmission of electrical impulses responsible for initiating depolarization of the atria and ventricles

2. When an ECG is recorded at the standard paper speed of 25 mm/sec, the dark vertical lines are _____ seconds apart and the light vertical lines are _____ seconds apart.
   A. 5: 1
   B. 20: 4
   C. 0.20: 0.4
   D. 0.20: 0.04

3. The sensitivity of the ECG machine is calibrated so that a _____ electrical signal produces a _____ deflection on the ECG.
   A. 0.5-mV: 1-mm
   B. 1-mV: 10-mm
   C. 5-mV: 10-mm
   D. 10-mV: 5-mm

4. The electric current generated by ventricular depolarization is recorded as the:
   A. P wave
   B. QRS complex
   C. atrial T wave (Ta)
   D. T wave

5. The electric current generated by ventricular repolarization is recorded as the:
   A. P wave
   B. QRS complex
   C. atrial T wave (Ta)
   D. T wave

6. Which of the following is the most common cause of ECG artifact?
   A. external chest compression
   B. muscle tremor
   C. poor electrode contact with the skin
   D. turning the gain up

7. An ECG lead composed of a single positive electrode and a zero reference point, the central terminal, is called a:
   A. bipolar lead
   B. MCL_1 lead
   C. multifocal lead
   D. unipolar lead

8. Monitoring lead II is obtained by attaching the negative electrode to the _____ and the positive electrode to the _____.
   A. left arm: left leg
   B. right arm: left arm
   C. right arm: left leg
   D. right arm: left upper chest

9. If the positive electrode is attached to the left leg or lower left anterior chest, all of the electric currents generated in the heart that flow toward the positive electrode will be recorded as a _____ (_____) deflection.
   A. negative (inverted)
   B. negative (upright)
   C. positive (inverted)
   D. positive (upright)

10. Monitoring lead MCL_1 is obtained by attaching the positive electrode from lead _____:
    A. II, to the left chest below the clavicle
    B. II, to the middle of the sternum at the level of the fourth intercostal space
    C. III, to the left side of the sternum in the fourth intercostal space
    D. III, to the right side of the anterior chest in the fourth intercostal space next to the sternum

3

Components of the Electrocardiogram

OBJECTIVES

Upon completion of all or part of this chapter, you should be able to complete the following objectives:

1. Define the following components of the electrocardiogram:
   - P wave
   - QRS complex
   - T wave
   - U wave
   - PR interval
   - QT interval
   - R-R interval
   - ST segment
   - PR segment
   - TP segment

2. Name and identify the components of the ECG, including the waves, complexes, segments, and intervals in an ECG.

3. Give the characteristics, description, and significance of the following waves and complexes:
   - Normal P wave
   - Abnormal P wave
   - Ectopic P wave
   - Normal QRS complex
   - Abnormal QRS complex
   - Normal T wave
   - Abnormal T wave
   - U wave

4. Give the characteristics, description, and significance of the following intervals and segments:
   - Normal PR interval
   - Abnormal PR interval
   - QT interval
   - R-R interval
   - Normal ST segment
   - Abnormal ST segment
   - PR segment
   - TP segment

5. Define the following
   - P pulmonale
   - P mitrale
   - Retrograde conduction
   - J point
   - Prime (′); double prime (″)
   - Notch in the R or S wave
   - Ventricular activation time (VAT)
   - Incomplete bundle branch block
   - Complete bundle branch block
   - Supraventricular arrhythmia
   - Aberrant ventricular conduction (aberrancy)
   - Ventricular preexcitation
   - Delta wave
   - Ectopy
   - QT_c
   - Torsades de pointes

27

WAVES

P Wave

NORMAL SINUS P WAVE

Characteristics

Pacemaker site. The pacemaker site is the sinoatrial (SA) node.

Relationship to cardiac anatomy and physiology. A normal sinus P wave (Figure 3-1) represents normal depolarization of the atria. Depolarization of the atria begins near the SA node and progresses across the atria from right to left and downward. The first part of the normal sinus P wave represents depolarization of the right atrium; the second part represents depolarization of the left atrium. During the P wave, the electrical impulse progresses from the SA node through the internodal atrial conduction tracts and most of the atrioventricular (AV) node.

Description

Onset and end. The onset of the P wave is identified as the first abrupt or gradual deviation from the baseline. The point where the wave flattens out to return to the baseline, joining with the PR-segment, marks the end of the P wave.

Direction. The direction is positive (upright) in lead II. This is due to the fact that the majority of the current is directed toward the positive electrode of lead II.

Duration. The duration is between 0.08 and 0.10 seconds.

Amplitude. The amplitude is 0.5 to 2.5 mm in lead II. The normal P wave is rarely over 2 mm high.

Shape. The shape is smooth and rounded.

P wave–QRS complex relationship. A QRS complex normally follows each sinus P wave, but in certain dysrhythmias, such as AV blocks (see Chapter 9), a QRS complex may not follow each sinus P wave.

PR interval. The PR interval may be normal (0.12 to 0.20 second) or abnormal (greater than 0.20 second or less than 0.12 second).

Significance

A normal sinus P wave indicates that the electrical impulse responsible for the P wave originated in the SA node and that normal depolarization of the right and left atria has occurred.

ABNORMAL SINUS P WAVE

Characteristics

Pacemaker site. The pacemaker site is the SA node.

Relationship to cardiac anatomy and physiology. An abnormal sinus P wave (Figure 3-2) represents depolarization of altered, damaged, or abnormal atria. Increased right atrial pressure and right atrial dilatation and hypertrophy—as found in chronic obstructive pulmonary disease and chronic congestive heart failure—may result in tall and symmetrically peaked P waves (P pulmonale). Over time the increased pressure of venous blood return to the right atria causes it to dilate and/or hypertrophy. Because there is more atrial muscle to depolarize, the total amount of current detected is equally increased resulting in a larger amplitude.

Increased left atrial pressure and left atrial dilatation and hypertrophy—as found in systemic hypertension, mitral and aortic valvular disease, acute myocardial infarction (MI), and pulmonary edema secondary to left heart failure—may cause wide, notched P waves (P mitrale). Besides the previously mentioned changes in amplitude, such notched P waves may also result from a delay or block of the progression of electrical impulses through the interatrial conduction tract between the right and left atria. In effect, the right atria depolarizes significantly sooner than the left atria and therefore the combined P waves take a longer period of time to occur.

Biphasic P waves can be seen in both right and left atrial dilatation and hypertrophy. Biphasic P waves are best detected in leads V_1 and V_2 because these two unipolar leads have direct views of the SA node from the front of the chest. They will have an initial positive deflection (right atrial depolarization) followed by a negative deflection (left atrial depolarization). Biphasic P waves are described in Chapter 15.

Description

Onset and end. The onset and end of the abnormal sinus P wave are the same as those of a normal P wave.

Direction. The direction is positive (upright) in lead II. May be biphasic (initially positive, then negative) in V_1 and V_2

Duration. The duration may be normal (0.08 to 0.10 second) but rarely greater than 0.16 second.

Amplitude. The amplitude may be normal (0.5 to 2.5 mm) or greater than 2.5 mm in lead II. By definition, a P pulmonale is 2.5 mm or greater in amplitude.

Shape. The abnormal sinus P wave may be tall and symmetrically peaked or may be wide and notched in lead II. By definition, the notched P wave equal to or greater than 0.12 seconds with the tops of each mound greater than 0.04 second apart is called P mitrale. Abnormal P waves may be biphasic in leads V_1 and V_2.

P wave–QRS complex relationship. The P wave-QRS complex relationship is the same as that of a normal sinus P wave.

PR interval. The PR interval may be normal (0.12 to 0.20 second) or abnormal (greater than 0.20 second or less than 0.12 second).

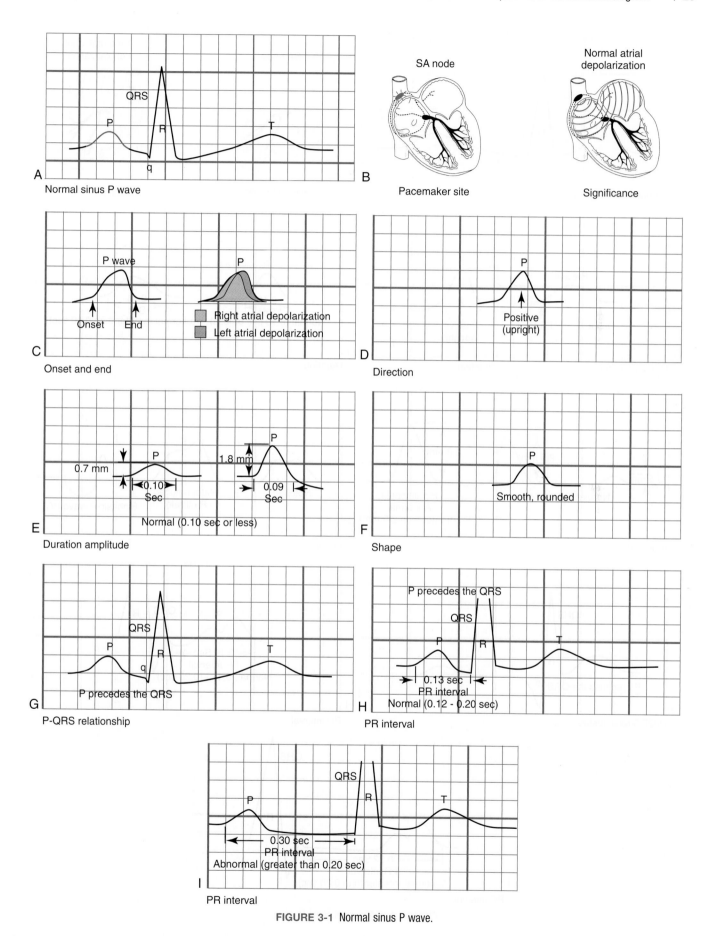

FIGURE 3-1 Normal sinus P wave.

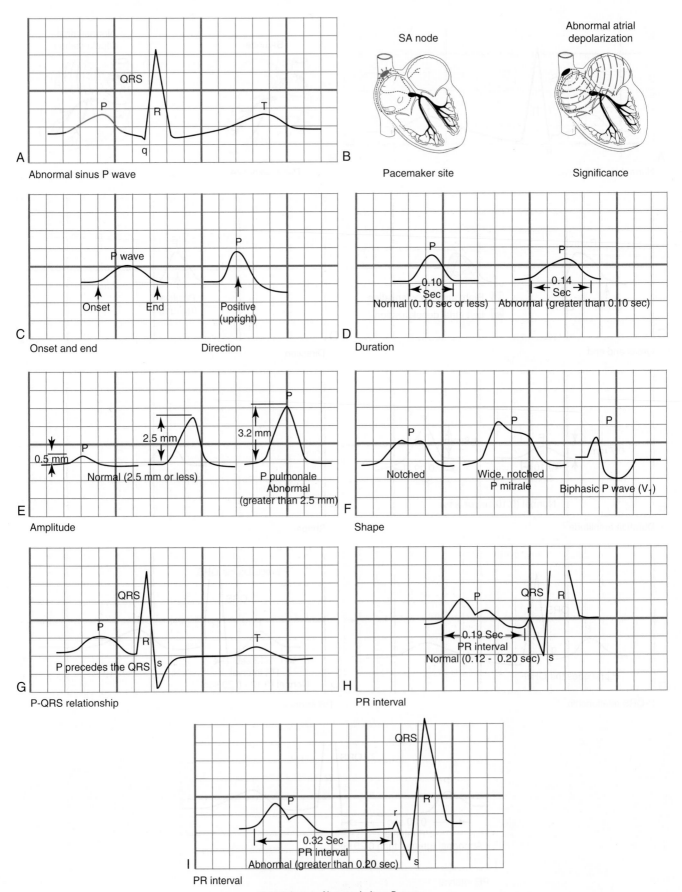

FIGURE 3-2 Abnormal sinus P wave.

Significance

An abnormal sinus P wave indicates that the electrical impulse responsible for the P wave originated in the SA node and that depolarization of altered, damaged, or abnormal atria has occurred.

Characteristics

Pacemaker site. The pacemaker site is an ectopic pacemaker in the atria outside of the SA node or in the AV junction.

Relationship to cardiac anatomy and physiology. An ectopic P wave (P′) (Figure 3-3) represents atrial depolarization

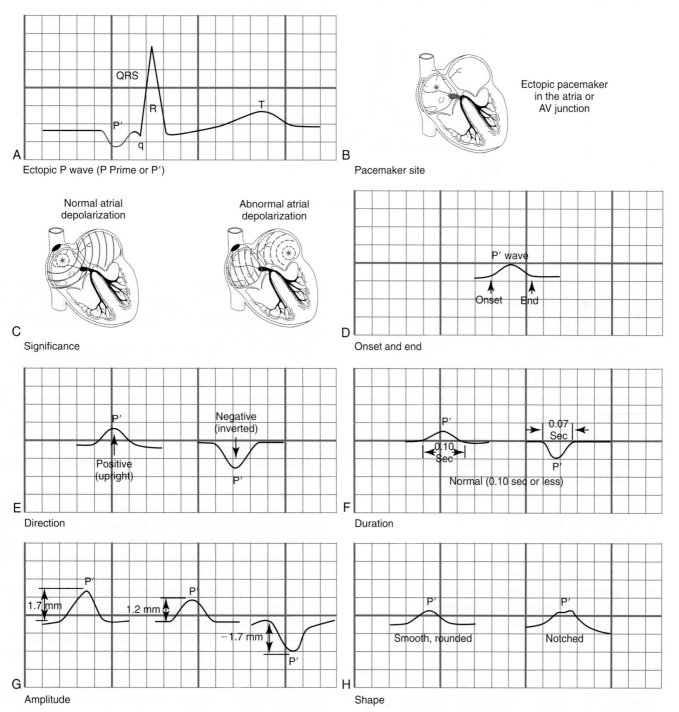

FIGURE 3-3 Ectopic P wave (P prime or P′).

Continued

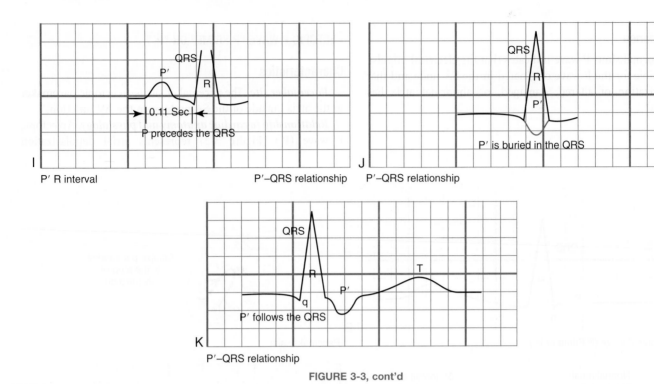

FIGURE 3-3, cont'd

occurring in an abnormal direction or sequence or both, depending on the ectopic pacemaker's location.

- If the ectopic pacemaker is in the upper or middle right atrium, depolarization of the atria occurs in a normal, antegrade, direction (right to left and downward)
- If the ectopic pacemaker is in the lower right atrium near the AV node or in the left atrium, depolarization of the atria occurs in a retrograde direction (left to right and upward)
- If the ectopic pacemaker is in the AV junction, the electrical impulse travels upward through the AV junction into the atria (retrograde conduction), causing retrograde atrial depolarization

Ectopic P waves occur in the following settings:
- Wandering atrial pacemaker
- Premature atrial complexes
- Atrial tachycardia
- Premature junctional complexes
- Junctional escape rhythm
- Nonparoxysmal junctional tachycardia
- Paroxysmal supraventricular tachycardia
- Atrial pacing by a cardiac pacemaker

Description

Onset and end. The onset and end of the abnormal ectopic P wave are the same as those of a normal P wave.

Direction. The ectopic P wave may be either positive (upright) or negative (inverted) in lead II if the ectopic pacemaker is in the atria. The P′ wave is always negative (inverted) in lead II if the ectopic pacemaker is in the AV junction or ventricles. Generally, if the ectopic pacemaker is in the upper part of the right atrium, the P′ wave is positive, resembling a normal sinus P wave.

If the ectopic pacemaker is in the middle of the right atrium, the P′ wave is less positive (upright) than one arising in the upper right atrium. If the ectopic pacemaker is in the lower right atrium near the AV node or in the left atrium or in the AV junction or the ventricles, the P′ wave is negative (inverted).

Duration. The duration may be normal or prolonged depending on the site of origin.

Amplitude. The amplitude is usually less than 2.5 mm in lead II, but it may be greater.

Shape. The ectopic P wave may be smooth and rounded, peaked, or slightly notched. Atrial pacemakers will have a sharp spike appearance and precede the QRS complex. See Chapter 14.

P′ Wave–QRS complex relationship. The ectopic P wave may precede, be buried in, or follow the QRS complex with which it is associated.

- If the ectopic pacemaker is in any part of the atria or in the upper part of the AV junction, the P′ wave generally precedes the QRS complex.
- If the ectopic pacemaker is in the lower part of the AV junction or in the ventricles, the P′ wave may occur either during or after the QRS complex.

If the P′ wave occurs during the QRS complex, it is buried in the QRS complex and is said to be hidden or invisible. If it follows the QRS complex, it becomes superimposed on the succeeding ST segment and/or T wave, distorting them.

P′R interval. The P′R (or RP′) interval varies depending on the location of the ectopic pacemaker.

- If the ectopic pacemaker is in the upper or middle right atrium, the P′R interval is generally normal (0.12 to 0.20 second).
- If the ectopic pacemaker is in the lower right atrium, close to the AV node, in the left atrium, or in the upper part of the AV junction, the ectopic P wave usually precedes the QRS complex with a P′R interval of less than 0.12 second.
- If the ectopic pacemaker is in the lower part of the AV junction or in the ventricles, the ectopic P wave may be buried in the QRS complex or follow it. In the latter case, the interval between the end of the QRS complex and the onset of the P′ is called the *RP′ interval.* It is usually less than 0.12 second.

Significance

An ectopic P wave indicates that the electrical impulse responsible for the ectopic P wave originated in part of the atria outside the SA node or in the AV junction or ventricles, and that depolarization of the right and left atria has occurred in an abnormal direction or sequence or both.

QRS Complex

KEY DEFINITION

A QRS complex represents depolarization of the right and left ventricles. There are two types of QRS complex:
- Normal QRS complex
- Abnormal QRS complex

NORMAL QRS COMPLEX

Characteristics

Pacemaker site. The pacemaker site of the electrical impulse responsible for a normal QRS complex is the SA node or an ectopic or escape pacemaker in the atria or AV junction.

Relationship to cardiac anatomy and physiology. A normal QRS complex (Figure 3-4) represents normal depolarization of the ventricles. Depolarization begins in the left side of the interventricular septum near the AV junction and progresses across the interventricular septum from left to right. Then, beginning at the endocardial surface of the ventricles, depolarization progresses through the ventricular walls to the epicardial surface.

The first short part of the QRS complex, usually the Q wave, represents depolarization of the interventricular septum; the rest of the QRS complex represents the simultaneous depolarization of the right and left ventricles. Because the left ventricle is larger than the right ventricle and has more muscle mass, the QRS complex represents, for the most part, depolarization of the left ventricle.

The electrical impulse that causes normal ventricular depolarization originates above the ventricles in the SA node or an ectopic or escape pacemaker in the atria or AV junction and has normal conduction down the right and left bundle branches to the Purkinje network. Also a relatively normal-appearing QRS complex may originate in an ectopic or escape pacemaker in the proximal left bundle branch. The QRS complex precedes ventricular systole.

Description

Onset and end. The onset of the QRS complex is identified as the point where the first wave of the complex just begins to deviate, abruptly or gradually, from the baseline. The end of the QRS complex is the point where the last wave of the complex begins to flatten out (sharply or gradually) at, above, or below the baseline. This point, the junction between the QRS complex and the ST segment, is called the *junction* or *J point.*

Components. The QRS complex consists of one or more of the following: positive (upright) deflections called *R waves* and negative (inverted) deflections called *Q, S,* and *QS waves.* The characteristics of the waves that make up the QRS complex in lead II are as follows:

- **Q wave:** The Q wave is the first negative deflection in the QRS complex not preceded by an R wave.
- **R wave:** The R wave is the first positive deflection in the QRS complex. Subsequent positive deflections are called *R prime (R′), R double prime (R″),* and so forth.
- **S wave:** The S wave is the first negative deflection in the QRS complex after an R wave. Subsequent negative deflections are called *S prime (S′), S double prime (S″),* and so forth.
- **QS wave:** A QS wave is a QRS complex that consists entirely of a single, large negative deflection.
- **Notch:** A notch in the R wave is a negative deflection that does not extend below the baseline; a notch in the S wave is a positive deflection that does not extend above the baseline.

> Although there may be only one Q wave, there can be more than one R and S wave in the QRS complex.

The waves comprising the QRS complex are usually identified by upper or lower case letters, depending on the relative size of the waves. The large waves that form the major deflections are identified by upper case letters (Q, R, S). The smaller waves that are less than half of the amplitude of the major deflections are identified by lower case letters (q, r, s). Thus the ventricular depolarization complex can be described more accurately by using upper and lower case letters assigned to the waves (e.g., qR, Rs, qRs). However, the complex is still referred to as the "QRS" complex when discussing it in general.

Direction. The direction of the QRS complex may be predominantly positive (upright), predominantly negative (inverted), or equiphasic (equally positive and equally negative). A predominantly positive QRS complex, for example, has more area encompassed by the R wave, the major deflection,

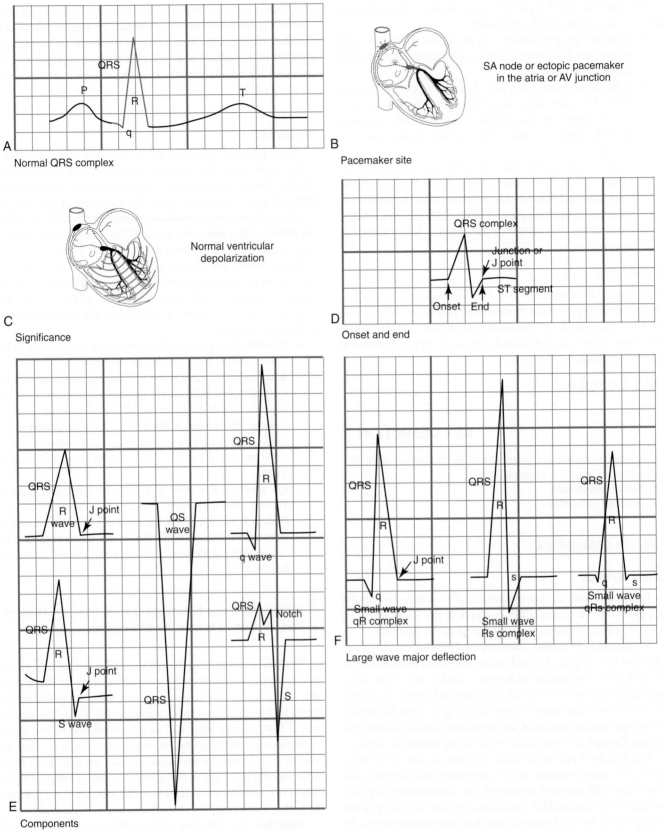

FIGURE 3-4 Normal QRS complex.

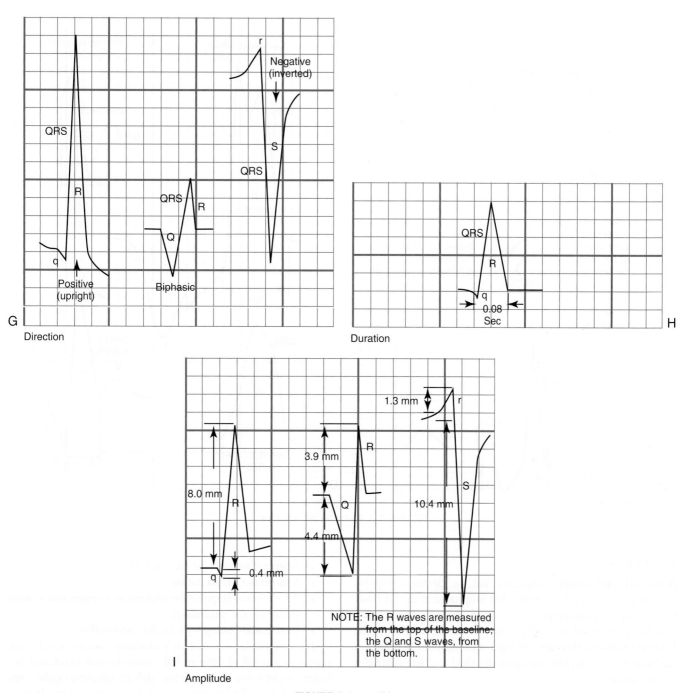

FIGURE 3-4, cont'd

than is encompassed by the Q and S waves. Usually this is easy to determine by simply looking at the QRS complex; however, if you are unsure, place a ruler at the baseline and estimate the number of small squares covered by the QRS complex above and below the baseline.

Duration. The duration of the normal QRS complex is 0.06 to 0.12 second in adults and 0.08 second or less in children. The QRS complex is measured from the onset of the Q or R wave to the end of the last wave of the complex; the J point. The duration of the Q wave does not normally exceed 0.04 second. The time from the onset of the QRS complex to the peak of the R wave is the ventricular activation time (VAT). The VAT represents the time taken for the depolarization of the interventricular septum plus depolarization of the ventricle from the endocardium to the epicardium under the facing lead. The upper limit of the normal VAT is 0.05 seconds.

Amplitude. The amplitude of the R or S wave in the QRS complex in lead II may vary from 1 to 2 mm to 15 mm or more. The normal Q wave is less than 25% of the height of the succeeding R wave.

Shape. The waves in the QRS complex are generally narrow and sharply pointed.

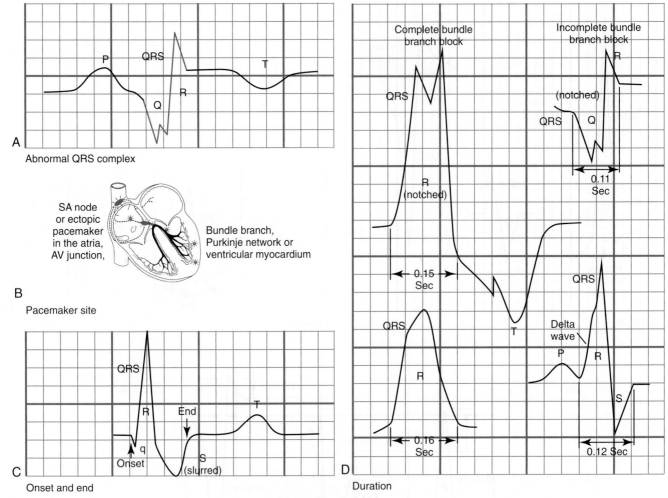

A
Abnormal QRS complex

B
Pacemaker site

SA node or ectopic pacemaker in the atria, AV junction,

Bundle branch, Purkinje network or ventricular myocardium

C
Onset and end

D
Duration

FIGURE 3-5 Abnormal QRS complex.

Significance

A normal QRS complex indicates that the electrical impulse responsible for the QRS complex has originated in the SA node or an ectopic or escape pacemaker in the atria or AV junction and has progressed normally from the bundle of His to the Purkinje network through the right and left bundle branches and that normal depolarization of the right and left ventricles has occurred.

ABNORMAL QRS COMPLEX

Characteristics

Pacemaker site. The pacemaker site of the electrical impulse responsible for an abnormal QRS complex is the SA node or an ectopic or escape pacemaker in the atria, AV junction, bundle branches, Purkinje network, or ventricular myocardium.

Relationship to cardiac anatomy and physiology. An abnormal QRS complex (Figure 3-5) represents abnormal depolarization of the ventricles. This may result from any one of the following:

- Intraventricular conduction disturbance (such as a bundle branch block)

- Aberrant ventricular conduction
- Ventricular preexcitation
- An electrical impulse originating in a ventricular ectopic site or escape pacemaker
- Ventricular pacing by a cardiac pacemaker

Intraventricular conduction disturbance occurs most commonly as a result of right or left bundle branch block and to a lesser extent from a nonspecific, diffuse intraventricular conduction defect (IVCD) seen in some acute coronary syndromes, fibrosis, and myocardial hypertrophy; electrolyte imbalances, such as hypokalemia and hyperkalemia; and excessive administration of such cardiac drugs as amiodarone, procainamide, and flecainide. Bundle branch block results from partial or complete block in the conduction of electrical impulses from the bundle of His to the Purkinje network through the right or left bundle branch while conduction continues uninterrupted through the unaffected bundle branch (see Chapter 13). A block in one bundle branch causes the ventricle on that side to be depolarized later than the other ventricle.

For example, in complete right bundle branch block, depolarization of the right ventricle is delayed because of a block in conduction through the right bundle branch. This results in an

1. Blockage of conduction of the electrical
impulse through a bundle branch

Block in
right bundle
branch

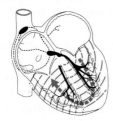

Right bundle branch block

Block in
left bundle
branch

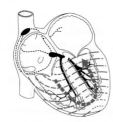

Left bundle branch block

Bundle branch block and aberrant ventricular conduction

Direction
of ventricular
depolarization

2. Conduction of the electrical impulse through
accessory conduction pathways

Ventricular
preexcitation

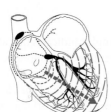

3. Ventricular ectopic or artificial cardiac pacemaker

Abnormal
ventricular
depolarization

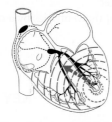

Ventricular
pacemaker

E

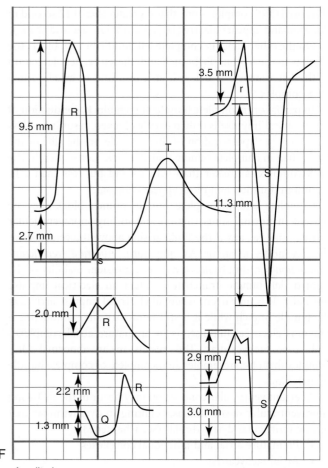

F

Amplitude

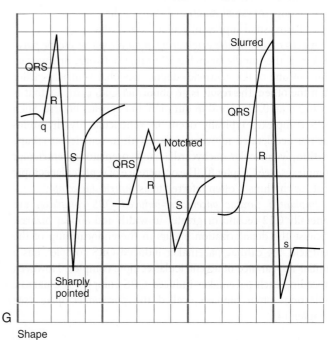

G

Shape

FIGURE 3-5, cont'd

abnormal QRS complex—one that is greater than 0.12 second in duration and appears bizarre (i.e., abnormal in size and shape).

On the other hand, in complete left bundle branch block, the block is in the left bundle branch and, therefore, depolarization of the left ventricle is delayed, also resulting in an abnormal QRS complex.

In partial or incomplete bundle branch block, conduction of the electrical impulse is only partially blocked, resulting in less of a delay in depolarization of the ventricle on the side of the block than in complete bundle branch block. Consequently, the QRS complex is greater than 0.10 second but less than 0.12 second in duration and often appears normal.

Complete and incomplete bundle branch block may be present in normal sinus rhythm and in any supraventricular arrhythmia (i.e., any arrhythmia arising above the ventricles in the SA node, atria, or AV junction). *Aberrant ventricular conduction* (or, simply, *aberrancy*) is a transient inability of the right or left bundle branch to conduct an electrical impulse normally. This may occur when an electrical impulse arrives at the bundle branch while it is still refractory after conducting a previous electrical impulse, as in premature atrial complexes and some tachycardias. This results in an abnormal QRS complex that often resembles an incomplete or complete bundle branch block.

Aberrant ventricular conduction may occur in the following supraventricular dysrhythmias, resulting in dysrhythmias that mimic ventricular dysrhythmias (see Chapter 8):

- Premature atrial and junctional complexes
- Atrial tachycardia
- Atrial flutter and fibrillation
- Nonparoxysmal junctional tachycardia
- Paroxysmal supraventricular tachycardia

An electrical impulse originating in an ectopic or escape pacemaker in the bundle branches, Purkinje network, or myocardium of one of the ventricles depolarizes that ventricle earlier than the other. The result is an abnormal QRS complex that is greater than 0.12 second in duration and appears bizarre. Such QRS complexes typically occur in ventricular dysrhythmias such as accelerated idioventricular rhythm, ventricular escape rhythm, ventricular tachycardia, and premature ventricular complexes (see Chapter 8). The occurrence of ventricular ectopic beats or rhythms is often referred to as *ventricular ectopy*.

Implanted cardiac pacemaker-induced QRS complexes are generally 0.12 second or greater in width and appear bizarre. Because the depolarization occurs in the endocardium of the ventricle, the cardiac pacemaker-induced QRS complex has a similar appearance of a ventricular ectopic complex. However, preceding each pacemaker-induced QRS complex is a narrow deflection, often biphasic, called the *pacemaker spike* (see Chapter 14).

Description

Onset and end. The onset and end of the abnormal QRS complex are the same as those of a normal QRS complex.

Direction. The direction of the abnormal QRS complex may be predominantly positive (upright), predominantly negative (inverted), or equiphasic (equally positive and equally negative).

Duration. The duration of the abnormal QRS complex is greater than 0.12 second. If a bundle branch block is present and the duration of the QRS complex is between 0.10 and 0.12 second, the bundle branch block is called *incomplete*. If the duration of the QRS complex is greater than 0.12 second, the bundle branch block is called *complete*. In ventricular preexcitation, the duration of the QRS complex is greater than 0.12 second.

The duration of a QRS complex caused by an electrical impulse originating in an ectopic or escape pacemaker in the Purkinje network or ventricular myocardium is always greater than 0.12 second; typically, it is 0.16 second or greater. However, if the electrical impulse originates in a bundle branch, the duration of the QRS complex may be only slightly greater than 0.10 second and appear normal.

Amplitude. The amplitude of the waves in the abnormal QRS complex varies from 1 to 2 mm to 20 mm or more.

Shape. An abnormal QRS complex varies widely in shape, from one that appears quite normal—narrow and sharply pointed (as in incomplete bundle branch block)—to one that is wide and bizarre, slurred and notched (as in complete bundle branch block and ventricular dysrhythmias). In ventricular preexcitation the QRS complex is wider than normal at the base because of an initial slurring or bulging of the upstroke of the R wave (or of the down stroke of the S wave, as the case may be)—the delta wave.

Significance

An abnormal QRS complex indicates that abnormal depolarization of the ventricles has occurred because of one of the following:

- A block in the progression of the electrical impulse from the bundle of His to the Purkinje network through the right or left bundle branch (bundle branch block and aberrant ventricular conduction)
- The progression of the electrical impulse from the atria to the ventricles through an abnormal accessory conduction pathway (ventricular preexcitation)
- The origination of the electrical impulse responsible for the ventricular depolarization in a ventricular ectopic or escape pacemaker
- The excitation of the ventricles by a cardiac pacemaker

T Wave

KEY DEFINITION

A T wave represents ventricular repolarization. There are two types of T waves:
- Normal T wave
- Abnormal T wave

NORMAL T WAVE

Characteristics

Relationship to cardiac anatomy and physiology. A normal T wave (Figure 3-6) represents normal repolarization of the ventricles. Normal repolarization begins at the epicardial surface of the ventricles and progresses inwardly through the ventricular walls to the endocardial surface. The T wave occurs during the last part of ventricular systole.

Description

Onset and end. The onset of the T wave is identified as the first abrupt or gradual deviation from the ST segment (or the point where the slope of the ST segment appears to become abruptly or gradually steeper). If the ST segment is absent, the T wave begins at the end of the QRS complex (or the J point). The point where the T wave returns to the baseline marks the end of the T wave. In the absence of an ST segment, the T wave is sometimes called the *ST-T wave.* Sometimes the onset and end of the T wave are difficult to determine with certainty.

Direction. The direction of the normal T wave is positive (upright) in lead II.

> The normal T wave is almost always in the same direction as the QRS complex.

Duration. The duration is 0.10 to 0.25 second or greater. The duration of the T wave alone is less important than the QT interval.

Amplitude. The amplitude is normally less than 5 mm.

> A good rule of thumb is that the normal T wave is never more than two-thirds the height of the R wave.

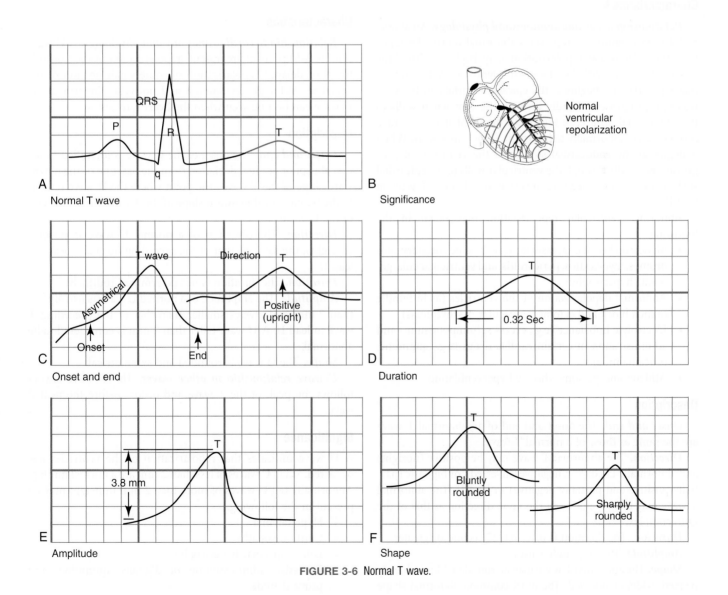

FIGURE 3-6 Normal T wave.

Shape. The normal T wave is sharply or bluntly rounded and asymmetrical. The first, upward part of the T wave is longer than the second, downward part.

> Symmetrical T waves almost always indicate some pathology such as ischemia or electrolyte imbalance.

T wave–QRS complex relationship. The T wave always follows the QRS complex.

Significance

The examination of T waves must also include the examination of the ST segment (to be discussed later). A normal T wave preceded by a normal ST segment indicates that normal repolarization of the right and left ventricles has occurred.

ABNORMAL T WAVE

Characteristics

Relationship to cardiac anatomy and physiology. An abnormal T wave (Figure 3-7) represents abnormal ventricular repolarization. Abnormal repolarization may begin at either the epicardial or endocardial surface of the ventricles. When abnormal repolarization begins at the epicardial surface of the ventricles, it progresses inwardly through the ventricular walls to the endocardial surface, as it normally does, but at a slower rate, producing an abnormally tall, upright T wave in lead II. When it begins at the endocardial surface of the ventricles, it progresses outwardly through the ventricular walls to the epicardial surface, producing a negative, inverted, or "flipped" T wave in lead II.

Abnormal ventricular repolarization may occur in the following:

- Myocardial ischemia, associated with acute coronary syndromes, myocarditis, pericarditis, and ventricular enlargement (hypertrophy)
- Abnormal depolarization of the ventricles (as in bundle branch block and ectopic ventricular dysrhythmias)
- Electrolyte imbalance (e.g., excess serum potassium) and administration of certain cardiac drugs (e.g., quinidine, procainamide)
- Athletes and persons who are hyperventilating

Description

Onset and end. The onset and end of an abnormal T wave are the same as those of a normal T wave.

Direction. The abnormal T wave may be positive (upright) and abnormally tall or low, negative (inverted), or biphasic (partially positive and partially negative) in lead II. The abnormal T wave may or may not be in the same direction as that of the QRS complex.

Duration. The duration is 0.10 to 0.25 second or greater.

Amplitude. The amplitude varies.

Shape. The abnormal T wave may be rounded, blunt, sharply peaked, wide, or notched. The most common abnormal shape

is a symmetrical T wave or reverse asymmetry where the first portion of the T wave is steep and short while the second portion is more gradual and long.

T wave–QRS complex relationship. The abnormal T wave always follows the QRS complex.

Significance

An abnormal T wave indicates that abnormal repolarization of the ventricles has occurred. An examination of the ST segment must also be taken into consideration to fully understand the clinical significance of the abnormal T wave.

U Wave

> **KEY DEFINITION**
>
> A U wave probably represents the final stage of repolarization of the ventricles.

Characteristics

Relationship to cardiac anatomy and physiology. A U wave (Figure 3-8) probably represents repolarization of the Purkinje fibers or delayed repolarization of some small portion of the ventricle. Although uncommon and not easily identified, the U wave can best be seen when the heart rate is slow.

Description

Onset and end. The onset of the U wave is identified as the first abrupt or gradual deviation from the baseline or the downward slope of the T wave. The point where the U wave returns to the baseline or downward slope of the T wave marks the end of the U wave.

Direction. The direction of a normal U wave is positive (upright), the same as that of the preceding normal T wave in lead II.

Duration. The duration is not determined routinely.

Amplitude. The amplitude of a normal U wave is usually less than 2 mm and always smaller than that of the preceding T wave in lead II. A U wave taller than 2 mm is considered to be abnormal.

Shape. The U wave is rounded and symmetrical.

U wave relationship to other waves. The U wave always follows the peak of the T wave and occurs before the next P wave.

Significance

A U wave indicates that repolarization of the ventricles has occurred. Small U waves of less than 2 mm are a normal finding. Abnormally tall U waves of more than 2 mm in height may be present in the following:

- Hypokalemia
- Cardiomyopathy
- Left ventricular hypertrophy
- Excessive administration of digitalis, quinidine, and procainamide

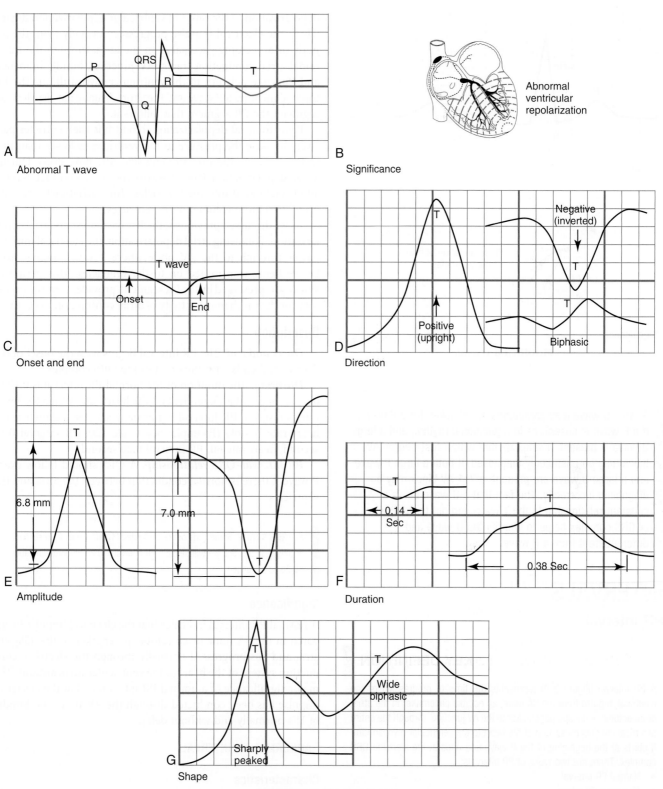

FIGURE 3-7 Abnormal T wave.

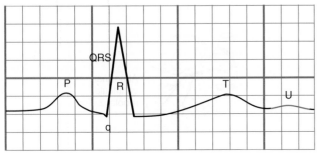

U wave

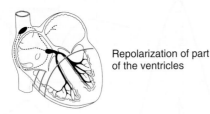

Repolarization of part of the ventricles

Significance

FIGURE 3-8 U wave.

> A large U wave may sometimes be mistaken for a P wave. If a P wave is absent, as in a junctional rhythm, and a large U wave is present, a sinus rhythm with a first-degree AV block may be mistakenly diagnosed. If both a large P wave and a large U wave are present, a 2:1 AV block may be diagnosed incorrectly. The fact that a U wave bears a constant relationship to the T wave and not to the P wave or QRS complex helps to identify the U wave and differentiate it from a P wave.

INTERVALS

PR Interval

KEY DEFINITION

A PR interval (Figure 3-9) represents the time of progression of the electrical impulse from the SA node, an ectopic pacemaker in the atria, or an ectopic or escape pacemaker in the AV junction, through the entire electrical conduction system of the heart to the ventricular myocardium. It starts at the beginning of the P wave and ends at the start the QRS complex. There are two types of PR intervals:
- Normal PR interval
- Abnormal PR interval

NORMAL PR INTERVAL

Characteristics

Relationship to cardiac anatomy and physiology. A normal PR interval represents the time from the onset of atrial depolarization to the onset of ventricular depolarization during which the electrical impulse progresses normally from the SA node or an ectopic pacemaker in the atria, through the internodal atrial conduction tracts, AV junction, bundle branches, and Purkinje network to the ventricular myocardium. The PR interval includes a P wave and the short, usually flat (isoelectric) segment, the PR segment that follows it.

Prior to atrial depolarization, blood fills the ventricles passively because the pressure in the ventricles is lower than that in the atria. As the pressure equalizes the flow stops. During atrial depolarization (the P wave) the atria contract forcing additional blood into the ventricles. This "atrial kick" can add up to 25% more volume to the ventricles.

As we discussed previously, the P wave represents atrial depolarization. Following atrial depolarization, the electrical impulse passes through to the AV node where it slows momentarily before being transmitted on to the ventricles. This period of slowing, represented by the PR segment, provides the time necessary for the mechanical activity of atrial contraction to occur.

Description

Onset and end. The PR interval begins with the onset of the P wave and ends with the onset of the QRS complex.

Duration. The duration of the normal PR interval is 0.12 to 0.20 second and is dependent on the heart rate. When the heart rate is fast, the PR interval is normally shorter than when the heart rate is slow (Example: heart rate 120, PR interval 0.16 second; heart rate 60, PR interval 0.20 second).

PR interval–QRS relationship. A QRS should follow every P wave if there is normal conduction between the atria and the ventricles.

> **AUTHOR'S NOTE** Some texts define prolonged PR interval as 0.20 second or longer. In this text we will define a PR interval = 0.20 as borderline and >0.20 as prolonged.

Significance

A normal PR interval indicates that the electrical impulse originated in the SA node or an ectopic pacemaker in the adjacent atria and has progressed normally through the electrical conduction system of the heart to the ventricular myocardium. The major significance of a normal PR interval is that the electrical impulse has been conducted through the AV node and bundle of His normally and without delay.

ABNORMAL PR INTERVAL

Characteristics

Relationship to cardiac anatomy and physiology. A PR interval greater than 0.20 second (Figure 3-10) represents delayed progression of the electrical impulse through the AV node, bundle of His, or, rarely, the bundle branches. A PR interval less than 0.12 second is commonly present when the electrical impulse originates in an ectopic pacemaker in the atria close to the AV node or in an ectopic or escape pacemaker in the AV

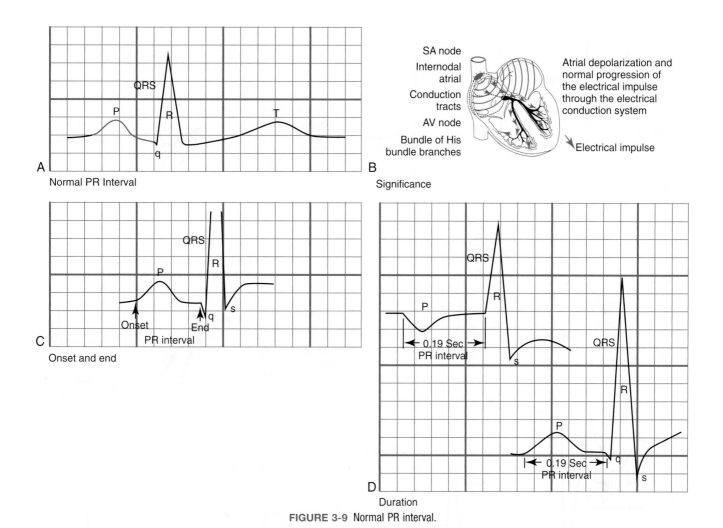

FIGURE 3-9 Normal PR interval.

junction. This occurs because the time for the impulse to reach the AV node is very short.

A negative (inverted) P wave in lead II is commonly associated with abnormally short PR intervals because the impulse is conducted in an antegrade fashion (from left to right and upward) from the AV node through the atria.

A positive and normal appearing P wave with a PR interval less than 0.12 second also occurs when the electrical impulse progresses from the atria to the ventricles through one of several accessory conduction pathways, which bypass the entire AV junction or just the AV node itself, depolarizing the ventricles earlier than usual. These anomalous conduction pathways include the following:

- **Accessory AV pathways (bundles of Kent)**: These abnormal AV conduction pathways that run from the atria to the ventricles bypass the AV junction, *causing ventricular preexcitation.* In this AV conduction anomaly, the short PR interval is commonly followed by a wide, abnormally shaped QRS complex with a delta wave (the slurring and sometimes notching at the onset of the QRS complex). This type of abnormal AV conduction is also called *Wolff-Parkinson-White syndrome* (WPW).

- **Atrio-His fibers (James fibers)**: This accessory conduction pathway, which extends from the atria to the lowermost part of the AV node near the onset of the bundle of His, bypassing the AV node, results in a short PR interval followed by a normal QRS complex. This anomalous AV conduction is called Lown-Ganong-Levine (LGL).

Description

Onset and end. The onset and end of the abnormal PR interval are the same as those of a normal PR interval.

Duration. The duration of the abnormal PR interval may be greater than 0.20 second or less than 0.12 second. PR intervals as long as 1 second have been reported; however, most commonly seen PR interval prolongation rarely exceeds 0.48 seconds. Additionally, the PR interval may vary from beat to beat or may be at time normal then progressively lengthen until there is no associated QRS complex.

Prolonged PR interval–QRS complex relationship. If a QRS complex is present following each P wave and prolonged PR interval then it can be assumed that the QRS complex resulted from the conducted originating in the P wave. However, if the PR interval continues to lengthen the conduction delay

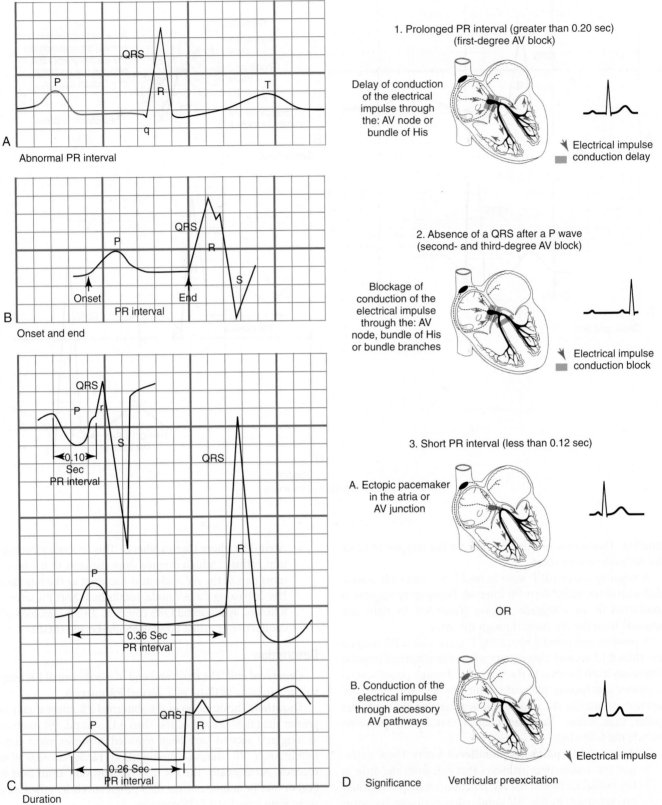

FIGURE 3-10 Abnormal PR interval.

can reach a point at which ventricular depolarization does not occur and subsequently no QRS complex is seen.

Significance

An abnormally prolonged PR interval indicates that a delay of progression of the electrical impulse through the AV node, bundle of His, or, rarely, the bundle branches is present. If the period or prolongation is constant, then the conduction delay is not changing. If the PR interval is changing constantly lengthening then the conduction delay is progressively worsening with each beat. This is classic of a second-degree heart block type I.

An abnormally short PR interval indicates one of the following:

- That the electrical impulse originated in an ectopic pacemaker in the atria near the AV node or in an ectopic or escape pacemaker in the AV junction
- That the electrical impulse originated in the SA node or atria and progressed through one of several abnormal accessory conduction pathways that bypass the entire AV junction or just the AV node

QT Interval

> ### KEY DEFINITION
>
> A QT interval represents the time between the onset of depolarization and the termination of repolarization of the ventricles.

Characteristics

Relationship to cardiac anatomy and physiology. The QT interval (Figure 3-11) represents the total time for the ventricles to depolarize and repolarize. It encompasses the QRS complex, the ST segment, and the T wave. An abnormally prolonged QT interval, one that exceeds the average QT interval for any given heart rate by 10%, represents a slowing in the repolarization of the ventricles. Abnormally prolonged QT intervals may occur in the following:

- Pericarditis, acute myocarditis, acute myocardial ischemia and infarction, left ventricular hypertrophy, and hypothermia
- Bradydysrhythmias (e.g., marked sinus bradycardia, third-degree AV block with slow ventricular escape rhythm)
- Electrolyte imbalance (hypokalemia and hypocalcemia) and liquid protein diets
- Medication effects (quinidine, procainamide, disopyramide, amiodarone, phenothiazines, and tricyclic antidepressants)
- Central nervous system disorders (e.g., cerebrovascular accident, subarachnoid hemorrhage, and intracranial trauma)
- Congenital prolonged QT syndrome

An abnormally short QT interval, one that is less than the average QT interval for any given heart rate by 10%, represents an increase in the rate of repolarization of the ventricles. This occurs in digitalis therapy and hypercalcemia.

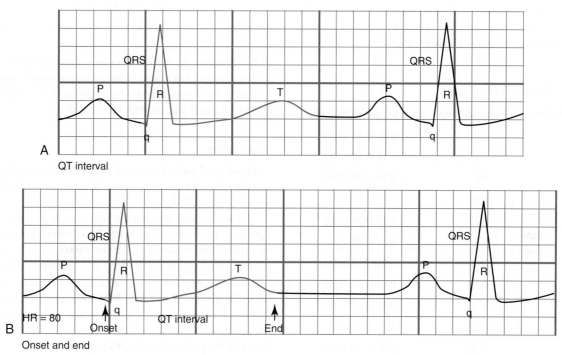

FIGURE 3-11 QT interval.

Description

Onset and end. The onset of the QT interval is identified as the point where the first wave of the QRS complex begins to deviate, abruptly or gradually, from the baseline. The end of the QT interval is the point where the T wave returns to the baseline.

> The determination of the QT interval should be made in the lead where the T wave is most prominent and not deformed by a U wave and should not include the U wave.

Duration. The duration of the QT interval is dependent on the heart rate. In general, a QT interval less than half the R-R interval is normal, one that is greater than half is abnormal, and one that is about half is "borderline." When the heart rate is fast, the QT interval is shorter than when the heart rate is slow (e.g., heart rate 120, QT interval about 0.29 second; heart rate 60, QT interval about 0.39 second). As the heart rate increases, the time for ventricular systole decreases and therefore the ventricles must depolarize and repolarize in a shorter amount of time. The reverse is true as the heart rate slows. The QT intervals may be equal or unequal in duration depending on the underlying rhythm. For example, if portions of the rhythm are fast, the QT interval will be shorter than those portions of the rhythm that are slower. In these instances it will be impossible to obtain an accurate measurement of the QT interval but you can estimate an average interval.

Because the QT interval is dependent on heart rate, "normal" is therefore dependent on heart rate and must be "corrected." This new value is termed QTc or QT corrected interval. The average duration of the QT interval normally expected at a given heart rate, the corrected QT interval (or QTc), and the normal range of 10% above and 10% below the average value are shown in Table 3-1. Regardless of heart rate, a QT interval of greater than 0.45 second is considered abnormal.

TABLE 3-1 QT_c Intervals

Heart Rate/min	R-R Interval (sec)	QT_c (sec) and Normal Range
40	1.5	0.46 (0.41–0.51)
50	1.2	0.42 (0.38–0.46)
60	1.0	0.39 (0.35–0.43)
70	0.86	0.37 (0.33–0.41)
80	0.75	0.35 (0.32–0.39)
90	0.67	0.33 (0.30–0.36)
100	0.60	0.31 (0.28–0.34)
120	0.50	0.29 (0.26–0.32)
150	0.40	0.25 (0.23–0.28)
180	0.33	0.23 (0.21–0.25)
200	0.30	0.22 (0.20–0.24)

> An easy way to calculate the QTc is as follows:
> QTc = QT (milliseconds) + 1.75 (ventricular rate −60)
> Example: HR = 100, QT = 330
> 1.75(100 − 60) =1.75 × 40 = 70
> 330 + 70 = 400 or 0.400 second, which is normal

Significance

A QT interval represents the time between the onset of ventricular depolarization until the end of ventricular repolarization. As discussed earlier, the ventricles are vulnerable during the relative refractory period of the T wave. A prolonged QT interval indicates slowing of ventricular repolarization and therefore a longer period of ventricular vulnerability.

Therefore, QT prolongation increases the potential for lethal ventricular dysrhythmias such as torsades de pointes. Short QT intervals are relatively rare but when found (often in infants and children) are due to genetic disorders that predispose them to sudden cardiac death and are treated with implantable defibrillators.

R-R Interval

> **KEY DEFINITION**
>
> An R-R interval represents the time between two successive ventricular depolarizations.
> There are 2 types of R-R intervals
> - Regular
> - Irregular

Characteristics

Relationship to cardiac anatomy and physiology. An R-R interval (Figure 3-12) normally represents one cardiac cycle during which the atria and ventricles contract and relax once.

> It is possible for there to be more than one atrial depolarization (P wave) between consecutive R waves. Noting the P waves and measuring the P-P interval will further assist your rhythm interpretation.

Description

Onset and end. The onset of the R-R interval is generally considered to be the peak of one R wave; the end is the peak of the succeeding R wave.

Duration. The duration is dependent on the heart rate. When the heart rate is fast, the R-R interval is shorter than when the heart rate is slow (e.g., heart rate 120, R-R interval 0.50 second; heart rate 60, R-R interval 1.0 second). The R-R intervals may be equal or unequal in duration, depending on the underlying rhythm. We refer to this equality as regularity. If the R-R intervals are equal, the ventricular rate is regular. If they are unequal, the rate is irregular. There are further subcategories that will be explored in later chapters. Examples of irregular rhythms include the following:

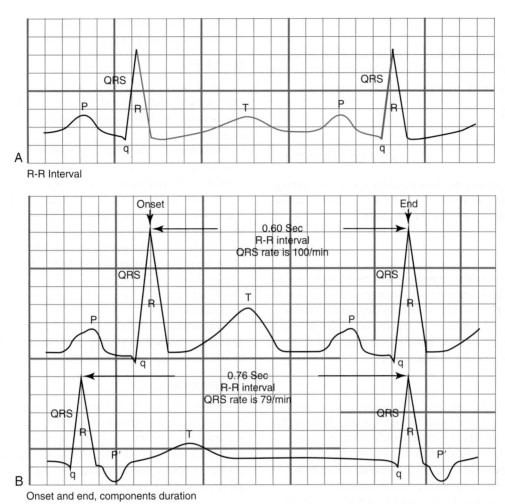

FIGURE 3-12 R-R interval.

- A regular rhythm interspersed with premature atrial, junctional, and ventricular premature beats
- Atrial fibrillation
- Second-degree AV blocks

Significance

An R-R interval represents the time between two successive ventricular depolarizations. Measuring the R-R interval and correlating it with the presence and timing of the P waves and other intervals is a crucial step in rhythm interpretation and should be mastered.

SEGMENTS
TP Segment

> **KEY DEFINITION**
>
> A TP segment is the interval between two successive P-QRST complexes, during which electrical activity of the heart is absent. This is referred to as the "Baseline."

Characteristics

Relationship to cardiac anatomy and physiology. A TP segment represents the time from the end of ventricular repolarization to the onset of the following atrial depolarization, during which electrical activity of the heart is absent. A TP segment may include a U wave after the T wave.

Description

Onset and end. The TP segment begins with the end of the T wave and ends with the onset of the following P wave.

Duration. The duration is 0.0 to 0.40 second or greater and is dependent on the heart rate and the configuration of the P waves and the QRS-T complexes. When the heart rate is fast, the TP segment is shorter than when the heart rate is slow. For example, when the heart rate is about 120 or greater, the TP segment is absent, with the P wave immediately following the T wave or buried in it. With a heart rate of 60 or less, the TP segment is about 0.4 second or greater.

Amplitude. Usually, the TP segment is flat (isoelectric).

Significance

A TP segment indicates the absence of any electrical activity of the heart. The TP segment is used as the baseline reference for the determination of ST-segment elevation or depression.

PR Segment

KEY DEFINITION

A PR segment represents the time of progression of the electrical impulse from the AV node through the bundle of His, bundle branches, and Purkinje network to the ventricular myocardium.

Characteristics

Relationship to cardiac anatomy and physiology. The PR segment (Figure 3-13) represents the time from the end of atrial depolarization to the onset of ventricular depolarization during which the electrical impulse progresses from the AV node through the bundle of His, bundle branches, and Purkinje network to the ventricular myocardium.

Description

Onset and end. The onset of the PR segment begins with the end of the P wave and ends with the onset of the QRS complex.

Duration. The duration normally varies from about 0.02 to 0.10 second. It may be greater than 0.10 second if there is a delay in the progression of the electrical impulse through the AV node, bundle of His, or rarely the bundle branches.

Amplitude. Normally the PR segment is flat (isoelectric).

Significance

A PR segment of 0.10-second duration or less indicates that the electrical impulse has been conducted through the AV junction normally and without delay or through an accessory conduction pathway. A PR segment exceeding 0.10 second in duration indicates a delay in the conduction of the electrical impulse through the AV junction or rarely the bundle branches.

ST Segment

KEY DEFINITION

An ST segment represents the early part of repolarization of the right and left ventricles. There are two types of ST segment:
- Normal ST segment
- Abnormal ST segment

NORMAL ST SEGMENT

Characteristics

Relationship to cardiac anatomy and physiology. The ST segment (Figure 3-14) represents the early part of ventricular repolarization. This is a period of electrical silence of the heart during which the mechanical contraction of the ventricles (ventricular systole) is reaching completion.

Description

Onset and end. The ST segment begins with the end of the QRS complex and ends with the onset of the T wave. The junction between the QRS complex and the ST segment is called the *junction or J point.*

Duration. The duration is 0.20 second or less and is dependent on the heart rate. When the heart rate is fast, the ST segment is shorter than when the heart rate is slow.

Amplitude. Normally, the ST segment is flat (isoelectric). Slight elevation or depression of less than 1.0 mm during the first 0.04 second (1 small square) after the J point of the QRS complex is considered normal. The TP segment is normally used as a baseline reference for the determination of the amplitude of the ST segment. However, if the TP segment is absent because of a very rapid heart rate, the PR segment is used instead.

Appearance. If slightly elevated, the ST segment may be flat, concave, or arched. If slightly depressed, the ST segment may be flat, upsloping, or downsloping.

Significance

A normal ST segment followed by a normal T wave indicates that normal repolarization of the right and left ventricles has occurred. Examination of the ST segment and its relationship with the T wave it critical when assessing for evidence of myocardial ischemia and/or infarction and will be explored in greater detail in Chapter 17.

ABNORMAL ST SEGMENT

Characteristics

Relationship to cardiac anatomy and physiology. An abnormal ST segment (Figure 3-15, p. 51) signifies abnormal ventricular repolarization, a common consequence of myocardial ischemia and injury. It occurs because the damaged myocardium begins to repolarize earlier than the normal myocardium and this electrical activity causes the ST segment to merge into the T wave. This can result in either ST segment elevation or depression depending on the area of the heart affected and the lead examined.

Description

Onset and end. The onset and end of the abnormal ST segment are the same as those of a normal ST segment.

Duration. The duration is 0.20 second or less.

Amplitude. An ST segment is abnormal when it is elevated or depressed 1.0 mm or more 0.04 second (1 small square) after the J point of the QRS complex.

Appearance. If elevated, the ST segment may be flat, concave, or arched. If depressed, the ST segment may be flat, upsloping, or downsloping.

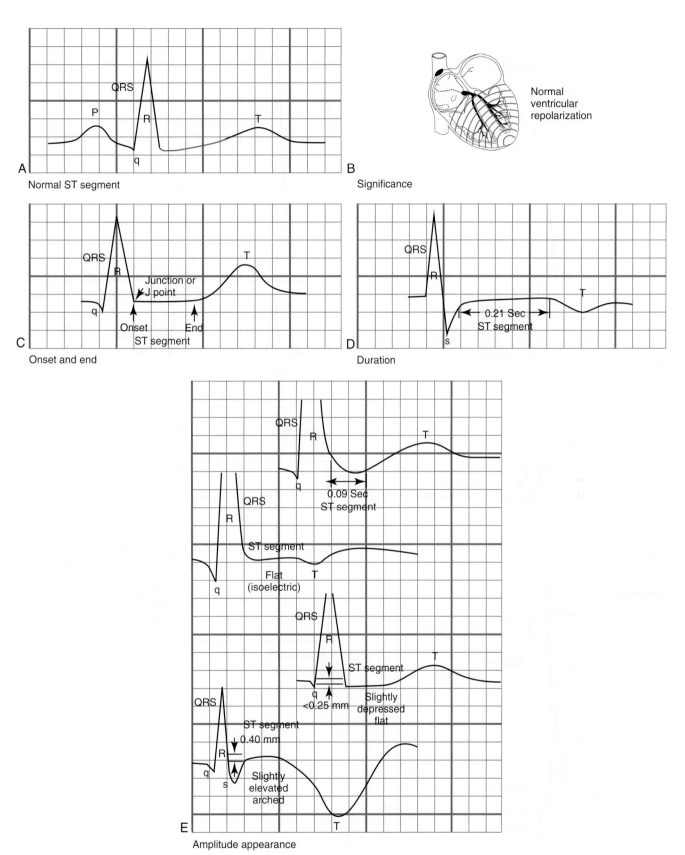

FIGURE 3-13 PR segment.

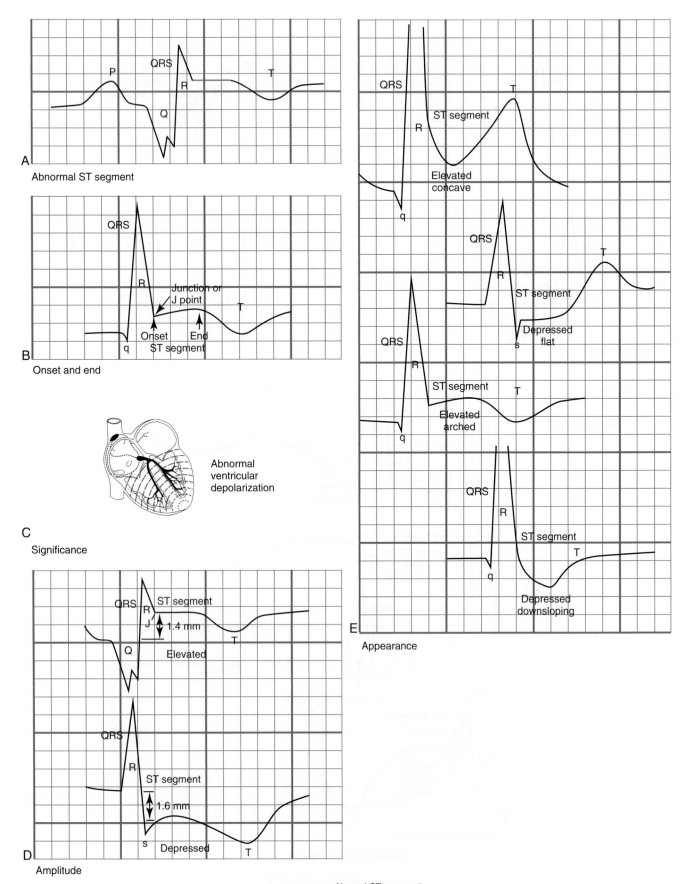

A Abnormal ST segment

B Onset and end

C Significance

D Amplitude

E Appearance

FIGURE 3-14 Normal ST segment.

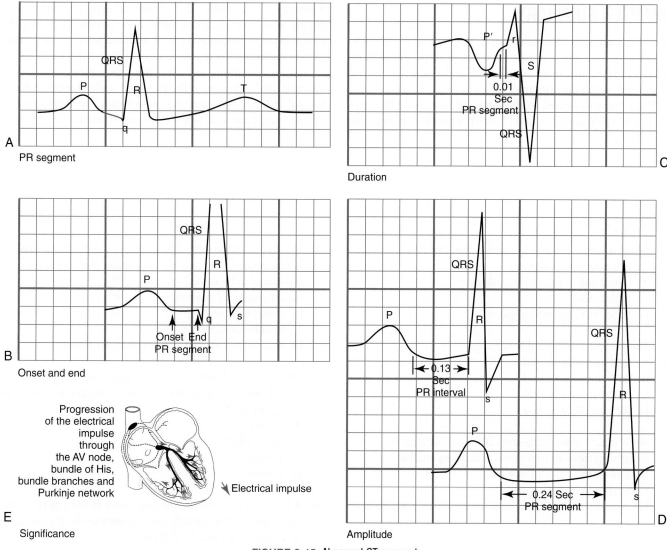

FIGURE 3-15 Abnormal ST segment.

Significance

An abnormal ST segment indicates that abnormal ventricular repolarization has occurred. Common causes of ST-segment elevation include the following:

- Acute myocardial infarction (cell death)
- Myocardial ischemia (hypoxia)
- Prinzmetal angina (severe transmural myocardial ischemia from coronary artery spasm)
- Ventricular aneurysm
- Acute pericarditis
- Early repolarization pattern (a form of myocardial repolarization seen in normal healthy people that produces ST-segment elevation closely mimicking that associated with ACS)
- Left ventricular hypertrophy and left bundle branch block (leads V_1-V_3)
- Hyperkalemia (leads V_1, V_2)
- Hypothermia (along with the J wave and Osborne wave)

Common causes of ST-segment depression include the following:

- Subendocardial myocardial infarction (non-ST elevation myocardial infarction)
- Angina pectoris (subendocardial myocardial ischemia)
- Reciprocal ECG changes in acute myocardial infarction
- Right and left ventricular hypertrophy ("strain" pattern)
- Right and left bundle branch block
- Digitalis effect
- Hypokalemia

Examination of the ST segment must take into consideration any changes in the T wave because both relate to repolarization of the ventricles. Therefore changes in either can affect the other.

CHAPTER SUMMARY

The ECG waveform consists of waves, intervals, and segments. Each has normal characteristics that define them. These characteristics relate to the function of the underlying area of the heart from which they originate.

The P wave is related to the electrical activity of the atria while the QRS complex and T wave provides information regarding the ventricles. The PR interval is that period of time during which the electrical signal is transmitted between the atria and the ventricles and the ST segment provides vital information regarding the depolarization of the ventricles.

Various conditions will affect the appearance of the waves, intervals, and segments of the ECG and understanding what is normal and the conditions that cause these abnormalities is key to successful cardiac dysrhythmia interpretation.

CHAPTER REVIEW

1. Wide, notched P waves are most often caused by:
   A. orthostatic hypotension
   B. mitral and aortic valvular disease
   C. pericarditis
   D. faster ECG recording speeds

2. The normal PR interval is between:
   A. 0.08 and 0.24 second
   B. 0.08 and 0.16 second
   C. 0.10 and 0.24 second
   D. 0.12 and 0.20 second

3. An ectopic P wave represents atrial depolarization:
   A. arising from an implanted cardiac pacemaker
   B. arising from the SA node
   C. arising from the ventricle
   D. occurring in an abnormal direction or sequence, or both

4. A normal QRS complex represents normal:
   A. depolarization of the atria
   B. depolarization of the ventricles
   C. repolarization of the atria
   D. repolarization of the ventricles

5. The time taken for the depolarization of the interventricular septum plus depolarization of the ventricle from the endocardium to the epicardium under the facing lead is called the:
   A. atrial repolarization phase
   B. QT interval
   C. septal excitation time
   D. ventricular activation time

6. Which one of the following accessory conduction pathways is not involved in causing ventricular preexcitation with associated delta waves?
   A. accessory AV pathways
   B. atrio-His fibers
   C. bundles of Kent
   D. nodoventricular/fasciculoventricular fibers

7. Myocardial ischemia, acute MI, excess serum potassium, and administration of procainamide can cause an abnormal _____ on the ECG.
   A. P wave
   B. QRS complex
   C. T wave
   D. U wave

8. A U wave indicates that repolarization of the ventricles has occurred. An abnormally tall U wave may be present in:
   A. cardiac tamponade, diabetes
   B. CVA, syncope
   C. hypokalemia, cardiomyopathy
   D. hypothermia, vertigo

9. A delay of progression of the electrical impulse through the AV node or bundle of His would show on an ECG as a(n):
   A. elevated ST segment
   B. peaked T wave
   C. prolonged PR interval
   D. prolonged QRS complex

10. An abnormal ST segment indicates:
    A. abnormal atrial repolarization
    B. abnormal ventricular contraction
    C. abnormal ventricular repolarization
    D. conduction delay in the AV node

Eight Steps to ECG Interpretation and Analysis

OBJECTIVES   *Upon completion of this chapter, you should be able to complete the following objectives:*

1. List the eight steps to interpret a dysrhythmia and its significance.
2. Define heart rate and describe the following methods of determining it:
   - 6-second count method
   - Heart rate calculator ruler method
   - R-R interval method
     ○ Seconds method
     ○ Small square method
     ○ Large square method
     ○ Conversion table method
   - The Rule of 300
3. List and describe two methods of determining the ventricular regularity.
4. Define the following terms as they apply to rhythm regularity:
   - Regular
   - Irregular
   - Occasional Irregularity
   - Regular (Patterned) Irregularity
   - Irregular (Total) Irregularity
5. List and describe the three steps in identifying and analyzing the P, P′, F, and f waves.
6. Define the basic differences between the following components of the ECG, including shape, width, height, relationship to the QRS complexes, and rate and rhythm:
   - Normal P wave
   - Abnormal P wave
   - Atrial flutter waves
   - Atrial fibrillation waves
   - "Coarse"
   - "Fine"
7. List and describe the steps in determining the PR intervals and the AV conduction ratio.
8. Define the following normal and abnormal PR intervals:
   - Normal and abnormal PR intervals
   - RP′ intervals
9. Give the causes of a PR interval less than 0.12 second in duration and greater than 0.20 second.

10. Define the following terms:
    - Atrioventricular (AV) block
    - Variable AV block
    - Isoelectric line
    - Incomplete AV block
    - Complete AV block
    - First-degree AV block
    - Second-degree AV block
    - Third-degree AV block
    - Dropped beat
    - Wenckebach AV block
    - AV dissociation
    - AV conduction ratio
    - Accessory conduction pathway

11. List and describe the three steps in identifying and analyzing the QRS complexes.

12. List the most likely site or sites of origin (or pacemaker sites) of dysrhythmias under the following circumstances:
    - Upright P waves preceding each QRS complex in lead II
    - Inverted P waves preceding each QRS complex in lead II
    - Inverted P waves following each QRS complex in lead II
    - QRS complexes occurring without any P waves
    - Atrial flutter waves
    - Atrial fibrillation waves
    - Normal QRS complexes with no set relationship to the P waves
    - Slightly widened QRS complexes (0.10 to 0.12 second in duration) with no set relationship to the P waves
    - Widened QRS complexes (greater than 0.12 second in duration and bizarre) with no set relationship to the P waves

SYSTEMATIC APPROACH TO ECG ANALYSIS

Regardless of one's proficiency at ECG analysis, using a systematic approach to the interpretation of any dysrhythmia is essential. Many dysrhythmias are easily recognized by their patterns but even the most common ones will present with variations that unless analyzed logically may lead to confusion. Another reason to use a systematic approach is to enable one to explain to or teach others how the interpretation was made. Each dysrhythmia has unique features which, even in the face of variation, will be seen when analyzed systematically. This will then allow the creation of a mental flowchart to follow to reach a confident conclusion.

> **AUTHOR'S NOTE** All ECG texts use systematic approaches and some may vary from the steps outlined here, but if examined closely are only slight variations on a common theme. No single system works for every one. As one's knowledge grows, learn, adapt, and adopt the best techniques.

Box 4-1 contains an outline of the steps used in interpreting an electrocardiogram (ECG) to determine the presence of a dysrhythmia and interpret it.

STEP ONE: DETERMINE THE HEART RATE

- Calculate the heart rate by determining the number of ventricular depolarizations (QRS complexes) that occur in the ECG in 1 minute. The heart rate can be determined by using

> **BOX 4-1** Dysrhythmia Interpretation
>
> **Step One**: Determine the heart rate
> **Step Two**: Determine the regularity
> **Step Three**: Identify and analyze the P, P′, F, or f waves
>   1. Identify the P, P′, F, or f waves
>   2. Determine the atrial rate and regularity
>   3. Compare and associate the atrial rate to the ventricular rate
> **Step Four**: Determine the PR or RP′ intervals and AV conduction ratio
>   1. Determine the PR intervals
>   2. Assess the equality of the PR intervals
>   3. Determine if all P waves are followed by a QRS complex
>   4. Determine the AV conduction ratio
> **Step Five**: Identify and analyze the QRS complexes
>   1. Identify the QRS complexes
>   2. Note the duration and shape of the QRS complexes
>   3. Assess the equality of the QRS complexes
>   4. Determine if there is a P wave associated with each QRS complex
> **Step Six**: Determine the site of origin of the dysrhythmia
> **Step Seven**: Identify the dysrhythmia
> **Step Eight**: Evaluate the clinical significance of the dysrhythmia

the 6-second count method, a heart rate calculator ruler, the R-R interval method, or the rule of 300.

> When referring to the heart rate as it relates to an ECG, it is vital to recognize that this is the rate of electrical impulses or "cardiac cycles" that are being counted. The physiologic heart rate may or may not be equal to the ECG "heart" rate because only by physically assessing the patient can you determine whether a given QRS complex is associated with a pulse. However, it is customary to refer to the rate on the ECG as the heart rate.

The 6-Second Count Method

The 6-second count method is the simplest and most common way of determining the heart rate and is generally considered the fastest, with the exception of the heart rate calculator ruler method. The 6-second count method, however, is the least accurate. This method can be used when the rhythm is either regular or irregular.

The short, vertical lines (or some other similar marking) at the top or bottom of most ECG papers divide the ECG strip into 3-second intervals (Figure 4-1) when the paper is run at a standard speed of 25 mm per second. Two of these intervals are equal to a 6-second interval. When the ECG strip is run at 50 mm per second, four of these "3-second" intervals are equal to a 6-second interval.

Calculate the heart rate by determining the number of QRS complexes in a 6-second interval and multiplying this number by 10 (Figure 4-2). The result is the heart rate in beats per minute. If premature complexes are present in the 6-second interval, they should be included in the QRS complex count.

The heart rate calculated by this method is a close approximation of the actual heart rate.

Example. If there are eight QRS complexes in a 6-second interval, the heart rate is:

$$8 \times 10 = 80 \text{ beats/min}$$

> **AUTHOR'S NOTE** Just as with heart rate and electrical rate, beats per minute implies that the complexes are conducted and generate a pulse. However, since rate is commonly referred to as "beats per minute" we will use that term, but remember in actuality you are calculating "complexes per minute."

To obtain a more accurate heart rate when the rate is extremely slow and/or the rhythm is grossly irregular, determine the number of QRS complexes in a longer interval, such as a 12-second interval, and adjust the multiplier accordingly.

Example. If there are six QRS complexes in a 12-second interval, the heart rate is:

$$6 \times 5 = 30 \text{ beats/min}$$

The Heart Rate Calculator Ruler Method

A heart rate calculator ruler, such as the one shown in Figure 4-3, is a device that can be used to determine the heart rate rapidly and accurately. This method is most accurate if the rhythm is regular. The directions printed on the ruler should be followed (e.g., "Third complex from arrow is rate per minute."). Premature complexes should not be included in the QRS complexes used in determining the heart rate by this method, if possible.

> **KEY DEFINITION**
>
> A premature complex is a QRS complex that occurs unexpectedly at some point in the P-QRS-T cycle or between cycles.

The R-R Interval Method

The R-R interval may be used four different ways to determine the heart rate. The rhythm must be regular if the calculation of the heart rate is to be accurate. The two R waves used for measuring the R-R interval should be those of the underlying rhythm and not those of premature complexes. The four methods are as follows:

Method 1

Measure the distance in seconds between the peaks of two consecutive R waves and divide this number into 60 to obtain the heart rate (Figure 4-4, p. 58).

Example. If the distance between the peaks of two consecutive R waves is 0.56 seconds, the heart rate is:

$$60/0.56 = 107 \text{ beats/min}$$

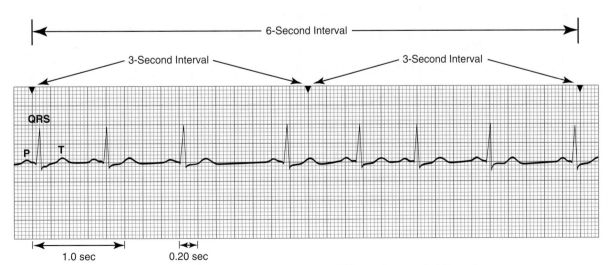

FIGURE 4-1 Intervals of 3 and 6 seconds at an ECG recording speed of 25 mm/sec.

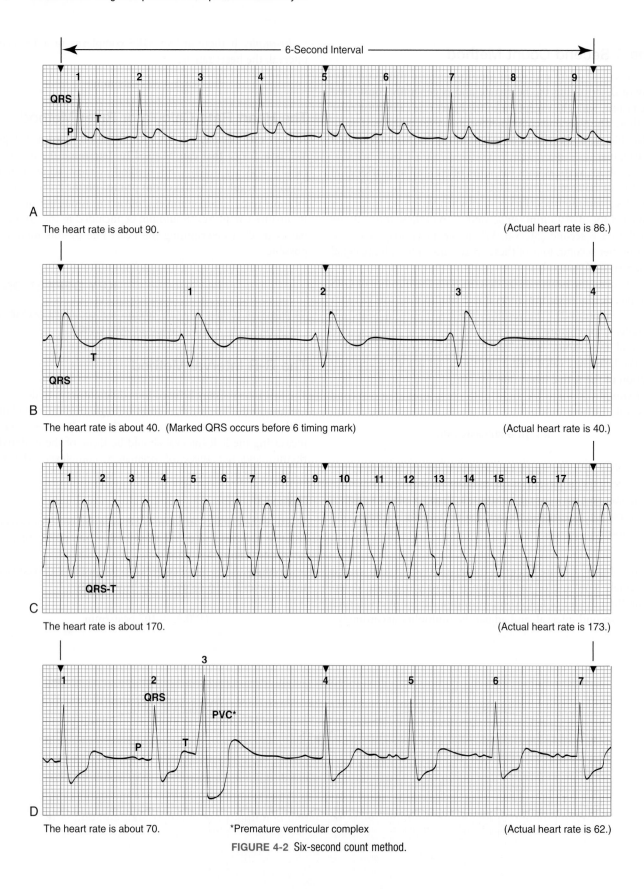

The heart rate is about 90.   (Actual heart rate is 86.)

The heart rate is about 40. (Marked QRS occurs before 6 timing mark)   (Actual heart rate is 40.)

The heart rate is about 170.   (Actual heart rate is 173.)

The heart rate is about 70.   *Premature ventricular complex   (Actual heart rate is 62.)

FIGURE 4-2 Six-second count method.

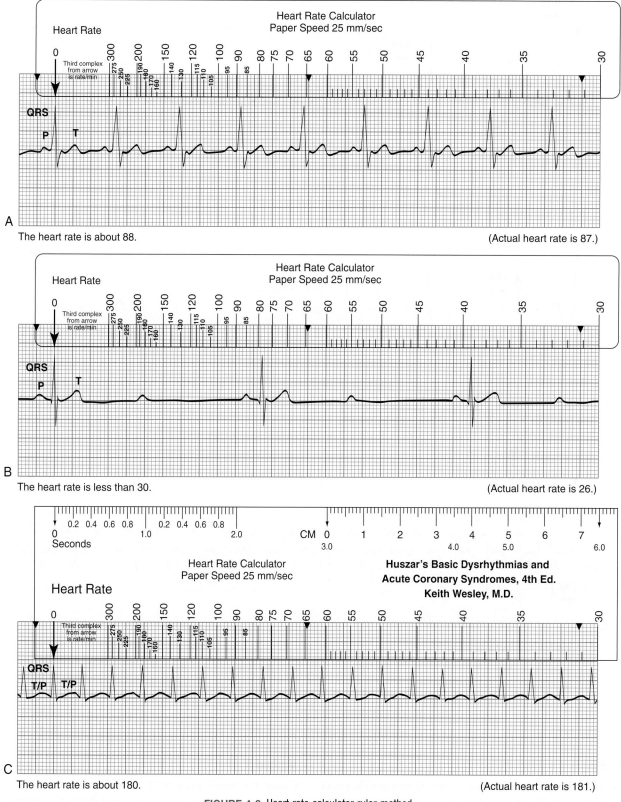

FIGURE 4-3 Heart rate calculator ruler method.

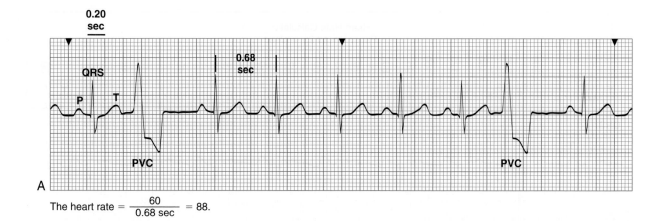

The heart rate = $\dfrac{60}{0.68 \text{ sec}}$ = 88.

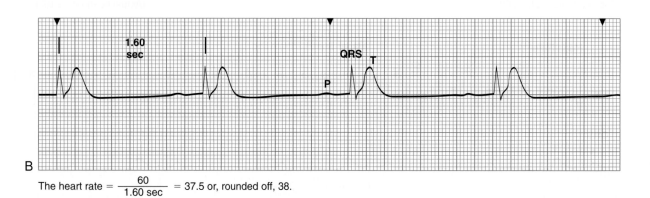

The heart rate = $\dfrac{60}{1.60 \text{ sec}}$ = 37.5 or, rounded off, 38.

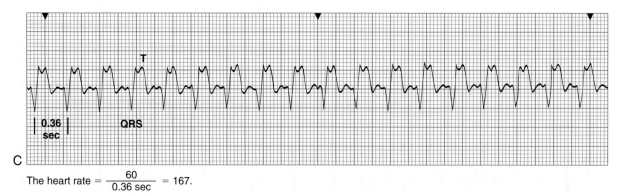

The heart rate = $\dfrac{60}{0.36 \text{ sec}}$ = 167.

FIGURE 4-4 R-R interval method 1.

Method 2

Count the large squares (0.20-second spaces) between the peaks of two consecutive R waves and divide this number into 300 to obtain the heart rate (Figure 4-5).

Example. If there are 2.5 large squares between the peaks of two consecutive R waves, the heart rate is:

$$300/2.5 = 120 \text{ beats/min}$$

Method 3

Count the small squares (0.04-second spaces) between the peaks of two consecutive R waves and divide this number into 1500 to obtain the heart rate (Figure 4-6).

Example. If there are 19 small squares between the peaks of two consecutive R waves, the heart rate is:

$$1500/19 = 78.9 \text{ or, rounded off, 79 beats/min}$$

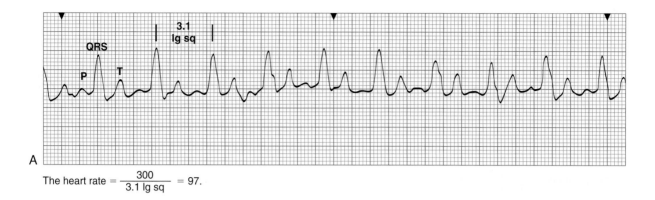

The heart rate = $\dfrac{300}{3.1 \text{ lg sq}}$ = 97.

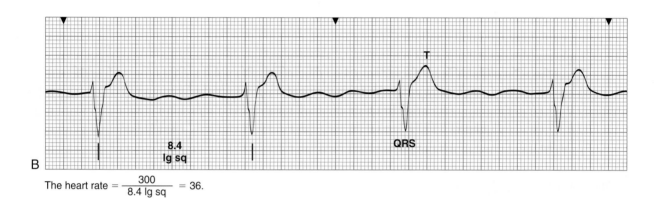

The heart rate = $\dfrac{300}{8.4 \text{ lg sq}}$ = 36.

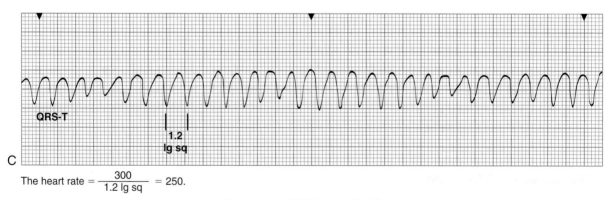

The heart rate = $\dfrac{300}{1.2 \text{ lg sq}}$ = 250.

FIGURE 4-5 R-R interval method 2.

Method 4

Count the small squares (0.04-second spaces) between the peaks of two consecutive R waves and, using a rate conversion table (Table 4-1), convert the number of small squares into the rate (Figure 4-7, p. 62).

Example. If there are 17 small squares between the peaks of two consecutive R waves, the heart rate is 88 beats/min.

> **AUTHOR'S NOTE** Methods 2 and 3 are more commonly used because they can be performed rapidly without the aid of tables.

The Rule of 300

The Rule of 300 for determining the heart rate will be accurate only if the rhythm is regular (Figure 4-8, p. 62). It is a result of the using method 2 of the previously described R-R interval method. It is calculated by dividing 300 by the number of large red boxes between consecutive QRS complexes. This creates a logical progression of numbers that can be memorized and placed on the graph paper. The numeric progression is 300, 150, 100, 75, 60, 50, 43, 38, 33, 30. If the QRS complex falls between lines, then estimate the rate based on which dark line is closest to the QRS complex.

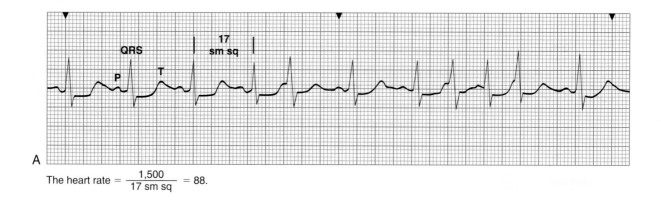

A

The heart rate = $\dfrac{1{,}500}{17 \text{ sm sq}}$ = 88.

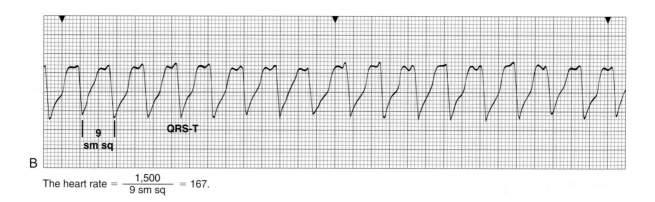

B

The heart rate = $\dfrac{1{,}500}{9 \text{ sm sq}}$ = 167.

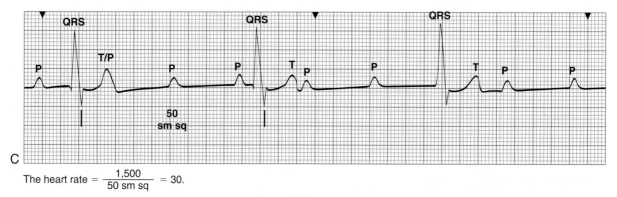

C

The heart rate = $\dfrac{1{,}500}{50 \text{ sm sq}}$ = 30.

FIGURE 4-6 R-R interval method 3.

The heart rate per minute is determined as follows:
1. Select an R wave that lines up with a dark vertical line, and label it "A."
2. Place 300 above the next dark line to the right of "A" and each of the subsequent numbers in the progression above the following dark lines.
3. Identify the first R wave to the right of the R wave labeled "A," and label this R wave "B."
4. Estimate the distance of the R wave labeled "B" to the nearest dark vertical lines (e.g., one quarter, one third, or one half of the total distance) and add that to 3.

5. Estimate the heart rate by equating the estimated distance of the R wave labeled "B" from the nearest adjacent numbered, dark vertical line to beats per minute.

Example. If the R wave labeled "B" is half way between the "150" dark vertical line and the "100" dark vertical line, the heart rate is about 125 beats/min.

Example. If the R wave labeled "B" is a third of the way between the "75" dark vertical line and the "60" dark vertical line, the heart rate is about 70 beats/min.

Instead of memorizing the progression, one can refer to method 2 or the R-R interval and perform the calculation.

TABLE 4-1 Conversion of the Number of Small Squares (0.04-Second Spaces) Between the Peaks of Two Consecutive R Waves Into the Heart Rate

0.04-sec Spaces	Heart Rate/Min	0.04-sec Spaces	Heart Rate/Min
5	300	27	56
6	250	28	54
7	214	29	52
8	188	30	50
9	167	31	48
10	150	32	47
11	136	33	45
12	125	34	44
13	115	35	43
14	107	36	42
15	100	37	41
16	94	38	40
17	88	39	39
18	84	40	38
19	79	41	37
20	75	42	36
21	72	43	35
22	68	44	34
23	65	45	33
24	63	47	32
25	60	48	31
26	58	50	30

For example, if there are 5.5 red boxes between two consecutive QRS complexes, the heart rate is 300/5.5 = 54.5 rounded up = 55 beats/min

> The same method of calculating rate can be used on the P waves. This is useful to determine if the atrial rate and ventricular rate are not the same.

STEP TWO: DETERMINE REGULARITY

Determine regularity by:

1. (a) Estimating the R-R intervals; (b) measuring them using EGG calipers or, if calipers are not available, use pencil and paper; or (c) counting the small squares between the R waves and then
2. Comparing the R-R intervals to each other

The simplest way to determine regularity is to first estimate the width of one of the R-R intervals, preferably one located on the left side of the EGG strip (Figure 4-9). Then visually compare the R-R intervals in the rest of the strip to the one first determined in a systematic way from left to right.

If EGG calipers are used, first place one tip of the calipers on the peak of one R wave; then adjust the EGG calipers so that the other tip rests on the peak of the next R wave to the right. Then, without changing the distance between the tips of the calipers, compare the other R-R intervals to the R-R interval first measured.

If pencil and paper are used, place the straight edge of the paper horizontally, close to the peaks of the R waves, and mark off the distance between two consecutive R waves (the R-R interval) with the pencil. Then compare this R-R interval to the other R-R intervals in the EGG strip.

The last method of determining regularity is to count the number of small squares (0.04 second/small square) between the R waves and then compare the width of the R-R intervals with each other.

The regularity as determined using one of the methods above may be regular or irregular.

Regular

In general, if the shortest and longest R-R intervals vary by less than 0.08 second (two small square) in a given EGG strip, the rhythm is considered to be "regular" (Figure 4-10, p. 64). (Thus the R-R intervals of an "essentially regular" rhythm may be precisely equal or slightly unequal.)

Irregular

If the shortest and longest R-R intervals vary by more than 0.08 second, the rhythm is considered to be irregular. (Figure 4-11, p. 65).

The rhythm may be *slightly irregular.* This means that over the length of the ECG the amount of R-R interval variation is rarely more than 0.08 seconds. This occurs in the following conditions:

- Sinus arrhythmia

> The degree of acceptable variability is related to the rate. The faster the rate, the less the acceptable variability that should be expected for a rhythm to be considered regular. A rule of thumb is that the variability of the R-R interval should not exceed 10% for any given rate for the rhythm to be considered regular.

The rhythm may be *occasionally irregular.* This occurs when premature complexes occur in an otherwise regular rhythm. This is seen in the following:

- Premature atrial complexes
- Premature ventricular complexes

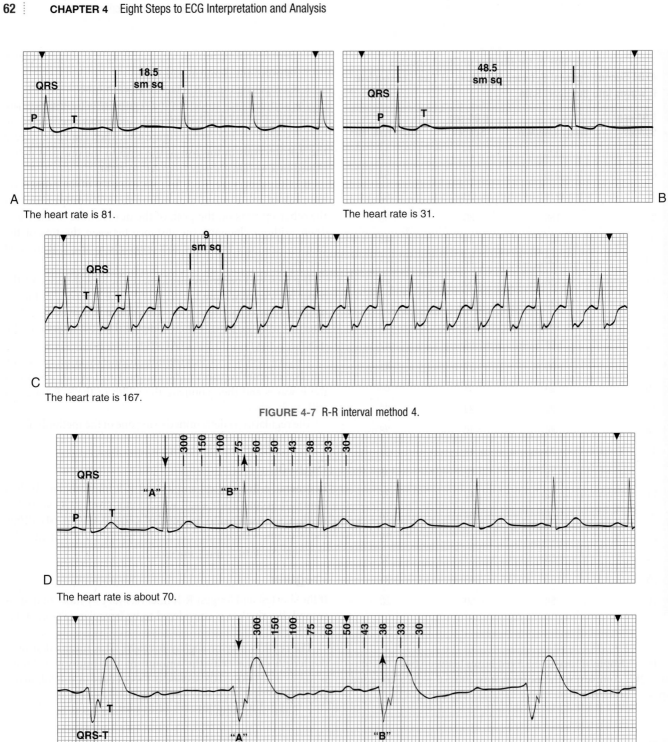

The heart rate is 81.

The heart rate is 31.

The heart rate is 167.

FIGURE 4-7 R-R interval method 4.

The heart rate is about 70.

The heart rate is about 38.

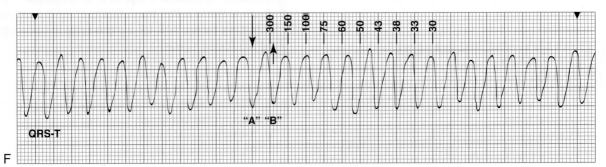

The heart rate is about 270.

FIGURE 4-8 Rule of 300.

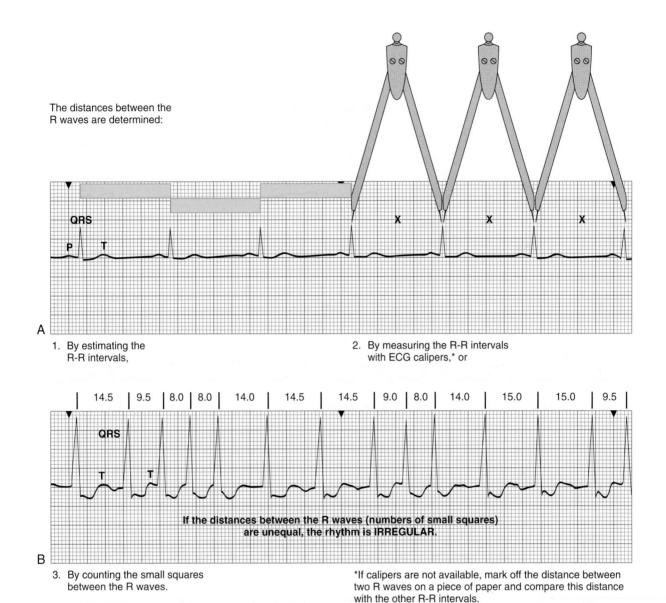

The distances between the R waves are determined:

A

1. By estimating the R-R intervals,

2. By measuring the R-R intervals with ECG calipers,* or

3. By counting the small squares between the R waves.

*If calipers are not available, mark off the distance between two R waves on a piece of paper and compare this distance with the other R-R intervals.

FIGURE 4-9 Determining the regularity.

The rhythm may be *regularly irregular.* Another term for this type of regularity is *patterned irregularity.* This occurs when there is a pattern seen between the measured R-R intervals. For example, the R-R interval may progressively lengthen in a predictable manner, or there may be a fixed ratio of short to long R-R intervals. This is seen in the following:

- Second-degree AV block type I (Wenckebach)
- Second-degree AV block type II
- Atrial flutter with variable conduction ratio

The rhythm may be *irregularly irregular.* Other terms used interchangeably to describe an irregularly irregular rhythm are *grossly* and *totally* irregular. When there appears to be no fixed pattern or ratio of the R-R intervals, the rhythm is considered to be totally irregular. This occurs in the following:

- Atrial fibrillation
- Multifocal atrial tachycardia
- Ventricular fibrillation

STEP THREE: IDENTIFY AND ANALYZE THE P, P′, F, OR f WAVES

- Identify the P, P′, F, or f waves
- Determine the atrial rate
- Compare and associate atrial rate with ventricular rate

A normal P wave is a positive, smoothly rounded wave in lead II (Figure 4-12, p. 66). It is 0.5 to 2.5 mm high and 0.10 second or less wide. It typically appears before each QRS complex, but it may occur singly without a QRS complex following it, as in atrioventricular (AV) block. An AV block is a condition in which there is a complete or incomplete (partial) block in the conduction of electrical impulses from the atria to

Regular Rhythms

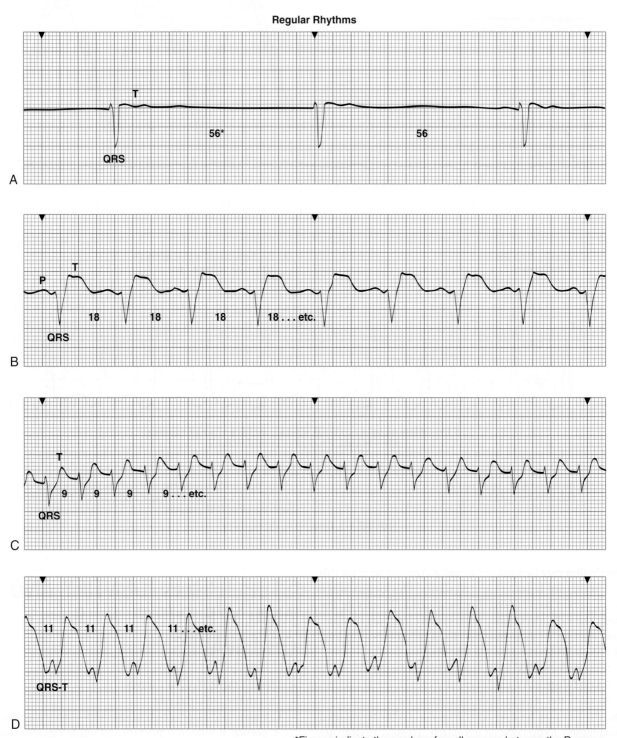

*Figures indicate the number of small squares between the R waves.

FIGURE 4-10 Regular rhythms.

Irregular Rhythms

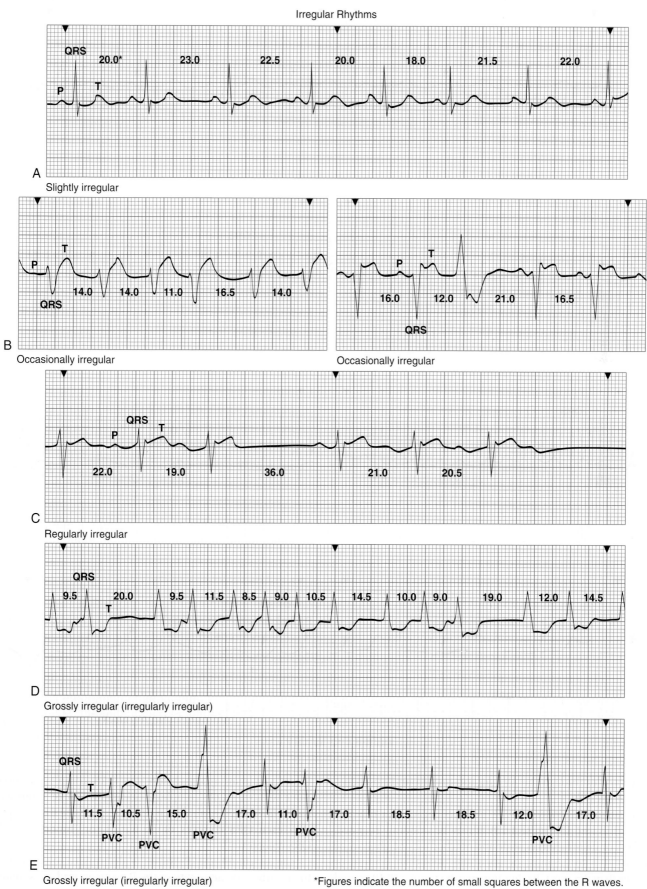

A Slightly irregular

B Occasionally irregular   Occasionally irregular

C Regularly irregular

D Grossly irregular (irregularly irregular)

E Grossly irregular (irregularly irregular)

*Figures indicate the number of small squares between the R waves.

FIGURE 4-11 Irregular rhythms.

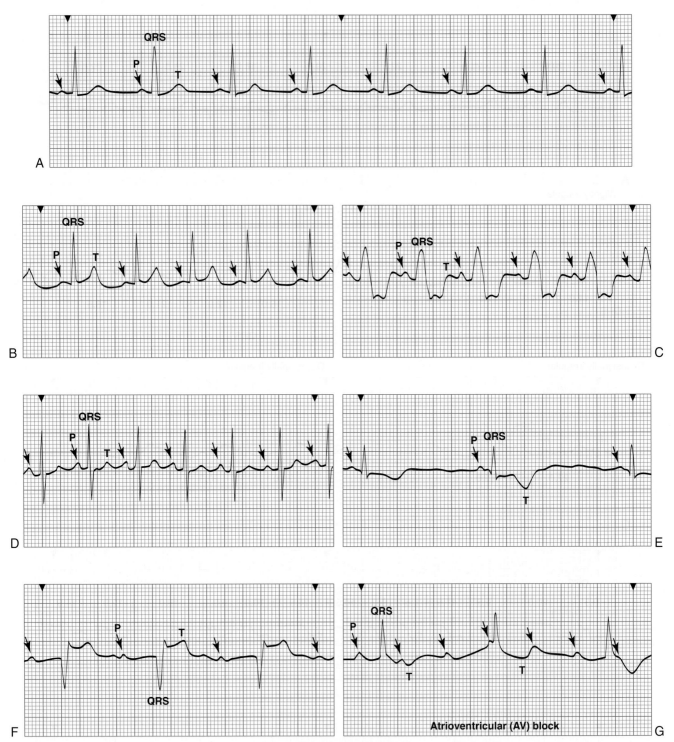

FIGURE 4-12 Normal P waves.

the ventricles through the AV junction or the bundle branches (see Chapter 9).

An abnormal P wave may be positive, negative, or flat (iso-electric) in lead II (Figure 4-13). It may be smoothly rounded, peaked, or deformed (i.e., wide and notched). Its height may be normal (0.5 to 2.5 mm) or abnormal (less than 0.5 mm or greater than 2.5 mm). Its duration may be normal (0.10 second or less) or abnormal (greater than 0.10 second). Like a normal

P wave, it may appear before the QRS complex or occur alone without a QRS complex following it. Unlike a normal P wave, however, an abnormal P wave may regularly appear after each QRS complex or be buried (or "hidden") in the QRS complex.

The origin of the P waves is determined by observing the positivity or negativity of the P waves in lead II as follows (Table 4-2):

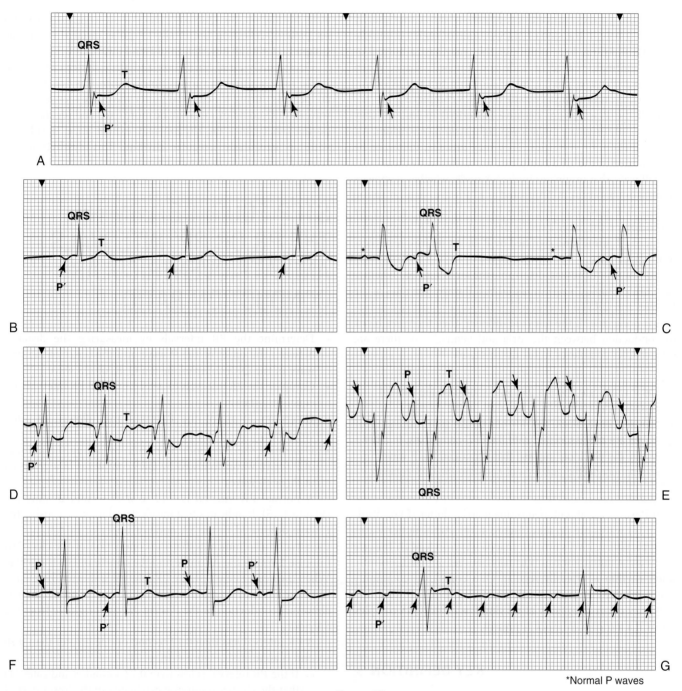

FIGURE 4-13 Abnormal P waves.

*Normal P waves

TABLE 4-2 Appearance of the P Waves Relative to Their Site of Origin

Site of Origin of the P Wave	Appearance in Lead II	P Wave Location
SA node (P wave)	Positive (upright)	Precedes the QRS complex
Upper or middle right atrium (P′ wave)	Normal, peaked, or wide and notched	
Lower right atrium or left atrium (P′ wave)	Negative (inverted)	Precedes the QRS complex
AV junction (P′ wave)		
Upper part	Negative (inverted)	Precedes the QRS complex
Middle or distal part	Absent	Is buried in the QRS complex
Distal part	Negative (inverted)	Follows the QRS complex

- If the P waves are positive (upright) in lead II, they usually originate in the sinoatrial (SA) node or upper or middle right atrium. Even if upright, they may have a normal or abnormal (peaked or wide and notched) shape. When such P waves have a set relationship to the QRS complexes, they always precede the QRS complexes.
- If the P waves are negative (inverted) in lead II, they usually originate in the lower right atrium, left atrium, AV junction, or ventricles. They may precede, follow, or be buried in the QRS complexes associated with them.

A P wave that originates in the SA node, whether it appears normal or abnormal, is designated as a "P wave" or a "P" in the figures. A P wave that originates in the atria, AV junction, or ventricles, on the other hand, is designated as a "P′ wave," pronounced "P prime" and signified by P′ in the figures, regardless of its appearance.

If P waves are present, determine the atrial rate and whether each QRS complex is accompanied by a P wave. The rates of the P waves and QRS complexes will be the same if normal conduction is occurring. If the rates are different then there is a block to conduction between the atria and ventricles or there are ectopic QRS complexes in the dysrhythmia.

> The P wave rate and the QRS rate should be the same if normal conduction occurs. However, in the case of complete heart block, the rate can be the same but the P waves are not associated with the QRS complexes. In other words, the electrical impulse that generated the P wave was not conducted and did not generate the QRS complex.

If P waves are absent, determine if atrial flutter (F) or fibrillation (f) waves are present (Figure 4-14). Atrial flutter waves are typically positive, sawtooth shaped waves in lead II. The rate of the atrial flutter F waves is usually between 240 and 350/min. Their rhythm is typically regular. QRS complexes commonly occur regularly after every other or every fourth F wave, but they may occur irregularly at varying F wave-to-QRS complex ratios if a *variable AV block* is present.

KEY DEFINITION

A fixed AV block is present when the ratio of F wave-to QRS complex is constant. When the ratio changes, a variable AV block is present.

Atrial fibrillation waves are irregularly shaped, chaotic waves, each dissimilar in configuration and amplitude to the other. If the f waves are less than 1 mm high, they are called *fine* fibrillatory waves; if they are greater than 1 mm high, they are called *coarse* fibrillatory waves. If the f waves are extremely fine, they may not be identified as such, and the sections of the EGG between the T waves and QRS complexes may appear only slightly wavy or even flat (isoelectric).

The rate of the f waves is usually between 350 and 600 (average 400)/min, and their rhythm is totally irregular. Typically, in atrial fibrillation, the QRS complexes occur irregularly with no set pattern, reflecting the totally irregular atrial rhythm. See Chapter 6 for a full description of F and f waves.

Occasionally atrial fibrillation and atrial flutter can coexist in the same rhythm at various times. When this occurs, there are periods during which atrial flutter waves are seen and the F wave to QRS complex ratio will be more fixed and regular. Then during other times the rhythm may exhibit atrial fibrillation with an irregularly irregular rhythm. This dysrhythmia is referred to as *atrial fib-flutter*.

STEP FOUR: DETERMINE THE PR OR RP′ INTERVALS AND ATRIOVENTRICULAR CONDUCTION RATIO

- Determine the PR intervals by measuring the distance between the onset of the P wave and the onset of the first wave of the QRS complex, be it a Q, R, or QS wave
- Compare the PR intervals to determine if all PR intervals are equal in duration
- Determine if all of the P waves are followed by QRS complexes
- Determine the AV conduction ratio by noting the number of P (or F) waves followed by QRS complexes in a given set of P (or F) waves

A normal PR interval is 0.12 to 0.20 second in duration (Figure 4-15). It indicates that the electrical impulse causing the P wave originated in the SA node or upper or middle part of the atria. It also indicates that the conduction of the electrical impulse through the AV node and the bundle of His is normal. When the heart rate is fast, the PR interval is shorter than when it is slow but it will remain within normal limits unless there is abnormal conduction or the P wave did not originate from the SA node.

A PR interval less than 0.12 second or one greater than 0.20 second is abnormal (Figure 4-16, p. 71).

- If the PR interval is less than 0.12 second, it indicates (1) that the electrical impulse originated in the lower part of the atria or in the AV junction or (2) that the electrical impulse progressed from the atria to the ventricles through an abnormal accessory conduction pathway and not through the AV node and bundle of His or the AV node alone.
- A PR interval greater than 0.20 seconds indicates a delay in the conduction of the electrical impulse through the AV node, bundle of His, or rarely the bundle branches. When this occurs and the PR intervals are all the same, a first-degree AV block is present (Table 4-3).

If a P wave follows the QRS complex, the P prime or P′ wave, an RP′ interval is present, indicating that the electrical impulse responsible for the P′ wave and QRS complex has originated in

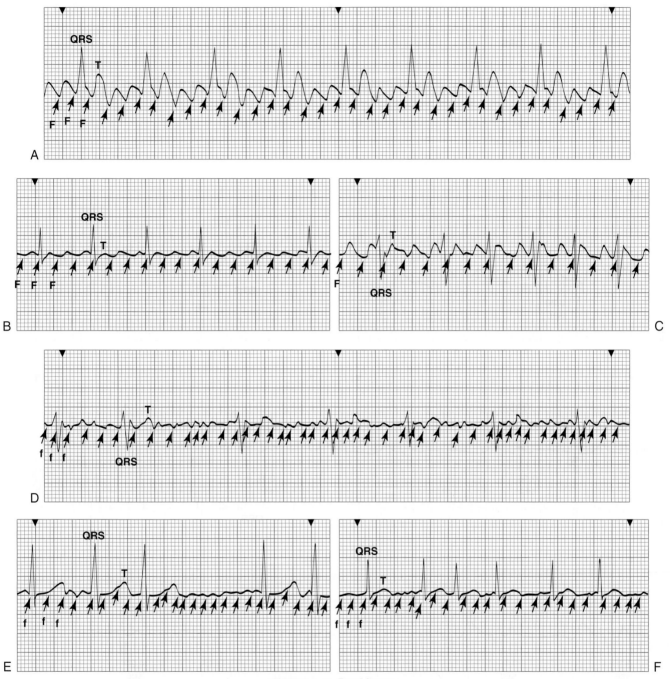

FIGURE 4-14 F and f waves.

the lower part of the AV junction or in the ventricles. An RP′ interval is usually 0.12 second or less but can be as long as 0.20 seconds. If a QRS complex does not follow a P wave, a PR interval is absent. This indicates a blockage of the conduction of the electrical impulse through the AV node, bundle of His, or bundle branches into the ventricles. If QRS complexes follow some P waves and not others, an incomplete AV block (second-degree AV block) is present. There are two kinds of second-degree AV blocks—type I AV block (Wenckebach AV block) and type II AV block. Often type I and type II AV blocks are referred to as *Mobitz type I* and *Mobitz type II* AV blocks, respectively (see Chapter 9).

- If the PR intervals are unequal, determine if there is an increase in their duration until a P wave is not followed by a QRS complex (nonconducted P wave or "dropped beat"). This indicates that there is, typically, a progressive delay in the conduction of the electrical impulse through the AV node (or, less commonly, the bundle of His or bundle branches) into the ventricles until conduction is completely blocked. This kind of second-degree AV block, which occurs cyclically, is called a type I AV block (Wenckebach AV block).

- If the PR intervals are equal, the second-degree AV block is a type II AV block. The type II AV block will have more

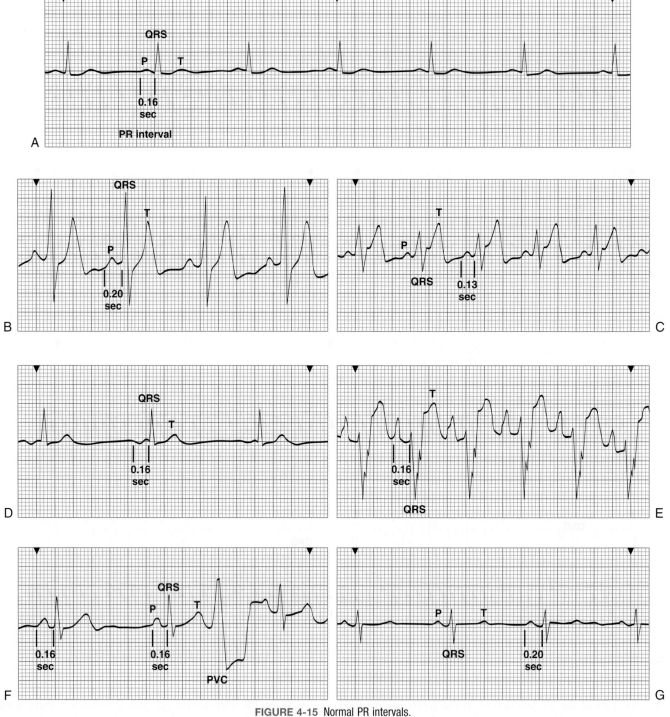

FIGURE 4-15 Normal PR intervals.

P waves than QRS complexes; the P to QRS ratio. This ratio is the AV conduction ratio of the block. The following are examples of AV conduction ratios (Figure 4-17).

- If all P waves are followed by QRS complexes, the AV conduction ratio is 1:1.
- If, for every two P waves one is followed by a QRS complex, the AV conduction ratio is 2:1.
- If, for every three P waves two are followed by QRS complexes, the AV conduction ratio is 3:2.

- If, for every four P waves three are followed by QRS complexes and one is not, the AV conduction ratio is 4:3.
- If, for every five P waves, one is followed by a QRS complex, the AV conduction ratio is 5:1.

If QRS complexes are present but do not regularly precede or follow the P waves, a complete AV block (third-degree AV block) is present. Another term used to describe the condition when QRS complexes occur totally unrelated to the P, P′, or F waves is *AV dissociation*.

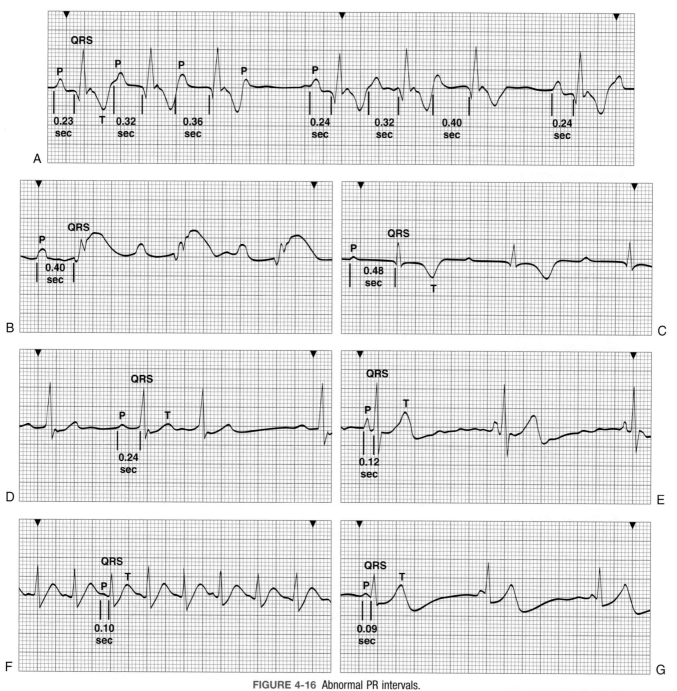

FIGURE 4-16 Abnormal PR intervals.

TABLE 4-3 PR Intervals and AV Conduction Ratios in Relation to AV Blocks

AV Block	PR Intervals	AV Conduction Ratio
First-degree AV block	Prolonged, equal	1:1
Second-degree AV block		
Type I AV block (Wenckebach)	Gradually lengthening	5:4, 4:3, 3:2 or 6:5, 7:6, etc.
Type II AV block	Equal	2:1, 3:1, 4:1, 5:1, etc.
Third-degree AV block	No relationship of P to R waves	None

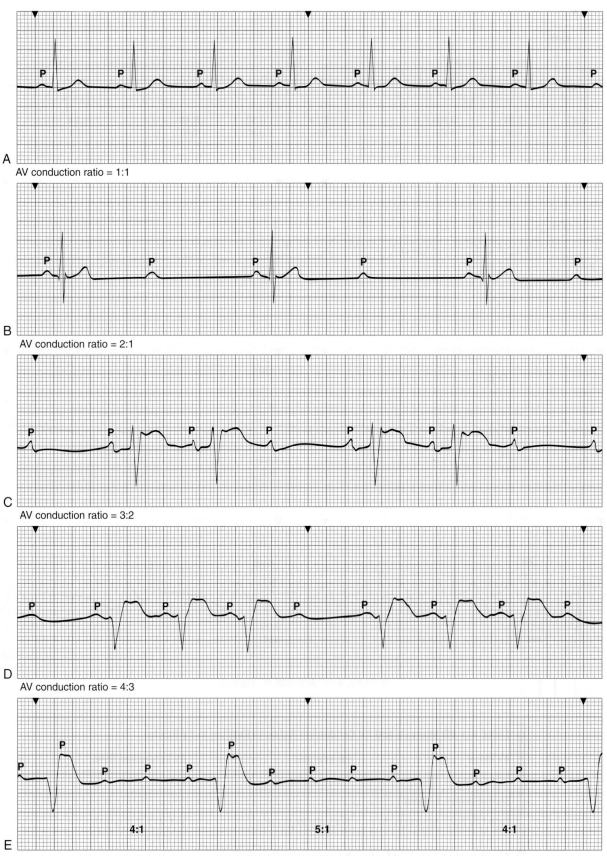

A

AV conduction ratio = 1:1

B

AV conduction ratio = 2:1

C

AV conduction ratio = 3:2

D

AV conduction ratio = 4:3

E

FIGURE 4-17 Examples of AV conduction ratios.

STEP FIVE: IDENTIFY AND ANALYZE THE QRS COMPLEXES

- Identify the QRS complexes.
- Note the duration of the QRS complexes. The duration of the QRS complexes may be normal (0.12 second or less) or long (greater than 0.12 second).
- Note the shape of the QRS complexes. The shape will be normal if conduction occurs through the normal pathway of the AV junction and bundle of His. The shape will be abnormal if there is a disturbance of the conduction pathway.
- Compare the QRS complexes to determine if all QRS complexes are equal in duration and shape or if one or more of the QRS complexes differ from the others.
- Determine if there is a P or P′ associated with the QRS.

A normal QRS complex, one that is 0.12 second or less in width (Figure 4-18), indicates that the electrical impulse progressed normally through the ventricles.

An abnormal QRS complex, one that is greater than 0.12 seconds in width and/or bizarre in appearance, indicates that the electrical impulse responsible for it progressed through the ventricles abnormally.

The cause may be one of the following dysrhythmias and associated conduction abnormalities:

- **Ventricular dysrhythmias.** Ectopic or escape complex and rhythms originating in the ventricles.
- **Supraventricular dysrhythmias.** Dysrhythmias originating in the SA node, atria, or AV junction with one of the following:
- **Bundle branch block.** A block in the conduction of electrical impulses through the right or left bundle branch.
- **Intraventricular conduction defect (IVCD).** A delay or blockage of conduction of electrical impulses through the myocardium caused by heart disease (myocardial infarction, fibrosis, and hypertrophy), electrolyte imbalance, and excessive administration of certain drugs.
- **Aberrant ventricular conduction (aberrancy).** A transient bundle branch block caused by the arrival of electrical impulses at a bundle branch while it is still in the refractory stage.
- **Ventricular preexcitation.** Disfigurement (slurring and sometimes notching) of the initial upstroke (or downstroke) of the QRS complex by a delta wave caused by premature depolarization of the ventricles. This results when an electrical impulse in the atria bypasses the AV junction or bundle of His, entering the ventricles via an abnormal accessory conduction pathway.

If all of the QRS complexes are equal and normal in duration and shape, they are most likely supraventricular in origin (i.e., originated from an impulse in the SA node, atria, or AV junction). If all of the QRS complexes are equal and abnormal in duration and shape, their origin may be either (1) ventricular or (2) supraventricular combined with a bundle branch block, intraventricular conduction defect, aberrancy, or ventricular preexcitation.

If, among QRS complexes that are equal and normal in duration and shape, QRS complexes occur that are abnormal in duration and shape, the origin of the abnormal QRS complexes may be either (1) ventricular (e.g., premature ventricular complexes) or (2) supraventricular with aberrancy (e.g., atrial and junctional premature complexes with aberrancy).

One of the clues as to whether the abnormal complexes are supraventricular or ventricular in origin are the presence of P waves. If P waves precede or immediately follow the abnormal QRS complexes, the origin of the electrical impulses responsible for the QRS complexes is most likely supraventricular. On the other hand, if no P waves are associated with the abnormal QRS complexes, these QRS complexes are most likely ventricular in origin.

STEP SIX: DETERMINE THE SITE OF ORIGIN OF THE DYSRHYTHMIA

- Determine the site of origin of the dysrhythmias by analyzing the P waves, the QRS complexes, and their association to each other.

The goal is to determine the source of the electrical discharge that generated the rhythm. Ventricular depolarization results in QRS complexes and physiologically in ventricular contractions in most cases. Therefore, when determining the origin of a dysrhythmia one concentrates on the electrical impulses that are driving the creation of QRS complexes.

If normal P waves are associated with the QRS complexes (i.e., the P waves regularly precede the QRS complexes), the site of origin of the dysrhythmia is that of the P waves (Figure 4-19). Conversely, if the P waves are not associated with the QRS complexes (i.e., the P waves follow the QRS complex or the P waves and QRS complexes occur independently of each other [AV dissociation]), or if the P waves are absent, the site of origin of the dysrhythmia is that of the QRS complexes (Figure 4-20, p. 76).

The electrical impulses causing the P waves may have originated in the SA node or an ectopic or escape pacemaker in the atria, AV junction, or ventricles. The site of origin of the electrical impulses responsible for the P waves can usually be deduced by noting the direction of the P waves in lead II and their relationship to the QRS complexes. Table 4-4 summarizes the determination of the pacemaker site of dysrhythmias with P waves associated with the QRS complexes.

- If the P waves are upright (positive) in lead II, the electrical impulses responsible for them may have originated either in the SA node or upper or middle right atrium. When upright P waves have a set relationship to the QRS complexes, they always precede the QRS complexes. The PR interval may be normal (0.12 to 0.20 second),

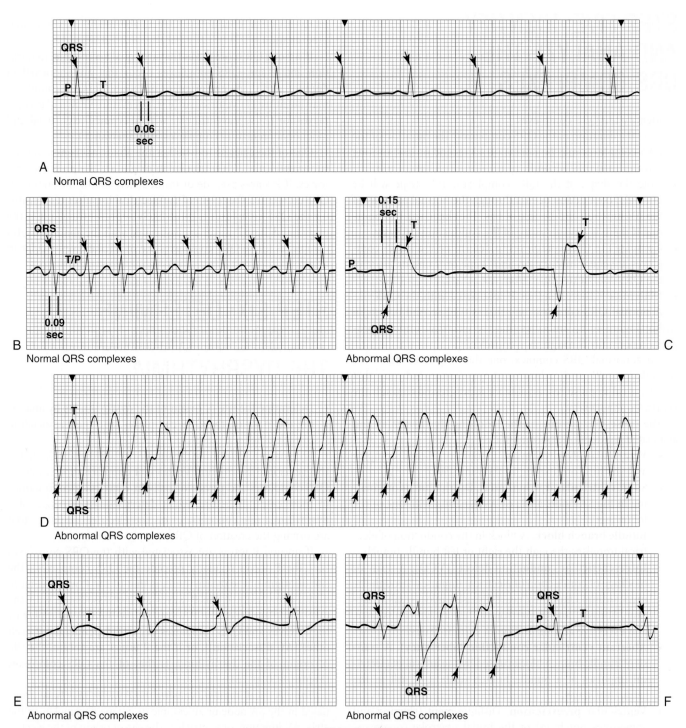

FIGURE 4-18 Identifying the QRS complexes.

prolonged (greater than 0.20 second, indicating first-degree AV block), or short (less than 0.12 second, indicating an accessory conduction pathway).

- If the P waves are negative (inverted) in lead II (P′), the electrical impulses responsible for them may have originated in the lower part of the atria near the AV junction, in the AV junction itself, or in the ventricles. The exact location of the site of origin of negative P′ waves can be deduced by analyzing their relationship to the QRS complexes in lead II as follows:

- If the negative P′ waves regularly precede the QRS complexes, the electrical impulses responsible for the P′ waves (and the QRS complexes as well) may have originated either in the lower part of the atria near the AV junction or in the proximal part of the AV junction itself. Typically, the P′R interval is less than 0.12 second, but it may be greater if first-degree AV block is present.

- If the negative P′ waves regularly follow the QRS complexes, the electrical impulses responsible for the P′ waves (and the QRS complexes as well) may have originated in

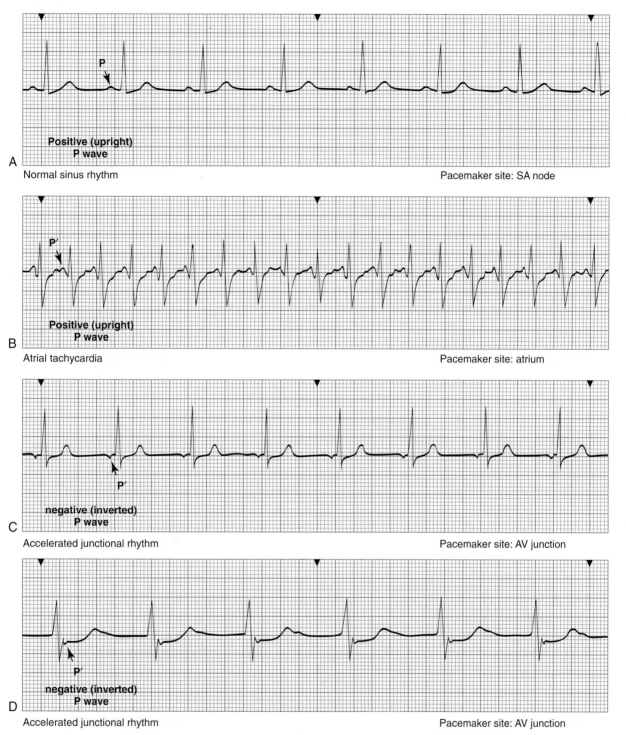

FIGURE 4-19 Examples of arrhythmias with P waves associated with the QRS complexes.

the distal part of the AV junction. If the QRS complexes are greater than 0.12 second in duration and appear bizarre, it is more likely that the P′ waves originated in the ventricles. The RP′ intervals are usually less than 0.20 second.

- If the negative P′ waves have no set relationship to the QRS complexes, occurring at a rate different from that of the QRS complexes (i.e., AV dissociation), the electrical impulses responsible for the P′ waves may have originated

either in the lower part of the atria near the AV junction or in the AV junction. The electrical impulses responsible for the QRS complexes may have originated in the AV junction or the ventricles.

- If atrial flutter or fibrillation waves are present, the electrical impulses responsible for them have originated in the atria.

If the QRS complexes have no set relationship to the P waves, occurring at a rate different from that of the P waves, or if P waves are absent, the electrical impulses causing the

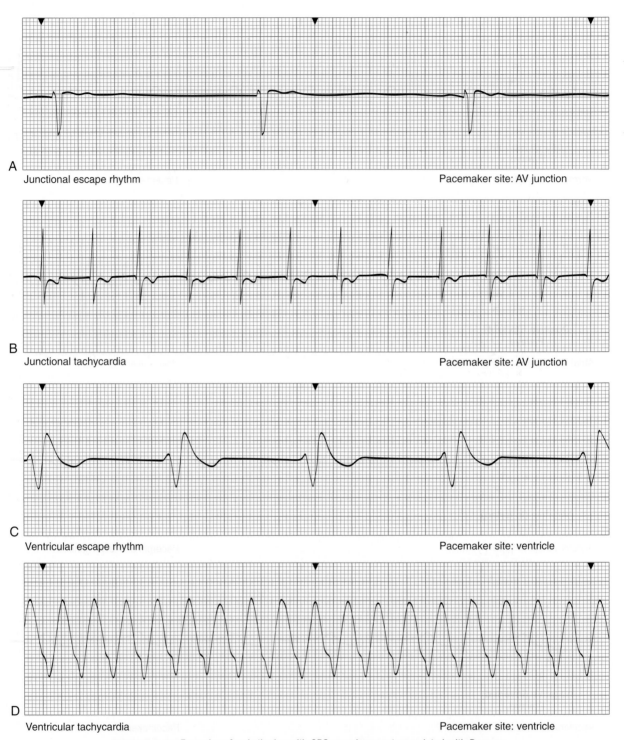

A
Junctional escape rhythm   Pacemaker site: AV junction

B
Junctional tachycardia   Pacemaker site: AV junction

C
Ventricular escape rhythm   Pacemaker site: ventricle

D
Ventricular tachycardia   Pacemaker site: ventricle

FIGURE 4-20 Examples of arrhythmias with QRS complexes not associated with P waves.

QRS complexes may have originated in an ectopic or escape pacemaker in the AV junction or the ventricles (i.e., bundle branch, Purkinje network, or ventricular myocardium).

The site of origin of the electrical impulses responsible for such QRS complexes can be deduced by noting the duration and shape of the QRS complex and whether or not a preexisting bundle branch block, an intraventricular conduction defect, or aberrant ventricular conduction is present. Often, the pacemaker site of wide and bizarre QRS complexes, occurring independently of the P waves or in their absence, cannot be determined with accuracy based on an EGG obtained from a single monitoring lead II. In such instances, a 12-lead EGG or lead MCL₁ is extremely helpful. Table 4-5 summarizes the origins of dysrhythmias with QRS complexes not associated with P waves.

- If the QRS complexes are 0.10 second or less in duration, the electrical impulses responsible for the QRS complexes most likely have originated in the AV junction or atrium.

TABLE 4-4 Origin of Dysrhythmias With P Waves Associated With the QRS Complexes

Origin	Direction of P Waves in Lead II	P/QRS Relationship	PR Interval
SA node *or* Upper or middle right atrium	Positive (upright)	P precedes QRS complex	0.12-0.20 sec or greater *or* less than 0.12 sec*
Lower atria *or* proximal AV junction	Negative (inverted)	P precedes QRS complex	Less than 0.12 sec
Distal AV junction	Negative (inverted)	P follows QRS complex	None (RP′ interval, <0.20 sec)

*In association with an accessory conduction pathway.

TABLE 4-5 Origin of Dysrhythmias With QRS Complexes Not Associated With P Waves

	QRS Complex	
Origin	Duration	Appearance
AV junction	0.12 sec or less	Normal
AV junction* *or*	0.10-0.12 sec	Normal
Proximal bundle branch AV junction† *or*	Greater than 0.12 sec	
Distal bundle branch, Purkinje network, or ventricular myocardium		Bizarre

*In association with a preexisting incomplete bundle branch block, an intraventricular conduction defect, or aberrant ventricular conduction.
†In association with a preexisting complete bundle branch block, an intraventricular conduction defect, or aberrant ventricular conduction.

- If the QRS complexes are between 0.10 and 0.12 second in duration and have a bizarre shape, the electrical impulses responsible for the QRS complexes may have originated in the AV junction (in which case, a preexisting incomplete bundle branch block, an intraventricular conduction defect, or aberrant ventricular conduction has to be present) or in the proximal part of a bundle branch in the ventricles near the bundle of His.
- If the QRS complexes are greater than 0.12 second in duration and appear bizarre, the electrical impulses responsible for the QRS complexes may have originated in the AV junction or in the distal part of a bundle branch, the Purkinje network, or ventricular myocardium.

STEP SEVEN: IDENTIFY THE DYSRHYTHMIA

Once each step has been performed sufficient information should be available to interpret the dysrhythmia. Each dysrhythmia has a unique feature or combination of features which once indentified will aid interpretation. These unique features will be presented in Chapters 5 through 9.

STEP EIGHT: EVALUATE THE SIGNIFICANCE OF THE DYSRHTHMIA

Once the dysrhythmia has been interpreted its clinical significance must be determined. Rhythm interpretation concentrates on the electrical activity in the heart while the clinical significance is a result of the mechanical pumping of the heart. Some dysrhythmias significantly diminish the hearts ability to contract efficiently while others don't. Additionally, some dysrhythmias provide clinically significant warning signs that the heart that may be suffering ischemia or the ill effects of medications or an electrolyte imbalance. The significance of each dysrhythmia will be presented following its presentation in Chapters 5 through 9.

CHAPTER SUMMARY

By using a systematic approach to the evaluation of a dysrhythmia an interpretation can be made. This systematic approach includes eight steps that include:
- Determining the rate
- Determining the regularity
- Identifying and analyzing the atrial activity
- Determining the P–R intervals and AV conduction ratio
- Identifying and analyzing the QRS complexes
- Determining the origin of the electrical activity of the dysrhythmia
- Creating a list of likely candidate dysrhythmias to choose from
- Assessing the clinical significance of the dysrhythmia

CHAPTER REVIEW

1. The most accurate regular heart rate is determined by
   A. the 6-second count method
   B. a heart rate calculator ruler
   C. the R-R interval method
   D. 300 rule

2. If the rhythm is irregular, use the _____ method to get an accurate calculation.
   A. 6-second method
   B. heart rate calculator
   C. R-R Interval
   D. rule of 300

3. If there are four large squares between the peaks of two consecutive R waves, the heart rate is _____ beats/min.
   A. 50
   B. 75
   C. 100
   D. 150

4. The rate of the P waves in a normally conducted rhythm is:
   A. unrelated to the rate of the QRS complexes
   B. sometimes less than the rate of QRS complexes
   C. greater than the QRS rate in AV block
   D. the same as that of the QRS complexes

5. If wide, bizarre-shaped QRS complexes are present but do not regularly precede or follow the P waves:
   A. a complete AV block is present
   B. the AV conduction ratio is fixed
   C. the P waves will be abnormal
   D. aberrant conduction can be excluded

6. If atrial flutter or fibrillation waves are present, the electrical impulses responsible for them have originated in the:
   A. ventricle
   B. atria
   C. septum
   D. bundle of His

7. The electrical origin of inverted P waves in lead II is in the:
   A. ventricles
   B. lower atria
   C. SA node
   D. bundle of His

8. A PR interval of less than 0.12 second indicates that the origin of the P wave is in all of the following except the:
   A. AV junction
   B. lower right atrium near the AV node
   C. upper right atrium with an accessory AV pathway present
   D. SA node

9. If the QRS complexes are 0.10 second or less in duration, the electrical impulses responsible for the QRS complexes could have originated in the:
   A. SA node
   B. Purkinje network
   C. AV junction in the presence of a right bundle branch block
   D. interventricular septum

10. A QRS that originates in the Purkinje network will have which of the following characteristics?
    A. bizarre shape and duration between 0.10. and 0.12 seconds
    B. normal shape and duration between 0.10 and 0.12 seconds
    C. normal shape and duration less than 0.12 seconds
    D. wide bizarre shape with duration greater than 0.12 seconds

5

Sinus Node Dysrhythmias

OBJECTIVES *Upon completion of this chapter, you should be able to complete the following objectives:*

1. Define and give the diagnostic characteristics, cause, and clinical significance of the following dysrhythmias:
   - Normal sinus rhythm (NSR)
   - Sinus arrhythmia
   - Sinus bradycardia
   - Sinus tachycardia
   - Sinus arrest
   - Sinoatrial (SA) exit block

NORMAL SINUS RHYTHM

KEY DEFINITION

Normal sinus rhythm (NSR) (Figure 5-1) is the normal rhythm of the heart, originating in the sinoatrial (SA) node, and characterized by a heart rate of 60 to 100 beats/min.

Diagnostic Characteristics (Table 5-1)

Rate. The rate is 60 to 100 beats/min. This is the normal resting heart rate.

Regularity. The rhythm is regular with equal R-R and P-P intervals. There are no dropped or blocked QRS complexes.

P waves. The P waves are identical and precede each QRS complex. They are positive (upright) in lead II, indicating that they originate in the SA node and that depolarization of the atria occurs normally.

PR intervals. The PR intervals are normal (less than 0.20 seconds) and constant but may vary slightly with the heart rate.

R-R and P-P intervals. The R-R intervals may be equal or vary slightly. The difference between the longest and shortest

TABLE 5-1 Diagnostic Characteristics of Normal Sinus Rhythm

Characteristic	Normal Sinus Ryhthm
Rate	60-100
Regularity	Regular
P waves	Upright, rounded
PR intervals	Normal, 0.12 < 0.20 sec.
P-P, R-R intervals	Equal
Conduction ratio	1:1
QRS complexes	Normal, wide if conduction delay exists
Site of origin	Sinoatrial node

R-R (or P-P) interval is usually less than 0.04 seconds in normal sinus rhythm.

Conduction ratio. There is a P wave before every QRS complex and a QRS complex following each P wave indicating that conduction is following the normal pathway and no blocks are occurring. This is a 1:1 ratio.

QRS complexes. A QRS complex follows each P wave. The duration of the QRS complexes may be normal (0.12 seconds

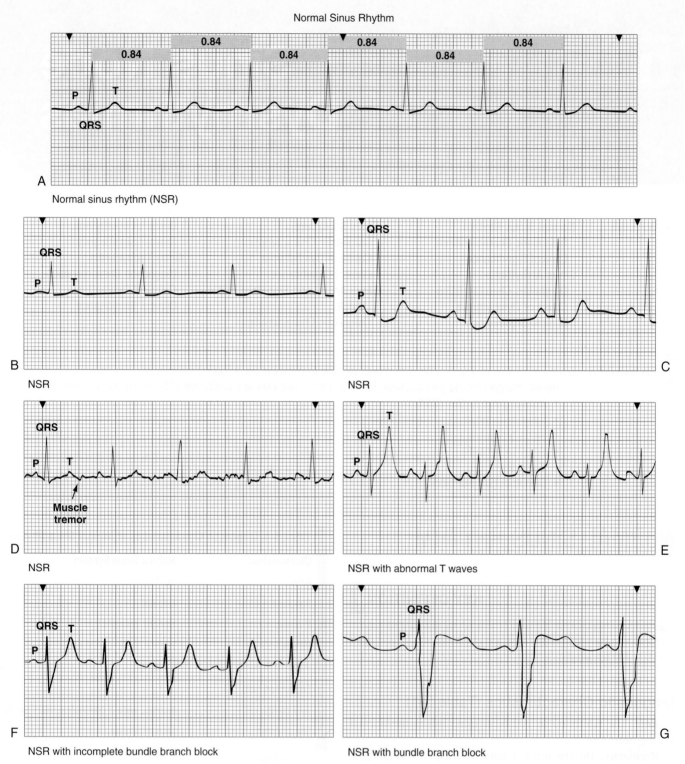

FIGURE 5-1 Normal sinus rhythm.

or less) or prolonged (greater than 0.12 seconds) if there is a preexisting intraventricular conduction disturbance (such as a bundle branch block).

Site of origin. Normal sinus rhythm originates from the sinus node.

Normal sinus rhythm (NSR) is the rhythm used to compare against all others. Dysrhythmia are defined as they differ from normal sinus rhythm. Being able to recognize variations of NSR is vital to ECG interpretation.

Clinical Significance

Normal sinus rhythm (NSR) with a palpable pulse occurring simultaneously with the QRS indicates that the heart is ejecting blood with each P-QRS-T cycle. However, the presence of a normal sinus rhythm on the cardiac monitor does not guarantee that a pulse is generated nor does it give any indication of the quality of that pulse (blood pressure). If a pulse is not palpable in the presence of a normal sinus rhythm as shown on the electrocardiogram (EGG), the treatment is that of pulseless electrical activity (PEA), which is described in Chapter 10.

> ### KEY DEFINITION
>
> Pulseless electrical activity (PEA) is not a cardiac rhythm but is instead a clinical condition. Whenever a pulseless patient has a rhythm, which under normal conditions would be expected to generate a pulse, the patient is said to be in PEA.

SINUS ARRHYTHMIA

> ### KEY DEFINITION
>
> Sinus arrhythmia (Figure 5-2) is an irregularity of the heart beat caused by a cyclical change in the rate of a sinus rhythm.

> **AUTHOR'S NOTE** Sinus arrhythmia is an old term and therefore while it is technically a dysrhythmia, we continue to refer to it by that title.

Diagnostic Characteristics (Table 5-2)

Rate. The rate is 60 to 100 beats/min. Occasionally, the rate may slow to slightly less than 60 and increase to slightly over 100 beats/min. Typically, the rate increases during inspiration and decreases during expiration.

Regularity. Sinus arrhythmia is regularly irregular as the heart rate gradually rises and falls; the changes in rate occur in cycles.

TABLE 5-2 Diagnostic Characteristics of Sinus Arrhythmia

Characteristic	Sinus Arrhythmia
Rate	60-100
Regularity	Cyclical irregularity
P waves	Upright, rounded
PR intervals	Normal, 0.12 < 0.20 sec
P-P, R-R intervals	Cyclical irregular
Conduction ratios	1:1
QRS complexes	Normal, wide if conduction delay exists
Site of origin	Sinoatrial node

Sinus Arrhythmia

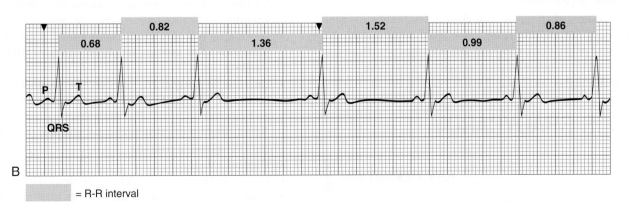

A

Sinus arrhythmia

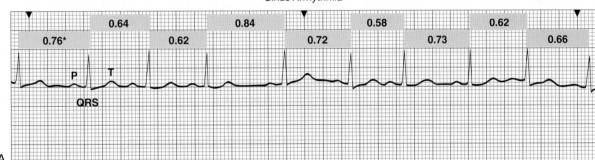

B

 = R-R interval

*Seconds

FIGURE 5-2 Sinus arrhythmia.

P waves. The sinus P waves are identical and precede each QRS complex. They are positive (upright) in lead II, indicating normal depolarization of the atria. The difference between the longest and shortest P-P (or R-R) interval is greater than 0.04 seconds.

PR intervals. The PR intervals are normal and constant.

R-R intervals. The R-R intervals are unequal. The most common type of sinus arrhythmia is related to respiration in which the R-R intervals become shorter during inspiration as the heart rate increases and longer during expiration as the heart rate decreases. In another, less common type of sinus arrhythmia, the R-R intervals become shorter and longer without any relation to respiration. The difference between the longest and shortest R-R interval is greater than 0.04 seconds in sinus arrhythmia.

Conduction ratio. There is a P wave before every QRS complex and a QRS complex following each P wave indicating that conduction is following the normal pathway and no blocks are occurring. This is a 1:1 ratio.

QRS complexes. A QRS complex normally follows each P wave. The QRS complexes are normal unless a preexisting intraventricular conduction disturbance (such as a bundle branch block) is present.

Site of origin. Sinus arrhythmia originates in the sinoatrial node.

Cause of Dysrhythmia

The most common type of sinus arrhythmia, the one related to respiration, is a normal phenomenon commonly seen in children, young adults, and elderly individuals. It is caused by the changes in vagal tone that occur during respiration. The vagal tone decreases during inspiration, causing the heart rate to increase, and increases during expiration, causing the heart rate to decrease.

The other, less common type of sinus arrhythmia is not related to respiration. It may occur in healthy individuals, but it is more commonly found in adult patients with heart disease, especially after acute inferior wall myocardial infarction, or in patients receiving certain drugs, such as digitalis and morphine.

Clinical Significance

Usually, sinus arrhythmia is of no clinical significance and generally does not require treatment. Marked sinus arrhythmia may cause palpitations, dizziness, and even syncope. However, the less common nonrespiration-related form has been associated with a higher incidence of sudden cardiac arrest.

SINUS BRADYCARDIA

KEY DEFINITION

Sinus bradycardia (Figure 5-3) is a dysrhythmia originating in the SA node, characterized by a rate of less than 60 beats/min.

TABLE 5-3 Diagnostic Characteristics of Sinus Bradycardia

Characteristic	Sinus Bradycardia
Rate	Less than 60
Regularity	Regular
P waves	Upright, rounded
PR intervals	Normal, 0.12 < 0.20 sec
P-P, R-R intervals	Regular and equal
Conduction ratio	1:1
QRS complexes	Normal, wide if conduction delay exists
Site of origin	Sinoatrial node

Diagnostic Characteristics (Table 5-3)

Rate. The rate is less than 60 beats/min.

Regularity. The rhythm is essentially regular, but it may be irregular if sinus arrhythmia is also present.

P waves. The sinus P waves are identical and precede each QRS complex. They are positive (upright) in lead II consistent with normal atrial depolarization.

PR intervals. The PR intervals are normal and constant. However, they tend to be at the upper limits of normal.

R-R intervals. The R-R intervals are equal but may vary slightly.

Conduction ratio. There is a P wave before every QRS complex and a QRS complex following each P wave, indicating that conduction is following the normal pathway and no blocks are occurring. This is a 1:1 ratio.

QRS complexes. A QRS complex normally follows each P wave. The QRS complexes are normal unless a preexisting intraventricular conduction disturbance (such as a bundle branch block) is present.

Site of origin. Sinus bradycardia originates in the sinoatrial node.

Cause of Dysrhythmia

Sinus bradycardia may be caused by any of the following:

- Excessive inhibitory vagal (parasympathetic) tone on the SA node as may be caused by carotid sinus stimulation, vomiting, Valsalva maneuvers, or neurocardiogenic (vasovagal) syncope, which causes a sudden loss of consciousness after extreme emotional stress or prolonged standing
- Decrease in sympathetic tone on the SA node as may be caused by beta-blockers (e.g., atenolol, metoprolol, propranolol)
- Administration of calcium channel blockers (e.g., diltiazem, verapamil, nifedipine)
- Digitalis toxicity
- Disease in the SA node, such as sick sinus syndrome
- Acute inferior wall and right ventricular myocardial infarctions
- Hypothyroidism (myxedema)

Sinus Bradycardia

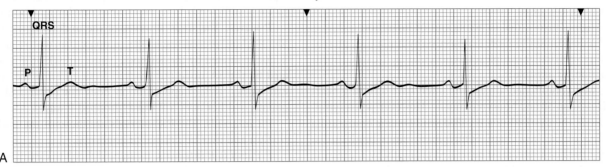

A

Sinus bradycardia

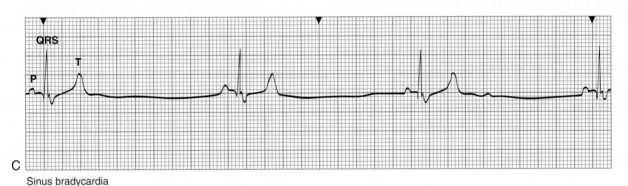

B

Sinus bradycardia with sinus arrhythmia

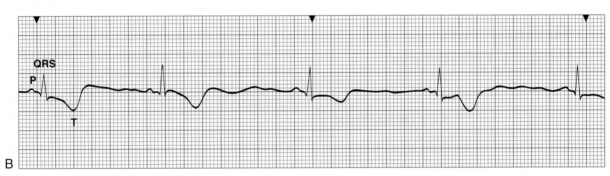

C

Sinus bradycardia

FIGURE 5-3 Sinus bradycardia.

- Hypothermia
- Hypoxia (especially in children)
- During sleep and in trained athletes

KEY DEFINITION

Valsalva maneuver is any forced expiratory effort against a closed airway, such as when an individual holds the breath and tightens the muscles in a concerted, strenuous effort to move a heavy object. It can also occur when straining during defecation. This causes a slowing of the heart rate due to increased vagal tone.

Clinical Significance

Sinus bradycardia with a heart rate between 50 to 59 beats/min (mild sinus bradycardia) usually does not produce symptoms

by itself. Such a bradycardia without symptoms is an *asymptomatic* bradycardia. In the presence of acute MI, mild sinus bradycardia may actually be beneficial in some patients because of decreased workload on the heart, which reduces the oxygen requirements of the myocardium, minimizes the extension of the infarction, and lessens the predisposition to certain dysrhythmias.

If the heart rate is 30 to 50 beats/min or less (marked sinus bradycardia), hypotension with a marked reduction in cardiac output and decreased perfusion of the brain and other vital organs may occur. This may result in the following signs, symptoms, and conditions:

- Dizziness, light-headedness, decreased level of consciousness, or syncope
- Shortness of breath
- Hypotension

- Shock
- Congestive heart failure
- Angina, myocardial ischemia and/or infarction
- Predisposition to more serious dysrhythmia (i.e., premature ventricular complexes, ventricular tachycardia, fibrillation, or asystole)

The well-conditioned athlete will often have a resting heart rate of less than 50 and be asymptomatic. However, when symptoms occur, the dysrhythmia is called *symptomatic* bradycardia regardless of the heart rate. Symptomatic sinus bradycardia, whatever the heart rate, must be treated promptly by addressing the underlying cause. Pharmacological and other treatments will be addressed in later chapters.

SINUS ARREST AND SINOATRIAL EXIT BLOCK

KEY DEFINITION

Sinus arrest (Figure 5-4) is a dysrhythmia caused by episodes of failure in the automaticity of the SA node, resulting in bradycardia, asystole, or both.

Sinoatrial (SA) exit block (see Figure 5-4) is a dysrhythmia caused by a block in the conduction of the electrical impulse from the SA node to the atria, resulting (like sinus arrest) in bradycardia, asystole, or both.

Diagnostic Characteristics (Table 5-4)

Rate. The rate is usually 60 to 100 beats/min but may be less.

Regularity. The rhythm is irregular when sinus arrest or SA exit block is present. The underlying rhythm will be seen then

TABLE 5-4 Diagnostic Characteristics of Sinus Arrest and Sinoatrial Exit Block

Characteristic	Sinus Arrest and Sinoatrial Exit Block
Rate	60-100
Regularity	Irregular when the block is present
P waves	Upright, rounded, no P wave when arrest/block occurs
PR intervals	Normal or Abnormal
P-P, R-R Intervals	Sinus Arrest: QRS following pause is NOT a multiple of P-P interval Sinoatrial Block: QRS following pause IS a multiple of P-P interval
Conduction ratio	1:1 Except if escape complexes are present
QRS complexes	Normal, wide if conduction delay exists
Site of origin	Sinoatrial node

a pause during which no QRS complex occurs. However, if the pause is sufficiently long, an escape complex may occur.

P waves. The sinus P waves of the underlying rhythm are identical and precede each QRS complex. If an electrical impulse is not generated by the SA node (sinus arrest), or if it is generated by the SA node but blocked from entering the atria (SA exit block), atrial depolarization does not occur and, consequently, neither does a P wave (dropped P wave).

PR intervals. The PR intervals are those of the underlying rhythm and may be normal or abnormal.

P-P and R-R intervals. It can be difficult to distinguish sinus arrest from SA block when a P wave does not occur. The difference between the two is that with sinus arrest, the SA node fails to fire and therefore the SA node does not reset, whereas with SA exit block the SA node fires and then does reset. This can be confirmed by measuring the P-P interval before and after the pause. When the SA node fails to fire, the next P wave (SA node firing) will not occur when expected. This can be determined by measuring the P-P interval before the pause. The long P-P interval following the SA block is twice (or a multiple of) the P-P interval of the underlying rhythm because the underlying rhythm remains undisturbed. This is because the SA node fired but the conduction to the atria was blocked. This is similar to a noncompensatory pause as described for PACs. (See p. 93)

The long P-P interval following the sinus arrest is typically not a multiple of the P-P interval of the underlying rhythm because the timing of the SA node is reset by the arrest. This is because the SA node did not fire.

Conduction ratio. When sinus arrest or SA exit block occurs there is no P wave. If a junctional escape complex occurs there may be an inverted P′ or only a narrow QRS complex with a retrograde P wave. A ventricular escape complex will have a wide QRS complex and no P wave. If there is no escape complex, the next complex to occur will be the underlying rhythm P-QRS-T. Therefore the conduction ratio is said to be 1:1 except for the period of the pause.

QRS complexes. A QRS complex normally follows each P wave. The QRS complexes are normal unless a preexisting intraventricular conduction disturbance (such as a bundle branch block) is present. A QRS complex is absent when a P wave does not occur.

Site of origin. The origin of the dysrhythmia is the SA node.

Cause of Dysrhythmia

Sinus arrest results from a marked depression in the automaticity of the SA node. SA exit block results from a block in the conduction of the electrical impulse from the SA node into the atria.

Sinus arrest or SA exit block may be precipitated by any of the following:

- Increase in vagal (parasympathetic) tone on the SA node
- Hypoxia
- Hyperkalemia
- Sleep apnea

Sinus Arrest and Sinoatrial Exit Block

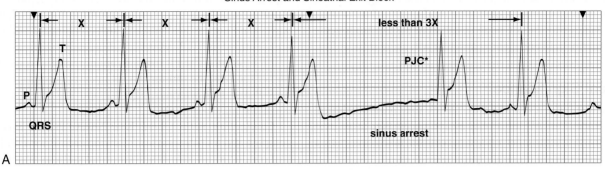

A

Sinus arrest

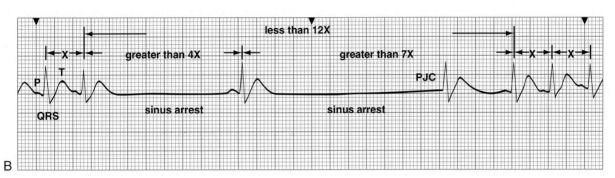

B

Sinus arrest

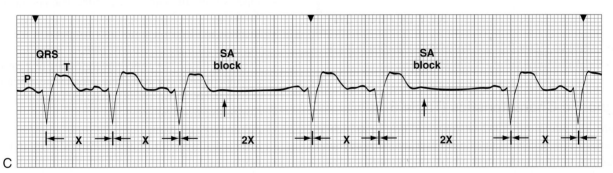

C

SA exit block

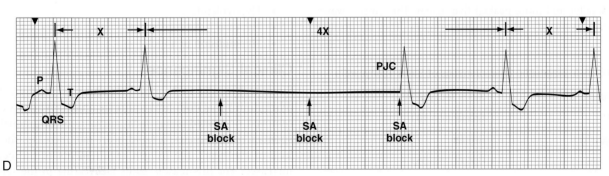

D

SA block
*Premature junctional contraction. See Chapter 7, Junctional Arrhythmias.

FIGURE 5-4 Sinus arrest and SA exit block.

- Excessive dose of digitalis, beta-blockers (e.g., atenolol, metoprolol, propranolol), or quinidine
- Damage to the SA node or adjacent atrium from acute inferior wall and right ventricular MI, acute myocarditis, or degenerative forms of fibrosis

Clinical Significance

Transient sinus arrest and SA exit block may have no clinical significance if an AV junctional escape pacemaker takes over promptly. If a ventricular escape pacemaker takes over with a slow heart rate or if an escape pacemaker does not take over at all, resulting in transient ventricular asystole, lightheadedness may occur, followed by syncope. The signs and symptoms, clinical significance, and management of sinus arrest and SA exit block with excessively slow heart rates are the same as those in symptomatic sinus bradycardia.

Intermittent sinus arrest or SA exit block can, however, progress to prolonged sinus arrest accompanied by lack of electrical activity of the atria (atrial standstill). If a junctional or ventricular escape pacemaker does not take over, asystole occurs, requiring immediate treatment.

SINUS TACHYCARDIA

> ### KEY DEFINITION
>
> Sinus tachycardia (Figure 5-5) is a dysrhythmia originating in the SA node, characterized by a rate of over 100 beats/min.

Diagnostic Characteristics (Table 5-5)

Rate. The rate is over 100 beats/min and may be as high as 180 beats/min or greater with extreme exertion. The onset and termination of sinus tachycardia are typically gradual.

Regularity. The rhythm is essentially regular.

P waves. The sinus P waves are usually normal but may be slightly taller and more peaked than usual. The sinus P waves are identical and precede each QRS complex. They are positive (upright) in lead II. When the heart rate is very rapid, the sinus P waves may be buried in the preceding T waves (buried P waves) and not easily identified. Such combined T and P waves are identified as "T/P" waves.

PR intervals. The PR intervals are normal and constant. The higher the rate, the shorter the PR interval becomes.

P-P and R-R intervals. The P-P and R-R intervals will be equal but may vary slightly.

Conduction ratio. There is a P wave before every QRS complex and a QRS complex following each P wave indicating that conduction is following the normal pathway and no blocks are occurring. The ratio is 1:1.

QRS complexes. The QRS complexes are normal unless a preexisting intraventricular conduction disturbance (such as a bundle branch block) or aberrant ventricular conduction is present. A QRS complex normally follows each P wave. Sinus tachycardia with abnormal QRS complexes may resemble ventricular tachycardia.

Site of origin. The origin of the dysrhythmia is the SA node.

Cause of Dysrhythmia

Sinus tachycardia in adults is a normal response of the heart to the demand for increased blood flow, as in exercise and exertion. It may also be caused by any of the following:

- Ingestion of stimulants (e.g., coffee, tea, and alcohol) or smoking
- Increase in catecholamines and sympathetic tone resulting from excitement, anxiety, pain, or stress
- Excessive dose of an anticholinergic drug (e.g., atropine), a sympathomimetic drug (e.g., dopamine, epinephrine, isoproterenol, or norepinephrine), or cocaine
- Congestive heart failure
- Pulmonary embolism
- Myocardial ischemia or acute myocardial infarction
- Fever
- Thyrotoxicosis
- Anemia
- Hypovolemia
- Hypoxia
- Hypotension or shock

Clinical Significance

Sinus tachycardia in healthy individuals is usually a benign dysrhythmia that does not require treatment. When its cause is removed or treated, sinus tachycardia resolves gradually and spontaneously. Because a rapid heart rate increases the workload of the heart, the oxygen requirements of the heart are increased. For this reason, sinus tachycardia in the setting of acute coronary syndrome may increase myocardial ischemia and the frequency and severity of chest pain, cause an extension of the infarct or even pump failure (e.g., congestive heart failure, hypotension, and/or cardiogenic shock), or predispose the patient to more serious dysrhythmias.

The primary issues to be concerned with when addressing any tachycardia are twofold. First, what is the effect on oxygen

TABLE 5-5 Diagnostic Characteristics of Sinus Tachycardia

Characteristic	Sinus Tachycardia
Rate	Greater than 100
Regularity	Regular
P waves	Upright, rounded
PR intervals	Normal or short
P-P, R-R intervals	Regular and equal
Conduction ratio	1:1
QRS complexes	Normal, wide if conduction delay exists
Site of origin	Sinoatrial node

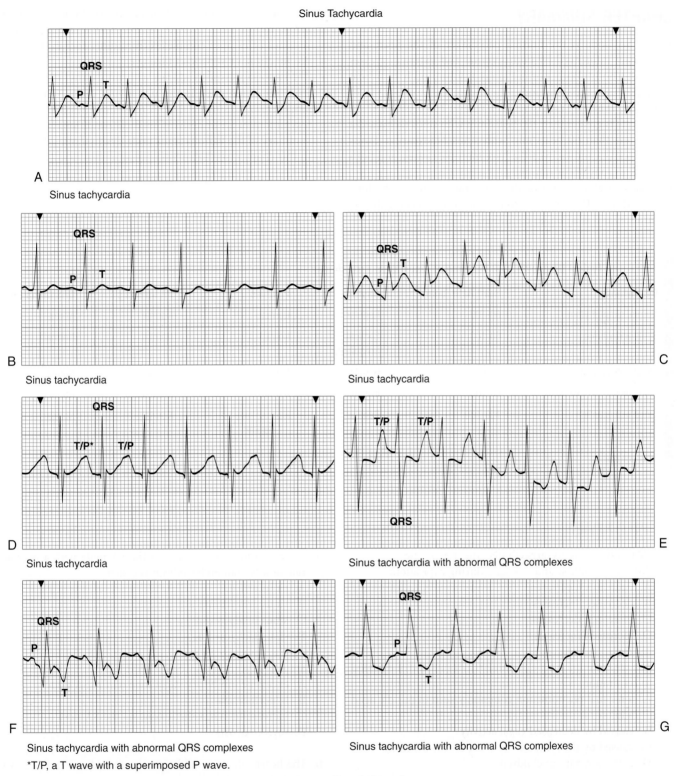

FIGURE 5-5 Sinus tachycardia.

demand in the heart? A heart with significant underlying cardiovascular disease will not tolerate the increased oxygen demand of the tachycardia and will be prone to ischemia, infarction, and potentially lethal dysrhythmias. The second and more common issue is that as the heart rate increases there is less time for the heart to relax (diastole) and fill completely. This can result in a significant decrease in the cardiac output leading to syncope and shock.

Treatment of sinus tachycardia should be directed to correcting the underlying cause of the dysrhythmia.

CHAPTER SUMMARY

- The SA node is the normal pacemaker of the heart and is easily influenced by both internal and external stresses on the body. With normal sinus rhythm, each heartbeat originates in the sinus node. The P wave is always positive in lead II. The heart rate is between 60 and 100 beats/min.
- The rate is greater than 100 beats/min with sinus tachycardia and less than 60 beats/min with sinus bradycardia. Sinus bradycardia and tachycardia have multiple causes, and both rhythms may occur normally.
- Beat-to-beat variation of the sinus rate occurs with sinus arrhythmia. The rate variation is typically cyclical with respiration and is a benign condition.

- SA node disease may lead to SA arrest. Prolonged sinus arrest causes fatal asystole unless normal sinus rhythm resumes or escapes complexes from other foci in the atria, AV junction, or ventricles take over.
- The important issue to address with any dysrhythmia arising from the sinus node is the underlying cause. Other than sinus arrest and sinoatrial block most sinus dysrhythmias are a symptom of an underlying medical condition. For a brief summary of the various sinus node dysrhythmias discussed in this chapter, see Table 5-6.

TABLE 5-6 Typical Diagnostic ECG Features of Sinus Node Arrhythmias

Dysrhythmia	Heart Rate (bpm)	Rhythm	P Waves	PR Intervals	QRS Complexes
Normal sinus rhythm	60-100	Regular	Normal	Normal	Normal
Sinus arrhythmia	60-100	Cyclical Irregularity	Normal	Normal	Normal
Sinus bradycardia	<60	Regular	Normal	Normal	Normal
Sinus arrest, SA exit block	60-100	Irregular	Normal	Normal	Normal
Sinus tachycardia	100-180	Regular	Normal; may be peaked	Normal	Normal

*SA, Sinoatrial.

CHAPTER REVIEW

1. Typically, in sinus arrhythmia, the heart rate _____ during inspiration and _____ during expiration.
   A. decreases; decreases
   B. decreases; increases
   C. increases; decreases
   D. increases; increases

2. The most common type of sinus arrhythmia, the one related to respiration, is:
   A. a normal phenomenon commonly seen in middle aged adults
   B. caused by decreased vagal activity
   C. caused by the sympathetic effect on the SA node
   D. extremely rare in children

3. Another less common type of sinus arrhythmia is not related to respiration. It is most commonly associated with the use of which of the following
   A. cocaine
   B. beta-blocker
   C. digitalis use
   D. calcium channel blockers

4. A dysrhythmia originating in the SA node with a regular rate of less than 60 beats/min is called:
   A. sinus arrest
   B. sinus arrhythmia
   C. sinus bradycardia
   D. sinus tachycardia

5. Sinus bradycardia may be caused by:
   A. excessive inhibitory vagal tone on the SA node
   B. hyperthermia
   C. increase in sympathetic tone on the SA node
   D. thyrotoxicosis

6. The heart rate in a mild sinus bradycardia is _____ to _____ beats/min.
   A. 30; 39
   B. 40; 49
   C. 50; 59
   D. 60; 69

7. A patient with marked sinus bradycardia who is symptomatic will likely have:
   A. hypertension and decreased cerebral perfusion
   B. hypotension and decreased cerebral perfusion
   C. hypothermia and chest pain
   D. hypoxia and increased central venous pressure (CVP)

8. Symptomatic sinus tachycardia is best treated by:
   A. addressing the underlying cause
   B. administering a beta-blocker
   C. administering oxygen
   D. performing vagal maneuvers

9. A dysrhythmia caused by episodes of failure in the automaticity of the SA node resulting in bradycardia or asystole is called:
   A. marked sinus arrhythmia
   B. marked sinus bradycardia
   C. sinus arrest
   D. Wenckebach phenomenon

10. Sinoatrial (SA) exit block may result from toxicity of the medication(s):
    A. amitriptyline
    B. digitalis
    C. epinephrine
    D. verapamil

6 Atrial Dysrhythmias

OBJECTIVES *Upon completion of this chapter, you should be able to complete the following objectives:*

1. Define and give the diagnostic characteristics, causes, and clinical significance of the following dysrhythmias:
   - Wandering atrial pacemaker (WAP)
   - Premature atrial complexes (PACs)
   - Atrial tachycardia
   - Ectopic atrial tachycardia
   - Multifocal atrial tachycardia (MAT)
   - Atrial flutter
   - Atrial fibrillation

WANDERING ATRIAL PACEMAKER

KEY DEFINITION

A wandering atrial pacemaker (WAP) (Figure 6-1) is a dysrhythmia originating in multiple pacemakers that shift back and forth between the sinoatrial (SA) node, ectopic pacemakers in the atria or atrioventricular (AV) junction, or between any of the three. It is characterized by P waves of varying size, shape, and direction in any one lead.

Diagnostic Characteristics (Table 6-1)

Rate. The rate is usually 60 to 100 beats/min but may be slower. Usually, the heart rate gradually slows slightly when the pacemaker site shifts from the SA node to the atria or AV junction and increases as the pacemaker site shifts back to the SA node.

Regularity. The rhythm is usually irregular.

P waves. The P waves change in size, shape, and direction over the duration of several beats. They vary in lead II from positive (upright) P waves to negative (inverted) P waves,

TABLE 6-1 Diagnostic Characteristics of Wandering Atrial Pacemaker

Characteristic	Wandering Atrial Pacemaker
Rate	60-100
Regularity	Irregular
P waves	Vary in size and shape
PR intervals	Normal to very short
P-P, R-R intervals	Unequal
Conduction ratio	1:1
QRS complexes	Normal, wide if conduction delay exists
Site of origin	SA node, ectopic atrial sites, AV junction (randomly)

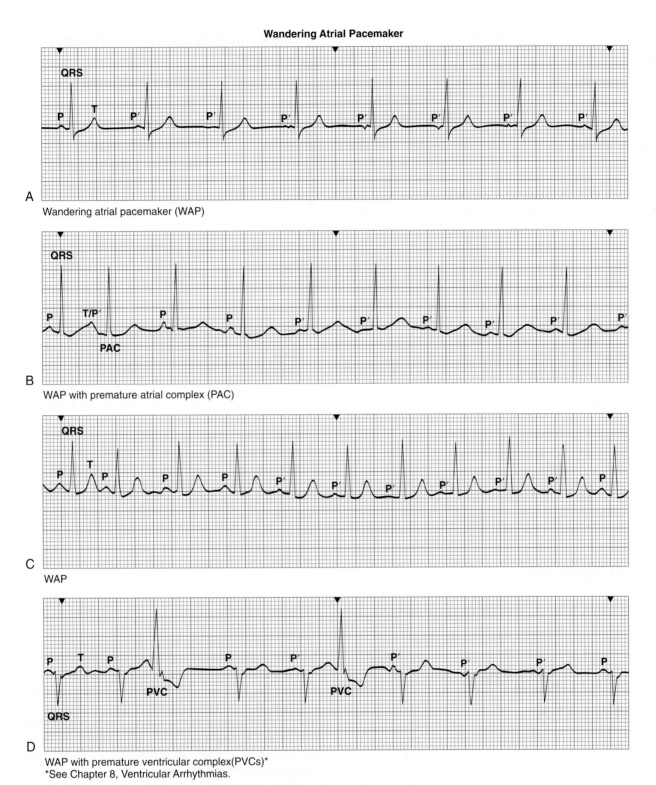

FIGURE 6-1 Wandering atrial pacemaker.

or even become buried in the QRS complexes as the pacemaker site shifts from the SA node to the atria or AV junction. These changes occur in reverse as the pacemaker site shifts back to the SA node. The ectopic P waves do not always originate from the AV junction and there are no rules for the progression of the movement of the ectopic site from one point to the other.

The shape of the P wave provides clues as to its source. The P waves, other than those arising in the SA node, are ectopic P waves (P′ waves). The changing configuration of the P waves distinguishes a WAP from a normal sinus rhythm in which the P waves remain constant in size, shape, and direction throughout a lead.

PR intervals. The duration of the PR intervals usually decreases gradually from about 0.20 second to about 0.12 second or less as the pacemaker site shifts from the SA node to the lower part of the atria or AV junction. The duration of the intervals will lengthen as the pacemaker site shifts back to the SA node.

P-P and R-R intervals. The P-P, and R-R intervals are usually unequal, but they may be equal particularly if the rate is fast. They usually increase in duration as the pacemaker site shifts from the SA node to the atria or AV junction and decrease as the pacemaker shifts back to the SA node.

Conduction ratio. There is a P wave before every QRS complex and a QRS complex following each P wave, indicating that conduction through to the AV node and no blocks are occurring. The ratio is 1:1.

QRS complexes. The QRS complexes are normal unless a preexisting intraventricular conduction disturbance (such as a bundle branch block) is present. A QRS complex follows each P wave.

Site of origin. The pacemaker site shifts back and forth between the SA node and one or more ectopic pacemakers in the atria or AV junction.

Cause of Dysrhythmia

A WAP may be a normal phenomenon seen in the very young or the elderly and in athletes. It is caused in the majority of cases by the inhibitory vagal (parasympathetic) effect of respiration on the SA node and AV junction. It may also be caused by the administration of digitalis.

Clinical Significance

A WAP is usually not clinically significant, and treatment is rarely indicated. When the heart rate slows excessively, the signs and symptoms, clinical significance, and management are the same as those in symptomatic sinus bradycardia.

PREMATURE ATRIAL COMPLEXES

KEY DEFINITION

A premature atrial complex (PAC) (Figure 6-2) is an extra P-QRS-T complex consisting of an abnormal (sometimes normal) P wave followed by a normal or abnormal QRS complex, occurring earlier than the next expected beat of the underlying rhythm, usually a sinus rhythm. A PAC is generally followed by a noncompensatory pause.

TABLE 6-2 Diagnostic Characteristics of Premature Atrial Complex

Characteristic	Premature Atrial Complex
Rate	Underlying rhythm
Regularity	Irregular at point of PAC
P waves	P′ waves, varying shapes
PR intervals	Normal (0.12-0.20 sec) to very short (<0.12 sec)
P-P, R-R intervals	P-P′ unequal. Noncompensatory pause. P-P and R-R intervals the same
Conduction ratio	1:1
QRS complexes	Normal, wide if conduction delay exists
Site of origin	Multiple sites in the atria or high in the AV junction

Diagnostic Characteristics (Table 6-2)

Rate. The rate is that of the underlying rhythm.

Regularity. The rhythm is irregular when PACs are present.

P waves. A PAC is diagnosed when a P wave accompanied by a QRS complex occurs earlier than the next expected sinus P wave. The premature P wave is called an *ectopic P wave (P′)*. Although the P′ waves of the PACs may resemble the normal sinus P waves, they are generally different. The size, shape, and direction of the P′ waves depend on the location of the ectopic site. For example, they may appear positive (upright) and quite normal in lead II if the ectopic site is near the SA node, but they may appear negative (inverted) if the ectopic site is near the AV junction—the result of retrograde atrial depolarization. P′ waves originating in the same atrial ectopic site are usually identical. The P′ waves precede the QRS complexes and are sometimes buried in the preceding T waves, distorting them and often making these T waves more peaked and pointed than the other nonaffected ones. A P′ wave followed by a QRS complex is said to be a *conducted* PAC.

If the atrial ectopic site discharges too soon after the preceding QRS complex—early in diastole, for example—the AV junction or bundle branches may not be repolarized sufficiently to conduct the premature electrical impulse into the ventricles normally. Thus being still refractory from conducting the previous electrical impulse, the AV junction or bundle branches may either slow the conduction of the premature electrical impulse, prolonging the PR interval (first-degree AV block), or block it completely (complete AV block).

When complete AV block occurs, the P′ wave is not followed by a QRS complex. Such a PAC is called a *nonconducted* or *blocked* PAC. Nonconducted PACs are commonly the cause of unexpected pauses in the electrocardiogram (ECG), suggesting sinus arrest or SA exit block. However, unlike sinus arrest or SA exit block, a P′ wave is present in a nonconducted PAC.

PR intervals. The PR intervals of the PACs may be normal but they usually differ from those of the underlying rhythm. The PR interval of a PAC varies from 0.12 to less than 0.20 second when the pacemaker site is near the SA node to less than 0.12 second when the pacemaker is near the AV junction.

P-P and R-R intervals. The interval between the P wave of the QRS complex preceding the PAC and the P′ wave of the PAC—the P-P′ interval—is typically shorter than the P-P interval of the underlying rhythm. Because the PAC usually depolarizes the SA node prematurely, the timing of the SA node is reset, causing the next cycle of the SA node to begin anew at this point. When this occurs, the next expected P wave of the underlying rhythm appears earlier than it would have if the SA node had not been reset. The resulting P′-P interval is called a *noncompensatory pause*. This interval may be equal to the P-P inter-

val of the underlying rhythm, or it may be slightly longer because of the depressing effect on the automaticity of the SA node brought on by its being depolarized prematurely. Because of the noncompensatory pause, the interval between the P waves of the underlying rhythm preceding and following the PAC is less than twice the P-P interval of the underlying rhythm.

Less commonly, the SA node is not depolarized by the PAC so that its timing is not reset, allowing the next P wave of the underlying rhythm to appear at the time expected. Such a P′-P interval is said to be a *compensatory pause*. In this case, the interval between the P waves of the underlying rhythm occurring before and after the PAC is twice the P-P interval of the

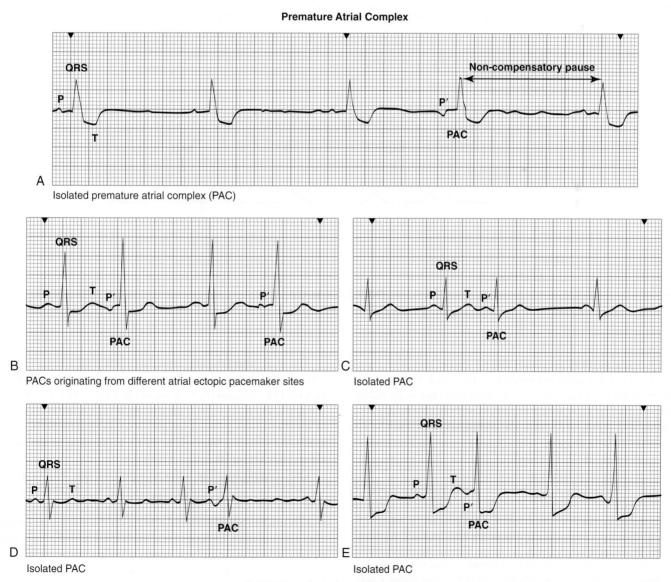

Premature Atrial Complex

A — Isolated premature atrial complex (PAC)

B — PACs originating from different atrial ectopic pacemaker sites

C — Isolated PAC

D — Isolated PAC

E — Isolated PAC

FIGURE 6-2 Premature atrial complexes.

Continued

Lead II

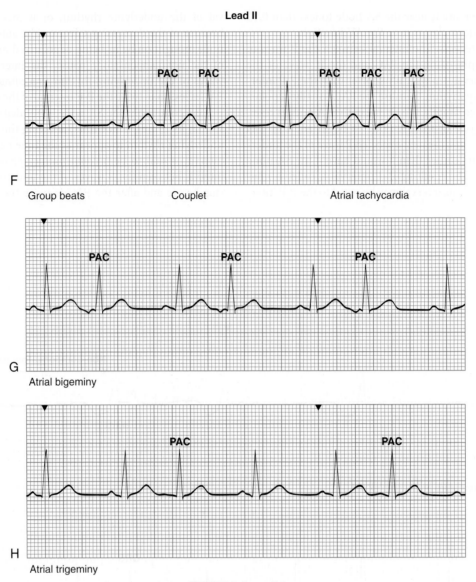

FIGURE 6-2, cont'd

underlying rhythm. A compensatory pause may also occur, even if the SA node is prematurely depolarized, if the automaticity of the SA node is excessively depressed after its premature depolarization. *Compensatory pauses* are more commonly associated with premature ventricular complexes, which will be discussed in a later chapter.

KEY DEFINITION

Compensatory pause: Pause is termed "compensatory" if the normal beat following a premature complex occurs when expected indicating that the SA node was not reset.

Noncompensatory pause: Pause is termed "noncompensatory" if the normal beat following the premature complex occurs before it was expected, indicating that the SA node was reset.

The R-R intervals are unequal when PACs are present. The interval between the P wave of the underlying rhythm preceding a PAC and the P′ wave of the PAC—the P-P′ interval (coupling interval)—varies depending on the ectopic site's rate of spontaneous depolarization and its location in the atria. Generally, the coupling intervals of PACs originating in the same ectopic site are equal.

QRS complexes. The QRS complex of the PAC usually resembles that of the underlying rhythm because the conduction of the electrical impulse through the bundle branches is usually unchanged. If the atrial ectopic site discharges very soon after the preceding QRS complex, the bundle branches may not be repolarized sufficiently to conduct the electrical impulse of the PAC normally. If this occurs, the electrical impulse may only be conducted down one bundle branch, usually the left one, and blocked in the other. The result is a wide and bizarre-appearing

QRS complex that resembles a right bundle branch block. Such a PAC, called a *premature atrial complex with aberrancy* (or with *aberrant ventricular conduction*), can mimic a premature ventricular complex (PVC) (see Premature Ventricular Complexes, p. 117).

Usually, a QRS complex follows each P′ wave (conducted PACs), but a QRS complex may be absent because of a temporary complete AV block (nonconducted PACs). A nonconducted PAC is also called a *blocked* or *dropped* PAC.

Frequency and pattern of occurrence of PACs. The following are the various forms in which PACs may appear:

- **Isolated:** PACs may occur singly (isolated complex).
- **Group beats:** The PACs may occur in groups of two or more consecutive complexes. Two PACs in a row are called a *couplet.* When three or more PACs occur in succession, atrial tachycardia is considered to be present.
- **Repetitive beats:** PACs may alternate with the QRS complexes of the underlying rhythm (atrial bigeminy) or occur after every two QRS complexes (atrial trigeminy) or after every three QRS complexes of the underlying rhythm (atrial quadrigeminy).

Site of origin. The origin of the PACs is an ectopic site in any part of the atria outside the SA node. PACs may originate from a single ectopic site or from multiple sites in the atria or high in the AV junction.

Cause of Dysrhythmia

Common causes of PACs include the following. Often, however, they appear without apparent cause.

- Increase in catecholamines and sympathetic tone
- Infections
- Emotional stress
- Stimulants (e.g., alcohol, caffeine, and tobacco)
- Sympathomimetic drugs (e.g., epinephrine, isoproterenol, and norepinephrine)
- Hypoxia
- Digitalis toxicity
- Cardiovascular disease (acute coronary syndromes [ACS], or early congestive heart failure)
- Dilated or hypertrophied atria resulting from increased atrial pressure commonly caused by mitral stenosis or an atrial septal defect

The electrophysiological mechanism responsible for PACs is either enhanced automaticity or reentry.

Clinical Significance

Isolated PACs may occur in persons with apparently healthy hearts and are not significant. In persons with heart disease, however, frequent PACs may indicate enhanced automaticity of the atria, or a reentry mechanism resulting from a variety of causes, such as congestive heart failure or acute myocardial infarction. In addition, such PACs may warn of or initiate more serious supraventricular dysrhythmias, such as atrial tachycardia, atrial flutter, atrial fibrillation, or paroxysmal supraventricular tachycardia (PSVT).

If nonconducted PACs are frequent and the heart rate is less than 50 beats/min, the signs and symptoms, clinical significance, and management are the same as those of symptomatic sinus bradycardia.

Because PACs with wide and bizarre-appearing QRS complexes (i.e., aberrancy) often resemble PVCs (see p. 117), care must be taken to identify such PACs correctly so as not to treat them inappropriately as PVCs.

ATRIAL TACHYCARDIA (ECTOPIC AND MULTIFOCAL)

KEY DEFINITION

Atrial tachycardia (Figure 6-3) is a dysrhythmia originating in an ectopic pacemaker in the atria with a rate between 160 to 240 beats/min. It includes ectopic atrial tachycardia and multifocal atrial tachycardia (MAT).

Diagnostic Characteristics (Table 6-3)

Rate. The atrial rate is usually 160 to 240 beats/min but may be slower, especially in MAT. The ventricular rate is usually the same as that of the atria, but it may be slower, often half the atrial rate because of a 2 : 1 AV block. Because atrial tachycardia commonly starts and ends gradually, it is called a *nonparoxysmal atrial tachycardia.* By definition, three or more consecutive PACs are considered to be atrial tachycardia.

Vagal maneuvers, such as carotid sinus massage, by increasing the parasympathetic (vagal) tone, do not terminate atrial tachycardia abruptly nor slow the atrial rate, but they do impede AV conduction and result in an AV block.

Regularity. The atrial rhythm is essentially regular. The ventricular rhythm is usually regular if the AV conduction ratio is constant, but it may be irregular if a variable AV block or MAT is present.

TABLE 6-3 Diagnostic Characteristics of Atrial Tachycardia

Characteristic	Atrial Tachycardia
Rate	160-240 (half the rate if 2 : 1 conduction ratio)
Regularity	Regular (usually)
P waves	P′ all the same in atrial tachycardia P′ vary in MAT
PR intervals	Normal, 0.12 <0.20 sec
P-P, R-R intervals	Equal
Conduction ratio	1 : 1, (2 : 1 or higher if AV conduction block)
QRS complexes	Normal, wide if conduction delay exists
Site of origin	Ectopic atrial sites outside of SA node

**Atrial Tachycardia
(Ectopic Atrial Tachycardia, Multifocal Atrial Tachycardia)**

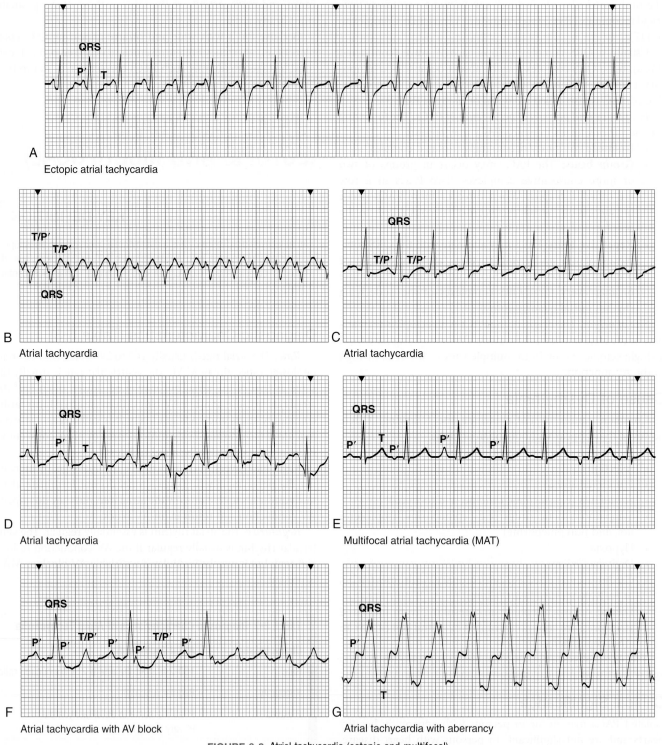

A

Ectopic atrial tachycardia

B

Atrial tachycardia

C

Atrial tachycardia

D

Atrial tachycardia

E

Multifocal atrial tachycardia (MAT)

F

Atrial tachycardia with AV block

G

Atrial tachycardia with aberrancy

FIGURE 6-3 Atrial tachycardia (ectopic and multifocal).

P waves. The ectopic P waves in atrial tachycardia usually differ from normal sinus P waves. The size, shape, and direction of the P′ waves vary, depending on the location of the pacemaker site. They may appear positive (upright) and quite normal in lead II if the pacemaker site is near the SA node, but negative (inverted) if they originate near the AV junction.

The P′ waves are usually identical in ectopic atrial tachycardia and precede each QRS complex. In MAT, on the other hand, the P′ waves usually vary in size, shape, and direction in each given lead. There must be at least 3 different P and P′ waves present to classify the rhythm as MAT. The P′ waves are often not easily identified because they are buried in the preceding T waves or QRS complexes. Normal sinus P waves are absent.

PR intervals. The PR intervals are usually normal and constant in ectopic atrial tachycardia. In MAT, the PR intervals usually vary slightly in each given lead. They may vary from 0.20 second to less than 0.12 second, depending on the pacemaker site. Occasionally, the PR intervals are prolonged (greater than 0.20 second), particularly when the atrial rate is extremely rapid. This occurs when the atrial impulses reach the AV junction while it is in the relative refractory period, thereby increasing the AV conduction time. In addition, a preexisting first-degree AV block may be present. A shorter than normal PR interval may be present when atrial tachycardia is relatively slow, when it occurs in healthy young individuals, or when ventricular preexcitation is present.

P-P and R-R intervals. The R-R intervals are usually equal in ectopic atrial tachycardia if the AV conduction ratio is constant. But if the AV conduction ratio varies (i.e., 3:1, 2:1, 4:1, 3:1, and so forth), the R-R intervals will be unequal.

Conduction ratio. In most untreated atrial tachycardias not caused by digitalis intoxication, and in which the atrial rate is less than 200/min, the AV conduction ratio is 1:1. When the atrial rate is greater than 200 per minute, a 2:1 AV conduction ratio is common. (A 2:1 AV conduction ratio indicates that for every two P′ waves, one is followed by a QRS complex.) When the AV block occurs only during the tachycardia, the arrhythmia is called *atrial tachycardia with block.*

The cause of the AV block is the relatively long refractory period of the AV junction, which prevents the conduction of all of the rapidly occurring atrial electrical impulses into the ventricles (*physiological AV block*).

If there is a preexisting AV block because of cardiac disease, if digitalis excess is the cause of the atrial tachycardia or if certain drugs (e.g., beta-blockers or calcium channel blockers) have been administered, 2:1 AV block may occur at atrial rates less than 200 per minute. Higher-degree AV block (e.g., 3:1, 4:1, and so forth) or variable AV block may also occur, particularly in atrial tachycardia caused by digitalis toxicity.

QRS complexes. The QRS complexes are normal unless a preexisting intraventricular conduction disturbance (such as a bundle branch block), aberrant ventricular conduction, or ventricular preexcitation is present. If the QRS complexes are abnormal only during the tachycardia, the arrhythmia is called *atrial tachycardia with aberrancy* (or *with aberrant ventricular conduction*). Atrial tachycardia with abnormal QRS complexes may resemble ventricular tachycardia (see p. 121).

Site of origin. Atrial tachycardia originates from an ectopic site in any part of the atria outside the SA node. Atrial tachycardia may occasionally originate in more than one atrial ectopic site. One that originates in a single ectopic site is called *ectopic atrial tachycardia;* one originating in three or more different ectopic atrial sites is called *multifocal atrial tachycardia (MAT).* The activity of the SA node is completely suppressed by atrial tachycardia.

Cause of Dysrhythmia

In general, the causes of atrial tachycardia are essentially the same as those of PACs. Like PACs, atrial tachycardia may occur in persons with apparently healthy hearts, and in those with diseased hearts.

Most often, atrial tachycardia occurs in patients with the following conditions:

- Digitalis toxicity
- Metabolic abnormalities (including acute alcohol abuse)
- Electrolyte disturbances
- Hypoxia
- Chronic lung disease
- Coronary artery disease (associated with acute coronary syndrome)
- Rheumatic heart disease

Atrial tachycardia caused by digitalis toxicity is often associated with a 2:1 or a varying AV block. Atrial tachycardia with AV block may also occur in patients with significant heart disease, such as coronary artery disease or lung disease. MAT is most often associated with respiratory failure, as in decompensated chronic obstructive pulmonary disease (COPD); it is rarely caused by digitalis excess. The electrophysiological mechanism responsible for atrial tachycardia is either enhanced automaticity or reentry.

Clinical Significance

The signs and symptoms of atrial tachycardia depend on the presence or absence of heart disease, the nature of the heart disease, the ventricular rate, and the duration of the dysrhythmia. Frequently, atrial tachycardia is accompanied by feelings of palpitations, nervousness, or anxiety.

When the ventricular rate is very rapid, the ventricles are unable to fill completely during diastole, resulting in a significant reduction of the cardiac output and a decrease in perfusion of the brain and other vital organs. This decrease in perfusion may cause confusion, dizziness, lightheadedness, shortness of breath, near-syncope, or syncope.

In addition, because a rapid heart rate increases the workload of the heart, the oxygen requirements of the myocardium are usually increased in atrial tachycardia. Because of this, in addition to the consequences of decreased cardiac output, atrial tachycardia in the setting of acute coronary syndrome may increase myocardial ischemia and the frequency and severity of chest pain; extend the size of the infarct; precipitate congestive heart failure; result in hypotension and cardiogenic shock; or predispose the patient to serious ventricular dysrhythmias.

Symptomatic atrial tachycardia must be treated promptly to reverse the consequences of the reduced cardiac output and increased workload of the heart and to prevent the occurrence of serious ventricular dysrhythmias. As noted earlier, atrial tachycardia with wide QRS complexes may resemble ventricular tachycardia. A 12-lead ECG (particularly lead V_1 or V_2) or lead MCL_1 may be useful in making a differentiation in this situation by helping to identify the presence or absence of P waves. P waves are best visualized in V_1, V_2, and MCL_1.

ATRIAL FLUTTER

KEY DEFINITION

Atrial flutter (Figures 6-4 and 6-5) is a dysrhythmia arising in an ectopic pacemaker or the site of a rapid reentry circuit in the atria, characterized by rapid atrial flutter (F) waves with a sawtooth appearance and, usually, a slower, regular ventricular response.

Diagnostic Characteristics (Table 6-4)

Rate. Usually, the atrial rate is between 240 and 360 (average, 300) per minute, but it may be slower or faster. The ventricular rate is commonly about 150 beats/min (half the atrial rate because of a 2:1 AV block) in an uncontrolled (untreated) atrial flutter and about 60 to 75 in a controlled (treated) one or one with a preexisting AV block. Rarely, the ventricular rate may be over 240 beats/min, the same as the atrial rate, if a 1:1 AV conduction ratio is present. When the ventricular rate is greater than 100, the dysrhythmia is referred to as atrial flutter with rapid ventricular response.

Regularity. The atrial rhythm is typically regular, but it may be irregular. The ventricular rhythm is usually regular if the AV conduction ratio is constant, but it may be grossly irregular if a variable AV block is present.

P waves. As discussed in Chapter 4, the P wave can assume many shapes. In atrial flutter, because of the rapid firing of the ectopic atrial, waveform takes on a unique configuration. This is termed the atrial flutter or "F" wave.

Characteristics of atrial flutter F waves. An atrial flutter F wave represents depolarization of the atria in an abnormal direction followed by atrial repolarization. Depolarization of the atria commonly begins near the AV node and progresses across the atria in a retrograde direction. The characteristics of atrial flutter F waves include the following:

- **Onset and end:** The onset and end of the F waves cannot be determined with certainty.
- **Components:** The F wave consists of an abnormal atrial depolarization wave corresponding to an ectopic P wave followed by an atrial T wave (Ta) of atrial repolarization.
- **Direction:** The first part of the F wave, corresponding to an ectopic P wave, is commonly negative (inverted) in lead II and followed by a positive (upright) wave, the atrial T wave. This results in a characteristic "sawtoothed" pattern.
- **Duration:** The duration of the F waves varies according to their rate.
- **Amplitude:** The amplitude, measured from peak to peak of the F wave, varies greatly from less than 1 mm to more than 5 mm.
- **Shape:** The atrial F waves have a sawtooth appearance. The typical F wave consists of a negative (inverted), V-shaped ectopic atrial wave immediately followed by an upright, peaked atrial T wave in lead II. An isoelectric line is seldom present between the waves. Typically, the first, downward part of the F wave is shorter and more abrupt than the second, upward part. F waves are generally identical in shape and size in any given lead but may occasionally vary slightly. Atrial fibrillation may occur during atrial flutter and vice versa. Such a mixture of atrial fibrillation and flutter is called *atrial fib-flutter.*

F wave-QRS complex relationship. The F waves precede, are buried in, and follow the QRS complexes and may be superimposed on the T waves or ST segments.

FR intervals. FR intervals are difficult to measure but are usually equal.

R-R intervals. The R-R intervals are equal if the AV conduction ratio is constant, but if the AV conduction ratio varies, the R-R intervals are unequal.

Conduction ratios. The AV conduction ratio in most instances of atrial flutter is commonly 2:1, which indicates that every other F wave is followed by a QRS complex. The conduction ratio of F waves and the QRS complexes is the result of the long refractory period of the AV junction, which prevents the conduction of all the rapidly occurring atrial electrical impulses into the ventricles (physiological AV block).

The AV block may be greater (i.e., 3:1, 4:1, and so forth) or even variable because of disease of the AV node, increased

TABLE 6-4 Diagnostic Characteristics of Atrial Flutter

Characteristic	Atrial Flutter
Rate	Atria 240-360 Ventricular ¹⁄₂ atrial rate or less
Regularity	Regular
P waves	Normal P wave absent F waves (sawtooth)
PR intervals	FR intervals difficult to measure
P-P, R-R intervals	No P-P, R-R intervals equal unless conduction ratio changes
Conduction ratio	Commonly 2:1, 3:1, 4:1. Rarely 1:1
QRS complexes	Normal, wide if conduction delay exists
Site of origin	Ectopic atrial sites outside of SA Node

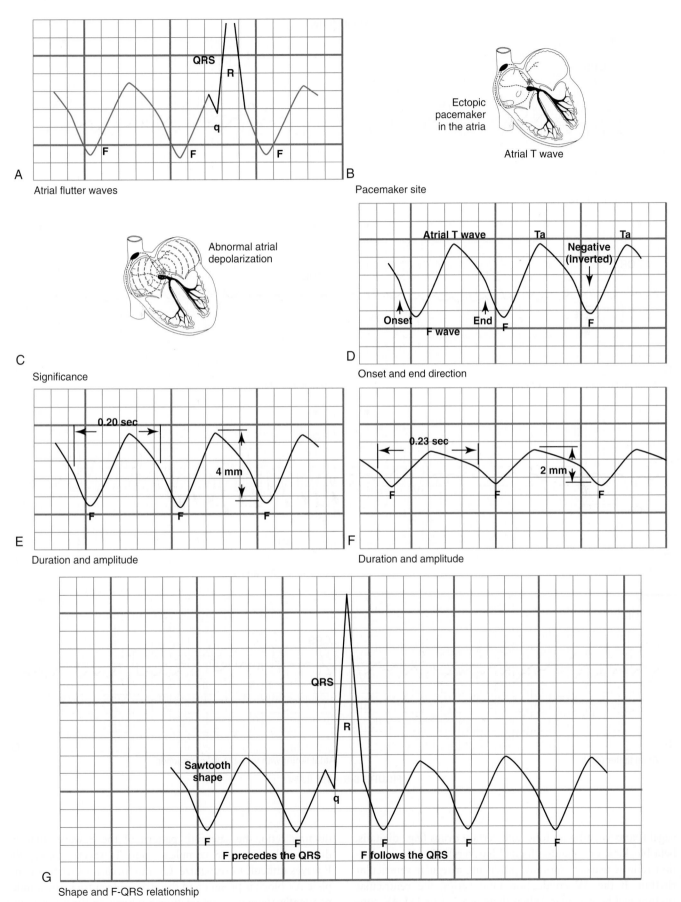

A Atrial flutter waves

B Ectopic pacemaker in the atria / Atrial T wave / Pacemaker site

C Abnormal atrial depolarization / Significance

D Atrial T wave / Ta / Ta / Negative (Inverted) / Onset / End / F wave / F / F / Onset and end direction

E 0.20 sec / 4 mm / F / F / F / Duration and amplitude

F 0.23 sec / 2 mm / F / F / F / Duration and amplitude

G Sawtooth shape / QRS / R / q / F / F / F / F / F / F precedes the QRS / F follows the QRS / Shape and F-QRS relationship

FIGURE 6-4 Atrial flutter F waves.

Atrial Flutter

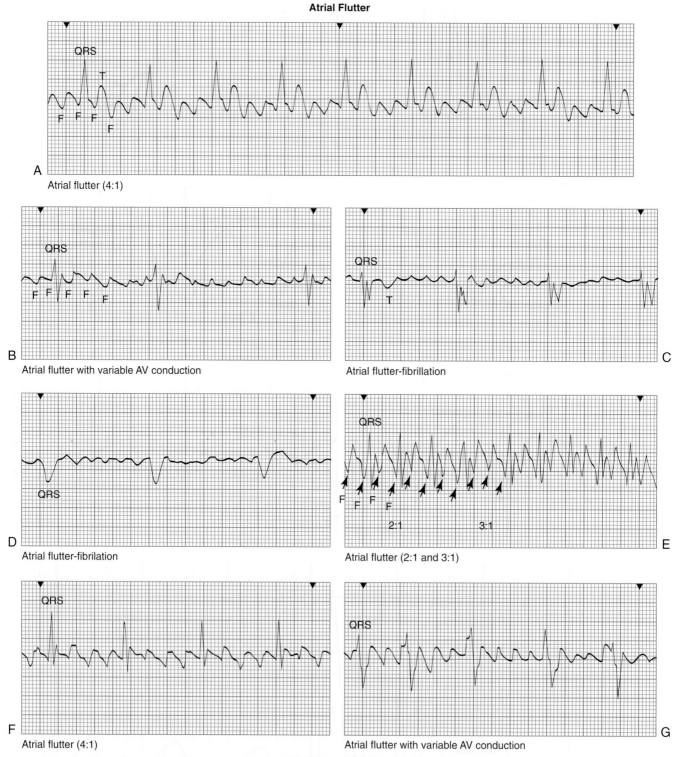

FIGURE 6-5 Atrial flutter.

vagal (parasympathetic) tone, and certain drugs (e.g., digitalis, beta-blockers, or calcium channel blockers). The AV conduction ratio is usually constant, producing a regular ventricular rhythm. If the AV conduction ratio varies, the ventricular rhythm will be irregular. When there is a 2:1 or 1:1 AV con-

duction ratio, the sawtooth pattern of the F waves may be distorted by the QRS complexes and T waves, making the F waves difficult to recognize. On rare occasions when a complete AV block is present and the atria and ventricles beat independently, there is no set relationship between the F waves and the QRS complexes. When this occurs, AV dissociation is present. Rarely, the AV conduction ratio in untreated atrial flutter is 1:1.

QRS complexes. The QRS complexes are normal unless a preexisting intraventricular conduction disturbance (such as a bundle branch block), aberrant ventricular conduction, or ventricular preexcitation is present. Atrial flutter with a rapid ventricular response and abnormal QRS complexes may resemble ventricular tachycardia.

Site of origin. The pacemaker site is an ectopic pacemaker in part of the atria outside of the SA node. Commonly, it is located low in the atria near the AV node. The activity of the SA node is completely suppressed by atrial flutter.

Cause of Dysrhythmia

Chronic (persistent) atrial flutter is most commonly seen in middle-aged and elderly persons with the following conditions:
- Advanced rheumatic heart disease, particularly if mitral or tricuspid valvular disease is present
- Coronary or hypertensive heart disease

Transient (paroxysmal) atrial flutter usually indicates the presence of cardiac disease; however, it may occasionally occur in apparently healthy persons. The dysrhythmia may also be associated with the following:
- Cardiomyopathy
- Atrial dilation from any cause
- Thyrotoxicosis
- Digitalis toxicity (rarely)
- Hypoxia
- Acute or chronic cor pulmonale
- Congestive heart failure
- Damage to the SA node or atria because of pericarditis or myocarditis
- Alcoholism

Atrial flutter may be initiated by a PAC. The electrophysiological mechanism responsible for atrial flutter is either enhanced automaticity or reentry.

Clinical Significance

The signs and symptoms and clinical significance of atrial flutter with a rapid ventricular response are the same as those of atrial tachycardia. In atrial flutter, the atria do not regularly contract and empty, as they normally do, during the last part of ventricular diastole, completely filling the ventricles just before they contract. The loss of this "atrial kick" may result in incomplete filling of the ventricles before they contract, causing a reduction of the cardiac output by as much as 25%. This can result in syncope, hypotension, and congestive heart failure.

Persons with atrial flutter are at risk for developing thrombi (clots), which attach themselves to the walls of the atria. Small portions of the thrombi may break free and travel up the aorta to the cerebrovascular circulation where they lodge resulting in a stroke.

ATRIAL FIBRILLATION

> ### KEY DEFINITION
>
> Atrial fibrillation (Figures 6-6 and 6-7) is a dysrhythmia arising in multiple ectopic atrial sites or sites of rapid reentry circuits in the atria, characterized by very rapid atrial fibrillation (f) waves and an irregular, often rapid ventricular response.

Diagnostic Characteristics (Table 6-5)

Rate. Typically, the atrial rate is 350 to 600 (average 400) per minute, but it can be as high as 700. The ventricular rate is commonly greater than 100 beats/min and is often about 160 to 180 (or as high as 200) beats/min in an uncontrolled (untreated) atrial fibrillation. The ventricular rate is less than 100 beats/min in a controlled (treated) one, or one with a preexisting AV block.

Regularity. The atrial rhythm is irregularly irregular. The ventricular rhythm is almost always irregularly irregular in untreated atrial fibrillation unless AV dissociation is present.

P waves. As discussed in Chapter 4 there are no normal P waves in atrial fibrillation. Instead, the chaotic rapid firing of the multiple ectopic atrial sites results in the characteristic atrial fibrillation "f" wave.

Characteristics of atrial fibrillation f waves. Atrial fibrillation f waves represent abnormal, chaotic, and incomplete depolarizations of small individual groups (or islets) of atrial muscle fibers. Because organized depolarizations of the atria are absent. P waves and organized atrial contractions are absent. Characteristics of atrial fibrillation f waves include the following:
- **Onset and end: The onset and end of the f waves** cannot be determined with certainty.

TABLE 6-5 **Diagnostic Characteristics of Atrial Fibrillation**

Characteristic	Atrial Fibrillation
Rate	Atrial 350-600 Ventricular >100 (uncontrolled) Ventricular <100 (controlled)
Regularity	Irregularly irregular
P waves	Normal P waves absent "f" waves present
PR Intervals	Absent
P-P, R-R Intervals	P-P absent R-R unequal
Conduction ratio	Random
QRS complexes	Normal, wide if conduction delay exists
Site of origin	Ectopic atrial sites outside of SA Node

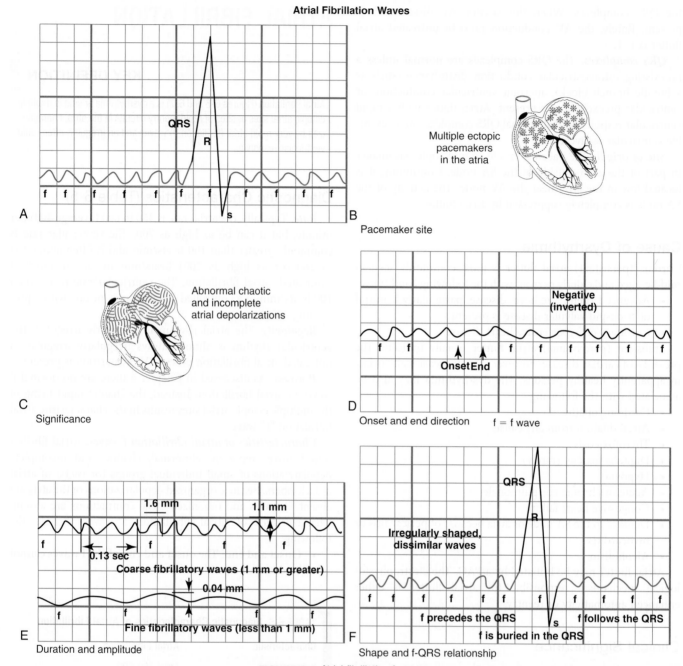

FIGURE 6-6 Atrial fibrillation f waves.

- **Direction:** The direction of the f waves varies from positive (upright) to negative (inverted) at random.
- **Duration:** The duration of the f waves varies greatly and cannot be determined with accuracy.
- **Amplitude:** The amplitude varies from less than 1 mm to several mm. If the f waves are small (less than 1 mm), they are called *fine* fibrillatory waves; if they are large (1 mm or greater), they are called *coarse* fibrillatory waves. If the f waves are so small or "fine" that they are not recorded, the sections of the ECG between

the QRS complexes may appear as a wavy or flat (isoelectric) line.
- **Shape**: The f waves are irregularly shaped, rounded (or pointed), and dissimilar.

f wave–QRS complex relationship. The f waves precede, are buried in, and follow the QRS complexes and are superimposed on the ST segments and T waves.

R-R intervals. The R-R intervals are typically unequal. When atrial fibrillation is complicated by a second-degree, type I AV block, the R-R intervals progressively decrease in duration over

Atrial Fibrillation

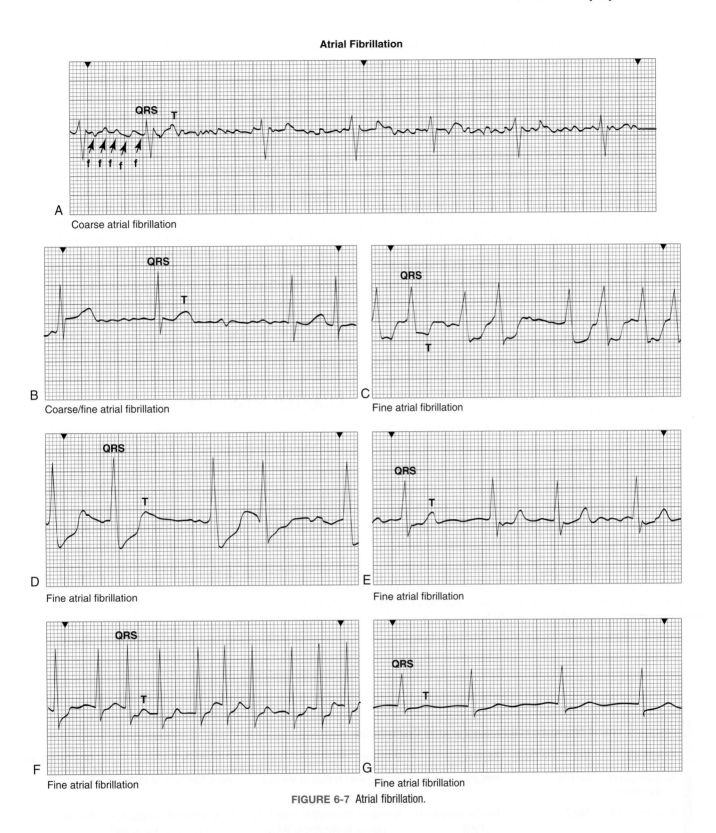

FIGURE 6-7 Atrial fibrillation.

a cycle of three or more R-R intervals, each cycle following an exceptionally wide R-R interval. When only two R-R intervals occur in a cycle, the ventricular rhythm assumes a roughly bigeminal appearance. If complete AV dissociation is present, a junctional or ventricular escape rhythm may result in a regular R-R interval.

Conduction ratio. Typically, in atrial fibrillation, fewer than one half to one third of the atrial electrical impulses are conducted through the AV junction into the ventricles, and these, at random. This results in a grossly irregular ventricular rhythm. This is due to the long refractory period of the AV junction, which prevents the conduction of all the rapidly occurring atrial electrical impulses into the ventricles (physiological AV block). When greater than 100 QRS complexes per minute are conducted, the rhythm is called *uncontrolled atrial fibrillation* or atrial fibrillation with rapid ventricular response. When less than 100 QRS complexes per minute are conducted the rhythm is termed *controlled atrial fibrillation* or atrial fibrillation with slow ventricular response.

QRS complexes. The QRS complexes are normal unless a preexisting intraventricular conduction disturbance (such as a bundle branch block), aberrant ventricular conduction, or ventricular preexcitation is present. Atrial fibrillation with a rapid ventricular response and abnormal QRS complexes may resemble ventricular tachycardia, except for the irregularity of the rhythm.

Site of origin. The origin of atrial fibrillation is from multiple ectopic sites in the atria outside of the SA node generating electrical impulses chaotically. The activity of the SA node is completely suppressed by atrial fibrillation.

Cause of Dysrhythmia

Atrial fibrillation is commonly associated with the following:
- Advanced rheumatic heart disease (particularly with mitral stenosis)
- Hypertensive or coronary heart disease (with or without acute MI)
- Thyrotoxicosis

Less commonly, atrial fibrillation may occur in the following:
- Cardiomyopathy
- Acute myocarditis and pericarditis
- Chest trauma
- Pulmonary disease
- Digitalis toxicity (rarely)

Whatever the underlying form of heart disease, atrial fibrillation is commonly associated with congestive heart failure. In a small percentage of cases, atrial fibrillation may occur in apparently normal individuals after excessive ingestion of alcohol and caffeine, during emotional stress, and sometimes without any apparent cause.

Atrial fibrillation may be intermittent, even occurring in short bursts or paroxysms, as does paroxysmal supraventricular tachycardia (PSVT), or it may be chronic (persistent). The electrophysiological mechanism responsible for atrial fibrillation is either enhanced automaticity or reentry.

Clinical Significance

The signs and symptoms and clinical significance of atrial fibrillation with a rapid ventricular response are the same as those of atrial tachycardia. In addition, in atrial fibrillation, the atria do not regularly contract and empty, as they normally do, during the last part of ventricular diastole, completely filling the ventricles just before they contract. The loss of this "atrial kick" may result in incomplete filling of the ventricles before they contract, causing a reduction of the cardiac output by as much as 25%. A small yet significant percentage of patients with persistent atrial fibrillation may develop atrial thrombi with peripheral arterial embolization resulting in stroke.

CHAPTER SUMMARY

- Atrial dysrhythmias are the result of either increased automaticity or reentry phenomenon causing an ectopic pacemaker in the atria to fire.
- The result can be as benign as a single premature atrial complex or as malignant as atrial fibrillation with rapid ventricular response.
- The primary concern when addressing atrial dysrhythmias is the resulting heart rate and cardiac output.
- In the presence of ventricular conduction delay it is vital to examine the rhythm closely to determine its origin as the treatment of atrial and ventricular dysrhythmias differs.
- Table 6-6 summarizes the diagnostic characteristics of the various atrial dysrhythmias discussed in this chapter.

TABLE 6-6 Typical Diagnostic ECG Features of Atrial Dysrhythmias

Arrhythmia	Heart Rate (bpm)	Rhythm	P Waves	P'R Intervals	QRS Complexes
Wandering atrial pacemaker	60-100	Irregular	Varying from normal to inverted	Varying from 0.20 to 0.12 sec	Normal
Atrial tachycardia	160-240	Regular (irregular in MAT)	Normal or abnormal (varying from normal to inverted in MAT)	Normal, constant (varying from 0.20 to ≤ 0.12 sec in MAT)	Normal
Atrial flutter	60-150	Usually regular; may be irregular	Atrial flutter F waves	FR intervals: usually equal	Normal
Atrial fibrillation	60-180	Irregular	Atrial fibrillation f waves	None	Normal

MAT, Multifocal atrial tachycardia.

CHAPTER REVIEW

1. A dysrhythmia originating in pacemakers that shift back and forth between the SA node and an ectopic pacemaker in the atria or AV junction is called a(n):
   A. alternating atrial flutter
   B. atrial fibrillation
   C. supraventricular tachycardia
   D. wandering atrial pacemaker

2. The dysrhythmia described in question No. 1 may be a normal phenomenon seen in:
   A. acute myocardial infarction
   B. digitalis toxicity
   C. during respiration
   D. the very young

3. An extra atrial complex consisting of a positive P wave in lead II followed by a normal or abnormal QRS complex, occurring earlier than the next beat of the underlying rhythm, is called:
   A. a premature atrial complex
   B. a premature junctional contraction
   C. a premature ventricular contraction
   D. intraventricular conduction delay

4. A nonconducted or blocked PAC is:
   A. always symptomatic in patients
   B. a P′ wave that is not followed by a QRS complex
   C. caused by ventricular conduction delay
   D. found in bradycardiac arrhythmias

5. The QRS complex of a PAC usually resembles that of:
   A. a left bundle branch block
   B. a premature ventricular complex
   C. a right bundle branch block
   D. the underlying rhythm

6. Two PACs in a row are called:
   A. atrial tachycardia
   B. a couplet
   C. a reentry rhythm
   D. bigeminy

7. A dysrhythmia originating in an ectopic pacemaker in the atria with an atrial rate between 160 and 240 beats/min and characterized differing P waves is called:
   A. atrial flutter
   B. atrial tachycardia
   C. junctional tachycardia
   D. sinus tachycardia

8. The symptoms associated with rapid atrial tachycardia are a result of:
   A. drug toxicity
   B. increased vagal tone
   C. palpitations
   D. reduced cardiac output

9. Atrial flutter is characterized by:
   A. an atrial rate between 160 and 240 beats/min
   B. an atrial rate slower than the ventricular rate
   C. varying and chaotic flutter waves
   D. waves with a sawtooth appearance

10. A dysrhythmia characterized by numerous dissimilar and chaotic atrial waves occurring at 350 or more beats/min is:
    A. atrial fibrillation
    B. atrial flutter
    C. ectopic atrial tachycardia
    D. multifocal atrial tachycardia

7 Junctional Dysrhythmias

OBJECTIVES *Upon completion of this chapter, you should be able to complete the following objective:*

1. Define and give the diagnostic characteristics, cause, and clinical significance of the following dysrhythmias:
   - Premature junctional complexes (PJCs)
   - Junctional escape rhythm
   - Nonparoxysmal junctional tachycardia
   - Accelerated junctional rhythm
   - Junctional tachycardia
   - Paroxysmal supraventricular tachycardia (PSVT)

PREMATURE JUNCTIONAL COMPLEXES

KEY DEFINITION

A premature junctional complex (PJC) (Figure 7-1) is an extraventricular complex that originates in an ectopic site within the atrioventricular (AV) junction and occurs before the next expected beat of the underlying rhythm. It consists of a normal or abnormal QRS complex with or without an inverted P wave. If a P wave is present, it may precede or follow the QRS complex.

Diagnostic Characteristics (Table 7-1)

Rate. The rate is that of the underlying rhythm.

Regularity. The rhythm is irregular when PJCs occur.

P waves. P waves may or may not be associated with the PJCs. If they are present, they are P′ waves, varying in size, shape, and direction from normal P waves. The P′ waves may precede, be buried in, or follow the QRS complexes of the PJCs (Box 7-1).

TABLE 7-1 Diagnostic Characteristics of Premature Junctional Complexes

Characteristic	Premature Junctional Complex
Rate	Underlying rhythm
Regularity	Irregular when PJC occur
P waves	P′ waves before or after QRS *P′ may be absent*
PR intervals	P′R intervals <0.12 sec
P-P, R-R intervals	Compensatory pause present
Conduction ratio	1:1
QRS complexes	Normal, wide if conduction delay exists
Site of origin	Ectopic pacemaker in AV junction

A P′ wave that occurs before the QRS complex has most likely originated in the proximal, upper part of the AV junction. A P′ wave that occurs during or after the QRS complex has most likely originated in the middle or distal part of the AV junction. If the P′ waves precede the QRS complexes, they may be buried in the preceding T waves, distorting them. If the P′ waves follow the QRS complexes, they are usually found in the ST segments. Because atrial depolarization occurs in a retrograde fashion, the P′ waves that precede or follow the QRS complexes are negative (inverted) in lead II.

Absent P′ waves indicate that either (1) retrograde atrial depolarizations occurred during the QRS complexes or (2) atrial depolarizations have not occurred because of a retrograde AV block between the ectopic pacemaker site in the AV junction and the atria.

Premature Junctional Complexes

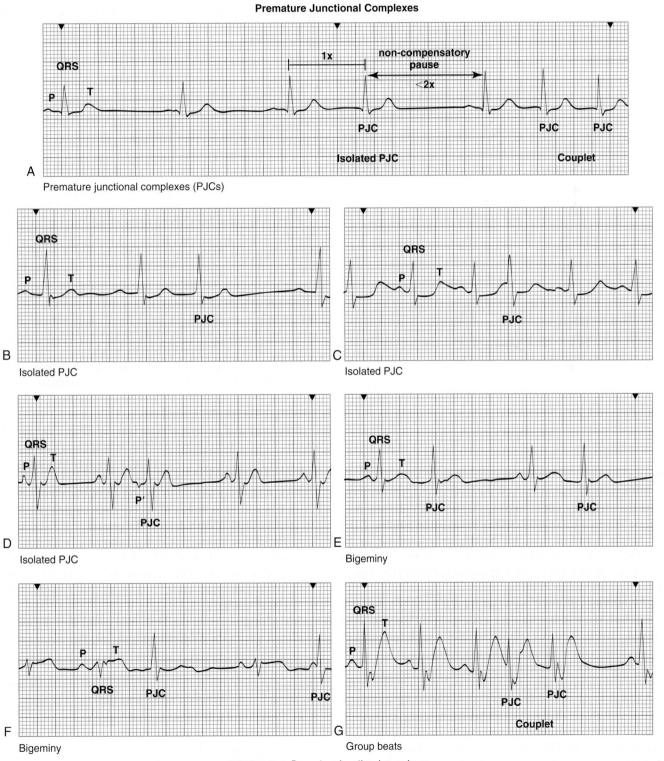

FIGURE 7-1 Premature junctional complexes.

Continued

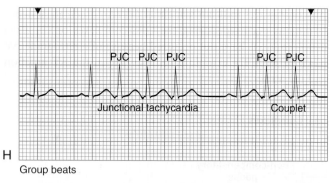

H

Group beats

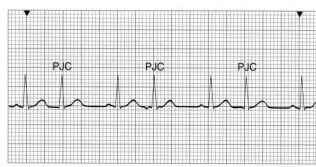

I

Junctional bigeminy

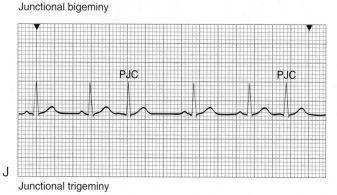

J

Junctional trigeminy

FIGURE 7-1, cont'd

BOX 7-1 Relationship of P′ Waves to the QRS Complexes Depending on Their Site of Origin

Site of Origin of the P′ Wave in the AV Junction	P′ Wave Location
Upper part	Precedes the QRS complex
Middle or distal part	Is buried in the QRS complex
Distal part	Follows the QRS complex

Conduction ratio. The impulse causing the PJC originates above the ventricles and is conducted down the bundle of His, resulting in ventricular depolarization. This is a 1:1 ratio. However, for the lone PJC the conduction ratio is not relevant clinically. Usually, a QRS complex follows each premature P′ wave (conducted PJC), but a QRS complex may be absent because of a transient complete AV block below the ectopic pacemaker site in the AV junction (nonconducted PJC).

QRS complexes. The QRS complex of the PJC usually resembles that of the underlying rhythm. If the ectopic pacemaker in the AV junction discharges too soon after the preceding QRS complex, the bundle branches may not be repolarized sufficiently to conduct the electrical impulse of the PJC normally. If this occurs, the electrical impulse may only be conducted down one bundle branch, usually the left one, and blocked in the other, producing a wide and bizarre-appearing QRS complex that resembles a right bundle branch block.

Such a bizarre-appearing PJC, called a *premature junctional complex with aberrancy* (or *with aberrant ventricular conduction*), can mimic a premature ventricular complex (PVC) (see Premature Ventricular Complexes, p. 117).

Frequency and pattern of occurrence of PJCs. The following are the various forms in which PJCs may appear:

- **Isolated**: PJCs may occur singly (isolated beats).
- **Group beats**: PJCs may occur in groups of two or more beats in succession. Two PJCs in a row are called a *couplet*. When three or more PJCs occur consecutively, *junctional tachycardia* is considered to be present.
- **Repetitive beats**: PJCs may alternate with the QRS complexes of the underlying rhythm (*bigeminy*) or occur after every two QRS complexes (*trigeminy*) or after every three QRS complexes of the underlying rhythm (*quadrigeminy*).

Site of origin. Premature junctional complexes originate in an ectopic site in the AV junction.

Cause of Dysrhythmia

Occasional PJCs may occur in a healthy person without apparent cause. Common causes of PJCs include the following:

- Digitalis toxicity (most common cause)
- Excessive dose of certain cardiac drugs (e.g., quinidine and procainamide)
- Excessive dose of sympathomimetic drugs (e.g., epinephrine, isoproterenol, and norepinephrine)

If the ectopic site in the AV junction discharges too soon after the preceding QRS complex, the premature P′ wave may not be followed by a QRS complex because the bundle of His or bundle branches may not be repolarized sufficiently to conduct an electrical impulse into the ventricles. When this occurs a P′ is seen but no accompanying QRS complex. This is termed a nonconducted PJC.

PR intervals. If the P′ waves of the PJCs precede the QRS complexes, the P′R intervals are usually short (less than 0.12 second). If the P′ waves follow the QRS complexes, the RP′ intervals are usually less than 0.12 second.

R-R intervals. The R-R intervals are unequal when PJCs are present. The interval between the PJC and the preceding QRS complex (the pre-PJC interval) is shorter than the R-R interval of the underlying rhythm. A compensatory pause commonly follows a PJC because the sinoatrial (SA) node is usually not depolarized by the PJC. (See the discussion of compensatory and noncompensatory pauses under Premature Atrial Complexes, p. 92.)

- Hypoxia
- Congestive heart failure
- Coronary artery disease (especially following an acute myocardial infarction)

The electrophysiological mechanism responsible for premature junctional complexes is either enhanced automaticity or reentry.

Clinical Significance

Isolated PJCs are not significant. However, if digitalis is being administered, PJCs may indicate digitalis toxicity and enhanced automaticity of the AV junction. Frequent PJCs, more than four to six per minute, may indicate an enhanced automaticity or a reentry mechanism in the AV junction and warn of the appearance of more serious junctional dysrhythmias.

Because PJCs with aberrancy resemble PVCs, such PJCs must be correctly identified so that the patient is not treated inappropriately.

JUNCTIONAL ESCAPE RHYTHM

KEY DEFINITION

Junctional escape rhythm (Figure 7-2) is a dysrhythmia originating in an escape pacemaker in the AV junction with a rate of 40 to 60 beats per minute. When less than three consecutive QRS complexes arising from the escape pacemaker are present, they are called junctional escape beats or complexes.

Diagnostic Characteristics (Table 7-2)

Rate. The rate is typically 40 to 60 beats/min, but it may be less.

Regularity. The ventricular rhythm is essentially regular.

P waves. Normal P waves are absent. Because the atria depolarize in a retrograde manner when the electrical impulses arise in the AV junction, the P′ waves are negative (inverted) in lead II. Therefore P′ waves are present.

If the P′ waves regularly precede or follow the QRS complexes and are identical, the electrical impulses responsible for them have originated in the pacemaker site of the junctional escape rhythm. Such P′ waves differ from normal P waves in size, shape, and direction.

P′ waves are absent in junctional escape rhythm if the P′ waves occur during the QRS complexes, if a complete AV block is present, or if atrial flutter or fibrillation is the underlying atrial rhythm.

If upright P waves are present but have no relation to the QRS complexes of the junctional escape rhythm, appearing independently at a rate different (typically faster) from that of the junctional rhythm, the pacemaker site of such P waves is the SA node. When the P waves occur independently of the QRS complexes, AV dissociation (third degree heart block) is present.

PR intervals. If the P′ waves regularly precede the QRS complexes, the P′R intervals are short (less than 0.12 second). If the P′ waves regularly follow the QRS complexes, the RP′ intervals are usually less than 0.12 second.

R-R intervals. The R-R intervals are equal.

Conduction ratio. The impulse causing the QRS originates above the ventricles and is conducted down the bundle of His, resulting in ventricular depolarization. This is a 1:1 ratio. While this was not clinically relevant in the lone PJC the presence of a junctional escape rhythm indicates that there is complete AV block or a failure of the SA node or any atrial pacemaker.

QRS complexes. The QRS complexes are normal unless a preexisting intraventricular conduction disturbance (such as a bundle branch block) is present. Junctional escape rhythm with abnormal QRS complexes may resemble ventricular escape rhythm. Three or more consecutive junctional escape complexes must be present to interpret the dysrhythmia as a junctional escape rhythm.

Site of origin. Junctional escape rhythm originates in a pacemaker in the AV junction.

Cause of Dysrhythmia

Junctional escape rhythm is a normal response of the AV junction under the following circumstances:

- When the rate of impulse formation of the dominant pacemaker (usually the SA node) drops below that of the escape pacemaker in the AV junction

OR

- When the electrical impulses from the SA node or atria fail to reach the AV junction because of sinus arrest, SA exit block, or third-degree (complete) AV block

Generally, when an electrical impulse fails to arrive at the AV junction within approximately 1.0 to 1.5 seconds, the escape pacemaker in the AV junction begins to generate electrical impulses at its inherent firing rate of 40 to 60 beats/min. The result is one or more junctional escape beats or a junctional escape rhythm.

TABLE 7-2 Diagnostic Characteristics of Junctional Escape Rhythm	
Characteristic	**Junctional Escape Rhythm**
Rate	40-60
Regularity	Regular
P waves	P′ waves before or after QRS P′ may be absent
PR intervals	P′R intervals <0.12 sec
P-P, R-R intervals	R-R interval equal
Conduction ratio	1:1
QRS complexes	Normal, wide if conduction delay exists
Site of origin	Ectopic pacemaker in AV Junction

Junctional Escape Rhythm

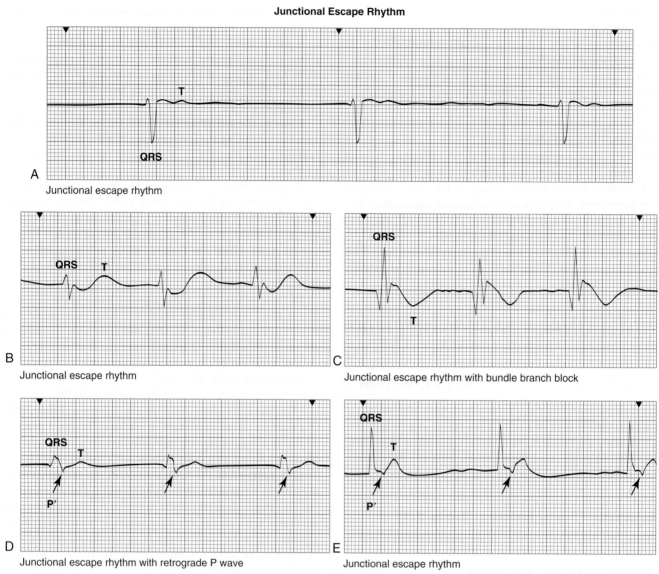

A
Junctional escape rhythm

B
Junctional escape rhythm

C
Junctional escape rhythm with bundle branch block

D
Junctional escape rhythm with retrograde P wave

E
Junctional escape rhythm

FIGURE 7-2 Junctional escape rhythm.

Clinical Significance

The signs, symptoms, and clinical significance of junctional escape rhythm are similar to those of symptomatic sinus brady-cardia. A junctional escape rhythm is often seen following successful cardiac arrest resuscitation as it is one of the first pacemakers to "awaken." However, because of its relatively slow rate and the fact that should it fail, the resulting rate would be even slower prompt therapy should be instituted to prevent the patient from suffering cardiovascular collapse. Treatments are aimed at increasing the rate of the ectopic pacemaker and treating any associated hypotension. Junctional escape rhythm may also be seen with new onset third-degree heart block. The patient may or may not be symptomatic and the treatment will be guided by the underlying cause. Often the therapy involves the placement of an electronic pacemaker.

NONPAROXYSMAL JUNCTIONAL TACHYCARDIA (ACCELERATED JUNCTIONAL RHYTHM, JUNCTIONAL TACHYCARDIA)

KEY DEFINITION

Nonparoxysmal junctional tachycardia (Figure 7-3) is a dysrhythmia originating in an ectopic pacemaker in the AV junction with a regular rhythm and a rate of 60 to 150 beats/min. It includes accelerated junctional rhythm and junctional tachycardia.

TABLE 7-3 Diagnostic Characteristics of Nonparoxysmal Junctional Tachycardia

Characteristic	Nonparoxysmal Junctional Tachycardia
Rate	60-100: *accelerated junctional rhythm* >100: *junctional tachycardia*
Regularity	Regular
P waves	P′ waves before or after QRS P′ may be absent
PR intervals	P′R intervals <0.12 sec
P-P, R-R intervals	R-R interval equal
Conduction ratio	1:1
QRS complexes	Normal, wide if conduction delay exists
Site of origin	Ectopic pacemaker in AV Junction

Diagnostic Characteristics (Table 7-3)

Rate. The rate is usually 60 to 130 beats/min, but it may be greater than 130 beats/min and as high as 150. Nonparoxysmal junctional tachycardia with a rate between 60 and 100 beats/min is called *accelerated junctional rhythm;* one with a rate greater than 100 beats/min is called *junctional tachycardia.* The onset and termination of nonparoxysmal junctional tachycardia is gradual.

Regularity. The rhythm is essentially regular.

P waves. Normal P waves are usually absent. If present, they may have no relation to the QRS complexes of the nonparoxysmal junctional tachycardia, appearing independently at a rate different from that of the junctional rhythm consistent with AV dissociation.

Instead, P′ waves are seen. Because the atria depolarize in a retrograde manner when the electrical impulses arise in the AV junction, the P′ waves are negative (inverted) in lead II. If the P′ waves are identical and regularly precede or follow the QRS complexes, the electrical impulses responsible for them have originated in the pacemaker site of the nonparoxysmal junctional tachycardia. Such P′ waves differ from normal P waves in size, shape, and direction.

P′ waves are absent in nonparoxysmal junctional tachycardia if the P′ waves occur during the QRS complexes, if a complete block in retrograde conduction is present, or if atrial flutter or atrial fibrillation is the underlying atrial rhythm.

PR intervals. If the P′ waves regularly precede the QRS complexes, the P′R intervals are abnormal (less than 0.12 second). If the P′ waves regularly follow the QRS complexes, the RP′ intervals are usually less than 0.12 second.

R-R intervals. The R-R intervals are equal.

Conduction ratio: The impulse causing the QRS originates above the ventricles and is conducted down the bundle of His, resulting in ventricular depolarization. This is a 1:1 ratio.

QRS complexes. The QRS complexes are normal unless a pre-existing intraventricular conduction disturbance (such as a bundle branch block) or aberrant ventricular conduction is present. If abnormal QRS complexes occur only when junctional tachycardia is present, the dysrhythmia is called *junctional tachycardia with aberrancy* (or *aberrant ventricular conduction*).

Nonparoxysmal junctional tachycardia with abnormal QRS complexes may resemble accelerated idioventricular rhythm if the heart rate is 60 to 100 beats/min (accelerated junctional rhythm), or it may resemble ventricular tachycardia if the heart rate is over 100 beats/min (junctional tachycardia).

Site of origin. Nonparoxysmal junctional tachycardia originates in an ectopic pacemaker in the AV junction.

Cause of Dysrhythmia

Common causes of nonparoxysmal junctional tachycardia include the following:

- Digitalis toxicity (most common cause)
- Excessive administration of catecholamines
- Damage to the AV junction from an acute inferior wall MI or rheumatic fever
- Electrolyte imbalance (especially hypokalemia)
- Hypoxia

The dysrhythmia may begin with one or more PJCs and becomes manifest when the rate of the sinus rhythm becomes slower than that of the ectopic pacemaker. The electrophysiological mechanism responsible for nonparoxysmal junctional tachycardia is most likely enhanced automaticity.

Clinical Significance

Nonparoxysmal junctional tachycardia is clinically significant because it commonly indicates digitalis toxicity. The signs, symptoms, and clinical significance of rapid nonparoxysmal junctional tachycardia are the same as those of atrial tachycardia.

In addition, in nonparoxysmal junctional tachycardia, the atria do not regularly contract and empty, as they normally do, during the last part of ventricular diastole, completely filling the ventricles just before they contract. The loss of this "atrial kick" may result in incomplete filling of the ventricles before they contract, causing a reduction of the cardiac output by as much as 25%.

Accelerated junctional tachycardia is also common following successful cardiac arrest resuscitation as a result of the catecholamines (epinephrine) administered. However, as the effects of these agents diminish, the rate of the rhythm slows and a junctional escape rhythm results which may or may not be symptomatic.

**Nonparoxysmal Junctional Tachycardia
(Accelerated Junctional Rhythm, Junctional Tachycardia)**

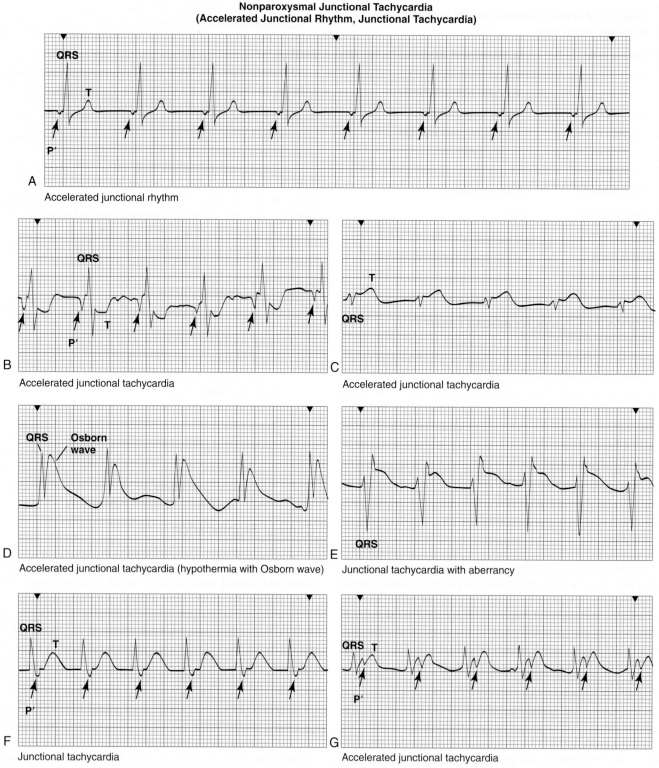

A
Accelerated junctional rhythm

B
Accelerated junctional tachycardia

C
Accelerated junctional tachycardia

D
Accelerated junctional tachycardia (hypothermia with Osborn wave)

E
Junctional tachycardia with aberrancy

F
Junctional tachycardia

G
Accelerated junctional tachycardia

FIGURE 7-3 Nonparoxysmal junctional tachycardia (accelerated junctional rhythm, junctional tachycardia).

PAROXYSMAL SUPRAVENTRICULAR TACHYCARDIA

KEY DEFINITION

Paroxysmal supraventricular tachycardia (PSVT) (Figure 7-4) is a dysrhythmia originating abruptly at the site of a rapid reentry circuit in the AV junction with a rate between 150 and 250 beats/min. The PSVT may present as an AV nodal reentry tachycardia (AVNRT) or an AV reentry tachycardia (AVRT).

TABLE 7-4 Diagnostic Characteristics of Paroxysmal Supraventricular Tachycardia

Characteristic	Paroxysmal Supraventricular Tachycardia
Rate	150-250
Regularity	Regular
P waves	Usually absent
PR intervals	P′R intervals <0.12 sec
P-P, R-R intervals	R-R interval equal
Conduction ratio	1:1
QRS complexes	Normal, wide if conduction delay exists
Site of origin	Reentry mechanism in the AV junction

Diagnostic Characteristics (Table 7-4)

Rate. The rate is usually 150 to 250 beats/min and constant. The rate may occasionally exceed 250 beats/min. The onset and termination of PSVT are typically abrupt, with the onset often being initiated by a premature atrial impulse. A brief period of asystole may follow the termination of the dysrhythmia. The rate may be slower during the few beats after onset and before termination.

Regularity. The rhythm is essentially regular.

P waves. P′ waves are usually absent, being buried in the QRS complex. If present, they are identical and typically follow the QRS complexes. Rarely, the P′ waves precede the QRS complexes. Because atrial depolarization occurs in a retrograde fashion, the P′ waves are negative (inverted) in lead II.

PR intervals. If the P′ waves precede the QRS complexes, the P′R intervals are short (less than 0.12 second). If the P′ waves follow the QRS complexes, the RP′ intervals are usually less than 0.12 second.

R-R intervals. The R-R intervals are usually equal.

Conduction ratio: The impulse causing the QRS complex originates above the ventricles and is conducted down the bundle of His, resulting in ventricular depolarization. This is a 1:1 ratio.

QRS complexes. The QRS complexes are normal unless a preexisting intraventricular conduction disturbance (such as a bundle branch block) or aberrant ventricular conduction is present. If abnormal QRS complexes occur only with the tachycardia, the arrhythmia is called *paroxysmal supraventricular tachycardia with aberrancy* (or *aberrant ventricular conduction*). PSVT with abnormal QRS complexes may resemble ventricular tachycardia.

Site of origin. Paroxysmal supraventricular tachycardia originates from a reentry mechanism in the AV junction that may involve the AV node alone or the AV node and an accessory conduction pathway located between the atria and ventricles, as described in Chapter 1. When the reentry mechanism involves only the AV node, the dysrhythmia is called AV *nodal reentry tachycardia (AVNRT).* When both the AV node and an accessory conduction pathway are involved in the reentry mechanism, the dysrhythmia is called *AV reentry tachycardia (AVRT).*

Any dysrhythmia that originates above the ventricles and results in a rate greater than 150 beats/min is termed supraventricular tachycardia. Therefore, atrial flutter with a 1:1 conduction ratio and multifocal atrial tachycardia are supraventricular tachycardias. While AVNRT and AVRT are both supraventricular in origin, they differ from other supraventricular dysrhythmias in that they are a result of a reentry mechanism that precipitates their paroxysmal (abrupt) onset. All supraventricular tachycardias can have wide QRS complexes, which makes distinguishing them from ventricular tachycardia difficult.

Cause of Dysrhythmia

PSVT may occur without apparent cause in healthy persons of any age with no apparent underlying heart disease. In susceptible persons, it may be precipitated by the following:

- Increase in catecholamine level and sympathetic tone
- Overexertion
- Stimulants (e.g., alcohol, coffee, and tobacco)
- Amphetamines and cocaine abuse
- Electrolyte or acid-base abnormalities
- Hyperventilation
- Emotional stress

The electrophysiological mechanism responsible for PSVT is a reentry mechanism involving the AV node alone, or the AV node in conjunction with an accessory conduction pathway as described above.

Clinical Significance

Any abnormally fast rhythm that arises above the level of the ventricles is technically speaking a supraventricular tachycardia (SVT). Therefore, atrial flutter with a 1:1 conduction is SVT as would be MAT or atrial tachycardia. However, these dysrhythmias do not typically present abruptly (paroxysmally) as do those listed above because their cause is not from a reentry phenomenon in the AV conduction.

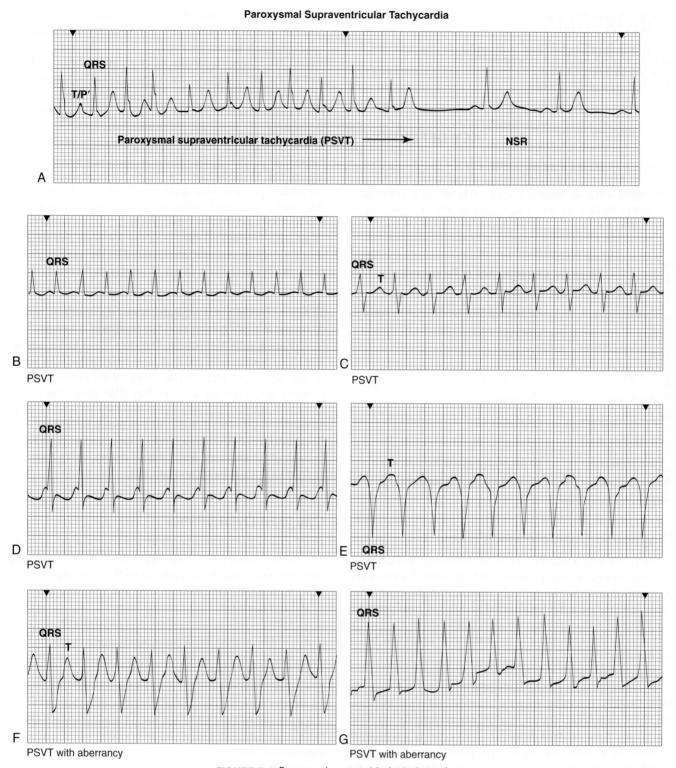

FIGURE 7-4 Paroxysmal supraventricular tachycardia.

PSVT is characterized by repeated episodes (paroxysms) of tachycardia that last from a few seconds to many hours or days and recur for many years. Vagal maneuvers, such as carotid sinus massage, usually terminate PSVT.

The signs and symptoms and clinical significance of PSVT are the same as those of atrial tachycardia. In addition, syncope may occur after the termination of PSVT because of the asystole that may follow its termination.

When PSVT with a wide QRS complex is encountered it may be difficult to distinguish from ventricular tachycardia. A discussion of this topic will be presented in the next chapter.

CHAPTER SUMMARY

- Junctional dysrhythmias are characterized by the presence of P′ waves that signify that atrial depolarization occurred in a retrograde fashion.

- Junctional dysrhythmias occur when there is a failure of the atrial impulse to reach the AV node or the SA node firing rate falls below that of the AV node causing an AV junction pacemaker to produce a junctional complex.
- The premature junctional complex is a lone complex while a series of PJCs is called junctional escape rhythm.
- The presence of a junctional dysrhythmia should prompt investigation of an underlying cause.
- If there is increased automaticity or a reentry pathway of stimulation to the AV node, the junctional pacemaker may fire continuously in either a paroxysmal or nonparoxysmal manner.
- Paroxysmal supraventricular tachycardia differs from supraventricular tachycardia in that it occurs abruptly and originates from a reentry mechanism.
- Distinguishing supraventricular tachycardia from ventricular tachycardia may be difficult.

Table 7-5 summarizes the diagnostic characteristics of the various junctional arrhythmias in this chapter.

TABLE 7-5 Typical Diagnostic ECG Features of Junctional Dysrhythmias

Arrhythmia	Heart Rate (bpm)	Rhythm	P Waves	P′R/RP′ Intervals	QRS Complexes
Junctional escape rhythm	40-60	Regular	Present or absent; if they precede or follow QRS complexes, negative; if no relation to QRS complexes usually normal	If P′R, <0.12 sec If RP′, <0.20 sec	Normal
Nonparoxysmal junctional tachycardia	60-150	Regular	Present or absent; if they precede or follow QRS complexes, negative; if no relation to QRS complexes, usually normal	If P′R, <0.12 sec If RP′, <0.20 sec	Normal
Paroxysmal supraventricular tachycardia	160-240	Regular	Present or absent; if they precede or follow QRS complexes, negative; if no relation to QRS complexes, usually normal	If P′R, <0.12 sec If RP′, <0.20 sec	Normal

CHAPTER REVIEW

1. Absent P′ waves in a junctional dysrhythmia indicate:
   A. atrial depolarizations have not occurred because of a retrograde AV block
   B. retrograde atrial depolarizations occurred after the QRS complexes
   C. the atrial depolarization was too weak to detect
   D. there was normal atrial depolarization

2. If the ectopic pacemaker (of a PJC) in the AV junction discharges too soon after the preceding QRS complex:
   A. a premature atrial complex with aberrancy occurs
   B. a premature ventricular complex will occur
   C. the premature P′ wave may not be followed by a QRS complex
   D. the QRS complex will be wide and bizarre

3. An extra QRS that originates from an ectopic pacemaker in the AV junction, occurring before the next expected beat of the underlying rhythm, is called:
   A. a premature atrial complex
   B. a premature junctional complex
   C. a premature ventricular complex
   D. nonconducted premature junctional complex

4. The QRS complex of a PJC:
   A. always follows the P′ wave associated with it
   B. is always narrow
   C. is present if the PJC is nonconducted
   D. resembles a premature ventricular contraction if aberrant ventricular conduction is present

5. The pause following a PJC is:
   A. a compensatory pause because the SA node *was* reset
   B. a noncompensatory pause because the SA node *was not* reset
   C. a compensatory pause because the SA node *was not* reset
   D. a noncompensatory pause because the SA node *was* reset

6. More than four to six PJCs per minute may indicate:
   A. a normal variant
   B. a reentry mechanism in the SA node
   C. enhanced automaticity in the AV junction
   D. that more serious ventricular dysrhythmias may occur

7. A dysrhythmia originating in an escape pacemaker in the AV junction with a regular rate greater than 100 beats/min is called a(n):
   A. junctional escape rhythm
   B. junctional tachycardia
   C. sinus bradycardia
   D. ventricular dysrhythmia

8. Any dysrhythmia that originates above the ventricles and results in a heart beat greater than 150/min is called:
   A. supraventricular tachycardia
   B. paroxysmal supraventricular tachycardia
   C. ventricular tachycardia
   D. ventricular fibrillation

9. Paroxysmal supraventricular tachycardia (PSVT) is characterized by:
   A. a heart rate between 60 and 130 beats/min
   B. a reentry mechanism in the bundle of His
   C. an abrupt onset and termination
   D. increased automaticity of the SA node

10. The dysrhythmia most difficult to distinguish from supraventricular tachycardia is:
    A. atrial flutter with 1:1 conduction
    B. atrial tachycardia
    C. ventricular fibrillation
    D. ventricular tachycardia

8

Ventricular Dysrhythmias

OBJECTIVES   *Upon completion of this chapter, you should be able to complete the following objective:*
1. Define and give the diagnostic characteristics, cause, and clinical significance of the following dysrhythmias:
   - Premature ventricular complexes (PVCs)
   - Ventricular tachycardia (V-Tach)
   - Ventricular fibrillation (VF)
   - Accelerated idioventricular rhythm (AIVR)
   - Ventricular escape rhythm
   - Asystole

PREMATURE VENTRICULAR COMPLEXES

KEY DEFINITION

A premature ventricular complex (PVC) (Figure 8-1) is an extra ventricular complex consisting of an abnormally wide and bizarre QRS complex that originates in an ectopic site in the ventricles, in the bundle branches, Purkinje network, or ventricular myocardium. It occurs earlier than the next expected beat of the underlying rhythm and is usually followed by a compensatory pause.

Diagnostic Characteristics (Table 8-1)

Rate. The rate is that of the underlying rhythm.
Regularity. The rhythm is irregular when PVCs occur.

TABLE 8-1 Diagnostic Characteristics of Premature Ventricular Complexes

Characteristic	Premature Ventricular Complexes
Rate	Underlying rhythm
Regularity	Irregular when PVC occurs
P waves	Of the underlying rhythm
PR intervals	Of the underlying rhythm
P-P, R-R Intervals	Unequal: compensatory pause
Conduction ratio	Not relevant
QRS complexes	Wide >0.12 sec
Site of origin	Ectopic site in the ventricles, in the bundle branches, Purkinje network, or ventricular myocardium

Premature Ventricular Complexes

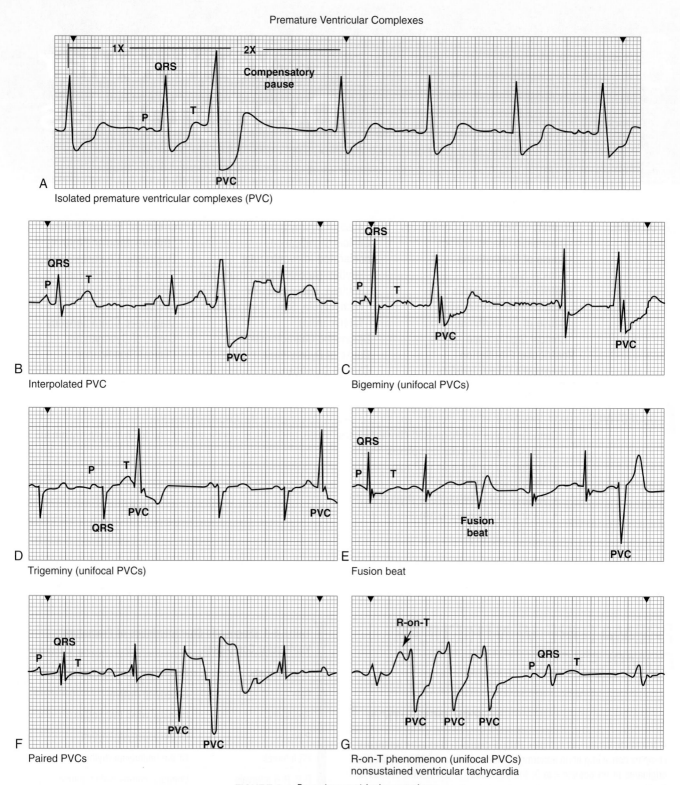

FIGURE 8-1 Premature ventricular complexes.

P waves. P waves may be present or absent. If present, they are of the underlying rhythm and have no relation to the PVCs. Typically, PVCs do not disturb the P-P cycle of the underlying rhythm, so the P waves continue without disruption during and after PVCs and occur at their expected time.

Often the P waves of the underlying rhythm are obscured by PVCs, but sometimes they appear as notches on the ST segment or T wave of PVCs. This provides a clue that the premature ectopic complex is a PVC and not a premature atrial contraction with aberrant ventricular conduction.

Various Forms of PVCs

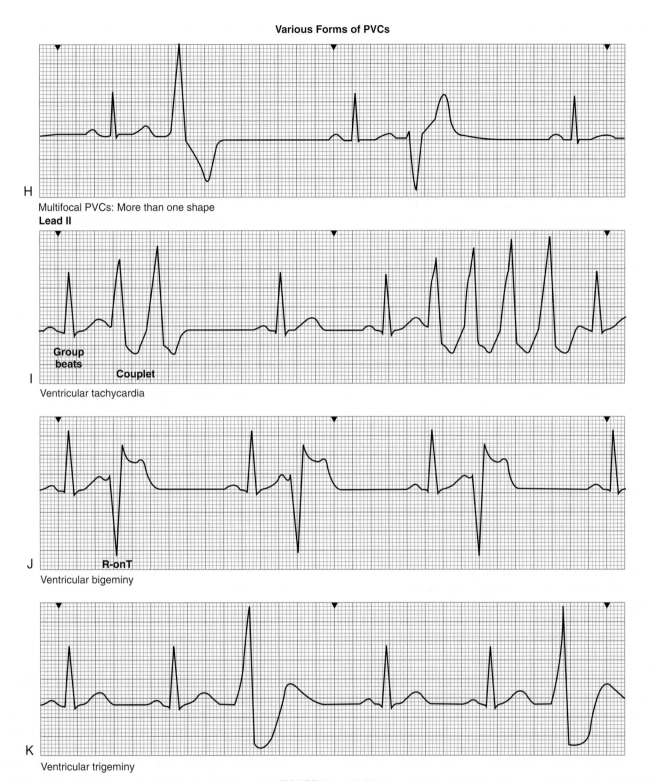

H
Multifocal PVCs: More than one shape
Lead II

I
Group
beats   **Couplet**
Ventricular tachycardia

J   **R-onT**
Ventricular bigeminy

K
Ventricular trigeminy

FIGURE 8-1, cont'd

PR intervals. No PR intervals are associated with PVCs.

R-R intervals. The R-R intervals are unequal when PVCs are present. The R-R interval between the PVC and the preceding QRS complex of the underlying rhythm is usually shorter than that of the underlying rhythm. This R-R interval is called the *coupling interval.* PVCs with the same coupling

interval in a given ECG lead usually originate from the same ectopic site.

A compensatory pause commonly follows a PVC because the SA node is not depolarized by the PVC (i.e., the P wave of the underlying rhythm that follows the PVC appears at the expected time). Consequently, the interval between the R waves of the underlying rhythm immediately before and after the PVC is twice the R-R interval of the underlying rhythm. Rarely, the SA node is depolarized by the PVC. When this occurs, a noncompensatory pause occurs. Refer to page 93 in Chapter 6 for discussion of compensatory and noncompensatory pauses.

A combination of a compensatory pause, an upright atrial P wave of the underlying rhythm superimposed on a premature ectopic beat, and a wide and bizarre QRS complex helps to confirm the interpretation of a PVC.

QRS complexes. The QRS complex of the PVC typically appears prematurely (and without a preceding ectopic P wave) before the next expected QRS complex of the underlying rhythm. The QRS complex is always greater than 0.12 seconds in duration. Because of the abnormal direction and sequence of ventricular depolarization, the QRS complex is also distorted and bizarre, often with notching, appearing different from the QRS complex of the underlying rhythm.

This abnormal QRS complex is usually followed by an abnormal ST segment (elevated or depressed) and a large T wave that is deflected opposite in direction to the major deflection of the QRS complex.

The shape of a PVC often resembles that of a right or left bundle branch block. For example, the QRS complex of a PVC originating from the left ventricle resembles that of a right bundle branch block. Likewise, a PVC originating in the right ventricle has a QRS complex resembling that of a left bundle branch block. A PVC originating from the ventricles near the bifurcation of the bundle of His may appear relatively normal, except that it will be greater than 0.12 second in duration. See Chapter 13 for discussion of bundle branch blocks.

PVCs that originate from the same ectopic pacemaker site (*unifocal*) usually have QRS complexes that are identical and are preceded by equal (constant) coupling intervals in any given lead. These PVCs are called *uniform PVCs.* Occasionally, PVCs originating from the same ectopic pacemaker site may differ from each other because of changing depolarization pathways within the ventricles—a common abnormality present in severe myocardial disease. Such PVCs with constant coupling intervals but differing QRS complexes are called *multiform PVCs.* When PVCs originate in two or more ectopic pacemaker sites (*multifocal*), they characteristically have different QRS complexes with varying coupling intervals in the same lead. Such PVCs, also commonly seen in severe myocardial disease, are also called *multiform PVCs.*

When a PVC occurs at about the same time that an electrical impulse of the underlying rhythm is activating the ventricles, depolarization of the ventricles occurs simultaneously in two directions. This results in a QRS complex that has the characteristics of both the PVC and the QRS complex of the underlying rhythm. Such a QRS complex is called a *ventricular fusion beat.* The presence of ventricular fusion beats provides evidence in favor of a premature ectopic complex being ventricular in origin and not supraventricular with aberrant ventricular conduction.

Frequency and pattern of occurrence of PVCs. The following are the various forms in which PVCs may appear:

- **Infrequent**: The PVCs may be infrequent (less than five per minute).
- **Frequent**: The PVCs may be frequent (five or more per minute).
- **Isolated**: The PVCs may occur singly (isolated).
- **Group beats**: The PVCs may occur in groups of two or more in succession. Groups of two or more PVCs are called *ventricular group beats* or *bursts* or *salvos of PVCs.* Two PVCs in a row are called *paired PVCs* or a *couplet.* A group of three or more consecutive PVCs is considered to be *ventricular tachycardia (V-Tach).*
- **Repetitive beats**: If PVCs alternate with the QRS complexes of the underlying rhythm, *ventricular bigeminy* is present. If, in ventricular bigeminy, the PVCs follow the QRS complexes of the underlying rhythm at precisely the same intervals, *coupling* is said to be present. *Ventricular trigeminy* occurs when there is one PVC for every two QRS complexes of the underlying rhythm, or one QRS complex of the underlying rhythm for every two PVCs. When there is one PVC for every three QRS complexes of the underlying rhythm, *quadrigeminy* is present.
- **R-on-T phenomenon**: The term *R-on-T phenomenon* is used to indicate that a PVC has occurred during the vulnerable period of ventricular repolarization—the relative refractory period of the ventricles that coincides with the downslope of the T wave. During this period, the myocardium is at its greatest electrical nonuniformity, a condition in which some of the ventricular muscle fibers may be completely repolarized, others may be only partially repolarized, and still others may be completely refractory. Stimulation of the ventricles at this point by an intrinsic electrical impulse such as that generated by a PVC or by an extrinsic impulse from a cardiac pacemaker or an electrical countershock may result in nonuniform conduction of the electrical impulse through the muscle fibers.
- In such nonuniform conduction of the electrical impulse through the muscle fibers, some of the fibers will be able to conduct the electrical impulse normally, whereas others will only be able to conduct them slowly or not at all. Thus a reentry mechanism will be established that may precipitate repetitive ventricular complexes resulting in ventricular tachycardia or ventricular fibrillation.
- **End-diastolic PVCs**: A PVC that occurs at about the same time that ventricular depolarization of the underlying rhythm is expected to occur is called an *end-diastolic PVC.* This usually results in a ventricular fusion beat. End-diastolic PVCs tend to occur when the underlying rhythm is relatively rapid.
- **Interpolated PVCs**: A PVC occurring between two normally conducted QRS complexes without greatly disturbing the underlying rhythm is called an *interpolated PVC.* This tends to occur when the underlying rhythm is relatively slow. The R-R interval that includes the PVC is often slightly greater than that of the underlying rhythm, but a compensatory pause does not occur.

Site of origin. The pacemaker site of the PVC is an ectopic site in the ventricles, in the bundle branches, Purkinje network, or ventricular myocardium. PVCs may originate from a single ectopic pacemaker site or from multiple sites in the ventricles.

Cause of Dysrhythmia

PVCs may occur in healthy persons with apparently healthy hearts and without apparent cause. PVCs, especially if they are frequent, may be caused by the following:

- Increase in catecholamines and sympathetic tone (as in emotional stress)
- Stimulants (alcohol, caffeine, and tobacco)
- Amphetamine and cocaine abuse
- Myocardial ischemia or infarction associated with acute coronary syndrome (ACS)
- Congestive heart failure
- Excessive administration of digitalis or sympathomimetic drugs (epinephrine, isoproterenol, and norepinephrine)
- Increase in vagal (parasympathetic) tone
- Hypoxia
- Acidosis
- Hypokalemia
- Hypomagnesemia

The electrophysiologic mechanism responsible for PVCs in the above conditions is either enhanced automaticity or reentry.

Clinical Significance

Isolated PVCs in patients with no underlying heart disease usually have no significance and usually require no treatment. However, in the presence of heart disease associated with acute coronary syndrome and/or drug toxicity (e.g., digitalis), PVCs may indicate the presence of enhanced ventricular automaticity, a reentry mechanism, or both, and may herald the appearance of such life-threatening dysrhythmia as ventricular tachycardia or ventricular fibrillation.

At times, premature atrial and junctional complexes with aberrant ventricular conduction may mimic PVCs because of the abnormally wide and bizarre-appearing QRS complexes that resemble right or left bundle branch block. The presence of P waves or a notch in the preceding T wave and a noncompensatory pause helps to differentiate PACs and PJCs with aberrant conduction from PVCs.

VENTRICULAR TACHYCARDIA

KEY DEFINITION

Ventricular tachycardia (VT or V-Tach) (Figure 8-2) is a dysrhythmia originating in an ectopic pacemaker in the bundle branches, Purkinje network, or ventricular myocardium with a rate between 100 and 250 beats/min. The QRS complexes are abnormally wide and bizarre.

TABLE 8-2 Diagnostic Characteristics of Ventricular Tachycardia

Characteristic	Ventricular Tachycardia
Rate	100-250, usually >150 and <200
Regularity	Regular
P Waves	Usually absent
PR Intervals	Not relevant
P-P, R-R Intervals	Equal
Conduction ratio	AV dissociation
QRS complexes	>0.12 sec
Site of origin	Ectopic pacemaker in the bundle branches, Purkinje network, or ventricular myocardium

Diagnostic Characteristics (Table 8-2)

Rate. The rate in ventricular tachycardia (V-Tach) is more than 100 beats/min, usually between 150 and 200 beats/min. V-Tach exists if three or more consecutive PVCs are present, occurring at a rate greater than 100 beats/min.

Regularity. The rhythm is usually regular.

P waves. Normal atrial P waves are usually absent. Rarely, identical P′ waves regularly follow the QRS complexes. The electrical impulses responsible for them originated in the ectopic pacemaker site of the V-Tach.

PR intervals. Since the ectopic pacemaker originates below the AV node the PR intervals are not relevant.

R-R intervals. The R-R intervals may be equal or vary slightly.

Conduction ratio. Ventricular tachycardia originates below the AV node, therefore there is AV dissociation.

QRS complexes. The QRS complexes exceed 0.12 second in duration and are usually distorted and bizarre, often with notching. They are followed by large T waves, opposite in direction to the major deflection of the QRS complexes. Usually, the QRS complexes are identical, but occasionally one or more QRS complexes differ in size, shape, and direction, especially at the onset or end of V-Tach. These are most likely fusion beats.

Occasionally, an electrical impulse of the underlying rhythm is conducted from the atria to the ventricles through the AV junction, producing a normal-appearing QRS complex (0.10 second or less) among the abnormal QRS complexes of the V-Tach. Such a QRS complex is called a *capture beat.* The R-R interval between the QRS complex of the V-Tach preceding the capture beat and the QRS complex of the capture beat is usually less than that of the V-Tach. The presence of capture or ventricular fusion beats provides evidence that the tachycardia is most likely ventricular in origin and not a supraventricular tachycardia with aberrant ventricular conduction.

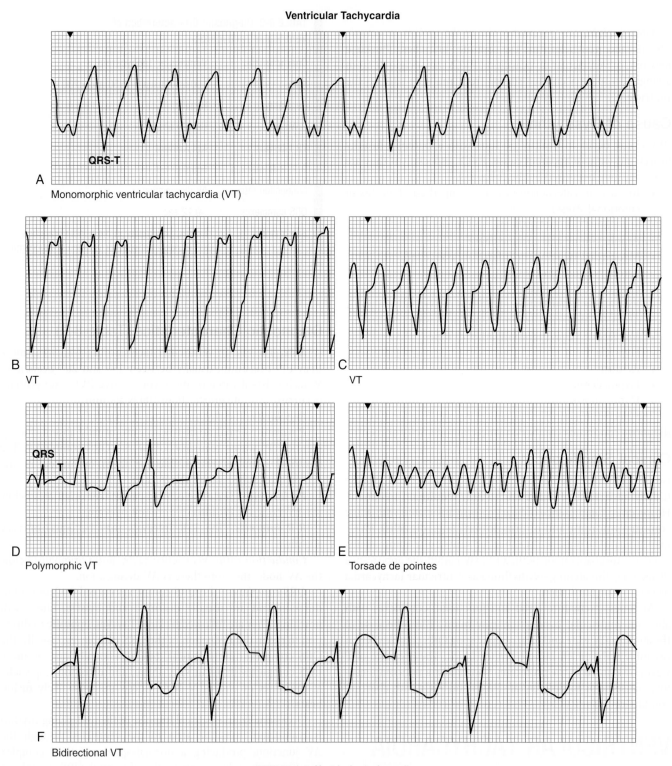

FIGURE 8-2 Ventricular tachycardia.

Differentiating Ventricular Tachycardia from Supraventricular Tachycardia with Wide QRS Complex

(Refer to 12-Lead section of text, Chapter 11, for additional information.)

At times, a supraventricular tachycardia (e.g., sinus, atrial, and junctional tachycardias, atrial flutter, and paroxysmal supraventricular tachycardia) with wide QRS complexes caused by a preexisting intraventricular conduction disturbance (such as a bundle branch block), aberrant ventricular conduction, or ventricular preexcitation may mimic V-Tach. Atrial fibrillation with wide QRS complexes and a rapid ventricular rate may also mimic V-Tach, but usually the grossly irregular rhythm of atrial fibrillation provides a clue to its true identity.

The presence of certain features common to V-Tach, namely AV dissociation, a QRS-complex duration greater than 0.12 second (and especially if it is greater than 0.14 second), and capture or ventricular fusion beats, helps to differentiate V-Tach from a supraventricular tachycardia with wide QRS complexes. A 12-lead ECG or lead MCL_1 is also useful in making a differentiation in this situation by helping to determine the presence or absence of P waves and, if present, their relationship to the QRS complexes. Analysis of specific QRS shapes can also be helpful in diagnosing V-Tach and localizing its site of origin. For example, QRS shapes suggesting V-Tach include left-axis deviation in the frontal plane and a QRS duration exceeding 0.14 seconds. In precordial leads with an RS pattern, the duration of the onset of the R to the bottom of the S exceeding 0.10 seconds suggests V-Tach as the diagnosis. During V-Tach with a right bundle branch block appearance, (1) the QRS complex is monophasic or biphasic in V_1, with an initial deflection different from that of the sinus-initiated QRS complex, (2) the amplitude of the R wave in V_1 exceeds the R′, and (3) a small R and large S wave or a QS pattern in V_6 may be present. With a V-Tach having a left bundle branch block contour, (1) the axis can be rightward, with negative deflections deeper in V_1 than in V_6, (2) a broad prolonged (more than 0.04 seconds) R wave can be noted in V_1, and (3) a small Q or QS pattern in V_6 can exist. A QRS complex that is similar in V_1 through V_6, either all negative or all positive, favors a ventricular origin.

Supraventricular QRS complexes with aberrant conduction often have a triphasic pattern in V_1. A grossly irregular, wide QRS tachycardia with ventricular rates exceeding 200 beats/min is more consistent with atrial fibrillation with conduction through an accessory pathway. In the presence of a preexisting bundle branch block, a wide QRS tachycardia with a QRS shape different from the shape during sinus rhythm is most likely V-Tach. Based on these criteria, several algorithms for distinguishing V-Tach from supraventricular tachycardia with aberrancy have been suggested, one of which is shown in Figure 8-3. Exceptions exist to all the aforementioned criteria, especially in patients who have preexisting conduction disturbances or preexcitation syndrome; when in doubt, rely on clinical judgment and consider the ECG only as one of several helpful ancillary tests.

Site of origin. Ventricular tachycardia originates in an ectopic pacemaker in the bundle branches, Purkinje network, or ventricular myocardium.

Cause of Dysrhythmia

V-Tach usually occurs in the presence of the following:

- Significant cardiac disease, such as the following:
  - Coronary artery disease, particularly in the setting of acute coronary syndrome especially if hypoxia or acidosis is present
  - Cardiomyopathy, mitral valve prolapse, and congenital heart disease
  - Left ventricular hypertrophy, valvular heart disease, and congestive heart failure
- Digitalis toxicity
- QT interval prolongation from various causes, including the following:
  - Excessive administration of quinidine, procainamide, disopyramide, sotalol, phenothiazines, and tricyclic antidepressants
  - Bradydysrhythmias (marked sinus bradycardia and third-degree AV block with slow ventricular escape rhythm)
  - Electrolyte disturbances (hypokalemia)
  - Liquid protein diets
  - Central nervous system disorders (subarachnoid hemorrhage and intracranial trauma)

The torsades de pointes form of V-Tach is particularly prone to occur following administration of such antiarrhythmic agents as disopyramide, quinidine, procainamide, and sotalol, or other agents that prolong the QT interval. It is also associated with low serum magnesium levels (hypomagnesemia). These conditions lead to enhanced automaticity as the precipitator to the onset of V-Tach.

Another electrophysiological mechanism responsible for V-Tach is triggered activity. When a PVC occurs during the vulnerable period of ventricular repolarization coinciding with the peak of the T wave (i.e., the R-on-T phenomenon, described in the section on PVCs) ventricular tachycardia may be

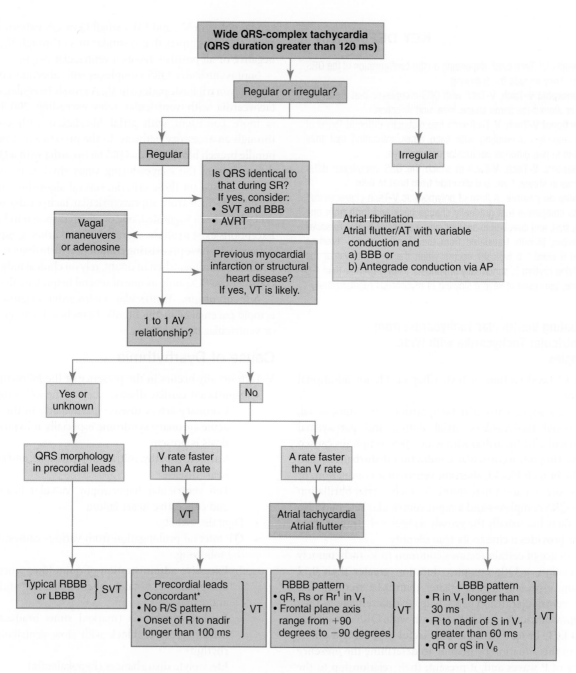

SR = Sinus rhythm, SVT = Supraventrenicular tachycardia, BBB = Bundle branch block, V = Ventricular
A = Atrial, AVRT = Atrioventricular reentrant tachycardia, AP = Accessory pathway

FIGURE 8-3 Algorithm for distinguishing SVT from VT. (Redrawn from Libby: *Braunwald's heart disease: A textbook of cardiovascular medicine*, ed 8, Philadelphia, 2008, Saunders.)

triggered. Often, V-Tach may occur without preexisting or precipitating PVCs.

Clinical Significance

The onset and termination of V-Tach may or may not be abrupt. V-Tach may occur in paroxysms of three or more consecutive PVCs, or it may persist for a long period. V-Tach lasting for three consecutive beats or less than 30 seconds is called *nonsustained* or *paroxysmal V-Tach*. When V-Tach lasts for more than 30 seconds, it is called *sustained V-Tach*.

Symptoms occurring during V-Tach depend on the ventricular rate, duration of tachycardia, and presence and extent of the underlying heart disease and peripheral vascular disease. V-Tach can occur in several forms: short, asymptomatic, nonsustained episodes; sustained, hemodynamically stable events, generally occurring at slower rates or in otherwise normal hearts; or unstable runs, often degenerating into ventricular fibrillation. In some patients who have nonsustained V-Tach initially, sustained episodes or ventricular fibrillation later develops.

The signs and symptoms in V-Tach vary, depending on the nature and severity of the underlying cardiac disease, such as acute MI or congestive heart failure. V-Tach may cause or aggravate existing angina pectoris, acute MI, or congestive heart failure; produce hypotension or shock; or terminate in ventricular fibrillation or asystole. The patient with V-Tach may often experience feelings of impending doom. The torsades de pointes form of V-Tach tends to terminate and recur spontaneously.

In V-Tach, there is little to no atrial contraction and this coupled with the fast rate results in a marked reduction in cardiac output, which compounds the already low cardiac output frequently seen in the diseased hearts in which V-Tach tends to occur. When the cardiac output is so low, it is unable to produce a blood pressure or palpable pulse, it is termed *pulseless ventricular tachycardia*.

Ventricular tachycardia is one of the three most common cardiac arrest dysrhythmias because it often presents without a pulse. Because V-Tach is considered a life-threatening dysrhythmia, often initiating or deteriorating into ventricular fibrillation (VF) or asystole, V-Tach and its underlying causes must be treated immediately. Pulseless V-Tach is treated the same as ventricular fibrillation in cardiac arrest.

VENTRICULAR FIBRILLATION

KEY DEFINITION

Ventricular fibrillation (VF or V-Fib) (Figures 8-4 and 8-5) is a dysrhythmia originating in numerous ectopic sites in the Purkinje network or in the ventricles, characterized by very rapid and chaotic fibrillatory waves and no QRS complexes.

Diagnostic Characteristics (Table 8-3)

Rate. No coordinated ventricular beats are present. The ventricles contract from 300 to 500 times a minute in an unsynchronized, uncoordinated, and haphazard manner. The fibrillating ventricles are often described as resembling a "bag of worms."

TABLE 8-3 **Diagnostic Characteristics of Ventricular Fibrillation**

Characteristic	Ventricular Fibrillation
Rate	300-500
Regularity	Totally irregular
P waves	Absent
PR Intervals	Absent
P-P, R-R intervals	Absent
Conduction ratio	Absent
QRS complexes	Chaotic, unorganized
Site of origin	Multiple ectopic sites in the Purkinje network and ventricular myocardium

Regularity. The rhythm is totally irregular.

PR intervals. PR intervals are absent.

R-R intervals. R-R intervals are absent.

Conduction ratio. Ventricular fibrillation originates below the AV node; therefore there is AV dissociation.

QRS complexes. QRS complexes are absent.

Characteristics of ventricular fibrillatory waves include the following:

- **Relationship to cardiac anatomy and physiology**: Ventricular fibrillatory waves represent abnormal, chaotic, and incomplete ventricular depolarizations caused by haphazard depolarization of small individual groups (or islets) of muscle fibers. Because organized depolarizations of the atria and ventricles are absent, distinct P waves, QRS complexes, ST segments, and T waves and consequentially organized atrial and ventricular contractions are absent.

- **Onset and end:** The onset and end of the fibrillatory waves often cannot be determined with certainty.

- **Direction:** The direction of the fibrillatory waves varies at random from positive (upright) to negative (inverted).

- **Duration:** The duration of fibrillatory waves cannot be measured with certainty.

- **Amplitude:** The amplitude varies from less than 1 mm to about 10 mm. Generally, if the fibrillatory waves of VF are small (less than 3 mm), the dysrhythmia is called *fine*

Ventricular Fibrillation Waves

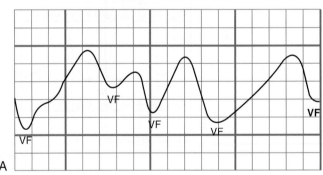

A

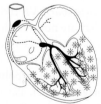

B

Multiple ectopic pacemakers in the ventricles

Pacemaker site

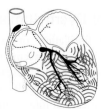

C

Abnormal, chaotic and incomplete ventricular depolarizations

Significance

FIGURE 8-4 Ventricular fibrillation waves.

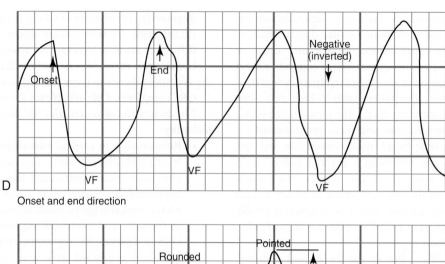

D

Onset and end direction

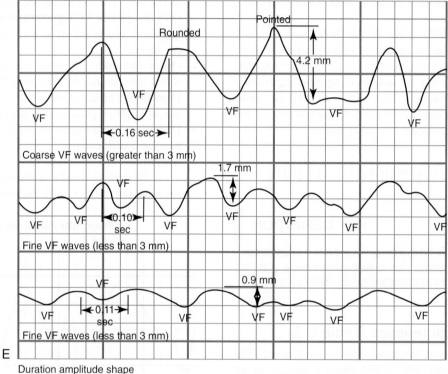

E

Duration amplitude shape

FIGURE 8-4, cont'd

VF. If the fibrillatory waves are large (greater than 3 mm), it is called *coarse VF.* If the VF waves are so small or "fine" that they are not recorded, the ECG appears as a wavy or flat (isoelectric) line resembling ventricular asystole.

- **Shape:** The VF waves are of varying shape, appearing bizarre, rounded or pointed, and markedly dissimilar.

Site of origin. Ventricular fibrillation originates in multiple ectopic sites in the Purkinje network and ventricular myocardium.

Cause of Dysrhythmia

Ventricular fibrillation, one of the most common causes of cardiac arrest, usually occurs in the following:

- Significant cardiac disease, such as the following:
  - Coronary artery disease (i.e., myocardial ischemia and myocardial infarction associated with ACS—the most common cause of VF)
  - Third-degree AV block with a slow ventricular escape rhythm
  - Cardiomyopathy, mitral valve prolapse, and cardiac trauma (penetrating or blunt)
- Cardiac, medical, and traumatic conditions as a terminal event
- Excessive dose of digitalis, quinidine, or procainamide
- Hypoxia
- Acidosis
- Electrolyte imbalance (hypokalemia and hyperkalemia)
- During anesthesia, cardiac and noncardiac operations, cardiac catheterization, and cardiac pacing
- Following cardioversion or accidental electrocution

The electrophysiological mechanism responsible for VF is either enhanced automaticity or reentry.

A PVC can initiate VF when the PVC occurs during the vulnerable period of ventricular repolarization coinciding with

Ventricular Fibrillation

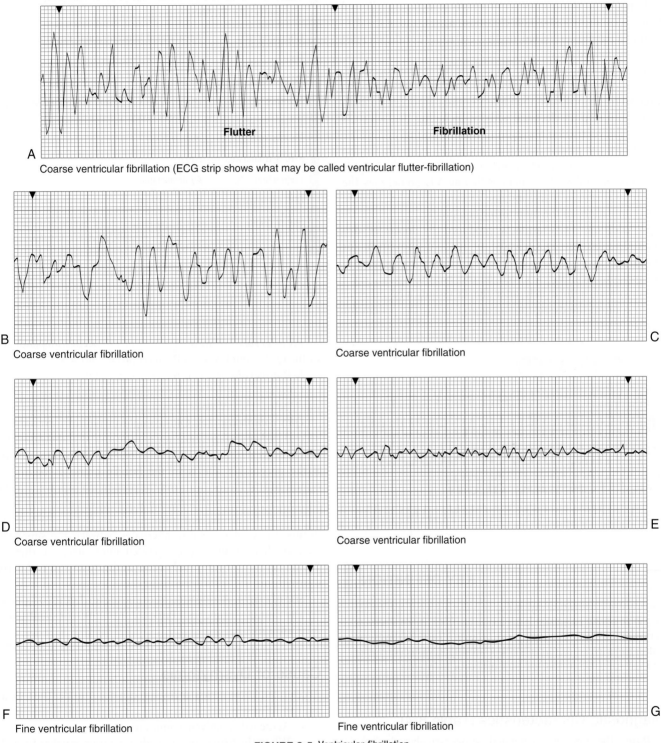

A   Coarse ventricular fibrillation (ECG strip shows what may be called ventricular flutter-fibrillation)

B   Coarse ventricular fibrillation

C   Coarse ventricular fibrillation

D   Coarse ventricular fibrillation

E   Coarse ventricular fibrillation

F   Fine ventricular fibrillation

G   Fine ventricular fibrillation

FIGURE 8-5 Ventricular fibrillation.

the peak of the T wave (i.e., the R-on-T phenomenon), particularly when electrical instability of the heart has been altered by ischemia or acute MI. Sustained V-Tach may also precipitate VF. Often, VF may begin without preexisting or precipitating PVCs or V-Tach.

Clinical Significance

Ventricular fibrillation is one of the three most common cardiac arrest dysrhythmias because organized ventricular depolarization and contraction and, consequently, cardiac output cease at the moment VF occurs, resulting in the sudden disappearance of the pulse and blood pressure. VF results in faintness, followed within seconds by loss of consciousness, apnea, and, if the dysrhythmia remains untreated, death. *Ventricular fibrillation must be treated immediately!*

The significance of coarse versus fine VF is that coarse VF, indicating a recent onset of the dysrhythmia, is more apt to be reversed by defibrillation than fine VF. The purpose of defibrillation is to stop all electrical activity, including that which is causing the ventricular fibrillation, so that a normal pacemaker can awaken and produce a rhythm that results in a pulse. Coarse VF is more likely to result in such a result because the heart is less hypoxic and acidotic than with fine VF. Sometimes the distinction between coarse and fine VF cannot be made because of the limitations of the monitoring equipment.

In addition, ECG artifacts produced by loose or dry electrodes, broken ECG leads, or patient movement or muscle tremor may also resemble VF. A rapid assessment of the patient, including a check of the patient's pulse, must be performed immediately after the ECG-indicated onset of VF to confirm the dysrhythmia before treating the patient for cardiac arrest.

ACCELERATED IDIOVENTRICULAR RHYTHM (ACCELERATED VENTRICULAR RHYTHM, IDIOVENTRICULAR TACHYCARDIA, SLOW VENTRICULAR TACHYCARDIA)

KEY DEFINITION

Accelerated idioventricular rhythm (Figure 8-6) is a dysrhythmia originating in an ectopic pacemaker in the bundle branches, Purkinje network, or ventricular myocardium with a rate between 40 and 100 beats/min. Other terms for this dysrhythmia include accelerated ventricular rhythm, idioventricular tachycardia, and slow ventricular tachycardia.

Diagnostic Characteristics (Table 8-4)

Rate. The rate in accelerated idioventricular rhythm is between 40 and 100 beats/min. The onset and termination of accelerated idioventricular rhythm are usually gradual, but the dysrhythmia may begin abruptly after a PVC.

Regularity. The rhythm is essentially regular.

P waves. P waves may be present or absent. If present, they have no relation to the QRS complexes of the accelerated idioventricular rhythm, appearing independently at a rate different from that of the QRS complexes (AV dissociation).

TABLE 8-4 Diagnostic Characteristics of Accelerated Idioventricular Rhythm

Characteristic	Accelerated Idioventricular Rhythm
Rate	40-100
Regularity	Regular
P waves	Usually absent *if present not related to QRS (AV Dissociation)*
PR Intervals	Usually absent
P-P, R-R Intervals	Equal
Conduction ratio	AV dissociation
QRS complexes	Wide >0.12 sec
Site of origin	Ectopic pacemaker in the bundle branches, Purkinje network, or ventricular myocardium

PR intervals. If P waves are present and occur independently of the QRS complexes, no PR intervals are present.

R-R intervals. The R-R intervals are equal.

Conduction ratio. Accelerated idioventricular rhythm originates below the AV node therefore there is AV dissociation.

QRS complexes. The QRS complexes typically exceed 0.12 second and are bizarre, but they may be only slightly wider than normal (greater than 0.12 second but less than 0.16 second) if the pacemaker site is in the bundle branches below the bundle of His. Fusion beats may be present if a supraventricular rhythm is present, and particularly if its rate is about the same as that of the accelerated idioventricular rhythm. When this occurs, the cardiac rhythm alternates between the supraventricular rhythm and the accelerated idioventricular rhythm. Fusion beats most commonly occur at the onset and end of the dysrhythmia.

Site of origin. Accelerated idioventricular rhythm originates in the bundle branches, Purkinje network, or ventricular myocardium.

Cause of Dysrhythmia

Accelerated idioventricular rhythm can occur under the following conditions:

- Acute MI (relatively common)
- When the firing rate of the dominant pacemaker (usually the SA node) or escape pacemaker in the AV junction becomes less than that of the ventricular ectopic pacemaker
- When a sinus arrest, SA exit block, or third-degree (complete) AV block develops
- Digitalis toxicity

The electrophysiologic mechanism responsible for accelerated idioventricular rhythm is probably enhanced automaticity.

Accelerated Idioventricular Rhythm (Accelerated Ventricular Rhythm, Idioventricular Tachycardia, Slow Ventricular Tachycardia)

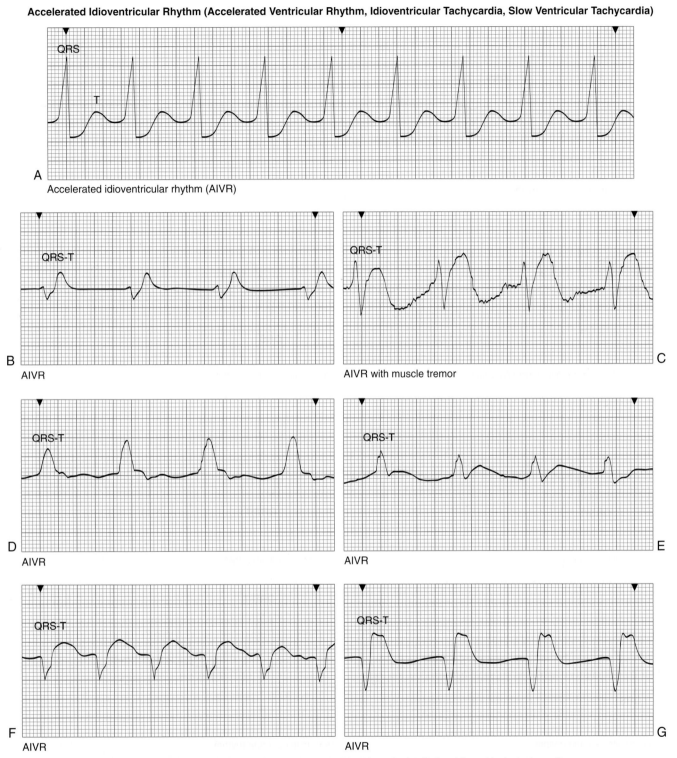

FIGURE 8-6 Accelerated idioventricular rhythm (accelerated ventricular rhythm, idioventricular tachycardia, slow ventricular tachycardia).

Clinical Significance

Accelerated idioventricular rhythm occurring in the setting of acute MI usually requires no treatment because it is self-limited in most cases. It is often seen following reperfusion of the occluded coronary artery. Because it does not affect the course or prognosis of the acute MI, it is considered relatively benign. In other settings addressing the underlying cause is appropriate and should resolve the dysrhythmia. If the patient does, however, become symptomatic (hypotensive), accelerated idioventricular rhythm should be treated as one would treat V-Tach.

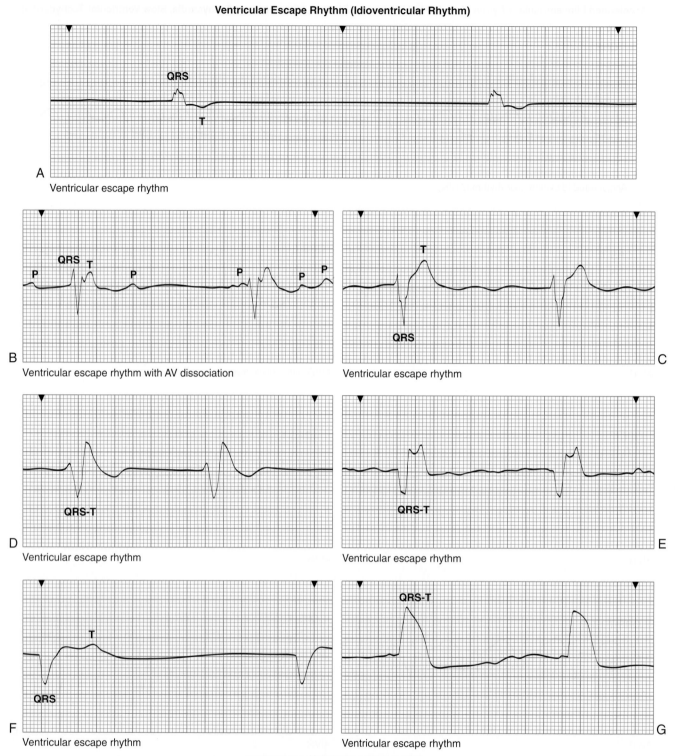

FIGURE 8-7 Ventricular escape rhythm.

VENTRICULAR ESCAPE RHYTHM (IDIOVENTRICULAR RHYTHM)

> ### KEY DEFINITION
>
> Ventricular escape rhythm (Figure 8-7) is a dysrhythmia originating in an ectopic pacemaker in the bundle branches, Purkinje network, or ventricular myocardium with a rate of less than 40 beats/min. When less than three consecutive QRS complexes originating from the escape pacemaker are present, they are called ventricular escape beats or complexes.

TABLE 8-5 Diagnostic Characteristics of Ventricular Escape Rhythm

Characteristic	Ventricular Escape Rhythm
Rate	Less than 40
Regularity	Regular
P waves	Usually absent *if present not related to QRS (AV dissociation)*
PR Intervals	Absent
P-P, R-R intervals	Equal
Conduction ratio	AV dissociation
QRS complexes	Wide >0.12 sec
Site of origin	Ectopic pacemaker in the bundle branches, Purkinje network, or ventricular myocardium

Diagnostic Characteristics (Table 8-5)

Rate. The rate is less than 40 beats/min, usually between 20 and 40 beats/min, but it may be less.

Regularity. The rhythm is usually regular.

P waves. P waves may be present or absent. If present, they have no set relation to the QRS complexes of the ventricular escape rhythm, appearing independently at a rate different from that of the QRS complexes consistent with AV dissociation.

PR intervals. PR intervals are absent.

R-R intervals. The R-R intervals may be equal or may vary.

Conduction ratio. The pacemaker is below the AV node, therefore there is AV dissociation.

QRS complexes. The QRS complexes exceed 0.12 second and are bizarre. Sometimes the shape of the QRS complexes varies from beat to beat.

Site of origin. Ventricular escape rhythm originates in an escape pacemaker in the bundle branches, Purkinje network, or ventricular myocardium.

Cause of Dysrhythmia

Ventricular escape rhythm can occur under either of the following conditions:

- When the rate of impulse formation of the dominant pacemaker (usually the SA node) and escape pacemaker in the AV junction becomes less than that of the escape pacemaker in the ventricles
- When the electrical impulses from the SA node, atria, and AV junction fail to reach the ventricles because of a sinus arrest, SA exit block, or third-degree (complete) AV block

Generally, when an electrical impulse fails to arrive in the ventricles within approximately 1.5 to 2.0 seconds, an escape pacemaker in the ventricles takes over at its inherent firing rate of 20 to 40 beats/min. The result is one or more ventricular escape beats or a ventricular escape rhythm.

Ventricular escape rhythm also occurs in advanced heart disease and is often the cardiac dysrhythmia that is present in a dying heart, the so-called *agonal rhythm*, just before the appearance of the final dysrhythmia—asystole.

Clinical Significance

In the hierarchy of cardiac pacemakers, the ventricular escape pacemaker is the lowest and slowest. If it fails to fire when needed the result is asystole. Even when called upon the ventricular escape rhythm is usually symptomatic because of its slow rate and the underlying condition of the heart. Hypotension with marked reduction in cardiac output and decreased perfusion of the brain and other vital organs usually occurs, resulting in syncope, shock, or congestive heart failure. Ventricular escape rhythm must be treated promptly, preferably with a transcutaneous pacemaker, to reverse the consequences of the reduced cardiac output.

ASYSTOLE

> ### KEY DEFINITION
>
> Asystole (Figure 8-8) is the absence of all electrical activity within the ventricles.

Diagnostic Characteristics (Table 8-6)

Rate. Heart rate is absent.

Regularity. There is no electrical activity to have a pattern.

TABLE 8-6 Diagnostic Characteristics of Asystole

Characteristic	Asystole
Rate	Absent
Regularity	None
P waves	Usually absent
PR Intervals	Absent
P-P, R-R intervals	Absent
Conduction ratio	None
QRS complexes	None
Site of origin	Total lack of ventricular electrical activity

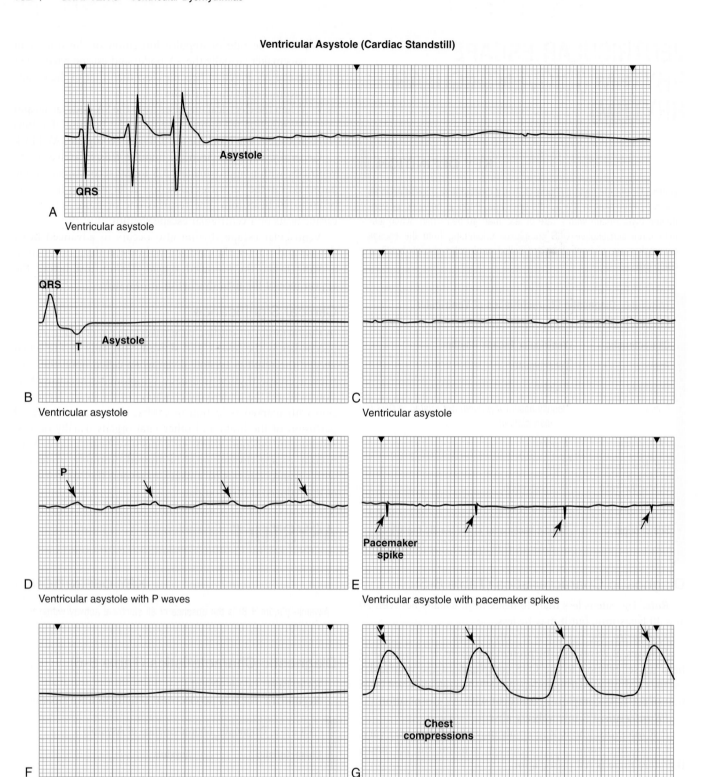

Ventricular Asystole (Cardiac Standstill)

A   Ventricular asystole

B   Ventricular asystole

C   Ventricular asystole

D   Ventricular asystole with P waves

E   Ventricular asystole with pacemaker spikes

F   Ventricular asystole

G   Ventricular asystole with chest compressions

FIGURE 8-8 Ventricular asystole.

P waves. P waves may be present or absent.

PR intervals. PR intervals are absent.

R-R intervals. R-R intervals are absent.

Conduction ratio. **No ventricular activity, therefore a conduction ratio is not clinically relevant.**

QRS complexes. QRS complexes are absent.

Site of origin. There is no rhythm, therefore no origin. If P waves are present, their pacemaker site is the SA node or an ectopic or escape pacemaker in the atria or AV junction.

Cause of Dysrhythmia

Asystole, sometimes referred to as ventricular asystole or ventricular standstill, is one of the three most common cardiac arrest rhythms. It is the only true arrhythmia as there is no electrical activity present. It may occur in advanced cardiac disease as a primary event in the following situations:

- When the dominant pacemaker (usually the SA node) and/or the escape pacemaker in the AV junction fail to generate electrical impulses
- When the electrical impulses are blocked from entering the ventricles because of a third-degree (complete) AV block and an escape pacemaker in the ventricles fails to take over
- In the dying heart, asystole is usually the final event that occurs after:
- V-Tach
- VF
- Ventricular escape rhythm

Asystole may also follow the termination of tachyarrhythmias by whatever means—drugs, defibrillation shocks, or synchronized cardioversion.

Clinical Significance

Organized ventricular depolarization, contraction and, consequently, cardiac output and a palpable pulse are absent in asystole. The occurrence of sudden asystole in a conscious person results in syncope, followed within seconds by loss of consciousness and, if the arrhythmia remains untreated, death. ***Asystole must be treated immediately***.

CHAPTER SUMMARY

The presence of any ventricular dysrhythmia is cause for concern.

- Ventricular dysrhythmias indicate an irritable foci in the bundle of His, Purkinje network, or myocardium.
- It may present with solitary premature ventricular complexes or multifocal PVCs.
- Ventricular tachycardia, fibrillation, and asystole are the primary presenting rhythms of cardiac arrest and have a high mortality.
- Ventricular tachycardia may be difficult to distinguish from supraventricular tachycardia with a wide QRS complex.
- If the ventricular foci generates an escape pacemaker, the rhythm is called an idioventricular escape rhythm and if greater than 40 beats/min, it is termed accelerated idioventricular rhythm.
- The idioventricular pacemaker is the last pacemaker of the heart in the chain of fail safes and should be treated promptly.
- Table 8-7 summarizes the diagnostic characteristics of the various ventricular arrhythmias discussed in this chapter.

TABLE 8-7 **Typical Diagnostic ECG Features of Ventricular Dysrhythmias**

Arrhythmia	Heart Rate (bpm)	Rhythm	P Waves	PR Intervals	QRS Complexes
Ventricular tachycardia	110-250	Regular	Present or absent; no relation to QRS complexes	None	Abnormal, >0.12 sec
Ventricular fibrillation	None	None	Present or absent	None	Ventricular fibrillation waves
Accelerated idioventricular rhythm	40-100	Regular	Present or absent; no relation to QRS complexes	None	Abnormal, >0.12 sec
Ventricular escape rhythm	<40	Regular	Present or absent; no relation to QRS complexes	None	Abnormal, >0.12 sec
Ventricular asystole	None	None	Present or absent	None	None

CHAPTER REVIEW

1. An unexpected abnormally wide and bizarre QRS complex originating in an ectopic site in the ventricles is called a:
   A. PAC
   B. PJC
   C. nonconducted PJC
   D. PVC

2. Identical PVCs that originate from a single ectopic site are called:
   A. isolated
   B. multifocal
   C. multiform
   D. unifocal

3. A PVC may:
   A. cause asystole
   B. depolarize the SA node, momentarily suppressing it, so that the next P wave of the underlying rhythm appears earlier than expected
   C. may occur simultaneously with a normal QRS forming an interpolated beat
   D. trigger ventricular fibrillation if it occurs on the T wave

4. A PVC is followed by a noncompensatory pause, which is _____ times the preceding R-R interval;
   A. 1
   B. 2
   C. 3
   D. variable

5. A QRS complex that has characteristics of both the PVC and a QRS complex of the underlying rhythm is called a(n):
   A. fascicular PVC
   B. isolated PVC
   C. multifocal PVC
   D. ventricular fusion beat

6. Groups of three PVCs in row are called:
   A. a burst of PVCs
   B. a couplet of PVCs
   C. a run of V-Tach
   D. a salvo of PVCs

7. A form of ventricular tachycardia characterized by QRS complexes that gradually change back and forth from one shape and direction to another over a series of beats is called:
   A. bigeminy
   B. multiform ventricular tachycardia
   C. torsades de pointes
   D. ventricular flutter

8. When the ventricles depolarize between 300 and 500 times a minute in an unsynchronized, chaotic manner the success of defibrillation is most dependent on:
   A. the rate of the fibrillatory waves
   B. the presence of P waves
   C. the size of the fibrillatory waves
   D. the underlying rhythm

9. The following is true of an asymptomatic accelerated idioventricular rhythm:
   A. it is often associated with acute myocardial infarction
   B. it should be treated immediately
   C. it usually develops during second-degree type II AV block
   D. the heart rate is usually more than 100 beats/min

10. A ventricular dysrhythmia with a rate of less than 40 beats/min is called:
    A. accelerated idioventricular rhythm
    B. pulseless electrical activity of the heart
    C. ventricular asystole
    D. ventricular escape rhythm

Atrioventricular Blocks

OBJECTIVES *Upon completion of this chapter, you should be able to complete the following objective:*

1. Define and give the diagnostic characteristics, cause, and clinical significance of the following dysrhythmias:
   - First-degree AV block
   - Second-degree, type I AV block (Wenckebach)
   - Second-degree, type II AV block
   - Second-degree, 2:1 and advanced AV block
   - Third-degree (complete AV block)

FIRST-DEGREE AV BLOCK

KEY DEFINITION

First-degree atrioventricular (AV) block (Figure 9-1) is a dysrhythmia in which there is a constant delay in the conduction of electrical impulses, usually through the AV node. It is characterized by abnormally prolonged PR intervals that are greater than 0.20 second and constant in duration.

Diagnostic Characteristics (Table 9-1)

Rate. The rate is that of the underlying sinus or atrial rhythm. The atrial and ventricular rates are typically the same. The rate may be slow, normal, or fast.

Regularity. The rhythm is regular because it originates from the sinus node or an atrial pacemaker.

TABLE 9-1 Diagnostic Features of First Degree AV Block

Characteristic	First-Degree Atrioventricular (AV) Block
Rate	Underlying rhythm
Regularity	Regular
P waves	Upright (lead II)
PR intervals	>0.20 sec
P-P, R-R intervals	Equal
Conduction ratio	1:1
QRS complexes	Normal unless conduction delay present
Site of origin	Sinus node or atrial pacemaker

P waves. The P waves are identical and precede each QRS complex. They are upright in lead II and have a normal shape and duration.

PR intervals. The PR intervals are prolonged (greater than 0.20 second) and are constant in duration.

First-Degree AV Block

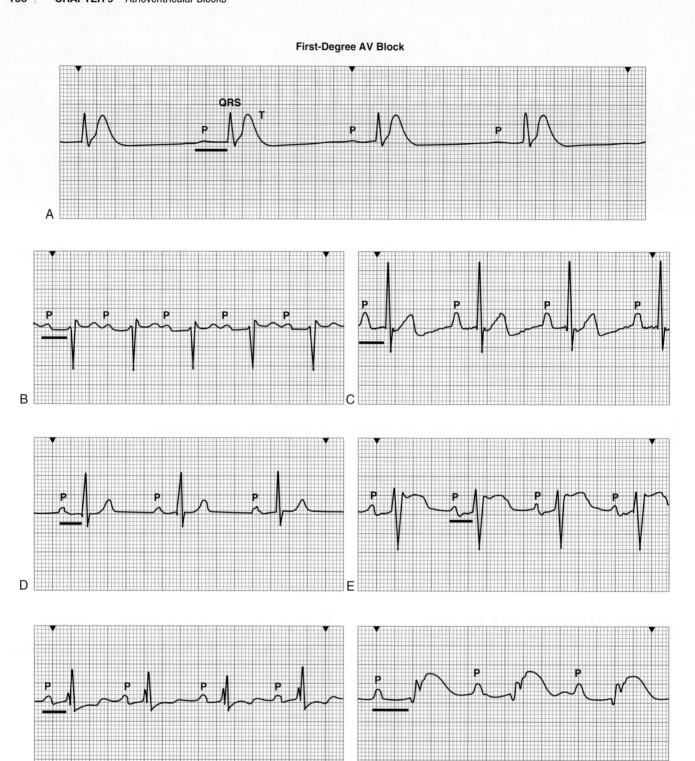

= PR interval

FIGURE 9-1 First-degree AV block.

R-R intervals. The R-R intervals are those of the underlying rhythm and regular.

Conduction ratio. There is a P wave for every QRS complex and a QRS complex for every P wave, therefore the conduction ratio is 1:1.

QRS complexes. The QRS complexes are usually normal, but they may be abnormal because of a preexisting intraventricular conduction disturbance (such as a bundle branch block).

Site of origin. The rhythm originates in the sinus node or an atrial pacemaker.

Cause of Dysrhythmia

First-degree AV block represents a delay in the conduction of the electrical impulses through the AV node and thus the QRS complexes are typically normal, unless a preexisting intraventricular conduction disturbance (such as a bundle branch block) is present. Infrequently, the AV block may occur below the AV node (infranodal AV block) in the His-Purkinje system of the ventricles (i.e., bundle of His or bundle branches).

Although first-degree AV block may appear without any apparent cause, it can occur in the following:

- Acute inferior wall or right ventricular myocardial infarction (MI) because of the effect of an increased vagal (parasympathetic) tone and/or ischemia in the AV node
- Ischemic heart disease in general
- Excessive inhibitory vagal (parasympathetic) tone from whatever cause
- Digitalis toxicity
- Administration of certain drugs, such as amiodarone, beta-blockers (e.g., atenolol, metoprolol, propranolol), or calcium channel blockers (e.g., diltiazem, verapamil, nifedipine)
- Electrolyte imbalance (e.g., hyperkalemia)
- Acute rheumatic fever or myocarditis

Clinical Significance

First-degree AV block produces no signs or symptoms and usually requires no specific treatment. However, any underlying cause should be corrected, if possible. Because it can progress to a higher-degree, AV block under certain conditions (e.g., excessive administration of beta-blockers or calcium channel blockers and acute inferior wall or right ventricular MI), the patient may require observation and ECG monitoring.

SECOND-DEGREE, TYPE I AV BLOCK (WENCKEBACH)

KEY DEFINITION

Second-degree, type I AV block (Wenckebach) (Figure 9-2) is a dysrhythmia in which there is a progressive delay following each P wave in the conduction of electrical impulses through the AV node until conduction is completely blocked. This dysrhythmia is characterized by progressive lengthening of the PR intervals until a QRS complex fails to appear after a P wave. The sequence of increasing PR intervals and an absent QRS complex is repetitive. Second-degree, type I AV block is also referred to as Mobitz I second-degree AV block.

Diagnostic Characteristics (Table 9-2)

Rate. The atrial rate is that of the underlying sinus or atrial rhythm. The ventricular rate is less than that of the atria because there are nonconducted beats.

TABLE 9-2 Second-Degree, Type I AV Block (Wenckebach)

Characteristic	Second-Degree, Type I AV Block
Rate	Underlying rhythm
Regularity	Patterned irregularity
P waves	Upright (lead II)
PR intervals	Progressively longer until dropped QRS complex
P-P, R-R intervals	Equal P-P, unequal R-R (progressively shorter)
Conduction ratio	Variable (commonly 5:4, 4:3, or 3:2)
QRS complexes	Normal unless conduction delay present
Site of origin	Sinus node or atrial pacemaker

Regularity. The sinus node impulse is slowed progressively with each complex resulting in each PR interval being longer than the one before until the AV node is completely blocked, resulting in a dropped QRS complex. This results in a pattern of grouped beats, which gives the dysrhythmia a patterned irregularity.

P waves. The P waves are identical and precede the QRS complexes when they occur.

PR intervals. The PR intervals gradually lengthen until a QRS complex fails to appear following a P wave (nonconducted P wave or dropped beat). Following the pause produced by the nonconducted P wave, the sequence begins anew. The PR interval following the nonconducted P wave is shorter than the previously conducted PR interval.

R-R intervals. The R-R intervals are unequal. As the PR intervals gradually lengthen, the R-R intervals typically decrease gradually until the P wave is not conducted. The cycle then repeats itself. The reason for the progressive decrease in the R-R intervals is that the PR intervals do not increase in such increments as to maintain the R-R intervals at the same duration as that of the first one immediately following the nonconducted P wave. This characteristic cyclic decrease in the R-R intervals may also be seen in atrial fibrillation complicated by a Wenckebach block.

Rarely, the R-R interval may remain constant until the nonconduction of the P wave. In this case the R-R interval that includes the nonconducted P wave is usually less than the sum of two of the R-R intervals of the underlying rhythm.

Conduction ratio. Commonly, the AV conduction ratio is 5:4, 4:3, or 3:2, but it may be 6:5, 7:6, etc. An AV conduction ratio of 5:4, for example, indicates that for every five P waves, four are followed by QRS complexes. The repetitive sequence of two or more beats in a row followed by a dropped beat is called *group beating.* The AV conduction ratio may be fixed or vary over time.

QRS complexes. The QRS complexes are typically normal in duration and shape, but they may be abnormal because of a preexisting intraventricular conduction disturbance (such as a bundle branch block).

Site of origin. The rhythm originates in the sinus node or an atrial pacemaker.

Second-Degree AV Block (Type I AV Block [Wenckebach])

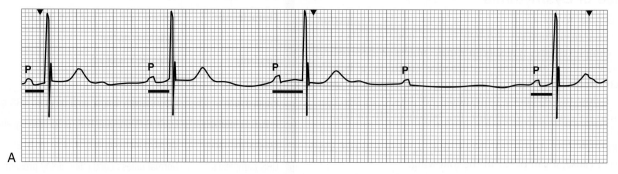

A

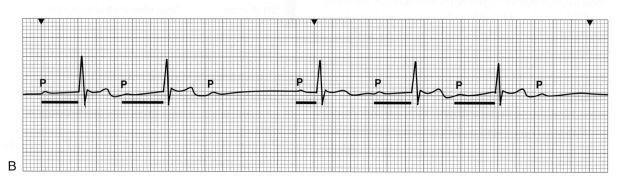

B

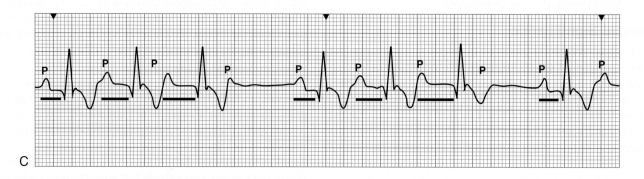

C

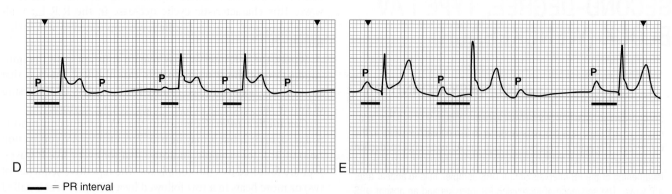

D

E

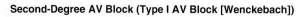 = PR interval

FIGURE 9-2　Second-degree, type I AV block (Wenckebach).

Cause of Dysrhythmia

Second-degree, type I AV block most commonly represents defective conduction of the electrical impulses through the AV node (nodal AV block), and thus the QRS complexes are typically normal unless a preexisting intraventricular conduction disturbance (such as a bundle branch block) is present. The AV block may infrequently occur below the AV node (infranodal AV block) in the His-Purkinje system of the ventricles (i.e., bundle of His or bundle branches). When this occurs the duration of the QRS complex will be 0.10 to 0.12 second, but it will have a bizarre shape.

Type I second-degree AV block often occurs, as does first-degree AV block, in the following:

- Acute inferior wall or right ventricular MI because of the effect of an increase in vagal (parasympathetic) tone and/or ischemia in the AV node
- Ischemic heart disease in general
- Excessive inhibitory vagal (parasympathetic) tone from whatever cause
- Digitalis toxicity
- Administration of certain drugs, such as amiodarone, beta-blockers (e.g., atenolol, metoprolol, propranolol), or calcium channel blockers (e.g., diltiazem, verapamil, nifedipine)
- Electrolyte imbalance (e.g., hyperkalemia)
- Acute rheumatic fever or myocarditis

Clinical Significance

Second-degree type I AV block is usually transient and reversible. Although it produces few if any symptoms, it can progress to a higher-degree AV block. For this reason, the patient requires observation and ECG monitoring. Type I AV block does respond to atropine if it is necessary to increase the heart rate.

SECOND-DEGREE, TYPE II AV BLOCK

> ### KEY DEFINITION
>
> Second-degree, type II AV block (Figure 9-3) is a dysrhythmia in which a complete block of conduction of the electrical impulses occurs in one bundle branch and an intermittent block in the other. This produces (1) an AV block characterized by regularly or irregularly absent QRS complexes, commonly producing an AV conduction ratio of 4:3 or 3:2, and (2) a bundle branch block. Second-degree, type II AV block is also referred to as Mobitz II second-degree AV block.

Diagnostic Characteristics (Table 9-3)

Rate. The atrial rate is that of the underlying sinus or atrial rhythm. The ventricular rate is less than the atrial rate since there are nonconducted P waves.

TABLE 9-3   Characteristics of Second-Degree Type II AV Block

Characteristic	Second-Degree, Type II AV Block
Rate	Underlying rhythm
Regularity	Patterned irregularity
P waves	Upright (lead II)
PR intervals	Normal or prolonged but constant until dropped QRS complex
P-P, R-R intervals	Equal P-P, unequal R-R
Conduction ratio	Variable (commonly 4:3, or 3:2)
QRS complexes	Usually greater than 0.12 sec
Site of origin	Sinus node or atrial pacemaker

Regularity. The atrial rhythm is essentially regular. The ventricular rhythm is irregular. This results in patterned irregularity of conducted and nonconducted QRS complexes.

P waves. The P waves are identical and precede the QRS complexes when they occur.

PR intervals. The PR intervals may be normal or prolonged (greater than 0.20 second). They are constant in duration when present.

R-R intervals. The R-R intervals are equal except for those that include the nonconducted P waves (dropped beats); these are equal to or slightly less than twice the R-R interval of the underlying rhythm.

Conduction ratio. Commonly, the AV conduction ratio is 4:3 or 3:2, but it may be 5:4, 6:5, 7:6, and so forth. More specifically, there is always one more P wave than QRS complexes. An AV conduction ratio of 4:3, for example, indicates that for every four P waves, three are followed by QRS complexes. The repetitive sequence of two or more beats in a row followed by a dropped beat is called *group beating*. The AV conduction ratio may be fixed, or it may vary over time.

> Second-degree, type II AV block in contrast to an advanced AV block always has only one more P wave than QRS complexes. This is secondary to the intermittent block of the remaining bundle branch conducting the electrical impulse.

QRS complexes. The QRS complexes are typically abnormal (greater than 0.12 second) because of a bundle branch block. Rarely, the QRS complex may be normal (0.12 second or less) if the AV block is at the level of the bundle of His and a preexisting intraventricular conduction disturbance (such as a bundle branch block) is not present.

Site of origin. The rhythm originates in the SA node or atrial pacemaker.

Cause of Dysrhythmia

Second-degree, type II AV block usually occurs below the bundle of His in the bundle branches (infranodal AV block). It

Second-Degree AV Block (Type II AV Block)

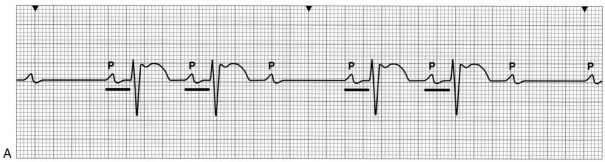

A

3:2 AV block

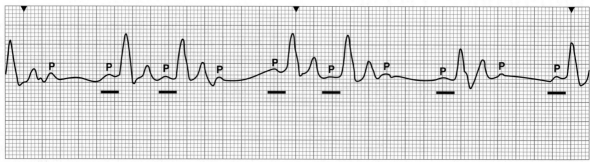

B

4:3 AV block

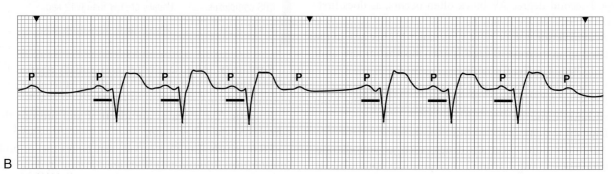

C

5:4 AV block

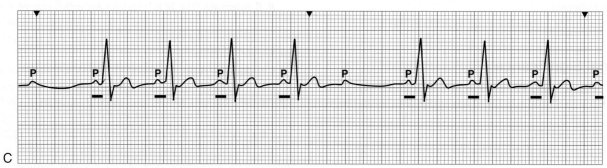

D

3:2 AV block with bundle branch block   2:1 AV block

━━ = PR interval

FIGURE 9-3 Second-degree, type II AV block.

represents an intermittent block of conduction of the electrical impulses through one bundle branch and a complete block in the other. This produces an intermittent AV block with an abnormally wide and bizarre QRS complex.

Commonly, second-degree type II AV block is the result of extensive damage to the bundle branches following an acute anterior wall MI. Rarely, the AV block occurs at the level of the bundle of His. When this occurs, the QRS complexes are normal (0.10 to 0.12 second). However, the QRS complex will have an abnormal shape.

Clinical Significance

The signs and symptoms of second-degree type II AV block with excessively slow heart rates are the same as those in symptomatic sinus bradycardia. Because second-degree type II AV block is more serious than type I AV block, often progressing to a third-degree AV block and even asystole, a standby cardiac pacemaker is indicated for asymptomatic patients, and temporary cardiac pacing is required immediately for symptomatic patients, especially in the setting of an acute anterior wall MI. Atropine is usually not effective in reversing a type II AV block.

SECOND-DEGREE 2:1 AND ADVANCED AV BLOCK

KEY DEFINITION

Second-degree 2:1 and advanced AV block (Figure 9-4) are dysrhythmias caused by the defective conduction of electrical impulses through the AV node or the bundle branches or both that produces a "high grade" AV block characterized by regularly or irregularly absent QRS complexes. The resulting AV conduction ratio of 2:1, 3:1, or greater characterizes second-degree 2:1 and advanced AV block separately from the classic second-degree type I and type II AV blocks.

Diagnostic Characteristics (Table 9-4)

Rate. The atrial rate is that of the underlying sinus or atrial rhythm. The ventricular rate is less than the atrial rate as a result of nonconducted P waves.

Regularity. The atrial rhythm is essentially regular. The ventricular rhythm may be regular or irregular. The ventricular rhythm is irregular when the AV block is intermittent, resulting in a varying AV conduction ratio.

P waves. The P waves are identical and precede the QRS complexes when they occur.

PR intervals. The PR intervals may be normal or prolonged (greater than 0.20 second); they are constant.

R-R intervals. The R-R intervals may be equal or may vary.

Conduction ratio. The AV conduction ratio is 2:1 with second-degree 2:1. Hence, the name. Commonly, the AV conduction ratios are even numbers, such as 4:1, 6:1, 8:1, and so forth with advanced AV block, but may be uneven numbers, such as 3:1 or 5:1. An AV conduction ratio of 4:1, for example,

TABLE 9-4 Characteristics of Second-Degree 2:1 and Advanced AVB

Characteristic	Second-Degree 2:1 and Advanced AVB
Rate	Underlying rhythm
Regularity	Patterned irregularity, regular with 2:1
P waves	Upright (lead II)
PR intervals	Normal or prolonged but constant until dropped QRS complex
P-P, R-R intervals	Equal P-P, unequal R-R
Conduction ratio	Variable (commonly 2:1, 3:1, 4:1) AVB: 2 or more consecutive nonconducted P waves
QRS complexes	Usually greater than 0.12 sec
Site of origin	Sinus node or atrial pacemaker

indicates for every four P waves, one is followed by a QRS complex. More specifically, it means that there are three consecutive P waves that are not followed by QRS complexes. This indicates a "high grade" AV block. The AV conduction ratio may be fixed, or it may vary in any given lead. The AV block is identified by the AV conduction ratio present (e.g., 2:1, 3:1, 4:1, or 6:1 AV block). An AV block with a 2:1 AV conduction ratio is termed a 2:1 AV *block*. A 3:1 or higher AV conduction ratio is called an *advanced AV block*.

Second-degree 2:1 can mimic second-degree type I AVB. The typical type I AVB will have a progressive lengthening of the PR such that the dropped QRS complex occurs after 3 to 6 cardiac cycles. If the PR is initially very long, the subsequent cycle may be sufficient to result in AV block, resulting in a dropped QRS complex. If the PR interval is normal and the conduction ratio is 2:1, then the dysrhythmia is more likely second-degree 2:1.

QRS complexes. The QRS complexes may be normal or abnormal because of a bundle branch block. In second-degree block the conduction delay resulting in the block usually occurs in the bundle branches, which results in a wider than normal QRS. If the block occurs in the bundle of His, the QRS complex will have a duration of 0.10 to 0.12 second but will have an abnormal shape.

Site of origin. The rhythm originates in the SA node or an atrial pacemaker.

Cause of Dysrhythmia

Narrow (<0.12 second) QRS 2:1 and advanced AV blocks with narrow QRS complexes usually represent defective conduction of the electrical impulses through the AV node (nodal AV block) and are often associated with a second-degree, type I AV block. They are commonly caused by the following:

Second-Degree AV Black (2:1 and High-Degree [Advanced] AV Block)

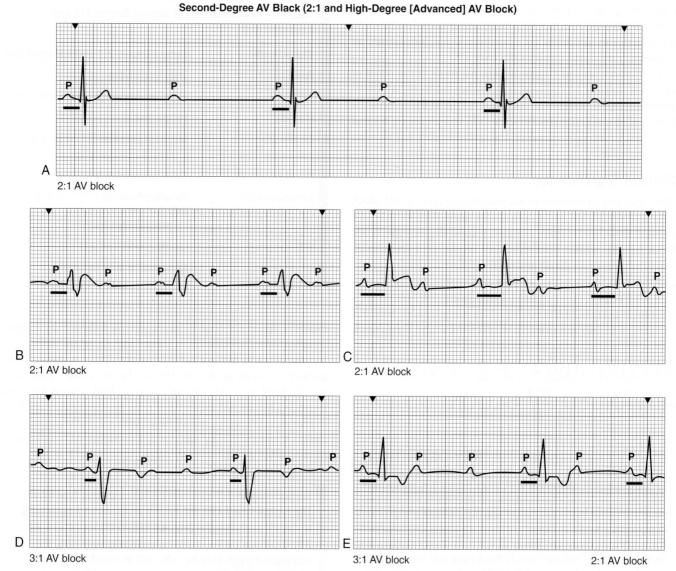

A 2:1 AV block

B 2:1 AV block

C 2:1 AV block

D 3:1 AV block

E 3:1 AV block   2:1 AV block

FIGURE 9-4 Second-degree, 2:1 and advanced AV block.

- Acute inferior wall or right ventricular MI because of the effect of an increase in vagal (parasympathetic) tone and/ or ischemia on the AV node
- Ischemic heart disease in general
- Excessive inhibitory vagal (parasympathetic) tone from whatever cause
- Digitalis toxicity
- Administration of certain drugs, such as amiodarone, beta-blockers (e.g., atenolol, metoprolol, propranolol), or calcium channel blockers (e.g., diltiazem, verapamil, nifedipine)
- Electrolyte imbalance (e.g., hyperkalemia)
- Acute rheumatic fever or myocarditis

Wide (>0.12 second) QRS Complex

2:1 and advanced AV blocks with wide QRS complexes usually represent defective conduction of the electrical impulses through the bundle branches (infranodal AV block) and are often associated with a second-degree, type II AV block. Acute anterior wall MI is commonly the cause of such AV blocks; 2:1 and advanced AV blocks with wide QRS complexes may also be the result of AV node dysfunction, as in type I AV block (nodal AV block), accompanied by a preexisting intraventricular conduction disturbance (such as a bundle branch block).

Clinical Significance

When the heart rate is excessively slow in 2:1 and advanced second-degree AV blocks, the signs and symptoms are the same as those in symptomatic sinus bradycardia. 2:1 and advanced AV blocks with normal QRS complexes may often be transient. Atropine may be effective in treating 2:1 AV block but is ineffective in advanced AV block.

Because 2:1 and advanced AV blocks with wide QRS complexes frequently progress to a third-degree AV block and even asystole, a standby cardiac pacemaker is indicated for asymptomatic patients, and temporary cardiac pacing is required immediately for symptomatic patients, especially in the setting of an acute anterior coronary syndrome. Atropine is usually not effective in reversing 2 : 1 or advanced AV blocks with wide QRS complexes.

THIRD-DEGREE AV BLOCK (COMPLETE AV BLOCK)

> ### KEY DEFINITION
>
> Third-degree AV block (Figure 9-5) is the complete absence of conduction of the electrical impulses through the AV node, bundle of His, or bundle branches, characterized by independent beating of the atria and ventricles.

Diagnostic Characteristics (Table 9-5)

Rate. The atrial rate is that of the underlying sinus or atrial rhythm. The ventricular rate is typically 40 to 60 beats/min, but it may be as slow as 20 to 40 or less. The ventricular rate is usually less than that of the atrial rate.

Regularity. The atrial rhythm may be regular or irregular, depending on the underlying sinus or atrial rhythm. The ventricular rhythm is essentially regular. The atrial and ventricular rhythms are independent of each other (AV dissociation).

P waves. P waves or atrial flutter or atrial fibrillation waves may be present. When present, they have no relation to the QRS complexes, appearing independently at a rate different from that of the QRS complexes (AV dissociation).

PR intervals. The PR intervals vary widely because the P waves and QRS complexes occur independently.

R-R and P-P intervals. The R-R intervals are usually equal and independent of the P-P intervals.

Conduction ratio. The atrial rate and the ventricular rate are independent of each other therefore there is no conduction ratio.

QRS complexes. The QRS complexes typically exceed 0.12 second and are bizarre if the escape pacemaker site is in the Purkinje network or ventricles or if the escape pacemaker site is in the AV junction and a preexisting intraventricular conduction disturbance (such as a bundle branch block) is present. The QRS complexes may be normal (0.12 to 0.10 second) if the pacemaker site is in the bundle of His or AV junction.

Site of origin. If P waves are present, they may have originated in the SA node or an ectopic or escape pacemaker in the atria. The pacemaker site of the QRS complexes is an escape pacemaker in the AV junction, bundle branches, Purkinje network, or ventricular myocardium.

Generally, if the third-degree AV block is at the level of the AV node, the escape pacemaker is usually infranodal, in the bundle of His. If the third-degree AV block is at the level of the bundle of His or bundle branches, the escape pacemaker is in the Purkinje network or ventricles distal to the site of the AV block. If the escape pacemaker is in the AV junction (i.e., junctional escape rhythm), the heart rate is 40 to 60 beats/min. If the escape pacemaker is in the ventricles (i.e., bundle branches, Purkinje network, or ventricular myocardium [ventricular escape rhythm]), the heart rate is 20 to 40 beats/min or less.

Cause of Dysrhythmia

Third-degree AV block represents a complete block of the conduction of the electrical impulses from the atria to the ventricles at the level of the AV node (nodal AV block) or bundle of His or bundle branches (infranodal AV block). It may be transient and reversible or permanent.

Transient and reversible third-degree AV block is usually associated with narrow QRS complexes and a heart rate of 40 to 60 beats/min (i.e., junctional escape rhythm). It is commonly caused by a complete block of conduction of the electrical impulses through the AV node. This can result from the following:

- Acute inferior wall or right ventricular myocardial infarction because of the effect of an increase in vagal (parasympathetic) tone and/or ischemia in the AV node
- Ischemic heart disease in general
- Excessive inhibitory vagal (parasympathetic) tone from whatever cause
- Digitalis toxicity
- Administration of certain drugs, such as amiodarone, beta-blockers (e.g., atenolol, metoprolol, propranolol), or calcium channel blockers (e.g., diltiazem, verapamil, nifedipine)
- Electrolyte imbalance (e.g., hyperkalemia)
- Acute rheumatic fever or myocarditis

Permanent or chronic third-degree AV block is usually associated with wide QRS complexes and a heart rate of 20 to 40 beats/min or less (i.e., ventricular escape rhythm). It is commonly caused by a complete block of conduction of electrical impulses through both bundle branches. The most likely causes include the following:

- Acute anterior wall myocardial infarction
- Chronic degenerative changes in the bundle branches present in the elderly

TABLE 9-5 Characteristics of Third-Degree Heart Block

Characteristic	Third-Degree Heart Block
Rate	Underlying rhythm
Regularity	Regular
P waves	Upright (lead II), f or F waves
PR Intervals	Variable
P-P, R-R intervals	Equal P-P, equal R-R
Conduction ratio	None. AV dissociation
QRS complexes	Usually greater than 0.12 sec
Site of origin	AV node or idioventricular

Third-Degree AV Block (Complete AV Block)

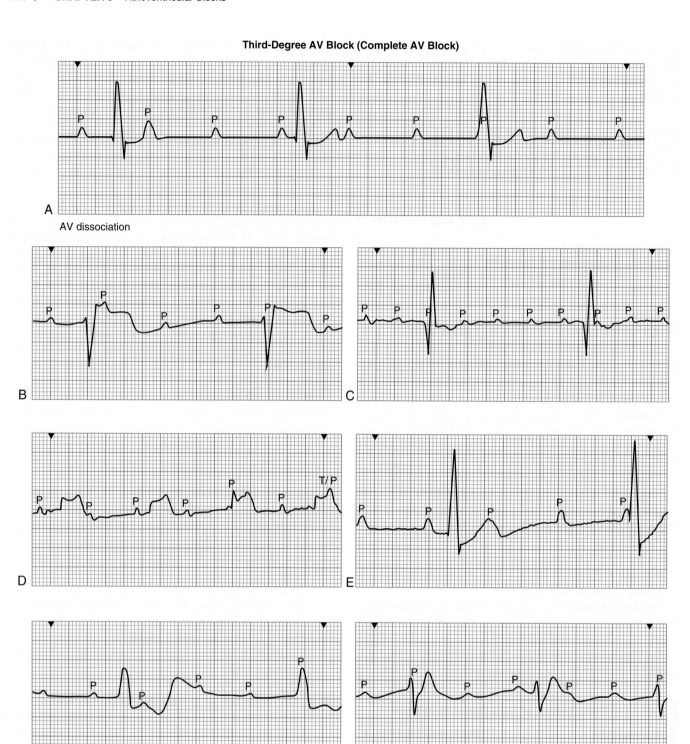

AV dissociation

FIGURE 9-5 Third-degree AV block (complete AV block).

Permanent third-degree AV block usually does not result from increased vagal (parasympathetic) tone or drug toxicity.

Clinical Significance

The signs and symptoms of third-degree AV block are the same as those in symptomatic sinus bradycardia, except that third-degree AV block can be more ominous, especially when it is associated with wide and bizarre QRS complexes. If an AV junctional or ventricular escape rhythm does not take over following a sudden onset of third-degree AV block, asystole will occur. This results in faintness, followed within seconds by loss of consciousness and death if an escape pacemaker does not respond.

Temporary cardiac pacing is required immediately for treatment of symptomatic third-degree AV block (regardless of cause) and for asymptomatic third-degree AV block in the setting of an acute anterior wall myocardial infarction. Third-degree AV block with narrow QRS complexes does respond to atropine occasionally if it is caused by an acute inferior wall or right ventricular myocardial infarction.

CHAPTER SUMMARY

- *Heart block* is the general term for atrioventricular (AV) conduction disturbance and occurs when transmission through the AV junction is impaired either transiently or permanently.

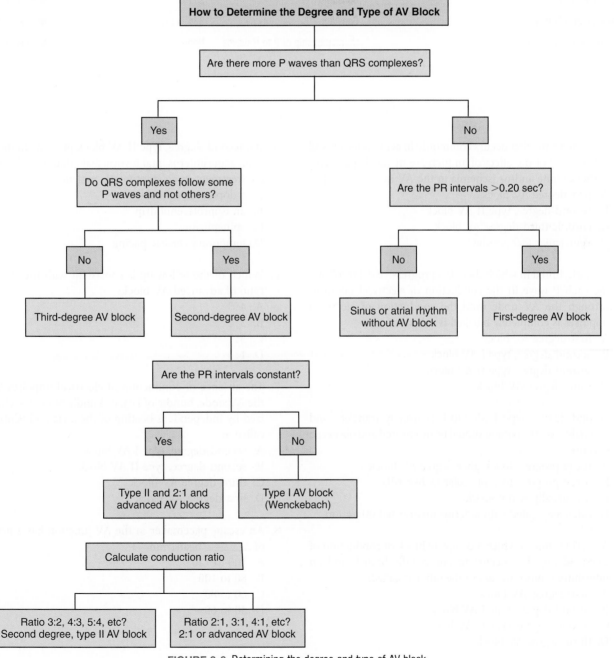

FIGURE 9-6 Determining the degree and type of AV block.

- The mildest form is called *first-degree heart block*. With first-degree heart block, the PR interval is uniformly prolonged beyond 0.20 second.
- *Second-degree heart block* is an intermediate grade of AV conduction disturbance in which impulse transmission between the atria and ventricles fails *intermittently*.

- The most extreme form of heart block is *third-degree* or *complete heart block*. In this case, the AV node does not conduct any stimuli between the atria and ventricles.
- Table 9-6 summarizes the characteristics of the heart blocks.

TABLE 9-6 Typical Diagnostic ECG Features of First-, Second-, and Third-Degree AV Blocks

AV Block	PR Intervals	AV Conduction Ratio	QRS Complex
First-degree AV block	Prolonged, constant	1:1	Usually normal
Second-degree AV block Type I AV block (Wenckebach)	Gradually lengthening	5:4, 4:3, 3:2 or 6:5, 7:6, etc.	Usually normal
Type II AV block	Constant	3:2, 4:3, 5:4, etc.	Typically abnormal
2:1 AV block	Constant	2:1	Normal or abnormal
Advanced AV block	Constant	3:1, 4:1, 5:1, etc.	Normal or abnormal
Third-degree AV block	No relationship of P to R waves	None	Normal or abnormal

CHAPTER REVIEW

1. A dysrhythmia that occurs commonly in acute inferior wall MI because of the effect of an increase in vagal (parasympathetic) tone and/or ischemia in the AV node is called:
   A. first-degree AV block
   B. second-degree, type II AV block
   C. chronic third-degree AV block
   D. ventricular tachycardia

2. A dysrhythmia in which there is a progressive delay following each P wave in the conduction of electrical impulses through the AV node until the conduction of electrical impulses is completely blocked is called:
   A. first-degree AV block
   B. second-degree, type I AV block
   C. second-degree, type II AV block
   D. third-degree AV block

3. Second-degree, type I AV block is usually transient and reversible, yet the patient should be monitored and observed because:
   A. it can progress to a higher degree AV block
   B. it can progress to ventricular tachycardia
   C. it is usually symptomatic
   D. often associated with anterior myocardial infarction

4. A dysrhythmia in which a complete block of conduction of electrical impulses occurs in one bundle branch and an intermittent block occurs in the other is called:
   A. first-degree, AV block
   B. second-degree, type I AV block
   C. second-degree, type II AV block
   D. third-degree AV block

5. If a second-degree, type II AV block presents in the setting of an acute anteroseptal myocardial infarction, the immediate treatment in a symptomatic patient is:
   A. a dopamine infusion
   B. an isoproterenol drip
   C. epinephrine
   D. temporary cardiac pacing

6. Which of the following is consistent with the conduction ratio of advanced AV block:
   A. 4:3
   B. 3:2
   C. 3:1
   D. 1:1

7. The absence of conduction of electrical impulses through the AV node, bundle of His, or bundle branches, characterized by independent beating of the atria and ventricles, is called a:
   A. second-degree, type I AV block
   B. second-degree, type II AV block
   C. third-degree AV block
   D. first-degree AV block

8. An escape pacemaker in the AV junction has a firing rate of _____ beats/min.
   A. 100 to 120
   B. 80 to 100
   C. 60 to 80
   D. 40 to 60

9. If a junctional or ventricular escape pacemaker does not take over following a sudden onset of third-degree AV block, asystole will occur, resulting in:
   A. cardiac arrest
   B. bundle branch block
   C. junctional escape rhythm
   D. ventricular escape rhythm

10. The clinical significance of atrioventricular heart block is primarily due to their effect on:
    A. rate of atrial response
    B. rate of ventricular response
    C. speed of electrical impulse conduction
    D. strength of cardiac muscle contraction

10

Clinical Significance and Treatment of Dysrhythmias

OBJECTIVES *Upon completion of this chapter, you should be able to complete the following objectives:*

1. Discuss the general approach to assessing and treating the patient with a dysrhythmia paying particular attention to the following:
   - Stable versus unstable
   - Role of electrical therapy
   - Role of pharmacologic therapy

2. List the general properties and indications for use of the following pharmacologic agents.
   - Atropine sulfate
   - Vasopressors
   - Epinephrine
   - Vasopressin
   - Norepinephrine
   - Dopamine
   - Dobutamine
   - Antidysrhythmics
   - Adenosine
   - Amiodarone
   - Lidocaine
   - Procainamide
   - Magnesium
   - Ibutilide
   - Calcium channel blockers
   - Beta-Blockers

3. Discuss the clinical significance of the following bradycardias, the indications for their treatment, and their treatment:
   - Sinus bradycardia
   - Sinus arrest/sinoatrial (SA) exit block
   - First-degree AV block
   - Second-degree, type I atrioventricular (AV) block (Wenckebach)
   - Second-degree, type II AV block
   - Second-degree, 2:1 and advanced AV block
   - With narrow QRS complexes
   - With wide QRS complexes
   - Third-degree AV block
   - With narrow QRS complexes
   - With wide QRS complexes
   - Junctional escape rhythm
   - Ventricular escape rhythm

4. Discuss the clinical significance of the following tachycardias, the indications for their treatment, and their treatment:
   - Sinus tachycardia
   - Atrial tachycardia with block
   - Narrow-QRS-complex tachycardia of unknown origin (with pulse)
5. Discuss the clinical significance of the following tachycardias, the indications for their treatment, and their treatment based on whether the patient is hemodynamically stable or unstable:
   - Atrial tachycardia without block
   - Atrial flutter with or without Wolff-Parkinson-White (WPW) syndrome or ventricular preexcitation
   - Atrial fibrillation with or without WPW syndrome or ventricular preexcitation
   - Less than 48 hours in duration
   - Greater than 48 hours in duration
   - Paroxysmal supraventricular tachycardia (PSVT) with narrow QRS complexes
   - Junctional tachycardia
6. Discuss the clinical significance of the following tachycardias, the indications for their treatment, and their treatment based on whether the patient is hemodynamically stable or unstable:
   - Wide-QRS-complex tachycardia of unknown origin (with pulse)
   - Ventricular tachycardia (VT), monomorphic (with pulse)
   - VT, polymorphic (with pulse)
   - Normal QT interval
   - Prolonged QT interval
   - Torsades de pointes (TdP) (with pulse)
7. Discuss the clinical significance of the following premature complexes, the indications for their treatment, and their treatment:
   - Premature atrial complexes (PACs)
   - Premature junctional complexes (PJCs)
   - Premature ventricular complexes (PVCs)
8. Discuss the clinical significance of the following dysrhythmias, the indications for their treatment, and their treatment based on whether the patient has suffered a monitored versus an unmonitored cardiac arrest: Ventricular fibrillation/pulseless ventricular tachycardia (VF/VT)
   - Asystole
   - Pulseless electrical activity

PART I

ASSESSING THE PATIENT

The first question to ask when assessing the patient with a dysrhythmia is whether or not the patient is symptomatic. Specifically, are the signs and symptoms they are exhibiting being caused by the dysrhythmia or is the dysrhythmia a symptom of an underlying condition. It is beyond the scope of this text to explore all the possible combinations of signs and symptoms a patient may present with so it will be assumed that any reference to being symptomatic is related to the dysrhythmia. The various symptoms associated with each dysrhythmia have been discussed in their respective chapters. Some are mild while others are profound. The question for the clinician is when to treat. Aggressive treatment of minimally symptomatic dysrhythmias will invariably lead to unwanted complications as the medications used to treat these conditions are not without their hazards. Therefore, for patients with milder symptoms, the prudent clinician will take a less aggressive approach while performing diagnostic testing and attempting to correct other underlying causes of the dysrhythmia. As the symptoms worsen, the level of urgency to treat them should be heightened. The decision then comes down to which of the two modalities, pharmacologic or electrical, the clinician should use as first-line therapy.

Stable Versus Unstable

Accepted practice is to use electrical therapy, transcutaneous pacing, cardioversion, or defibrillation, to treat dysrhythmias in the unstable patient and reserve pharmacologic agents for the stable patient. However, the question is what defines unstable? The typical list of signs and symptoms of the unstable patient include the following:

- Signs and symptoms of decreased cardiac output (e.g., decreased level of consciousness)
- Chest pain or dyspnea
- Hypotension (systolic blood pressure less than 90 mm Hg)
- Congestive heart failure or pulmonary edema

While it is true that each of these signs and symptoms represents the potential for significant deterioration of the patient's condition, they do not take into the account the clinical context of the patient's care. Is the patient being cared for in the prehospital setting far from a fully staffed emergency department or are they in an intensive care unit surrounded by a resuscitation team? As described later, the use of electrical therapy often requires the administration of sedation and therefore the need for diligent airway management. Additionally there is a risk that following cardioversion, the patient's condition will deteriorate or in the worst-case scenario be in cardiac arrest and will require more resources than are immediately available. Therefore, the degree of patient stability to which a clinician is willing to accept depends on many factors and is not always simply a matter of whether or not a set of symptoms exists.

In the end, each clinician, whether he/she is a prehospital provider, emergency physician, or intensivist, must decide what constitutes unstable based on available resources and protocol.

TREATING THE PATIENT

Once the dysrhythmia has been interpreted and the stability of the patient determined, the decision must be made as to what modality to use to treat that dysrhythmia. There are essentially two modalities to choose from: electrical or pharmacologic therapy. For some dysrhythmias (i.e., ventricular fibrillation), electrical therapy is the only option whereas for the majority of dysrhythmias a decision must be made between the relative merits of electrical versus pharmacologic therapy.

Electrical Therapy
Cardioversion and Defibrillation

It is beyond the scope of this text to describe the procedure for performing cardioversion and defibrillation because it differs with the make and model of each device despite some universal similarities. Regardless, the fundamental goal of both cardioversion and defibrillation is to momentarily stop all electrical activity in the heart to allow for the normal pacemaker to resume control of the heart's rhythm. The primary difference between cardioversion and defibrillation is the energy involved and the timing of the energy delivery. While there will be continued debate on the optimal energy to use to terminate a particular dysrhythmia, the following guidelines are consistent with current literature:

Defibrillation

Pulseless VT/VF	360 J monophasic, 120-200 J biphasic
Sustained polymorphic VT	360 J monophasic, 120-200 J biphasic
Synchronized cardioversion	
Narrow complex-QRS tachycardia	50 J, 100 J, 100 J, 200, 300 J, 360 J*
Atrial flutter with RVR	50 J, 100 J, 100 J, 200, 300 J, 360 J*
Atrial fibrillation with RVR	100-120 J, 200 J, 300 J, 360 J*
VT with a pulse	100-120 J, 200 J, 300 J, 360 J*

*Or biphasic equivalent

> **AUTHOR'S NOTE** Synchronized cardioversion will be referred simply as cardioversion throughout the text. Unsynchronized cardioversion is defibrillation.

Defibrillation is unsynchronized in that the energy is delivered when the discharge (shock) button of the defibrillator is pushed. Synchronized cardioversion occurs following the refractory period of the QRS-T complex by sensing the R and T waves. The operator pushes the discharge button and the machine delivers the energy at the proper time. For this reason, cardioversion is generally used when there is an underlying organized rhythm while defibrillation is reserved for a more life-threatening condition. As can be seen by the list of energies employed, those for cardioversion are less than that of defibrillation for the same reasons.

Sedation

When performing cardioversion it is important to remember that this procedure will cause the patient pain and anxiety and therefore vascular access will be required to administer analgesics and sedatives. In addition, they will usually require higher doses than were used for transcutaneous pacing. The following are agents to consider for sedation;

Administer 2 to 4 mg of midazolam IV slowly and repeat every 3 to 5 minutes, titrated to produce sedation/amnesia.

OR

Administer 5 to 10 mg diazepam IV repeated every 3 to 5 minutes, titrated to produce sedation/amnesia

OR

Administer 6 mg etomidate IV (0.2 to 0.6 mg/kg), repeated every 3 to 5 minutes, titrated to produce sedation/amnesia

In addition to any of the above if the patient is in pain, consider the following agents:

Administer 2 to 5 mg morphine IV slowly to produce analgesia

OR

Administer 1 μg/kg fentanyl IV to produce analgesia, may repeat 0.5 μg/kg fentanyl if sufficient analgesia not produced within 5 to 10 minutes.

Transcutaneous Pacing

Transcutaneous pacing (TCP) is usually effective in the treatment of all symptomatic bradycardias, regardless of cause.

The indications for TCP are as follows:

- TCP is indicated in the treatment of all symptomatic bradycardias resistant to pharmacologic therapy
- TCP is indicated in the initial treatment of the following symptomatic bradycardias with wide QRS complexes, when vascular access is delayed or dysrhythmia is resistant to pharmacologic therapy:
  - Second-degree, type II AV block
  - Second-degree, 2 : 1 and advanced AV block with wide QRS complexes
  - Third-degree AV block with wide QRS complexes
- TCP should be considered in the initial treatment of symptomatic bradycardias associated with acute coronary syndromes and in situations in which vascular access is difficult or delayed
- TCP is the treatment of choice in symptomatic bradycardias in patients with heart transplants because atropine sulfate is usually ineffective in such patients

Contraindications for TCP:

- TCP is not indicated in bradycardia caused by hypothermia

It is reasonable to attempt a trial of a pharmacologic agent to treat the bradycardia while preparing the transcutaneous pacemaker.

Transcutaneous pacing may also be used for the control of polymorphic ventricular tachycardia with prolonged QT interval such as torsades de pointes. Once capture is obtained, the rate of the pacer is lowered to a sustainable rate. This process is referred to as *overdrive pacing*.

Pharmacologic Therapy

Atropine Sulfate

Atropine sulfate, generically referred to as atropine, is a parasympatholytic, which means it blocks the parasympathetic nervous system influence on the heart. The vagus nerve provides this influence by inhibiting the SA node. Therefore atropine increases heart rate (positive chronotropic effect) by accelerating SA node firing rate and blocking the vagus nerve. Atropine also increases conduction velocity (positive dromotropic effect) through the atrioventricular pathways and to some degree in the upper portions of the AV node.

Administration of atropine is by intravenous bolus. Never administer atropine slowly as it may cause paradoxical slowing of the heart, which can last several minutes.

Atropine may or may not be effective or indicated in the treatment of symptomatic bradycardias, depending on the cause of the bradycardia and the site of the AV block. The effectiveness of and indications for atropine are as follows:

- Atropine is usually effective in the treatment of the following symptomatic bradycardias and is indicated in their initial treatment:
  - Sinus bradycardia and sinus arrest/SA exit block resulting from an increase in vagal (parasympathetic) tone on the SA node secondary to an inferior or right ventricular wall MI and/or SA node dysfunction usually caused by an acute right ventricular wall MI.
  - Second-degree, type I AV block (Wenckebach); second-degree, 2 : 1 and advanced AV block *with narrow QRS complexes*; and third-degree AV block *with narrow QRS complexes*. The cause of these AV blocks is commonly an increase in vagal (parasympathetic) tone on the AV node and/or an AV node dysfunction secondary to an acute inferior or right ventricular wall MI.
- Atropine is usually not effective (nor indicated) in the treatment of the following bradycardias that result from disruption of the electrical conduction system below the AV node, secondary to an acute anterior wall MI involving the interventricular septum:
  - Second-degree, type II AV block
  - Second-degree, 2 : 1 and advanced AV block with *wide QRS complexes*
  - Third-degree AV block *with wide QRS complexes*

In such second-degree AV blocks (which have a propensity to progress rapidly to complete third-degree AV block without warning) and third-degree AV blocks, particularly in the setting of an acute anterior wall MI involving the interventricular septum, the attachment of a transcutaneous pacemaker is indicated immediately, whether or not the bradycardia is symptomatic.

- Atropine should be used with caution in patients with acute MI because of the possibility of an excessive increase in the heart rate, with the potential of increasing myocardial ischemia and precipitating ventricular tachycardia or ventricular fibrillation. TCP is preferred in such patients and in those in which IV access is difficult or delayed.
- Atropine is usually ineffective in the treatment of bradycardia in patients with heart transplants because parasympathetic activity has no role in the production of bradycardia in such patients whose transplanted hearts have been denervated and are not connected to their own parasympathetic nervous system. TCP is the treatment of choice in symptomatic bradycardias in such patients. Catecholamines such as dopamine and epinephrine are also effective in treating symptomatic bradycardias in patients with transplanted hearts.

Vasopressors

Vasopressors are agents that cause vasoconstriction in the arteriole and venous circulatory system, resulting in an increase in peripheral vascular resistance—which can improve blood pressure, and coronary and cerebral blood flow. They also increase cardiac output by increasing heart rate (positive chronotropic effect) and increase the strength of cardiac contraction (positive inotropic effect).

Epinephrine. Epinephrine (adrenaline) is a naturally occurring catecholamine resulting from the degradation of norepinephrine. The sympathetic nervous system is mediated by the release of norepinephrine from the adrenal gland. In addition, sympathetic nerves release norepinephrine to exert their adrenergic (adrenaline-like) effect. There are two different adrenergic receptors: alpha and beta. Stimulation of alpha-receptors in the peripheral vasculature results in arteriole constriction. There are two types of beta-receptors. Beta$_1$-receptors in heart muscle are stimulated by epinephrine to increase the force of muscular contraction (positive inotropic effect) and also their spontaneous rate of discharge (positive chronotropic effect). Beta$_2$-receptors in the pulmonary, cerebral, and coronary arteries are stimulated to a lesser degree by epinephrine to dilate.

Epinephrine may be considered for the treatment of symptomatic bradycardias when atropine is ineffective. TCP should be prepared in the event epinephrine is also ineffective. However, it must be used cautiously because epinephrine stimulates the heart muscle directly and may result in too fast a heart rate. Furthermore, since this stimulation increases myocardial oxygen demand, which can result in irritability, PVCs or lethal dysrhythmias such as ventricular tachycardia or fibrillation may occur.

Administration of epinephrine for symptomatic bradycardias should be via a diluted infusion. High concentration bolus administration is more likely to precipitate complications.

Vasopressin. Vasopressin is a nonadrenergic peripheral vasoconstrictor that also causes coronary and renal vasoconstriction. Vasopressin has been found to be equivalent to epinephrine in the treatment of the following conditions:

- Shock-refractory VF/VT
- Asystole
- PEA

Vasopressin is administered as a single dose of 40 units IV or IO and may replace the first or second dose of epinephrine in the cardiac arrest treatment algorithms.

Dopamine. Dopamine is a naturally occurring precursor of norepinephrine in the body. At medium (5 to 10 µg/kg/min) doses, it stimulates the beta$_1$-receptors resulting in increased SA node discharge, improved myocardial contractility, and faster impulse conduction through the myocardium. At high doses (10 to 20 µg/kg/min) dopamine stimulates both alpha$_1$ (arteriole) and alpha$_2$ (venule) receptors resulting in vasoconstriction and increased heart rate.

Dopamine may be considered for the treatment of symptomatic bradycardias. Caution must be taken to avoid causing tachycardia, which will increase myocardial oxygen demand.

Administration of dopamine is by intravenous infusion only.

Norepinephrine. Norepinephrine is a naturally occurring potent vasoconstrictor and inotropic agent. It may be effective for management of patients with severe hypotension (e.g., systolic blood pressure <70 mm Hg) and a low total peripheral resistance who fail to respond to less potent adrenergic drugs, such as dopamine or epinephrine.

Norepinephrine is relatively contraindicated in patients with hypovolemia. It may increase myocardial oxygen requirements and therefore should be used with caution in patients with ischemic heart disease.

Dobutamine. Dobutamine hydrochloride is a synthetic catecholamine and potent inotropic agent useful for treatment of severe systolic heart failure. Dobutamine works well in conditions where the goal is to reduce left ventricular filling pressure (pulmonary edema). In addition to its direct inotropic effects, dobutamine may further increase stroke volume through reflex peripheral vasodilation (baroreceptors mediated), reducing ventricular afterload, so that arterial pressure is unchanged or may fall even though cardiac output increases. Hemodynamic end points rather than a specific dose should be used to optimize treatment with dobutamine.

Isoproterenol. Isoproterenol is a β-adrenergic agent with beta$_1$ and beta$_2$ effects that increases heart rate and, to a lesser extent, causes vasodilation in the pulmonary and coronary arteries. An infusion of 2 to 10 µg/min is titrated to heart rate.

Antidysrhythmics

Adenosine. Adenosine is an endogenous purine nucleoside that briefly depresses AV node and sinus node activity. Adenosine is indicated for the following conditions:

- Narrow-complex AV nodal or sinus nodal reentry tachycardias (SVT)
- SVT while preparing for cardioversion
- Undefined, stable, narrow-complex SVT as a combination therapeutic and diagnostic maneuver
- Stable, wide-complex tachycardias in patients with a recurrence of a known reentry pathway that has been previously defined
- Stable, regular, monomorphic, wide complex tachycardia as a therapeutic and diagnostic maneuver

It is important to realize that adenosine will not terminate dysrhythmias such as atrial flutter, atrial fibrillation, or atrial or ventricular tachycardias because these dysrhythmias are not due to reentry involving the AV or sinus node. However, while adenosine will not terminate these dysrhythmias, it may produce transient AV block resulting in a slowing of the rate and thus reveal the underlying rhythm.

Amiodarone. IV amiodarone affects sodium, potassium, and calcium channels and possesses alpha and beta-adrenergic blocking properties. It is indicated in the following conditions.

Tachycardias

- For narrow-complex tachycardias that originate from a reentry mechanism (SVT) if the rhythm remains uncontrolled by adenosine and vagal maneuvers
- Control of hemodynamically stable, monomorphic VT, polymorphic VT with a normal QT interval, and wide-complex tachycardia of uncertain origin

Cardiac Arrest

- Treatment of VF or pulseless VT unresponsive to defibrillation, CPR, and a vasopressor

The major adverse effects of amiodarone are hypotension and bradycardia, which can be prevented by slowing the rate of drug infusion.

Lidocaine. Lidocaine is an alternative antidysrhythmic of long standing and widespread familiarity with fewer immediate side effects than may be encountered with other antiarrhythmics. However, little scientific evidence exists to support its use. Regardless it continues to be included in treatment algorithms. The indications for the use of lidocaine include:

- *Stable monomorphic VT* (alternative agents are preferred)
- *Polymorphic VT* with *normal baseline QT interval* when ischemia is treated and electrolyte imbalance is corrected

Toxic reactions and side effects include slurred speech, altered consciousness, muscle twitching, seizures, and bradycardia.

Procainamide. Procainamide hydrochloride suppresses both atrial and ventricular dysrhythmias by slowing conduction through myocardial tissue. Procainamide may be considered in the following conditions:

- Stable monomorphic ventricular tachycardia
- Control of heart rate in atrial fibrillation or atrial flutter with rapid ventricular response
- Conversion of rhythm in atrial fibrillation or atrial flutter in patients with known preexcitation (WPW) syndrome
- AV reentrant, narrow-complex tachycardias (PSVT) if rhythm is uncontrolled by adenosine and vagal maneuvers in patients with preserved ventricular function

The administration of procainamide must be stopped when specific end points have been reached. These are listed in Box 10-1.

Magnesium. Magnesium is an electrolyte required for normal physiologic function and is a cofactor in neurochemical transmission and muscular excitability. It is indicated in the treatment of

- Polymorphic VT with a prolonged baseline QT interval that suggests torsades de pointes.

Magnesium is not likely to be effective in the treatment of polymorphic VT if the underlying QT interval is normal. However, until the VT is converted, the length of the QT interval may not be known.

Ibutilide. Ibutilide is a short-acting antidysrhythmic that acts by prolonging the action potential duration and increasing the refractory period of the myocardium. Ibutilide may be used in the following conditions:

- Acute pharmacologic rhythm conversion of atrial fibrillation or atrial flutter in stable patients when duration of the dysrhythmia is <48 hours
- Rate control in atrial fibrillation or atrial flutter in patients when calcium channel blockers or β-blockers are ineffective
- Acute pharmacologic rhythm conversion of atrial fibrillation or atrial flutter in stable patients with WPW syndrome when the duration of the dysrhythmia is <48 hours (the intervention of choice for this indication is DC cardioversion).

Ibutilide has minimal effects on blood pressure and heart rate. Its major limitation is a relatively high incidence of ventricular dysrhythmia (polymorphic VT, including torsades de pointes). Before administering ibutilide hyperkalemia or hypomagnesaemia must be corrected. Monitor patients receiving ibutilide *continuously* for dysrhythmias at the time of its administration and for *at least 4 to 6 hours* thereafter. Ibutilide is contraindicated if the baseline QT interval is greater than 440 msec.

Calcium Channel Blockers: Diltiazem and Verapamil

Verapamil and diltiazem are calcium channel blocking agents that slow conduction and increase the conduction time through the AV node. These actions may terminate reentrant dysrhythmias and control the ventricular response rate in patients with a variety of atrial tachycardias. These medications are indicated in the following circumstances:

- Stable, narrow-complex, reentry mechanism tachycardias (SVT) if rhythm remains uncontrolled or unconverted by adenosine or vagal maneuvers
- Stable, narrow-complex, ectopic focus tachycardias (junctional, ectopic, multifocal) if the rhythm is not controlled or converted by adenosine or vagal maneuvers
- Atrial fibrillation or atrial flutter with rapid ventricular response

Verapamil and, to a lesser extent, diltiazem may decrease myocardial contractility and critically reduce cardiac output in patients with severe left ventricular dysfunction and result in hypotension. Calcium channel blockers should not be given to patients with atrial fibrillation or atrial flutter associated with known preexcitation (WPW) syndrome because it may result in complete heart block. Box 10-2 lists other contraindications for the administration of calcium channel blockers.

BOX 10-1 Procainamide End Point

- Tachycardia is suppressed
- A total dose of 17 mg/kg of procainamide has been administered (1.2 g of procainamide for a 70-kg patient)
- Side effects from the procainamide appear (such as hypotension)
- The QRS complex widens by 50% of its original width

BOX 10-2 Administration of Calcium Channel Blockers

Calcium channel blockers are contraindicated:

- If hypotension or cardiogenic shock is present
- If second- or third-degree AV block, sinus node dysfunction, atrial flutter or fibrillation associated with ventricular or atrio-His preexcitation or a wide-QRS-complex tachycardia is present
- If beta-blockers are being administered intravenously, or
- If there is a history of bradycardia
- Calcium channel blockers should be used cautiously, if at all, in patients with congestive heart failure and those receiving oral beta-blockers. The patient's blood pressure and pulse must be monitored frequently during and after the administration of a calcium channel blocker.

If hypotension occurs with a calcium channel blocker, place the patient in a Trendelenburg position and administer 1 g of calcium chloride IV slowly, IV fluids, and a vasopressor.

If bradycardia, AV block, or asystole occurs, refer to the appropriate treatment protocol.

AUTHOR'S NOTE Diltiazem is used as the calcium channel blocker of choice throughout this text. However, some clinicians prefer verapamil. In those instances the initial dose of verapamil is 2.5 to 5 mg IV given over 2 minutes. In the absence of a therapeutic response or a drug-induced adverse event, repeat doses of 5 to 10 mg may be administered every 15 to 30 minutes to a total dose of 20 mg. An alternative dosing regimen is to give a 5 mg bolus every 15 minutes to a total dose of 30 mg.

CLINICAL NOTE In the guidelines and algorithms that follow the route of administration of all medications is listed as IV. Depending on the clinical scenario, vascular access may be obtained via a peripheral or central vein (IV) or through the insertion of an intraosseous needle (IO). All the agents listed may be administered by IO without a change in concentration or dose. The administration of medication via the endotracheal tube is not recommended.

Beta-Adrenergic Blockers

Beta-blocking agents (atenolol, metoprolol, esmolol) reduce the effects of circulating catecholamines and decrease heart rate and blood pressure. For acute tachydysrhythmias, these agents are indicated for rate control in the following conditions:

- Stable, narrow-complex tachycardias that originate from either a *reentry mechanism* (SVT) or an *ectopic focus* (junctional, ectopic, or multifocal tachycardia) uncontrolled by vagal maneuvers and adenosine
- Rate control in atrial fibrillation and atrial flutter in the stable patients

Side effects related to beta-blockade include bradycardias, AV conduction delays, and hypotension. Contraindications to the use of beta-adrenergic blocking agents are listed in Box 10-3.

Oxygen

All cells require oxygen and glucose to perform their metabolic activities. The application of high-flow oxygen has been the traditional therapy for all ill patients regardless of cause. However, recent research has revealed that high concentrations of oxygen in the human body can cause harm. It has been proposed that hypoxemia (elevated levels of oxygen saturation) worsens neurologic outcome from cardiac arrest and may extend the size of myocardial ischemia. The mechanism of harm is not fully known but is thought to relate to the creation of "free radicals," which are solitary oxygen atoms that are highly disruptive to cellular metabolism.

The current guidelines for oxygen administration are:
- Supplemental oxygen via nasal cannula at 4 L/min only if the patient is in respiratory distress, heart failure, cyanotic, or has documented hypoxemia with an oxygen saturation less than 94%.
- Titration of oxygen concentration following return of spontaneous circulation in cardiac arrest to a saturation of 94% to 98%.

BRADYCARDIAS

Clinical Significance of Bradycardias

A bradycardia with a heart rate between 50 to 59 beats/min (*mild bradycardia*) usually does not produce symptoms by itself. If the heart rate slows to 30 to 45 beats/min or less (*marked bradycardia*), the cardiac output may drop significantly, causing the systolic blood pressure to fall to 80 to 90 mm Hg or less and signs and symptoms of decreased perfusion of the body, especially of the vital organs, to appear. The skin may become pale, cold, and clammy; the pulse may be weak or absent; and the patient may be agitated, lightheaded, confused, or unconscious. The patient may experience chest pain and also become dyspneic.

In the setting of acute coronary syndrome (ACS), mild bradycardia may actually be beneficial to some patients because of the decrease in the workload of the heart, which reduces the oxygen requirements of the myocardium, minimizes the extension of the infarction, and lessens the predisposition to certain dysrhythmias. This is referred to a "cardio-protective" characteristic. Marked bradycardia, however, may result in hypotension, with a marked reduction of cardiac output leading to congestive heart failure, loss of consciousness, and shock, and predispose the patient to more serious dysrhythmias (i.e., premature ventricular complexes [PVCs], ventricular tachycardia or fibrillation, or asystole).

If sinus arrest or sinoatrial (SA) exit block is prolonged or second-degree atrioventricular (AV) block suddenly progresses to a third-degree AV block, and if an escape pacemaker in the AV junction (junctional escape rhythm) or ventricles (ventricular escape rhythm) does not take over, asystole will follow.

Indications for Treatment of Bradycardias

Treatment may not be indicated even if the heart rate falls below 60 beats/min if the systolic blood pressure remains greater than 100 mm Hg and the patient is stable; if congestive heart failure, chest pain, and dyspnea are not present; if agitation, lightheadedness, confusion, and loss of consciousness are absent; and if frequent PVCs do not occur. Such a bradycardia is considered to be an *asymptomatic bradycardia.*

However, treatment of bradycardia, regardless of cause, is indicated immediately if the heart rate is less than 60 beats/min and the patient is unstable (such a bradycardia is considered *symptomatic bradycardia*):

Occasionally, treatment to increase the heart rate may also be indicated if the heart rate is somewhat above 60 beats/min and the patient is symptomatic. This may result if the heart rate is too slow relative to the existing metabolic needs. This is called *"relative" bradycardia.*

Sinus Bradycardia
Sinus Arrest/SA Exit Block
First-Degree AV Block
Second-Degree, Type I AV Block (Wenckebach)
Second-Degree, 2:1 and Advanced AV Block With Narrow QRS Complexes
Third-Degree AV Block With Narrow QRS Complexes
(Figure 10-1)

Treatment
A. 1. Oxygen if indicated.
   2. If the bradycardia is symptomatic:
      Administer atropine 0.5 to 1 mg IV. Repeat every 3 to 5 minutes until the heart rate increases to 60 to 100 beats/min or the maximum dose of 3 mg of atropine has been administered.
      AND/OR
      Initiate TCP. If the patient is unable to tolerate TCP, consider sedation and analgesia.
   3. If the bradycardia, hypotension, or both persist:
      Start an IV infusion of epinephrine at an initial rate of 2 to 10 μg/min, and adjust the rate of infusion to increase the heart rate to 60 to 100 beats/min and the systolic blood pressure to within normal limits.
      OR
      Start an IV infusion of dopamine at an initial rate of 2 to 10 μg/kg/min, and adjust the rate of infusion up to 20 μg/kg/min to increase the heart rate to 60 to 100 beats/min and the systolic blood pressure to within normal limits.
      OR
B. 4. Insert a temporary transvenous pacemaker as soon as possible.

Second-Degree, Type II AV Block
Second-Degree, 2:1 and Advanced AV Block With Wide QRS Complexes
Third-Degree AV Block With Wide QRS Complexes (Figure 10-2)

Treatment. If the bradycardia is asymptomatic and the cause of the second- or third-degree AV block with wide QRS complexes is an acute anterior wall MI involving the interventricular septum:

A. 1. Oxygen if indicated.
   2. Attach a transcutaneous pacemaker, test for ventricular capture and patient tolerance, and put on standby.
      If the bradycardia is or becomes symptomatic:
   3. Initiate TCP. If the patient is unable to tolerate TCP, consider sedation and analgesia.
      Note: If TCP is not available, consider the administration of atropine; however, it is usually not effective in second- and third-degree AV blocks with wide QRS complexes.
      If the bradycardia, hypotension, or both persist:
      Start an IV infusion of dopamine at an initial rate of 2 to 10 μg/kg/min and adjust the rate of infusion up to 20 μg/kg/min to increase the heart rate to 60 to 100 beats/min and the systolic blood pressure to within normal limits.
      OR
      Start an IV infusion of epinephrine at an initial rate of 2 to 10 μg/min and adjust the rate of infusion to increase the heart rate to 60 to 100 beats/min and the systolic blood pressure to within normal limits.
      OR
B. 4. Insert a temporary transvenous pacemaker as soon as possible.

Junctional Escape Rhythm
Ventricular Escape Rhythm (Figure 10-3)

Treatment
A. 1. Oxygen if indicated.
     If the bradycardia is symptomatic:
   2. Initiate TCP. If the patient is unable to tolerate TCP, consider sedation and analgesia.
     If the bradycardia, hypotension, or both persist:
   3. Start an IV infusion of dopamine at an initial rate of 2 to 10 μg/kg/min and adjust the rate of infusion up to 20 μg/kg/min to increase the heart rate to 60 to 100 beats/min and the systolic blood pressure to within normal limits.
      OR
      Start an IV infusion of epinephrine at an initial rate of 2 to 10 μg/min and adjust the rate of infusion to increase the heart rate to 60 to 100 beats/min and the systolic blood pressure to within normal limits.
      OR
B. 4. Insert a temporary transvenous pacemaker as soon as possible.

TACHYCARDIAS

Clinical Significance of Tachycardias

The signs and symptoms in a tachycardia depend on the presence or absence of heart disease, the nature of the heart disease, the ventricular rate, and the duration of the tachycardia.

Frequently, a tachycardia is accompanied by feelings of palpitations, nervousness, or anxiety.

A tachycardia with a heart rate over 150 beats/min may cause the cardiac output to drop significantly because of the inability of the ventricles to fill completely during the extremely short diastole that results from the very rapid beating of the heart. Consequently, the systolic blood pressure may fall to 80 to 90 mm Hg or less, and signs and symptoms of decreased perfusion of the body, especially of the brain and other vital organs, may occur. The skin may become pale, cold, and clammy; the pulse may become weak or disappear; and the patient may become agitated, confused, lightheaded, or unconscious, or may experience chest pain and become dyspneic.

In addition, because a rapid heart rate increases the workload of the heart, the oxygen requirements of the myocardium are usually increased in a tachycardia. Thus in addition to the consequences of decreased cardiac output, a tachycardia in the setting of acute coronary syndrome may increase myocardial ischemia and the frequency and severity of chest pain; bring about the extension of the infarct; cause congestive heart failure, hypotension, or cardiogenic shock; or predispose the patient to serious ventricular dysrhythmias.

Contributing to the low cardiac output in certain tachycardias (atrial flutter, atrial fibrillation, supraventricular tachycardia [SVT]) is the loss of the normal atrial contraction which precedes each ventricular contraction (the so-called "atrial kick"). The ventricles do not fill completely during diastole, resulting in a drop in the cardiac output by as much as 25%.

Indications for Treatment of Tachycardias

Specific treatment of atrial tachycardia without block, atrial flutter, atrial fibrillation, PSVT, and junctional tachycardia is indicated if the heart rate is greater than 150 beats/min or even as low as 120 beats/min, particularly, if signs and symptoms of decreased cardiac output or increased workload of the heart are associated with the tachycardia.

Treatment of ventricular tachycardia, however, is indicated immediately, regardless of whether signs and symptoms of decreased cardiac output are present because of its potential for initiating or degenerating into ventricular fibrillation.

No specific treatment of sinus tachycardia and atrial tachycardia with block is indicated.

Sinus Tachycardia (Figure 10-4)

Treatment

No specific treatment of sinus tachycardia is indicated.
1. Treat the underlying cause of the tachycardia (anxiety, exercise, pain, fever, congestive heart failure, hypoxemia, hypovolemia, hypotension, or shock).
If excessive amounts of drugs, such as atropine, epinephrine, or a vasopressor, have been administered:
2. Discontinue such drugs.

Atrial Tachycardia With Block (Figure 10-5)

Treatment. No specific treatment of atrial tachycardia with block is indicated.

1. Treat the underlying cause of the tachycardia.
If digitalis toxicity is suspected:
2. Discontinue digitalis.
If digitalis toxicity is confirmed:
3. Administer Digibind if appropriate

Narrow-QRS-Complex Tachycardia of Unknown Origin (With Pulse) (Figure 10-6)

Treatment

A. 1. Oxygen if indicated.
   2. Attempt vagal maneuvers.

> ### KEY DEFINITION
>
> Vagal maneuvers are performed to stimulate baroreceptors in the internal carotid artery and the aortic arch. This stimulation produces a reflexive slowing of the heart rate. Examples of vagal maneuvers include:
> - Gagging
> - Having the patient bear down as if having a bowel movement (Valsalva maneuver)
> - Cold stimulation to the face with an ice water soaked washcloth or ice pack
> - Coughing, squatting, or breath-holding
> - Carotid sinus pressure applied at the angle of the jaw, preferably on the right, for 5 seconds
>
> Use *extreme caution* when applying carotid sinus pressure to older patients because it may result in stroke. *Never* apply bilateral carotid pressure or exceed 10 seconds in duration. Be prepared with vascular access, continuous ECG monitoring, and have a defibrillator ready.

If the vagal maneuvers are unsuccessful and the patient remains stable:

Administer an AV node depressant such as adenosine.

Administer a 6 mg bolus of adenosine IV rapidly over 1 to 3 seconds followed immediately by 10-cc saline bolus. If the initial dose is not immediately effective, administer in 1 to 2 minutes a 12-mg bolus of adenosine IV rapidly over 1 to 3 seconds followed immediately by a 10-cc saline bolus. Repeat the 12-mg bolus of adenosine a second time in 1 to 2 minutes if needed.

Note: Follow each dose of adenosine with a 10-cc saline bolus.

If the dysrhythmia converts to a sinus rhythm at any time, indicating that PSVT is present, continue with the appropriate step in the section on Paroxysmal Supraventricular Tachycardia With Narrow QRS Complexes, p. 157

If the heart rate slows at any time, indicating that an atrial or junctional tachycardia is present, continue with the treatment plans outlined in either the section on Atrial Tachycardia Without Block (p. 157) or Junctional Tachycardia (p. 158) as appropriate.

If the heart rate slows at any time, indicating an underlying atrial fibrillation or atrial flutter rhythm, continue with the treatment plans outlines in the section on Atrial Flutter/Fibrillation (p. 158) as appropriate.

Atrial Tachycardia Without Block (Figure 10-7)

Treatment

A. 1. Oxygen if indicated.

2. Administer a calcium channel blocker such as diltiazem.

    Administer a 20 mg (0.25 mg/kg) dose of diltiazem IV slowly over 2 minutes. If the initial dose is not effective in 15 minutes and no adverse effects have occurred, repeat a second 25 mg (0.35 mg/kg) dose of diltiazem IV slowly over 2 minutes.

    Note: In elderly patients (>60 years of age), the dose of diltiazem should be administered slowly over 3 to 4 minutes.

    AND

    Start a maintenance IV infusion of diltiazem at a rate of 5 to 15 mg/hr to maintain the heart rate within normal limits.

    OR

3. Administer a beta-blocker.

    Administer a 0.5 mg/kg dose of esmolol IV over 1 minute, followed by an IV infusion of esmolol at 0.05 mg/kg/min and repeat the 0.5 mg/kg dose of esmolol IV twice at 5-minute intervals while increasing the IV infusion of esmolol 0.05 mg/kg/min after each dose of esmolol if the response is inadequate to a maximum infusion of 0.2 mg/kg/min, if necessary, and then titrate the esmolol infusion to maintain the heart rate within normal limits. Do not exceed the maximum infusion of 0.2 mg/kg/min.

    OR

    Administer 2.5 mg to 5 mg atenolol IV over 5 minutes and repeat every 10 minutes as needed to a total dose of 10 mg, if needed.

    OR

    Administer 5 mg metoprolol IV over 2 to 5 minutes and repeat twice at 5-minute intervals to a total dose of 15 mg, if needed.

    AND

    Monitor the pulse, blood pressure, and EGG while administering the drug. Stop the administration of the beta-blocker if the systolic blood pressure falls below 100 mm Hg.

    OR

4. Administer an antidysrhythmic drug such as amiodarone.

    Administer a loading dose of 150 mg of amiodarone IV over 10 minutes.

    AND

    Start an IV infusion of amiodarone at a rate of 1 mg/min for 6 hours then decrease to 0.5 mg/min for 18 hours.

Paroxysmal Supraventricular Tachycardia With Narrow QRS Complexes (Without Wolff-Parkinson-White Syndrome or Ventricular Preexcitation) (Figure 10-8)

Treatment

A. 1. Oxygen if indicated.

2. Attempt vagal maneuvers. If the vagal maneuvers are unsuccessful and the patient remains stable:

C. Administer an AV node depressant such as adenosine.

Administer a 6 mg bolus of adenosine IV rapidly over 1 to 3 seconds followed immediately by a 10-cc saline bolus. If the initial dose is not immediately effective, administer in 1 to 2 minutes a 12-mg bolus of adenosine IV rapidly over 1 to 3 seconds followed immediately by a 10-cc saline bolus. Repeat the 12-mg bolus of adenosine a second time in 1 to 2 minutes if needed.

Note: Follow each dose of adenosine with a 10-cc saline bolus.

If vagal maneuvers and adenosine are not effective and the patient continues to be stable:

OR

4. Administer a calcium channel blocker such as diltiazem.

    Administer a 20 mg (0.25 mg/kg) dose of diltiazem IV slowly over 2 minutes. If the initial dose is not effective in 15 minutes and no adverse effects have occurred, repeat a second 25 mg (0.35 mg/kg) dose of diltiazem IV slowly over 2 minutes.

    Note: In elderly patients (>60 years of age) the dose of diltiazem should be administered slowly over 3 to 4 minutes.

    AND

    Start a maintenance IV infusion of diltiazem at a rate of 5 to 15 mg/hr to maintain the heart rate within normal limits.

    OR

5. Administer a beta-blocker.

    Administer a 0.5 mg/kg dose of esmolol IV over 1 minute, followed by an IV infusion of esmolol at 0.05 mg/kg/min and repeat the 0.5 mg/kg dose of esmolol IV twice at 5-minute intervals while increasing the IV infusion of esmolol 0.05 mg/kg/min after each dose of esmolol if the response is inadequate to a maximum infusion of 0.2 mg/kg/min, if necessary, and then titrate the esmolol infusion to maintain the heart rate within normal limits. Do not exceed the maximum infusion of 0.2 mg/kg/min.

    OR

    Administer 2.5 mg to 5 mg atenolol IV over 5 minutes and repeat every 10 minutes as needed to a total dose of 10 mg, if needed.

    OR

    Administer 5 mg metoprolol IV over 2 to 5 minutes and repeat twice at 5-minute intervals to a total dose of 15 mg, if needed.

    AND

    Monitor the pulse, blood pressure, and EGG while administering the drug. Stop the administration of the beta-blocker if the systolic blood pressure falls below 100 mm Hg.

    AND

6. Administer an initial digitalization dose of 0.5 mg digoxin IV over 5 minutes.

    If vagal maneuvers, adenosine, diltiazem, or a beta-blocker, and digoxin are not effective, or the patient becomes unstable, proceed to cardioversion.

Junctional Tachycardia (Figure 10-9)

Treatment

A. 1. Oxygen if indicated.
   2. Administer an antidysrhythmic drug such as amiodarone.

   Administer a loading dose of 150 mg of amiodarone IV over 10 minutes.

   AND

   Start an IV infusion of amiodarone at a rate of 1 mg/min for 6 hours then decrease to 0.5 mg/min for 18 hours.

   OR

   3. Administer a beta-blocker.

   Administer a 0.5 mg/kg dose of esmolol IV over 1 minute, followed by an IV infusion of esmolol at 0.05 mg/kg/min and repeat the 0.5 mg/kg dose of esmolol IV twice at 5-minute intervals while increasing the IV infusion of esmolol 0.05 mg/kg/min after each dose of esmolol if the response is inadequate to a maximum infusion of 0.2 mg/kg/min, if necessary, and then titrate the esmolol infusion to maintain the heart rate within normal limits. Do not exceed the maximum infusion of 0.2 mg/kg/min.

   OR

   Administer 2.5 mg to 5 mg atenolol IV over 5 minutes and repeat every 10 minutes as needed to a total dose of 10 mg, if needed.

   OR

   Administer 5 mg **metoprolol IV** over 2 to 5 minutes and repeat twice at 5-minute intervals to a total dose of 15 mg, if needed.

   AND

   Monitor the pulse, blood pressure, and EGG while administering the drug. Stop the administration of the beta-blocker if the systolic blood pressure falls below 100 mm Hg.

Atrial Flutter/Atrial Fibrillation (Without Wolff-Parkinson-White Syndrome or Ventricular Preexcitation) (Figure 10-10)

Treatment to Control the Heart Rate

A. 1. Oxygen if indicated.
   2. Administer a beta-blocker.

   Administer a 0.5 mg/kg dose of esmolol IV over 1 minute, followed by an IV infusion of esmolol at 0.05 mg/kg/min. Repeat the 0.5 mg/kg dose of esmolol IV twice at 5-minute intervals while increasing the IV infusion of esmolol 0.05 mg/kg/min after each dose of esmolol, if the response is inadequate, to a maximum infusion of 0.2 mg/kg/min (if necessary). Then titrate the esmolol infusion to maintain the heart rate within normal limits. Do not exceed the maximum infusion of 0.2 mg/kg/min.

   OR

   Administer 2.5 mg to 5 mg atenolol IV over 5 minutes and repeat every 10 minutes as needed to a total dose of 10 mg, if needed.

   OR

Administer 5 mg metoprolol IV over 2 to 5 minutes and repeat twice at 5-minute intervals to a total dose of 15 mg, if needed.

AND

Monitor the pulse, blood pressure, and EGG while administering the drug. Stop the administration of the beta-blocker if the systolic blood pressure falls below 100 mm Hg.

OR

   3. Administer a calcium channel blocker such as diltiazem.

   Administer a 20-mg (0.25 mg/kg) dose of diltiazem IV slowly over 2 minutes. If the initial dose is not effective in 15 minutes and no adverse effects have occurred, repeat a second 25 mg (0.35 mg/kg) dose of diltiazem IV slowly over 2 minutes.

   Note: In elderly patients (>60 years of age), the doses of diltiazem should be administered slowly over 3 to 4 minutes.

   AND

   Start a maintenance IV infusion of diltiazem at a rate of 5 to 15 mg/hr to maintain the heart rate within normal limits.

> **CLINICAL NOTE** Calcium channel blockers are contraindicated for the treatment of atrial fibrillation and atrial flutter in the presence of Wolf-Parkinson-White syndrome.

   4. Administer an initial digitalization dose of 0.5 mg digoxin IV over 5 minutes.

Treatment to Convert the Rhythm. Atrial Fibrillation <48 Hours

A. 1. Oxygen if indicated.
   2. Administer a short-acting antidysrhythmic such as ibutilide.

   If the patient weighs 60 kg (132 lb), administer 1 mg of ibutilide IV over 10 minutes and repeat in 10 minutes if necessary after completion of the first infusion.

   If the patient weighs less than 60 kg (<132 lb), administer 0.1 mg/kg of ibutilide IV over 10 minutes and repeat in 10 minutes, if necessary, after completion of the first infusion.

   Maximum dose of ibutilide is 2 mg.

   OR

   3. Administer an antidysrhythmic drug such as amiodarone.

   Administer a loading dose of 150 mg of amiodarone IV over 10 minutes.

   AND

   Start an IV infusion of amiodarone at a rate of 1 mg/min for 6 hours then decrease to 0.5 mg/min for 18 hours.

   OR

   4. Administer an antidysrhythmic drug such as procainamide.

Start an IV infusion of procainamide at a rate of 20 to 30 mg/min (up to 50 mg/min, if necessary). Continue the infusion of procainamide until reaching the endpoint listed in Box 10-1.

OR

5. Perform immediate synchronized cardioversion.

Cardiovert at 100 to 200 J (monophasic or biphasic equivalent)

Atrial fibrillation >48 hours or of unknown duration

A. 1. Oxygen if indicated.

2. Rhythm conversion is contraindicated until the patient has been anticoagulated with heparin. There is an increased risk of a thromboembolic event resulting in stroke because of thrombus formation that may have occurred during the period of atrial fibrillation.

If patient becomes unstable or amiodarone fails to convert rhythm perform immediate synchronized cardioversion.

For Atrial Fib:

Cardiovert at 100 to 200 J with a monophasic waveform.

Cardiovert at 100 to 120 J with a biphasic waveform. Escalate subsequent shock doses as required.

For Atrial Flutter:

Cardiovert at 50 to 100 J with a monophasic waveform. Escalate subsequent shock doses as required.

AND

Administer an antidysrhythmic drug such as amiodarone (if not already administered).

Administer a loading dose of 150 mg of amiodarone IV over 10 minutes.

AND

Start an IV infusion of amiodarone at a rate of 1 mg/min for 6 hours then decrease to 0.5 mg/min for 18 hours.

Atrial Flutter/Atrial Fibrillation (With Wolff-Parkinson-White Syndrome or Ventricular Preexcitation) (Figure 10-11)

Treatment to Control the Heart Rate and/or Convert the Rhythm. Atrial fibrillation <48 hours and atrial flutter of any duration

Patient hemodynamically stable:

A. 1. Oxygen if indicated.

2. Administer an antidysrhythmic drug such as amiodarone.

• Administer a loading dose of 150 mg of amiodarone IV over 10 minutes.

AND

Start an IV infusion of amiodarone at a rate of 1 mg/min for 6 hours then decrease to 0.5 mg/hr for 18 hours.

If one of the antidysrhythmic drugs is unsuccessful in converting atrial flutter or atrial fibrillation:

3. Perform immediate synchronized cardioversion.

For Atrial Fib:

Cardiovert at 100 to 200 J with a monophasic waveform.

Cardiovert at 100 to 120 J with a biphasic waveform.

Escalate subsequent shock doses as required.

For Atrial Flutter:

Cardiovert at 50 to 100 J with a monophasic or biphasic waveform. Escalate subsequent shock doses as required.

Wide-QRS-Complex Tachycardia of Unknown Origin (With Pulse) (Figure 10-12)

Treatment

A. 1. Oxygen if indicated.

2. If unstable

Consider immediate cardioversion or administration of an antidysrhythmic drug.

Deliver a cardioversion (100 J). Repeat the cardioversion as often as necessary at progressively increasing energy levels (200 J, 300 J, and 360 J).

OR

3. Administer an antidysrhythmic drug such as amiodarone

Administer a loading dose of 150 mg of amiodarone IV over 10 minutes.

AND

Start an IV infusion of amiodarone at a rate of 1 mg/min for 6 hours then decrease to 0.5 mg/min for 18 hours

OR

C. 2. If the wide-QRS-complex tachycardia persists and the patient is or becomes hemodynamically unstable and has a pulse:

Continue with an antidysrhythmic drug such as amiodarone while continuing the delivery of cardioversions.

If the wide-QRS-complex tachycardia persists and the patient becomes pulseless at any time:

Continue with section B, Monitored Cardiac Arrest under Ventricular Fibrillation/Pulseless Ventricular Tachycardia, p. 167.

If electrical or pharmacologic therapy is successful in terminating the wide-QRS-complex tachycardia:

Continue or start a maintenance IV infusion of amiodarone or procainamide as appropriate.

Ventricular Tachycardia, Monomorphic (With Pulse) (Figure 10-13)

Treatment

A. 1. Oxygen if indicated.

2. If unstable

Consider immediate **cardioversion** or administration of an antidysrhythmic drug.

Deliver a cardioversion (100 J). Repeat the cardioversion as often as necessary at progressively increasing energy levels (200 J, 300 J, and 360 J).

If ventricular tachycardia persists and the patient is or becomes hemodynamically unstable and has a pulse:

Administer an antidysrhythmic drug such as **amiodarone, lidocaine, or procainamide**, as in Step 3 below while continuing the delivery of cardioversions.

If ventricular tachycardia persists and the patient becomes pulseless at any time:

Continue with section B, Monitored Cardiac Arrest under Ventricular Fibrillation/Pulseless Ventricular Tachycardia, p. 167.

3. If stable, administer an antidysrhythmic drug such as amiodarone, lidocaine, or procainamide:
   - Administer a loading dose of 150 mg of amiodarone IV over 10 minutes, and repeat two to three times, if necessary, allowing 10 to 15 minutes between infusions.
     AND
     Start an IV infusion of amiodarone at a rate of 1 mg/min for 6 hours then decrease to 0.5 mg/min for 18 hours
     OR
   - Administer a 1.0 to 1.5-mg/kg bolus (75 to 100 mg) of lidocaine IV slowly, and repeat a 0.5 to 0.75-mg/kg bolus (25 to 50 mg) of lidocaine IV slowly every 5 to 10 minutes until the ventricular tachycardia is suppressed or a total dose of 3 mg/kg of lidocaine has been administered.
     If lidocaine is successful in suppressing the ventricular tachycardia:
     Start a maintenance infusion of lidocaine at a rate of 1 to 4 mg/min to prevent the recurrence of the ventricular tachycardia.
     OR
     Start an IV infusion of procainamide at a rate of 20 to 30 mg/min (up to 50 mg/min, if necessary) and continue until reaching end point listed in Box 10-1.
     If procainamide is successful in suppressing ventricular tachycardia:
     Start a maintenance IV infusion of procainamide at a rate of 1 to 4 mg/min.
     If amiodarone, lidocaine, or procainamide is unsuccessful in suppressing ventricular tachycardia, or if at any time the patient's condition becomes hemodynamically unstable and cardioversions were not delivered initially:
     Immediately deliver a cardioversion (100 J)
     AND
     Repeat the cardioversion as often as necessary at progressively increasing energy levels (200 J, 300 J, and 360 J).
     If one of the shocks or medications is successful in terminating ventricular tachycardia:
     Continue or start a maintenance IV infusion of amiodarone, lidocaine, or procainamide as appropriate.

Ventricular Tachycardia, Polymorphic (With Pulse) Normal Baseline QT Interval (Figure 10-14)

Treatment

A. 1. Oxygen if indicated.
      AND

Consider immediate DC cardioversion outlined in step 2 or administration of an antidysrhythmic drug outlined in step 3 while correcting any electrolyte imbalance.

2. Deliver a cardioversion (100 J).
   AND
   Repeat the cardioversion as often as necessary at progressively increasing energy levels (200 to 300 J and 360 J).
   If the polymorphic ventricular tachycardia persists and the patient remains hemodynamically stable and has a pulse:
   Administer a beta-blocker or an antidysrhythmic drug such as amiodarone, lidocaine, or procainamide as in Step 3 below while continuing the delivery of cardioversions.
   If the polymorphic ventricular tachycardia persists and the patient is or becomes hemodynamically unstable and has a pulse:
   Administer an antidysrhythmic drug such as amiodarone, lidocaine, or procainamide as in Step 3 below while continuing the delivery of cardioversions.
   If the polymorphic ventricular tachycardia persists and the patient becomes pulseless at any time:
   Continue with section B, Monitored Cardiac Arrest under Ventricular Fibrillation/Pulseless Ventricular Tachycardia, p. 167.

3a. If the polymorphic ventricular tachycardia is associated with an acute coronary syndrome:
    Treat the acute coronary syndrome (see Chapter 19). Administer a beta-blocker.
    Administer a 0.5 mg/kg dose of esmolol IV over 1 minute, followed by an IV infusion of esmolol at 0.05 mg/kg/min and repeat the 0.5 mg/kg dose of esmolol IV twice at 5-minute intervals while increasing the IV infusion of esmolol 0.05 mg/kg/min after each dose of esmolol if the response is inadequate to a maximum infusion of 0.2 mg/kg/min, if necessary, to suppress the polymorphic ventricular tachycardia, and then titrate the esmolol infusion to maintain the heart rate within normal limits. Do not exceed maximum infusion of 0.2 mg/kg/min.
    OR
    Administer 2.5 mg to 5 mg atenolol IV over 5 minutes and repeat every 10 minutes to a total dose of 10 mg, if needed.
    OR
    Administer 5 mg metoprolol IV over 2 to 5 minutes and repeat twice at 5-minute intervals to a total dose of 15 mg, if needed.
    AND
    Monitor the pulse, blood pressure, and ECG while administering the drug. Stop the administration of the beta-blocker if the systolic blood pressure falls below 100 mm Hg.
    OR

3b. If the polymorphic ventricular tachycardia is not associated with an acute coronary syndrome, administer an antidysrhythmic drug if not contraindicated.

Administer an antidysrhythmic drug such as amiodarone.

Administer a loading dose of 150 mg of amiodarone IV over 10 minutes and repeat two to three times if necessary, allowing 10 to 15 minutes between infusions.

AND

Start an IV infusion of amiodarone at a rate of 1 mg/min for 6 hours, then decrease to 0.5 mg/min for 18 hours.

OR

Administer an antidysrhythmic drug such as lidocaine.

Administer a 1 to 1.5 mg/kg bolus (75 to 100 mg) of lidocaine IV slowly, and repeat a 0.5 to 0.75-mg/kg bolus (25 to 50 mg) of lidocaine IV slowly every 5 to 10 minutes until the ventricular tachycardia is suppressed or a total dose of 3 mg/kg of lidocaine has been administered.

If lidocaine is successful in suppressing the ventricular tachycardia:

Start a maintenance infusion of lidocaine at a rate of 1 to 4 mg/min of lidocaine to prevent the recurrence of the ventricular tachycardia.

OR

Administer an antidysrhythmic drug such as procainamide.

Start an IV infusion of procainamide at a rate of 20 to 30 mg/min (up to 50 mg/min, if necessary). Continue the infusion of procainamide until reaching endpoint.

If procainamide is successful in suppressing ventricular tachycardia:

Start a maintenance IV infusion of procainamide at a rate of 1 to 4 mg/min.

If a beta-blocker, amiodarone, lidocaine, or procainamide is unsuccessful in suppressing the polymorphic ventricular tachycardia, or if, at any time while administrating the beta-blocker, procainamide, amiodarone, or lidocaine, the patient's condition becomes hemodynamically unstable and cardioversions were not delivered initially:

Immediately deliver a cardioversion (200 J), premedicating the patient first, if necessary

AND

Repeat the cardioversion as often as necessary at progressively increasing energy levels (200 to 300 J and 360 J).

If one of the shocks or is successful in terminating the polymorphic ventricular tachycardia:

Continue or start a maintenance IV infusion of the beta-blocker, amiodarone, lidocaine, or procainamide as appropriate.

Ventricular Tachycardia, Polymorphic (With Pulse) Prolonged Baseline QT Interval Torsades de Pointes (TdP) (With Pulse) (Figure 10-15)

Treatment

A. 1. Oxygen if indicated.
   2. If magnesium deficiency is present or suspected, and the patient is not hypotensive:
      - Administer a dose of 1 to 2 g (8 to 16 mEq) of magnesium sulfate, diluted with 50 to 100 mL of D_5W, IV over 5 to 60 minutes.
      AND
      Follow with a maintenance IV infusion of 0.5 to 1 g (4 to 8 mEq) of magnesium sulfate, diluted with 100 mL of D_5W, IV to run for 1 hour.
   3. Initiate transcutaneous overdrive pacing, if appropriate.
      AND
      Consider the administration of a beta-blocker if not contraindicated and hypotension not present.
      - Administer a 0.5 mg/kg dose of esmolol IV over 1 minute, followed by an IV infusion of esmolol at 0.05 mg/kg/min. Repeat the 0.5 mg/kg dose of esmolol IV twice at 5-minute intervals while increasing the IV infusion of esmolol 0.05 mg/kg/min after each dose of esmolol, if the response is inadequate, to a maximum infusion of 0.2 mg/kg/min (if necessary) to suppress the ventricular tachycardia. Then titrate the esmolol infusion to maintain the heart rate within normal limits. Do not exceed maximum infusion of 0.2 mg/kg/min.
      OR
      Administer 5 mg metoprolol IV over 5 minutes and repeat in 10 minutes to a total dose of 10 mg, if needed.
      OR
      Administer 2.5 mg to 5 mg atenolol IV over 2 to 5 minutes and repeat at 5-minute intervals to a total dose of 15 mg, if needed.
      AND
      Monitor the pulse, blood pressure, and ECG while administering the drug. Stop the administration of the beta-blocker if the systolic blood pressure falls below 100 mm Hg.
   4. Withhold administration of such antidysrhythmic agents as amiodarone, disopyramide, procainamide, quinidine, and sotalol or other agents that prolong the Q–T interval, such as phenothiazines and tricyclic antidepressants.
      AND
      Correct any electrolyte imbalance.
      If polymorphic ventricular tachycardia or torsades de pointes persists and the patient is or becomes unstable:
      Deliver a defibrillation (360 J)
      AND
      Repeat the defibrillation as often as necessary at 360 J.

If polymorphic ventricular tachycardia or torsades de pointes degenerates into ventricular fibrillation at any time:

- Continue with section B, Monitored Cardiac Arrest under Ventricular Fibrillation/Pulseless Ventricular Tachycardia, p. 167.

PREMATURE ECTOPIC BEATS

Premature Atrial Complexes (Figure 10-16)

Clinical Significance

Single, isolated premature atrial complexes (PACs) are not significant. Frequent PACs may indicate the presence of enhanced atrial automaticity, an atrial reentry mechanism, or both, and herald impending atrial dysrhythmia (such as atrial tachycardia, atrial flutter, and atrial fibrillation) and PSVT. The most common cause is elevated sympathetic tone from stress, pain, anxiety, or stimulant drugs or agents. Hypoxia must also be considered.

Indications for Treatment

Treatment may be indicated if the premature atrial complexes are frequent (8 to 10 per minute), occur in groups of two or more, or alternate with the QRS complexes of the underlying rhythm (bigeminy).

Treatment. If stimulants (such as caffeine, tobacco, or alcohol) or excessive amounts of sympathomimetic drugs (such as epinephrine or dopamine) have been administered:

1. Discontinue the stimulants and sympathomimetic drugs.
   If digitalis toxicity is suspected:
2. Withhold digitalis
   Once digitalis toxicity is confirmed:
3. Administer Digibind if indicated

Premature Junctional Complexes (Figure 10-16)

Clinical Significance

Single, isolated premature junctional complexes (PJCs) are not significant. Frequent PJCs may indicate the presence of enhanced AV junctional automaticity, an AV junctional reentry mechanism, or both, and herald an impending junctional tachycardia. The most common caused is elevated sympathetic tone from stress, pain, anxiety, or stimulant drugs or agents. Hypoxia must also be considered.

Indications for Treatment

Treatment is indicated if the premature junctional complexes are frequent (4 to 6 per minute), occur in groups of two or more, or alternate with the QRS complexes of the underlying rhythm (bigeminy).

Treatment. If stimulants (such as caffeine, tobacco, or alcohol) or excessive amounts of sympathomimetic drugs (such as epinephrine or dopamine) have been administered:

1. Discontinue the stimulants and sympathomimetic drugs.
   If digitalis toxicity is suspected:
2. Withhold digitalis.
   Once digitalis toxicity is confirmed:
3. Administer Digibind if indicated

Premature Ventricular Complexes (Figure 10-17)

Clinical Significance

Single premature ventricular complexes (PVCs), especially in patients who have no heart disease, are generally not significant. In patients with an acute coronary syndrome or an ischemic episode, PVCs may indicate the presence of enhanced ventricular automaticity, a ventricular reentry mechanism, or both, and herald the appearance of a life-threatening dysrhythmia, such as ventricular tachycardia or fibrillation. Although these lethal dysrhythmias may occur without warning, they are often initiated by PVCs, especially if the PVCs:

- Are frequent (six or more per minute)
- Occur in groups of two or more (group beats)
- Have different QRS configurations (multiform)
- Arise from different ventricular ectopic pacemakers (multifocal)
- Are close coupled
- Fall on the T wave (R-on-T phenomenon)

Indications for Treatment

Treatment should be considered for PVCs in patients in whom an acute MI or ischemic episode is suspected, except for those that occur in conjunction with bradycardias. In such circumstances, first treat the underlying bradycardia. Refer to the appropriate bradycardia treatment. If feasible, identify and correct the following underlying causes of PVCs:

- Hypoxia
- Acute coronary syndrome
- Congestive heart failure
- Digitalis toxicity
- Excessive administration of sympathomimetic drugs (e.g., cocaine, epinephrine, and dopamine)
- Low serum potassium (hypokalemia)
- Acidosis
- Low serum magnesium (hypomagnesemia)

Treatment. If the PVCs are associated with an acute coronary syndrome:

- Treat the acute coronary syndrome (see Chapter 19) AND
- Withhold administration of antidysrhythmic drugs
- If the PVCs *are not associated with an acute coronary syndrome*:
- Identify and correct any underlying causes of the PVCs. AND
- Consider the administration of an antidysrhythmic drug such as amiodarone, procainamide, or lidocaine

PART II

CARDIAC ARREST

Clinical Significance

Ventricular fibrillation is a life-threatening dysrhythmia, resulting in chaotic beating of the heart and the immediate end of organized ventricular contractions, cardiac output, and death.

Pulseless ventricular tachycardia, like ventricular fibrillation, becomes a life-threatening dysrhythmia when the ventricular contractions are unable to maintain an adequate cardiac output and a pulse.

At the moment ventricular fibrillation or pulseless ventricular tachycardia occurs and cardiac output stops, clinical death is present. Biological death occurs within a matter of minutes unless cardiopulmonary resuscitation (CPR) and defibrillation are administered.

Indications for Treatment

Treatment of ventricular fibrillation and pulseless ventricular tachycardia is indicated immediately.

Treatment

A. Unmonitored Cardiac Arrest (Figure 10-18)

If the cardiac arrest is unwitnessed by the resuscitation team, or if cardiac arrest occurred before the arrival of the team and the patient is not being monitored, the following procedures should be performed:

Rescuer One:

1. Assess the patient's responsiveness.
2. If unresponsive, perform CPR until the defibrillation pads are applied.

Rescuer Two:

1. Apply the defibrillation pads.
2. Determine the ECG rhythm on the ECG monitor. Verify ventricular fibrillation/tachycardia
3. Defibrillate at 360 J monophasic (120 to 200 J biphasic).
4. Resume CPR for five cycles.
5. Check rhythm. Check pulse. If pulse present, go to post resuscitation management.
6. If VF/VT persists, defibrillate at 360 J monophasic (120 to 200 J biphasic).
7. If asystole, go to asystole management
8. If pulseless electrical activity present go to PEA management.
9. Resume CPR for five cycles. Repeat steps 3-7 while accomplishing the following:
10. Secure airway and confirm placement with minimal interruptions to CPR.
11. Establish vascular (*IV,* intravenous; *IO,* intraosseous) access; with minimal interruptions to CPR.
12. Administer vasopressin 40 U IV/IO; one time only.
    OR

Administer epinephrine 1 mg IV/IO; repeat every 3 to 5 min

13. Continue CPR for 30 to 60 seconds after each drug administration before defibrillation. Give drug early in chest compression cycle to ensure sufficient time for drug to enter circulatory system.
14. Consider using antidysrhythmics:
    Amiodarone (300 mg IV/IO once, then repeat additional 150 mg IV/IO in 5 minutes)
15. If vasopressin is used initially and patient remains in VF/VT after 15 to 20 minutes of resuscitation, consider administration of epinephrine per step 12.
16. Consider the administration of magnesium sulfate.
    - Administer a dose of 1 to 2 g (8 to 16 mEq) of magnesium sulfate diluted with 10 mL D_5W, IV over 1 to 2 minutes followed by a 20-mL flush of IV fluid.
    - Continue CPR for 30 to 60 seconds to circulate the drug.
    - Deliver a defibrillation (360 J) and check the patient's ECG rhythm and pulse.

B. Monitored Cardiac Arrest (Figure 10-18)

If the patient is being monitored and ventricular fibrillation/pulseless ventricular tachycardia occurs:

1. Apply the defibrillator paddles or defibrillation pads to the patient.
   AND
   Defibrillate at (360 J) immediately.
2. Perform CPR for five cycles.
3. Continue with Step 5 in section A, Unmonitored Cardiac Arrest under Ventricular Fibrillation/Pulseless Ventricular Tachycardia (see above).

ASYSTOLE (FIGURE 10-19)

Clinical Significance

Asystole is a life-threatening dysrhythmia resulting in the absence of ventricular contractions, cardiac output, and death. At the moment ventricular asystole occurs in a person with an adequate circulation, cardiac output stops, and clinical death occurs. Biological death follows within minutes unless asystole is reversed.

Indications for Treatment

Treatment of ventricular asystole is indicated immediately.

Treatment

Rescuer One:

1. Assess the patient's responsiveness.
2. If unresponsive, perform CPR until the defibrillation pads are applied.

Rescuer Two:

1. Apply the defibrillation pads.
2. Determine the ECG rhythm on the ECG monitor. Verify asystole in a second lead if possible.
3. Resume CPR for five cycles.

4. Analyze rhythm. Check pulse. If pulse present, go to post resuscitation management.
5. If asystole, resume CPR for five cycles
6. If VF/VT present, go to VF/VT management
7. If pulseless electrical activity present, go to PEA management.
8. Repeat steps 3-7 while accomplishing the following:
9. Secure airway and confirm placement with minimal interruptions to CPR.
10. Establish vascular (*IV,* intravenous; *IO,* intraosseous) access with minimal interruptions to CPR.
11. Administer vasopressin 40 U IV/IO, one time only
    OR
    Administer epinephrine 1 mg IV/IO; repeat every 3 to 5 min.
12. Continue CPR for 30 to 60 seconds after each drug administration before defibrillation. Give drug early in chest compression cycle to ensure sufficient time for drug to enter circulatory system.
13. Analyze rhythm.
14. Search for underlying cause (6Hs and 5Ts)
    - **Hypovolemia**—administer 250 to 500 cc of normal saline bolus, repeat as needed
    - **Hypoxia**—ensure adequate oxygenation
    - **Hydrogen Ion-Acidosis**—ensure adequate ventilation
    - **Hyperkalemia/Hypokalemia**—correct with appropriate electrolyte
    - **Hypothermia**—rewarming
    - **Hypoglycemia**
    - **Toxins/Drug overdose**—administer antidote
    - **Tamponade-cardiac**—pericardiocentesis
    - **Tension pneumothorax**—needle decompression
    - **Thrombosis**—myocardial infarction or pulmonary embolism
    - **Trauma**

PULSELESS ELECTRICAL ACTIVITY (FIGURE 10-20)

Clinical Significance

Pulseless electrical activity (PEA)—the absence of a detectable pulse and blood pressure in the presence of electrical activity of the heart as evidenced by some type of an ECG rhythm other than ventricular fibrillation or ventricular tachycardia—is a life-threatening condition. At the moment pulseless electrical activity occurs in a person, cardiac output ceases and clinical death occurs. Biological death follows within minutes unless pulseless electrical activity is reversed.

Pulseless electrical activity is commonly the result of a marked decrease in cardiac output because of (1) hypovolemia, (2) obstruction to blood flow, or (3) dysfunction of the myocardium or electrical conduction system or both from a variety of causes, resulting in ventricular contractions too weak to produce a detectable pulse and blood pressure (pseudo-electromechanical dissociation).

The ECG rhythms encountered in pulseless electrical activity include:
- Organized electrical activity with narrow QRS complexes
- Wide-QRS-complex dysrhythmia, such as idioventricular rhythms and ventricular escape rhythms
- Significant bradycardias

Pulseless electrical activity can occur in the following conditions:

Narrow-QRS-Complex:
- Hypovolemia from acute blood loss (hemorrhagic shock secondary to trauma or other causes, such as ruptured abdominal aortic aneurysm or gastrointestinal hemorrhage) or from anaphylaxis-related vasodilation
- Obstruction of blood flow to or from the heart (tension pneumothorax or severe pulmonary embolization)
- Cardiac tamponade
- Cardiac rupture
- Drug overdose from tricyclic antidepressants, beta-blockers, and calcium channel blockers

Wide-QRS-Complex:
Massive acute MI
Following cardiac defibrillation (postdefibrillation idioventricular rhythms)
- Hypoxemia
- Severe acidosis
- Excessive vagal tone or loss of sympathetic tone
- Digitalis toxicity
- Hyperkalemia
- Hypothermia

Indications for Treatment

Treatment of pulseless electrical activity is indicated immediately.

Treatment

Rescuer One:
1. Assess the patient's responsiveness.
2. If unresponsive, perform CPR until the defibrillation pads are applied.

Rescuer Two:
1. Apply the defibrillation pads.
2. Determine the ECG rhythm on the ECG monitor. Verify that pulseless rhythm exists (PEA). If the PEA dysrhythmia is a tachycardia, then cardioversion or defibrillation is indicated (follow V-Tach algorithm).
3. Resume CPR for five cycles.
4. Analyze rhythm. Check pulse. If pulse present, go to post resuscitation management.
5. If PEA present, resume CPR for five cycles
6. If VF/VT present, go to VF/VT management

7. If asystole is present, go to asystole management.
8. Repeat steps 3-7 while accomplishing the following:
9. Secure airway and confirm placement with minimal interruptions to CPR.
10. Establish vascular (*IV,* intravenous; *IO,* intraosseous) access; with minimal interruptions to CPR.
11. Attempt to determine the cause (6Hs and 5Ts) of the pulseless electrical activity and treat it, if possible:
    - **Hypovolemia**—administer 250 to 500 cc of **normal saline** bolus, repeat as needed
    - **Hypoxia**—ensure adequate oxygenation
    - **Hydrogen Ion-Acidosis**—ensure adequate ventilation
    - **Hyperkalemia/Hypokalemia**—correct with appropriate electrolyte
    - **Hypothermia**—rewarming
    - **Hypoglycemia**
    - **Toxins/drug overdose**—administer antidote
    - **Tamponade-cardiac**—pericardiocentesis
    - **Tension pneumothorax**—needle decompression
    - **Thrombosis**—myocardial infarction or pulmonary embolism
    - **Toxins**—antidote if available
12. Administer vasopressin 40 U IV/IO; one time only
    OR
    Administer epinephrine 1 mg IV/IO; repeat every 3 to 5 min.
13. Continue CPR for 30 to 60 seconds after each drug administration before defibrillation. Give drug early in chest compression cycle to ensure sufficient time for drug to enter circulatory system.
14. If hyperkalemia, acidosis, or tricyclic antidepressant overdose suspected:
    Administer 1 mEq/kg sodium bicarbonate IV/IO bolus, repeat 0.5 mEq/kg boluses of sodium bicarbonate IV/IO every 10 minutes as needed based on blood gas analysis.

POSTRESUSCITATION MANAGEMENT

Once a pulse is regained following cardiac arrest, it is imperative that the patient be treated aggressively to prevent them from suffering another arrest. The greatest period for another arrest is during the minutes following a successful resuscitation.

When return of spontaneous circulation (ROSC) occurs, the initial objectives of postresuscitation care are to:
- Optimize cardiopulmonary function and systemic perfusion, especially perfusion to the brain
- Transport the victim of out-of-hospital cardiac arrest or hospital emergency department (ED) to an appropriately equipped critical care unit

- Try to identify the precipitating causes of the arrest.
- Institute measures to prevent recurrence
- Institute measures that may improve long-term, neurologically intact survival

Airway
- Ensure airway is properly secured and patient is easy to ventilate
- Assess pulse oximetry continuously
- Maintain end-tidal CO_2 between 35 to 45 mm Hg. If less than 35, slow ventilation rate. If greater than 45, increase ventilation rate.

Circulation
- Assess presence of pulses and attempt to obtain blood pressure
- If hypotension and *signs and symptoms of shock are present*:
Systolic blood pressure less than 70 mm Hg:
Start an IV infusion of norepinephrine at an initial rate of 0.5 to 1 µg/min and adjust the rate of infusion up to 8 to 30 µg/min to increase the systolic blood pressure to 70 to 100 mm Hg.
OR
Systolic blood pressure 70 to 100 mm Hg:
Start an IV infusion of dopamine at an initial rate of 2 to 10 µg/kg/min, and adjust the rate of infusion up to 20 µg/kg/min to increase the systolic blood pressure to 90 to 100 mm Hg or greater.
- If hypertensive, monitor frequently

Neurologic
- Assess level of consciousness
- Sedate patient if combative and in danger of dislodging airway

Metabolic
- Obtain blood glucose and administer D50 if less than 70, administer insulin if greater than 200.

Temperature Control
- Do not attempt to warm patient unless severe hypothermia is the suspected cause of the arrest
- Consider induced hypothermia if hospital is equipped to perform

Rate and Rhythm Control
- If a symptomatic postdefibrillation dysrhythmia is present:
- Refer to the appropriate algorithm for treatment
- If rhythm was converted with the administration of an antidysrhythmic, consider continuation of an infusion of that agent.
- Consider prophylactic administration of an antidysrhythmic agent.

SUMMARY OF DYSRHYTHMIA TREATMENT

Part I

Bradycardias
Sinus Bradycardia
Sinus Arrest/Sinoatrial (SA) Exit Block
Second-Degree, Type I AV Block (Wenckebach)
Second-Degree, 2:1 and Advanced AV Block With Narrow QRS Complexes
Third-Degree AV Block With Narrow QRS Complexes
1. Oxygen
2. Atropine sulfate
AND/OR
Transcutaneous pacing
3. Dopamine or epinephrine infusion
4. Transvenous pacemaker
Second-Degree, Type II AV Block
Second-Degree, 2:1 and Advanced AV Block With Wide QRS Complexes
Third-Degree AV Block With Wide QRS Complexes
1. Oxygen
2. Transcutaneous pacing
3. Dopamine or epinephrine infusion
4. Transvenous pacemaker
Junctional Escape Rhythm
Ventricular Escape Rhythm
1. Oxygen
2. Transcutaneous pacing
3. Dopamine or epinephrine infusion
Tachycardias
Sinus Tachycardia
Atrial Tachycardia With Block
1. No specific treatment
2. Treat underlying cause
3. Discontinue any responsible drugs
Narrow-QRS-Complex Tachycardia of Unknown Origin (With Pulse)
1. Oxygen
2. Vagal maneuvers
3. Adenosine
4. Determine if dysrhythmia is:
   - Paroxysmal supraventricular tachycardia (PSVT)
   - Atrial tachycardia without block
   - Junctional tachycardia
   - Atrial flutter/fibrillation
Atrial Tachycardia Without Block
1. Oxygen
2. Diltiazem or beta-blocker (esmolol, atenolol, or metoprolol), or amiodarone
Paroxysmal Supraventricular Tachycardia (PSVT) With Narrow QRS Complexes
1. Oxygen
2. Vagal maneuvers

3. Adenosine, diltiazem, or beta-blocker (esmolol, atenolol, or metoprolol)
4. Digoxin
5. Cardioversion
Junctional Tachycardia
1. Oxygen
2. Amiodarone or beta-blocker (esmolol, atenolol, or metoprolol)
Atrial Flutter/Atrial Fibrillation
Treatment to Control the Heart Rate
1. Oxygen
2. Beta-blocker (esmolol, atenolol, or metoprolol) or diltiazem
3. Digoxin
Treatment to Convert the Rhythm
Atrial Fibrillation <48 Hours
1. Oxygen
2. Ibutilide, amiodarone, or procainamide
3. Cardioversion
Atrial Fibrillation >48 Hours or of Unknown Duration
1. Oxygen
2. Delay cardioversion until the patient is anticoagulated and atrial thrombi are excluded
3. Cardioversion and amiodarone if patient unstable
Wide-QRS-Complex Tachycardia of Unknown Origin (With Pulse)
1. Oxygen
2. Cardioversion
3. Adenosine or amiodarone
Ventricular Tachycardia (VT), Monomorphic (With Pulse)
1. Oxygen
2. Cardioversion
3. Amiodarone, lidocaine, or procainamide
Ventricular Tachycardia (VT), Polymorphic (With Pulse)-Normal Baseline QT Interval
1. Oxygen
2. Correct any electrolyte imbalance
3. Cardioversion
4. Beta-blocker (esmolol, atenolol, or metoprolol) (if ventricular tachycardia is associated with an acute coronary syndrome)
5. Amiodarone, lidocaine, or procainamide
Ventricular Tachycardia (VT), Polymorphic (With Pulse)-Prolonged Baseline QT Interval Torsades de Pointes (TdP) (With Pulse)
1. Oxygen
2. Correct any electrolyte imbalance
3. Magnesium sulfate
4. Transcutaneous overdrive pacing and beta-blocker (esmolol, atenolol, or metoprolol)
5. Defibrillation
6. Defibrillation
7. Discontinue amiodarone, procainamide, beta-blockers, or agents that prolong QT interval
Premature Ectopic Beats
Premature Atrial Complexes (PACs) Premature Junctional Complexes (PJCs)

1. Discontinue any stimulants and sympathomimetic drugs.
2. Withhold digitalis (if digitalis toxicity is suspected)
3. Digibind if digitalis toxicity confirmed

Premature Ventricular Complexes (PVCs)
1. Oxygen
2. Identify and correct any underlying causes of the PVCs.
3. Consider one of the following:
   - Beta-blocker (esmolol, atenolol, or metoprolol) (if PVCs are associated with an acute coronary syndrome)
   - Amiodarone
   - Lidocaine
   - Procainamide

Part II

Cardiac Arrest
Ventricular Fibrillation/Pulseless Ventricular Tachycardia (VF/VT)
   Unmonitored/monitored cardiac arrest:
1. CPR
2. Defibrillation

3. Vasopressin or epinephrine
4. Amiodarone
5. Magnesium sulfate (if torsades de pointes is present and/or hypomagnesemia suspected)

Ventricular Asystole
   Unmonitored/monitored cardiac arrest:
1. CPR
2. Vasopressin or epinephrine

Pulseless Electrical Activity
   Unmonitored/monitored cardiac arrest:
1. CPR
2. Vasopressin or epinephrine
3. Treat underlying cause, if known

Drugs Used to Treat Dysrhythmias
(Table 10-1)

TABLE 10-1 **Drugs Used to Treat Dysrhythmias**

Drug	Class
Adenosine (Adenocard)	Antidysrhythmic agent
Amiodarone (Cordarone)	Antidysrhythmic agent
Atropine sulfate	Anticholinergic agent
Beta-blocker Atenolol (Tenormin), esmolol HCL (Brevibloc), metoprolol (Toprol, Lopressor)	Beta-adrenergic blocking agent
Diazepam (Valium)	Tranquilizer, amnesiac, sedative
Digoxin (Lanoxin)	Antidysrhythmic agent, inotropic agent, digitalis glycoside
Diltiazem (Cardizem)	Calcium channel blocker
Dobutamine (Dobutrex)	Adrenergic agent
Dopamine (Intropin)	Adrenergic (sympathomimetic) agent
Epinephrine (Adrenalin Chloride)	Adrenergic (sympathomimetic) agent
Ibutilide (Corvert)	Antiadysrhythmic agent
Lidocaine (Xylocaine)	Antidysrhythmic agent
Magnesium sulfate	Electrolyte
Midazolam (Versed)	Sedative, tranquilizer, amnesiac
Morphine sulfate	Narcotic, analgesic
Nitroglycerin (Nitrostat, Nitrol, Tridil, etc.)	Antianginal agent, vasodilator
Norepinephrine (Levophed)	Adrenergic (sympathomimetic) agent
Procainamide (Pronestyl)	Antidysrhythmic agent
Vasopressin	Vasoconstrictor

DYSRHYTHMIA TREATMENT ALGORITHMS

Part I

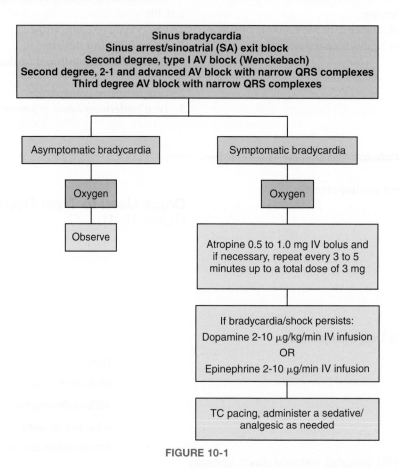

FIGURE 10-1

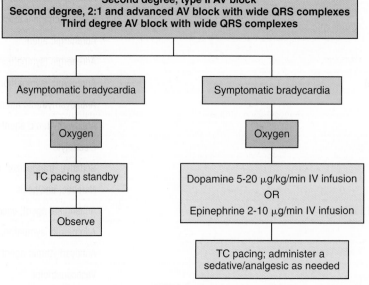

FIGURE 10-2

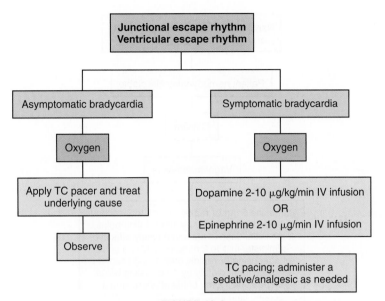

FIGURE 10-3

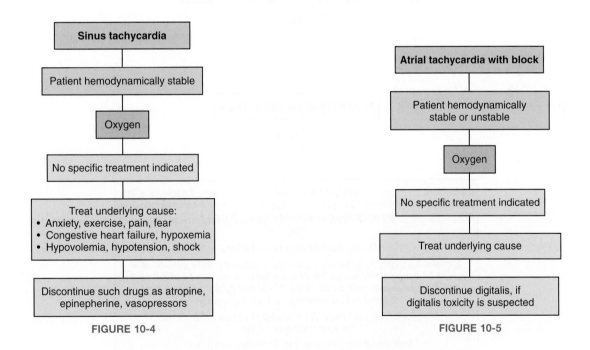

FIGURE 10-4

FIGURE 10-5

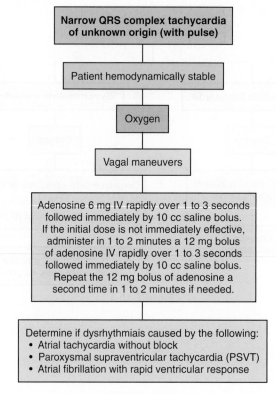

FIGURE 10-6

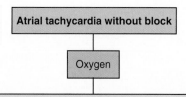

FIGURE 10-7

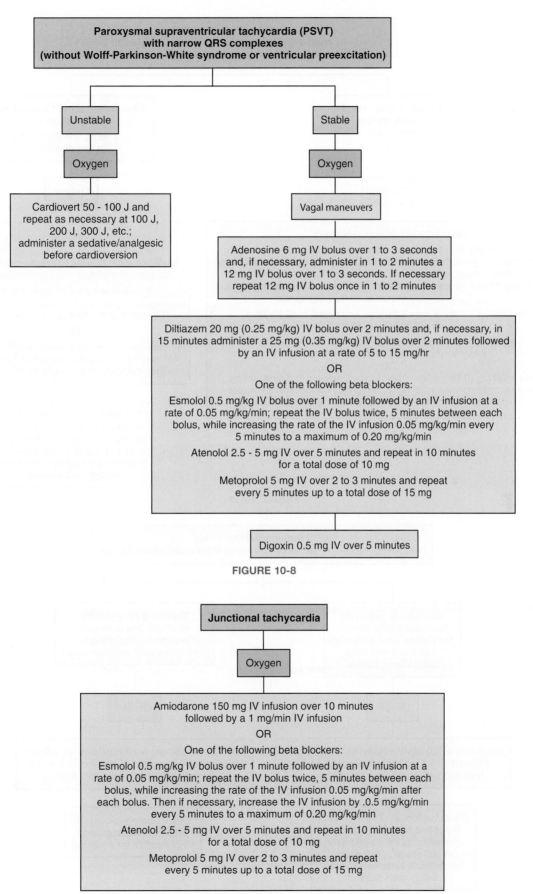

FIGURE 10-8

FIGURE 10-9

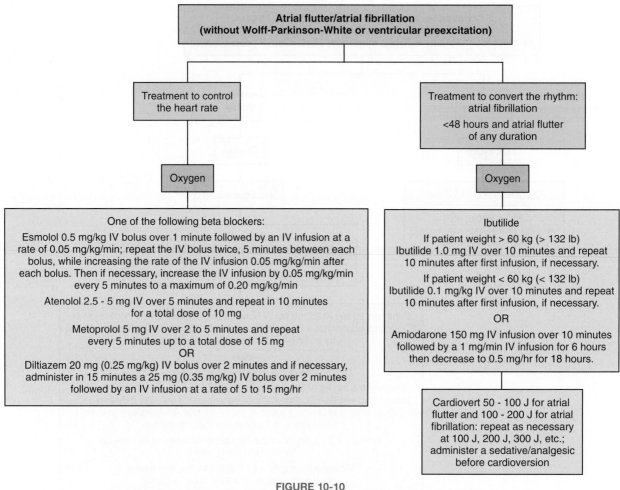

FIGURE 10-10

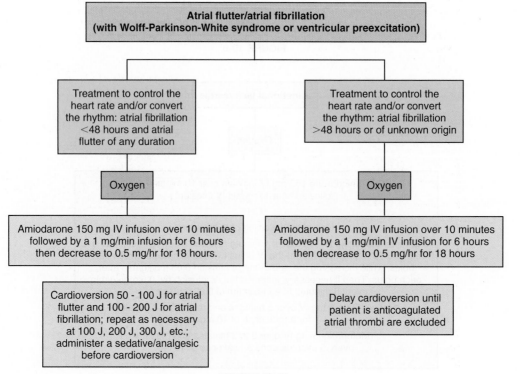

FIGURE 10-11

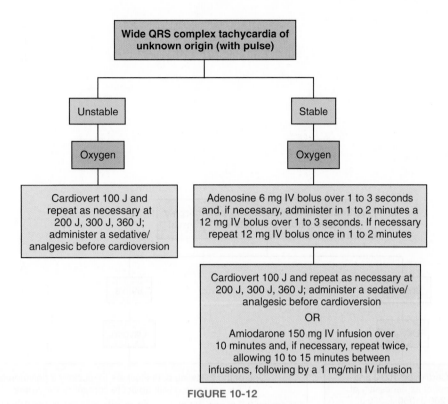

FIGURE 10-12

FIGURE 10-13

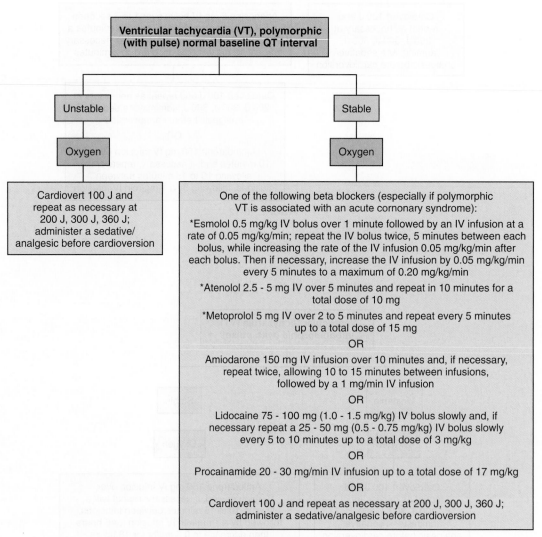

Ventricular tachycardia (VT), polymorphic (with pulse) normal baseline QT interval

Unstable

Oxygen

Cardiovert 100 J and repeat as necessary at 200 J, 300 J, 360 J; administer a sedative/ analgesic before cardioversion

Stable

Oxygen

One of the following beta blockers (especially if polymorphic VT is associated with an acute coronary syndrome):

*Esmolol 0.5 mg/kg IV bolus over 1 minute followed by an IV infusion at a rate of 0.05 mg/kg/min; repeat the IV bolus twice, 5 minutes between each bolus, while increasing the rate of the IV infusion 0.05 mg/kg/min after each bolus. Then if necessary, increase the IV infusion by 0.05 mg/kg/min every 5 minutes to a maximum of 0.20 mg/kg/min

*Atenolol 2.5 - 5 mg IV over 5 minutes and repeat in 10 minutes for a total dose of 10 mg

*Metoprolol 5 mg IV over 2 to 5 minutes and repeat every 5 minutes up to a total dose of 15 mg

OR

Amiodarone 150 mg IV infusion over 10 minutes and, if necessary, repeat twice, allowing 10 to 15 minutes between infusions, followed by a 1 mg/min IV infusion

OR

Lidocaine 75 - 100 mg (1.0 - 1.5 mg/kg) IV bolus slowly and, if necessary repeat a 25 - 50 mg (0.5 - 0.75 mg/kg) IV bolus slowly every 5 to 10 minutes up to a total dose of 3 mg/kg

OR

Procainamide 20 - 30 mg/min IV infusion up to a total dose of 17 mg/kg

OR

Cardiovert 100 J and repeat as necessary at 200 J, 300 J, 360 J; administer a sedative/analgesic before cardioversion

FIGURE 10-14

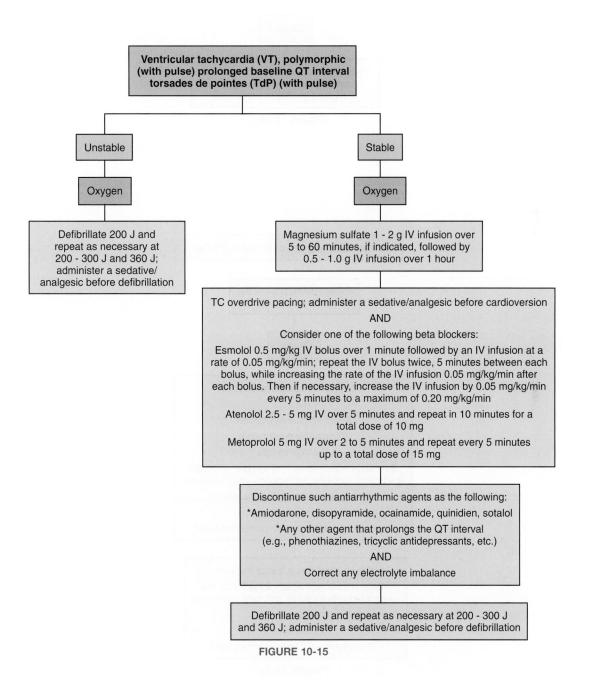

FIGURE 10-15

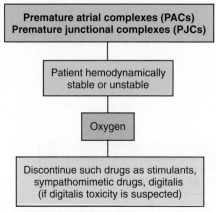

FIGURE 10-16

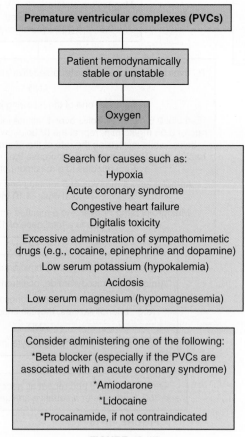

FIGURE 10-17

Part II

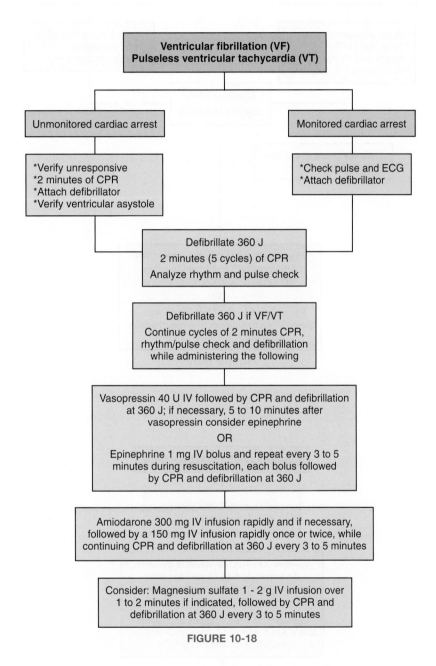

FIGURE 10-18

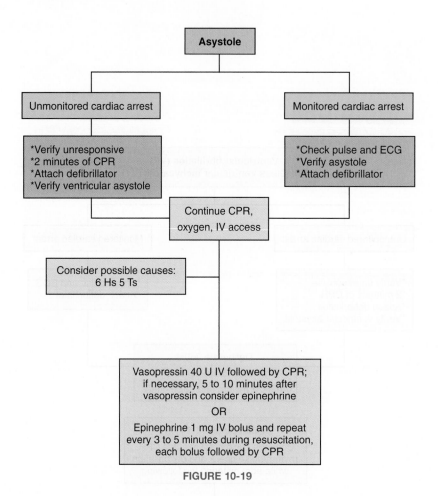

FIGURE 10-19

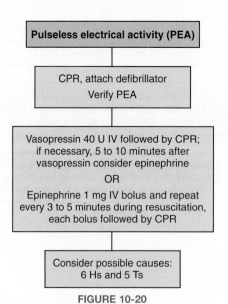

FIGURE 10-20

CHAPTER REVIEW

1. In an unstable patient with symptomatic bradycardia and an ECG showing a second-degree, type II AV block, you should administer oxygen, start an IV line, and administer or begin:
   A. a dopamine drip
   B. atropine
   C. lidocaine
   D. transcutaneous pacing

2. Patients with symptomatic sinus tachycardia should be treated with:
   A. appropriate treatment for the underlying cause of the tachycardia
   B. diltiazem
   C. dopamine
   D. epinephrine

3. If a patient is stable with an ECG showing PSVT after administering oxygen and starting an IV line, you should:
   A. administer adenosine
   B. administer diazepam
   C. administer diltiazem
   D. attempt vagal maneuvers

4. Your patient presents with chest pain and signs and symptoms of an acute MI. His ECG shows atrial tachycardia without a block. After administering oxygen and starting an IV line you should immediately consider:
   A. a cardioversion of 50 J
   B. a loading dose of amiodarone
   C. an adenosine bolus
   D. transcutaneous pacing

5. The administration of adenosine for a narrow complex tachycardia
   A. may reveal the underlying rhythm to be atrial fibrillation or atrial flutter
   B. must be administered slowly to avoid hypotension
   C. should only be performed if the diagnosis of SVT is known
   D. will always convert SVT to normal sinus rhythm

6. A patient with atrial fibrillation of less than 48 hours in duration, who is hemodynamically unstable and hypotensive, should be treated as follows:
   A. amiodarone alone
   B. ibutilide followed by DC cardioversion
   C. immediate DC cardioversion and amiodarone
   D. immediate DC cardioversion or amiodarone

7. Your patient is conscious and hemodynamically stable with a pulse and an ECG showing monomorphic ventricular tachycardia. After administering oxygen and starting an IV you should:
   A. administer 1 mg of epinephrine
   B. administer a 150-mg loading dose of amiodarone IV
   C. deliver a cardioversion of 100 J
   D. start an infusion of epinephrine

8. If your patient in question No. 7 begins to complain of chest pain and then becomes pulseless, you should immediately:
   A. administer a lidocaine bolus
   B. begin transcutaneous pacing
   C. deliver a cardioversion of 100 J biphasic
   D. deliver defibrillation of 360 J monomorphic or 200 J biphasic

9. Pulseless electrical activity may occur with which of the following rhythms:
   A. asystole
   B. sinus tachycardia
   C. ventricular fibrillation
   D. ventricular tachycardia

10. Once return of spontaneous circulation has been restored following a successful cardiac arrest resuscitation the primary goal becomes:
    A. ensuring a patent airway is present
    B. obtaining additional vascular access
    C. rapid rewarming
    D. treatment of the underlying cause of the arrest to prevent recurrence

The 12-Lead Electrocardiogram

OBJECTIVES *Upon completion of this chapter, you should be able to complete the following objectives:*

1. Discuss the purpose of the 12-lead ECG and the clinical role it plays.
2. List the leads of a 12-lead ECG and indicate which are unipolar and which are bipolar.
3. Define the following terms:
   - Lead
   - Lead axis
   - Perpendicular axis
   - Frontal and horizontal planes
4. Describe how the 6 limb leads of a 12-lead ECG are obtained.
5. Identify the sites of attachment of the electrodes for the 6 precordial leads of a 12-lead ECG on an anatomical drawing of the chest, and indicate over which region of the heart each electrode lies.
6 Explain how (1) the triaxial reference figures for the standard (bipolar) limb leads and the augmented (unipolar) leads, (2) the hexaxial reference figure, and (3) the precordial reference figure are derived.
7. Identify the right-sided chest leads, the sites of their attachment, and the indication for their use.
8. List the facing leads that view the following surfaces of the heart:
   - Anterior
   - Lateral
   - Inferior (or diaphragmatic)
   - Right ventricle

THE 12-LEAD ECG

The 12-lead ECG is used to obtain additional information from the electrical activity of the heart, discussed in previous chapters, to diagnose the presence of cardiac dysrhythmias. The 12-lead ECG, as its name implies, consist of 12-leads that examine the heart simultaneously from multiple angles. This allows the clinician to more closely examine the electrical activity of the heart and the various conditions that can alter it.

The primary role of the 12-lead ECG is to detect the presence of myocardial ischemia and infarction. The specific 12-lead ECG finding associated with these conditions will be discussed in chapter 17.

Another role of the 12-lead ECG is to assist in the differentiation of certain dysrhythmias, which can have very similar appearances in lead II (the most common lead used to interpret dysrhythmias).

THE 12-LEAD ECG LEADS

KEY DEFINITION

A 12-lead (or conventional) echocardiogram (ECG) consists of the following:
- Six limb or extremity leads
  - Three standard (bipolar) limb leads: leads I, II, and III
  - Three augmented (unipolar) leads: leads aVR, aVL, and aVF
- Six precordial (unipolar) leads: leads V_1, V_2, V_3, V_4, V_5, and V_6

The monitoring of leads I, II, and III was discussed in Chapter 2. The same three leads are used in a 12-lead ECG (Figure 11-1) and are obtained using a *positive electrode* and a *negative electrode* to detect the electrical current generated by the depolarization and repolarization of the heart. An additional electrode, the *ground electrode*, is often attached to the right leg (or any other location on the body) to provide a path of least resistance for electrical interference in the body. The three bipolar limb leads—I, II, and III—detect the heart's electrical activity by using two electrodes, one positive and the other negative, attached to the extremities (Figure 11-2, *A*). A bipolar lead thus represents the difference in electrical potential (or voltage) between the two electrodes.

Unipolar Leads

A lead that has only one electrode (which is positive) is called a *unipolar lead*. It does not have a corresponding negative lead but instead the "view" of the electrode is in relation to a reference point calculated by the ECG machine. This point is located in the center of the heart's electrical field and is referred to as the *central terminal*. It is theoretically located in the heart, left of the interventricular septum and below the atrioventricular (AV) junction.

> The central terminal is *not* an actual lead or electrode but is instead an imaginary point of "electrical neutrality" calculated by the ECG machine. It is the sum of the electrical activity of the leads *not* being examined and therefore can be considered a reference point. While it may appear labeled on figures, it is not an actual physical location or lead.

The three unipolar augmented limb leads—aVR, aVL, and aVF—detect the electrical potential between a positive electrode attached to one of three extremities and the central terminal (Figure 11-2, *B*). The central terminal used in the augmented leads (the "a" in these leads stands for "augmented") is one obtained by combining the electrical currents from the two electrodes other than the one being used as the positive electrode. For example, when the patient's right arm electrode is used as the positive electrode, the central terminal is formed by joining, or augmenting, the electrical currents obtained from the electrodes on the patient's left arm and left leg. These three unipolar leads thus measure the difference in electrical potential between a positive electrode and the common terminal.

The six unipolar precordial, or chest, leads—V_1, V_2, V_3, V_4, V_5, and V_6—detect the heart's electrical current using a positive electrode attached to one of six specified locations on the anterior chest wall and the central terminal (Figure 11-2, *C*). The central terminal used in the precordial leads, unlike that in the augmented limb leads, is obtained by combining the electrical currents from the electrodes attached to the right and left arms and left leg.

> The limb leads *must* be attached to the patient to record the precordial leads. If the electrodes are loose, the central terminal cannot be calculated by the machine.

Lead Axis

Each lead of the 12-lead ECG measures the difference in electrical potential between the positive and negative electrodes or central terminal. Thus each lead has a positive and negative pole.

A hypothetical line joining the poles of a lead is known as the axis of the lead (or lead axis) (Figure 11-3, p. 184). The axis runs from the negative to the positive pole of the lead. The location of the positive and negative poles in a lead determines the orientation (or direction) of the axis of the lead.

In addition, each lead axis has a perpendicular axis, or, simply, the *perpendicular*. It is usually depicted as a line intersecting or connecting with the lead axis at ± 90 degrees (or a right angle), midway along the axis between the two poles. This is considered the "zero" point of the lead axis. The perpendicular divides the lead axis into two halves or quadrants. The positive quadrant is that half on the side of the perpendicular closest to the positive pole. The negative quadrant is that half on the side closest to the negative pole. This will become important when examining QRS complexes and deciding which side of the lead axis perpendicular they are pointing to obtain the electrical axis of the heart. This will be discussed in chapter 12.

Frontal and Horizontal Planes

The three standard limb leads (I, II, and III) and the three augmented leads (aVR, aVL, and aVF) measure the electrical activity of the heart in the two-dimensional *frontal plane* (i.e., viewed from the front of the patient's body) (Figure 11-4, p. 183). The six precordial leads (V_1, V_2, V_3, V_4, V_5, and V_6) measure the electrical activity of the heart at a right angle to the frontal plane, the *horizontal plane*. The center of each of the radiating points on both the frontal and horizontal planes is the previously described central terminal.

Standard (Bipolar) Limb Leads

Each of the standard limb leads I, II, and III is obtained using a positive electrode attached to one of two extremities (left arm or left leg) and a single negative electrode attached to another extremity (right or left arm) (Figure 11-5, p. 184). Thus each standard limb lead measures the difference in electrical potential between two extremity electrodes.

The electrodes are attached as follows to obtain the three standard limb leads:

- Lead I: The positive electrode is attached to the left arm and the negative electrode to the right arm
- Lead II: The positive electrode is attached to the left leg and the negative electrode to the right arm
- Lead III: The positive electrode is attached to the left leg and the negative electrode to the left arm

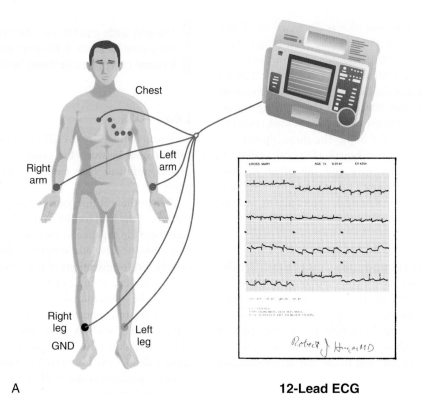

A

12-Lead ECG

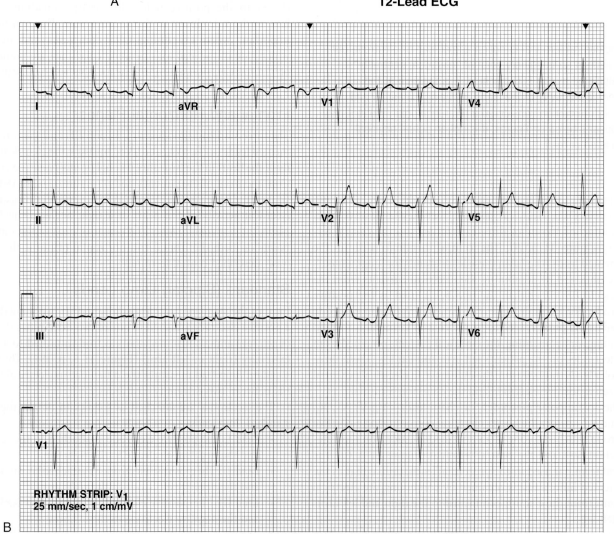

B

FIGURE 11-1 **A,** The 12-lead ECG. **B,** 12-lead ECG printout with a lead V₁, rhythm strip.

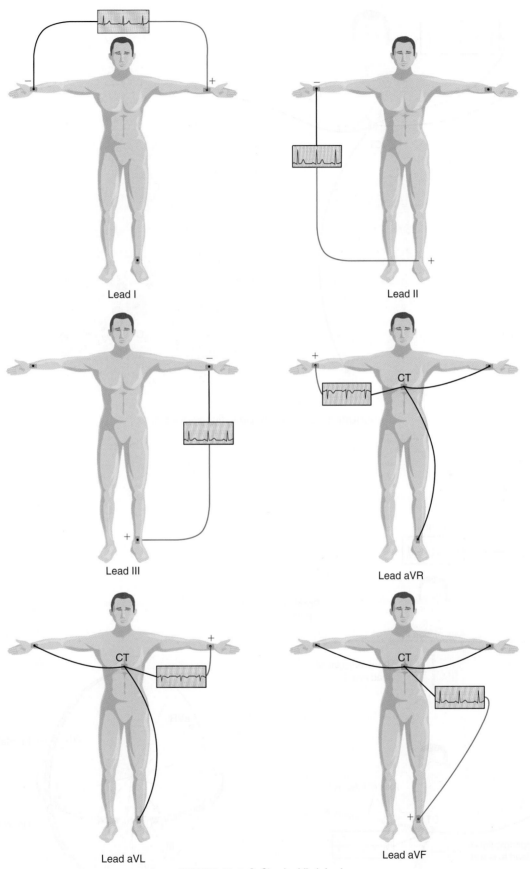

FIGURE 11-2 A, Standard limb leads.

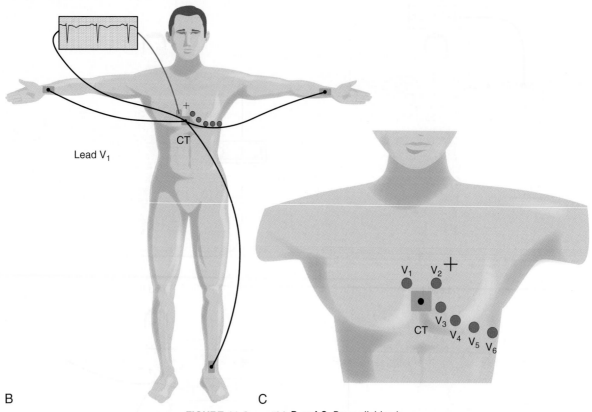

B

C

FIGURE 11-2, cont'd B and C, Precordial leads.

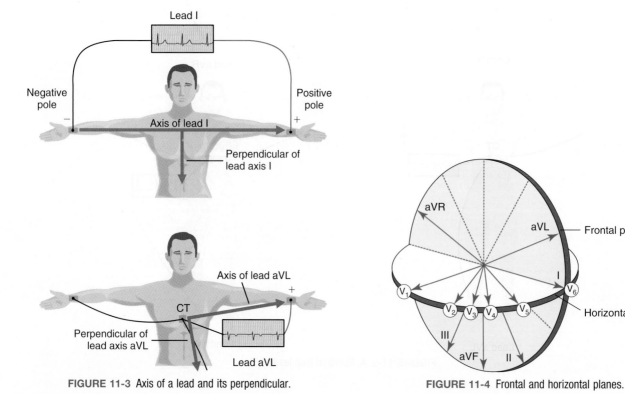

FIGURE 11-3 Axis of a lead and its perpendicular.

FIGURE 11-4 Frontal and horizontal planes.

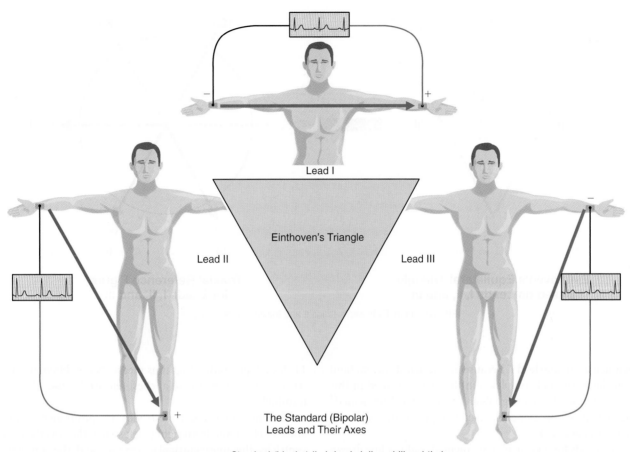

FIGURE 11-5 Standard (bipolar) limb leads I, II, and III and their axes.

The lead axis for each standard limb lead is a line drawn between the two extremity electrodes, with one electrode designated as the negative pole and the other as the positive pole. The perpendicular divides the lead axis into a positive and a negative half.

The relationships of the standard limb leads are such that the sum of the electrical currents recorded in leads I and III equals the sum of the electrical current recorded in lead II. This is called *Einthoven's law*, named after the developer of three-lead electrocardiography.

Einthoven's law is expressed mathematically as follows:

$$\text{Lead I} + \text{Lead III} = \text{Lead II}$$

Because the positive electrodes of the three standard limb leads are electrically about the same distance from the zero reference point in the heart, an equilateral triangle (Einthoven's equilateral triangle) can be depicted in the body's frontal plane using the three lead axes, with the heart and its zero reference point in the center (Figure 11-6). The three sides of the equilateral triangle can be shifted to the right, left, and down without changing the angle of their orientation until their midpoints intersect at the same point. This creates a standard limb lead triaxial reference figure, with each of the lead axis of the standard limb leads forming a 60-degree angle with its neighbors. The positive terminal of Lead I is 0°, Lead II is +60°, and Lead

III is +120°. The negative halves of the lead axis are usually depicted as dotted or dashed lines as shown in Figure 11-6.

Augmented (Unipolar) Leads

The augmented leads aVR, aVL, and aVF are obtained using a positive electrode attached to one of three extremities (right arm, left arm, or right leg) and the central terminal obtained from the other two extremity electrodes (Figure 11-7, *A*). Thus an augmented lead measures the difference in electrical potential between one of three extremity electrodes and the central terminal.

The three extremity electrodes are attached as follows to obtain the three augmented leads:

- Lead aVR: The positive electrode is attached to the right arm and the negative electrode to the central terminal (left arm and left leg)
- Lead aVL: The positive electrode is attached to the left arm and the negative electrode to the central terminal (right arm and left leg)
- Lead aVF: The positive electrode is attached to the left leg and the negative electrode to the central terminal (right and left arms)

In reality the augmented unipolar leads are the perpendicular lead axis of the limb leads. aVR is perpendicular to limb lead III. aVL is perpendicular to limb lead II. And, aVF is

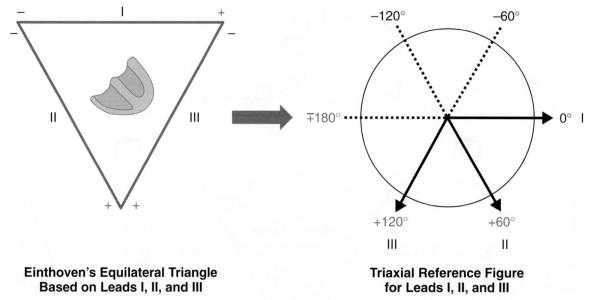

**Einthoven's Equilateral Triangle
Based on Leads I, II, and III**

**Triaxial Reference Figure
for Leads I, II, and III**

FIGURE 11-6 Einthoven's triangle and triaxial reference figure.

perpendicular to limb lead I. Because the electrical current (and size) of the waves and complexes in the ECG obtained in this manner are so small, these signals are increased or "augmented" by the ECG machine. Hence the name "augmented," for the "a" in aVR, aVL, and aVF.

The lead axis for a particular augmented lead is a line drawn between the central terminal and its extremity electrode, with the central terminal designated as the negative pole and the extremity electrode as the positive pole.

The positive electrodes of the three augmented leads, like those of the three standard limb leads, are also electrically equidistant from the zero reference point in the heart. The augmented lead triaxial reference figure (Figure 11-7, *B*) formed in the body's frontal plane by the axes of the three augmented leads is similar to that of the standard limb leads, with its lead axes 60 degrees apart but oriented around the zero reference point at slightly different angles. The augmented lead axis is usually depicted with its negative half extended as a dotted, dashed, or shaded line.

When the triaxial reference figures of the standard limb leads and the augmented leads are superimposed, they form a hexaxial reference figure (Figure 11-8). Each augmented lead axis is perpendicular to a standard limb lead axis, so that each lead axis is spaced 30 degrees apart. Chapter 12 will present a more comprehensive discussion of the electrical axis of the heart of methods to calculate it.

Precordial (Unipolar) Leads

The precordial leads V_1, V_2, V_3, V_4, V_5, and V_6 are unipolar leads obtained by attaching the positive electrode to prescribed areas over the anterior chest wall (Figure 11-9, *A*) and the negative lead of the central terminal, which in this case is made by combining all three extremity electrodes together: the right and left arm electrodes and the left leg electrode as shown in Figure

11-2, *C*. A precordial lead thus measures the difference in electrical potential between a chest electrode and the central terminal.

The individual chest electrodes are positioned across the anterior chest wall from right to left so that they overlie the right ventricle, the interventricular septum, and the anterior and lateral surfaces of the left ventricle. The placement of the chest electrodes is as follows:

- V_1: Right side of the sternum in the fourth intercostal space
- V_2: Left side of the sternum in the fourth intercostal space
- V_3: Midway between V_2 and V_4
- V_4: Left midclavicular line in the fifth intercostal space
- V_5: Left anterior axillary line at the same level as V_4
- V_6: Left midaxillary line at the same level as V_4

The chest electrodes for leads V_1 and V_2 (the right precordial [or septal] leads) overlie the right ventricle; the electrodes for leads V_3 and V_4 (the mid-precordial [or anterior] leads) overlie the interventricular septum and part of the left ventricle; and those for leads V_5 and V_6 (the left precordial [or lateral] leads) overlie the rest of the left ventricle.

The lead axis for each precordial lead is drawn from the central terminal to the specific chest electrode, with the central terminal designated as the negative pole, and the electrode as the positive pole (Figure 11-9, *B*). A transverse (cross-sectional) outline of the chest wall showing the central terminal, the six chest electrodes, and the six precordial lead axes is called a *precordial reference figure*. It is used in plotting the heart's electrical activity in the body's horizontal plane.

Right-Sided Chest Leads

The precordial leads of the 12-lead ECG record the heart's electrical activity primarily over the left ventricle. To determine the electrical activity over the right ventricle, right-sided chest leads

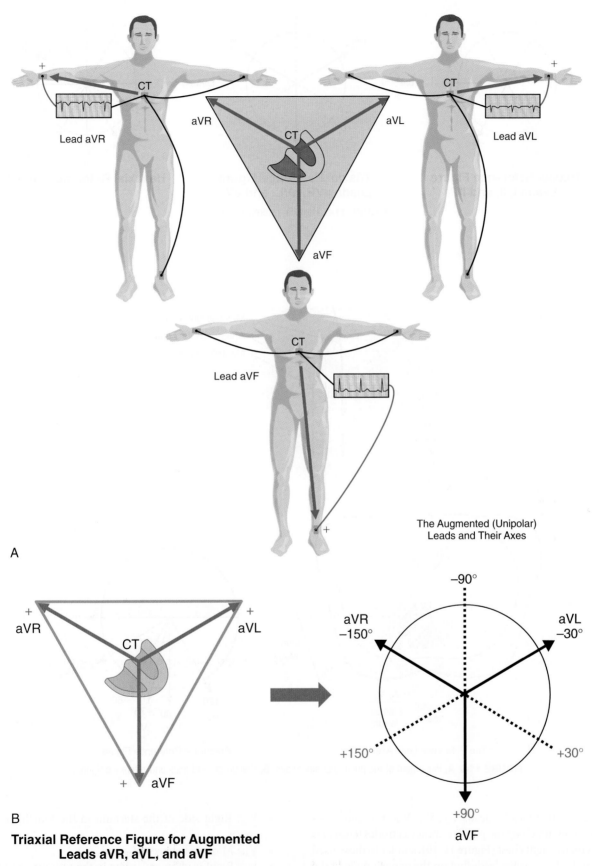

The Augmented (Unipolar)
Leads and Their Axes

A

B

**Triaxial Reference Figure for Augmented
Leads aVR, aVL, and aVF**

FIGURE 11-7 **A,** Augmented leads aVR, aVL, and aVF and their axes. **B,** Triaxial reference figure for the augmented leads.

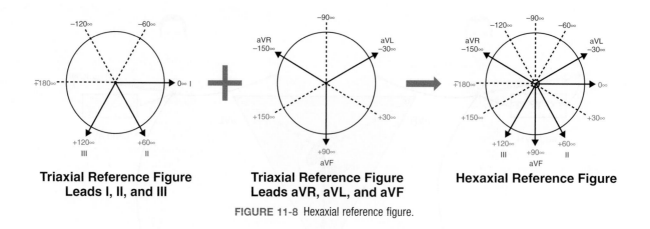

**Triaxial Reference Figure
Leads I, II, and III**

**Triaxial Reference Figure
Leads aVR, aVL, and aVF**

Hexaxial Reference Figure

FIGURE 11-8 Hexaxial reference figure.

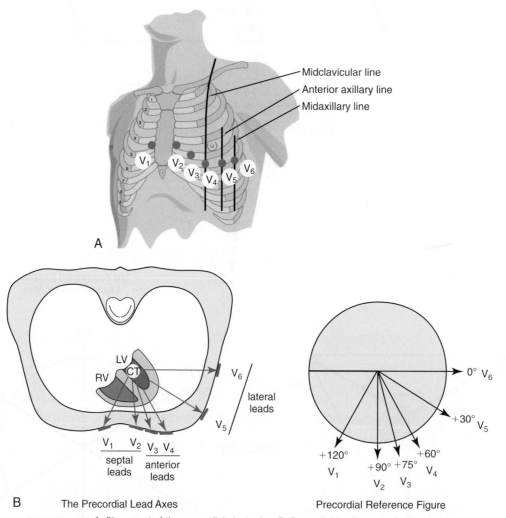

B   The Precordial Lead Axes

Precordial Reference Figure

FIGURE 11-9 A, Placement of the precordial electrodes. **B,** Precordial lead axes and reference figure.

must be used. These leads—leads V_{2R}, V_{3R}, V_{4R}, V_{5R}, and V_{6R}—are obtained by attaching the positive chest electrodes to various locations on the right chest (Figure 11-10), similar to those used in the standard precordial leads, but on the opposite side of the chest. The placement of the positive right-sided chest electrodes is as follows:

- V_{2R}: Right side of the sternum in the fourth intercostal space
- V_{3R}: Midway between V_{2R} and V_{4R}
- V_{4R}: Right midclavicular line in the fifth intercostal space
- V_{5R}: Right anterior axillary line at the same level as V_{4R}
- V_{6R}: Right midaxillary line at the same level as V_{4R}

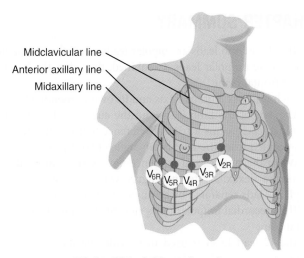

Midclavicular line
Anterior axillary line
Midaxillary line

V₂R
V₆R V₅R V₄R V₃R

Right-Sided Chest Leads

FIGURE 11-10 Right-sided chest leads.

Right-sided chest leads are used to rule out a right ventricular myocardial infarction after the initial finding of an inferior myocardial infarction. In the majority of instances, only one right-sided chest lead, lead V_{4R}, is needed to make the diagnosis. This will be discussed in greater detail in chapter 17.

Facing Leads

A 12-lead ECG provides 12 different views of the electrical activity of the heart, each view looking from the outside of the chest toward the zero reference point within the chest (Table 11-1). Because the left ventricle comprises the largest muscle mass of the heart and represent the predominant electrical component of the QRS complex, the views are referred to from the perspective of the left ventricle.

Leads I and aVL and the precordial leads V_5 and V_6 view the lateral wall of the left ventricle; leads II, III, and aVF view the inferior (diaphragmatic) wall; and leads V_1 through V_4 view the anterior wall of the left ventricle. The right-sided precordial lead—lead V_{4R}—views the right ventricle. No leads face the posterior surface of the heart.

The leads that view specific surfaces of the heart are termed *facing* leads in this book (Figure 11-11). These include all of the

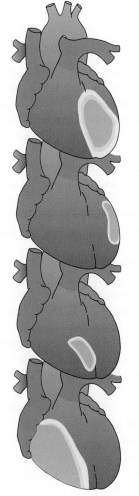

Surface of the Heart Viewed	Facing Leads
Anterior	V_1-V_4
Lateral	I, aVL, V_5-V_6
Inferior	II, III, aVF
Right ventricle	V_{4R}

FIGURE 11-11 The facing leads.

TABLE 11-1 Facing Leads

Facing Leads	Surface of the Heart Viewed
V_1-V_4	Anterior
I, aVL, V_5-V_6	Lateral
II, III, aVF	Inferior (or diaphragmatic)
V_{4R}	Right ventricle

leads except aVR, which faces the interior, endocardial surface of the ventricles.

It is important to know the facing leads in determining the location of an acute myocardial infarction!

CHAPTER SUMMARY

- The three limb leads are bipolar leads while the augmented leads are unipolar leads. Combined, they view the heart in the frontal plane
- Each lead has a unique axis and its own perpendicular
- The axis of the limb leads and the augmented leads when joined each forms a triaxial reference figure with each lead separated from the next by an angle of 60 degrees
- When the two triaxial reference figures are combined they form a hexaxial reference figure with each of the frontal plane leads separated by an angle of 30 degrees
- The precordial unipolar leads view the heart in the horizontal plane
- The 12-lead ECG is used to provide specific views of the heart

CHAPTER REVIEW

1. The electrode attached to the right leg is usually used as the _____ electrode.
   A. ground
   B. negative
   C. probing
   D. sensing

2. A _____ lead represents the difference in electrical potential between a positive and a negative electrode.
   A. bipolar
   B. central
   C. terminal
   D. unipolar

3. In leads aVR, aVL, and aVF, the "a" stands for:
   A. alternative
   B. arterial
   C. atrial
   D. augmented

4. The relationships of the standard limb leads are such that the electrical currents of lead _____ + lead _____ = lead _____.
   A. I, II, III
   B. I, III, II
   C. II, III, I
   D. II, III, IV

5. To obtain lead aVL, the positive electrode is attached to the _____ arm and the other two electrodes to the _____, which, when combined, form the central terminal.
   A. left, right and left arms
   B. left, right arm and left leg
   C. right, left arm and left leg
   D. right, right and left legs

6. A _____ lead measures the difference in electrical potential between a chest electrode and the central terminal.
   A. bipolar
   B. precordial
   C. terminal
   D. unipolar, augmented

7. The placement of the V_4 positive chest electrode is:
   A. in the anterior axillary line at the fifth intercostal space
   B. in the midaxillary line at the sixth intercostal space
   C. left side of the sternum in the fourth intercostal space
   D. midclavicular line in the fifth intercostal space

8. The placement of the V_2 positive chest electrode is:
   A. anterior axillary line at the same level as V_1
   B. left side of the sternum in the fourth intercostal space
   C. midway between V_1 and V_3
   D. right side of the sternum in the fourth intercostal space

9. Correct placement of the V_{6R} positive right-sided chest electrodes is:
   A. midway between V_{2R} and V_{6R}
   B. on the right side of the sternum in the fourth intercostal space
   C. right midaxillary line at the same level as V_{4R}
   D. right midclavicular line in the right fifth intercostal space

10. The _____ surface of the heart is viewed by ECG leads II, III, and aVF.
    A. anterior
    B. inferior
    C. lateral
    D. posterior

12 Electrical Axis and Vectors

OBJECTIVES *Upon completion of this chapter, you should be able to complete the following objectives:*

1. Define the following terms:
   - Vector
   - Mean vector
   - Biphasic deflection
   - Equiphasic deflection
   - Predominantly positive deflection
   - Predominantly negative deflection
2. Define the following terms:
   - Instantaneous electrical axis or vector
   - Cardiac vector
   - Mean QRS axis
   - P axis
   - T axis
3. Identify and label on a hexaxial figure (1) the 12 spokes of the hexaxial figure according to their polarity and degree and (2) the four quadrants.
4. Identify and label the lead axis of the six limb leads, their negative and positive poles, their direction in degrees, and their perpendiculars on a hexaxial figure in the frontal plane.
5. Define the following terms:
   - Normal QRS axis
   - Left axis deviation (LAD)
   - Right axis deviation (RAD)
   - Indeterminate axis (IND)
6. List the cardiac and pulmonary causes of left and right axis deviation.
7. List three major reasons for determining the QRS axis in an emergency situation.
8. List six important points to remember in the process of determining the QRS axis using leads I, II, III, and aVF.
9. List the basic steps in determining the QRS axis using leads I, II, III, and aVF.

ELECTRICAL AXIS AND VECTORS

The electrical current generated by the depolarization or repolarization of the atria or ventricles at any given moment produces an *instantaneous cardiac vector*. It is commonly visualized graphically as an arrow that has magnitude, direction, and polarity (Figure 12-1). The length of the shaft of the arrow represents the magnitude of the electrical current; the orientation or position of the arrow indicates the direction of flow of the electrical current; the tip of the arrow represents the positive pole of the electrical current, and the tail is the negative pole.

The sequence of electrical currents produced by the depolarization of the ventricles during one cardiac cycle, for example, can be depicted as a series of cardiac vectors, each representing

The Cardiac Vector

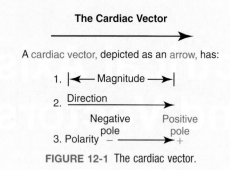

A cardiac vector, depicted as an arrow, has:

1. |◄— Magnitude —►|

2. Direction

3. Polarity

Negative pole　　Positive pole

FIGURE 12-1 The cardiac vector.

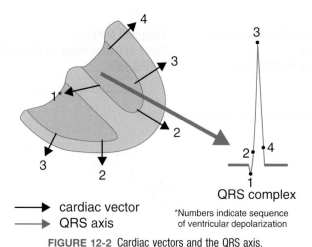

➤ cardiac vector
➤ QRS axis

*Numbers indicate sequence of ventricular depolarization

QRS complex

FIGURE 12-2 Cardiac vectors and the QRS axis.

the moment-to-moment electrical current generated by depolarization of a small segment of the ventricular wall. (Figure 12-2)

The first cardiac vector represents the depolarization of the interventricular septum (1) and is directed from left to right. This is followed immediately by a sequence of vectors flowing from the endocardial to epicardial depolarization of segments of the ventricular wall, beginning in the right and left ventricles in the apical region of the heart near the septum (2), continuing through the thin wall of the right ventricle and the thick lateral wall of the left ventricle (3), and ending in the lateral and posterior aspect of the left ventricle near its base (4).

The vectors arising in the right ventricle are directed mostly to the right when viewed in the frontal plane; those in the left ventricle are directed mostly to the left. The left ventricular vectors are larger and persist longer than those of the smaller right ventricle, primarily because of the greater thickness of the left ventricular wall.

The mean (or average) of all vectors that result from ventricular depolarization is a single large vector depicted as an arrow having a magnitude and a direction—the **mean QRS axis** or, simply, the **QRS axis**. Normally, the QRS axis points to the left and downward, reflecting the dominance of the left ventricle over the right.

The mean of all vectors generated during the depolarization of the atria is the *P axis*; those generated during repolarization of the ventricles are the *T axis* (Figure 12-3).

The P axis is rarely determined. The T axis is determined in certain conditions, such as myocardial ischemia and acute myocardial infarction, in which there is a significant shift in the direction of the T axis. Determination of the shift in the T axis helps to localize the affected area of the myocardium. The QRS axis is the most important and the most frequently determined axis. Commonly, when the term *axis* is used alone, it refers to the QRS axis.

THE ELECTRICAL CURRENT, VECTORS, AND THE LEAD AXIS

An electrical current flowing parallel to or along the axis of a lead, the hypothetical line joining the negative and positive poles of a lead, produces either a positive or negative deflection on an electrocardiogram (ECG), depending on the direction of its flow. An electrical current flowing toward the positive pole produces a positive deflection on the ECG; one that flows toward the negative pole produces a negative deflection. The greater the magnitude of the electrical current, the larger the deflection, and vice versa. When the flow of electrical current is perpendicular to the axis of a lead, no deflection is produced. Figure 12-4, *A* shows the relationship between the direction of flow of an electrical current, as represented by a vector, and the deflection it produces on an ECG.

When an electrical current flows in a direction that is somewhere between being parallel and perpendicular (i.e., oblique), the deflection is smaller than when the same electrical current flows parallel to the axis of a lead. The more parallel the electrical current is to the axis of the lead, the larger is the deflection; the more perpendicular, the smaller the deflection. This is true whether the electrical current is flowing toward or away from the positive pole (Figure 12-4, *B*).

Another way to think of this is to imagine yourself standing on the edge of a train track. As the approaching train sounds its horn, the sound grows loudest if you are directly in the path of the train. The further you move perpendicular to the track and away from the train the sound of the approaching train and the receding train cancel out and the net change in the level of the train noise is zero.

In the heart, there are numerous vectors of current firing in many directions throughout the cardiac cycle. The placement of the lead is analogous to the person standing directly on or at some angle to the track. The difference is that in the heart because there are multiple simultaneous horns sounding (vectors), the ECG lead measures the resulting average of all the vectors (noise) it detects.

When an electrical current flows partly toward and partly away from the positive pole over time, a bidirectional electrical current is present. It is represented by a single mean vector that is an average of all the positive and negative electrical currents (or vectors) present. Such an electrical current produces a biphasic deflection on the ECG, one that is partly positive and

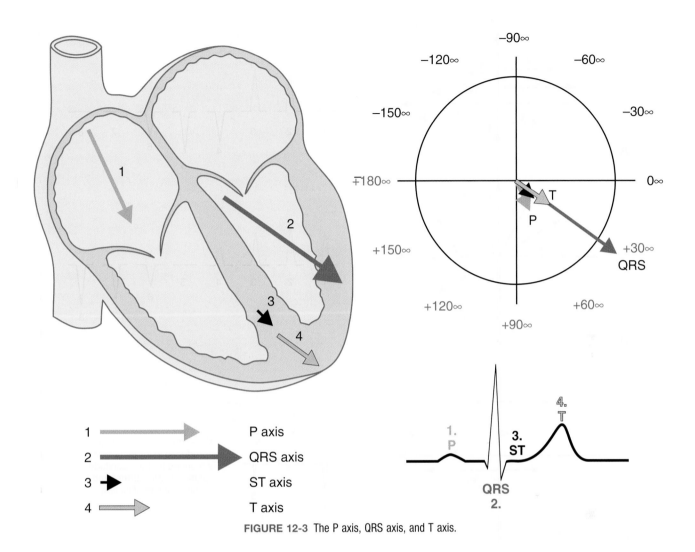

FIGURE 12-3 The P axis, QRS axis, and T axis.

partly negative. The size of the components of the deflection depends on the magnitude of the individual electrical currents. If the mean (or average) direction of the biphasic deflection in an ECG is positive, no matter by how much, the deflection is predominantly positive; if the mean direction is negative, the deflection is predominantly negative.

Using the train example, if at first a train comes toward me, I record the loud rising sound of the approaching train. As it passes, a second train on a nearby track moves away from me and I record the sound of the receding horn. If three trains come toward me and one away, then over the course of the period of observation I have recorded more approaching trains.

The QRS extends normally over a period of 0.12 seconds. During that period the vector of currents move through many directions of the compass; however, the average of the vectors is recorded and results in the deflection of the QRS complex. This average will be either positive, negative, or biphasic (both positive and negative).

Figure 12-4, *C* shows the relationship between a bidirectional electrical current, as represented by a mean vector, and the biphasic deflections on an ECG.

The more parallel the mean vector of a biphasic deflection is to the axis of the lead, the more positive is the biphasic deflection; the closer the orientation of the mean vector is to the perpendicular, the less positive is the biphasic deflection. When the positive and negative deflections are equal in magnitude, an equiphasic deflection is present, and the sum of the deflections is zero. In this case, the mean vector is perpendicular to the lead axis (Figure 12-4, *D*).

It is important to understand the significance of the relationship between the predominant direction of the deflections of the QRS complexes in a given lead, the perpendicular of the related lead axis, and the QRS axis. A predominantly positive QRS complex in a given lead indicates that the positive pole of the vector of the QRS axis lies somewhere on the positive side of the perpendicular to that lead axis. Conversely, a predominantly negative QRS complex in a lead indicates that the positive pole of the vector of the QRS axis lies somewhere on the negative side of the perpendicular (Figure 12-4, *E*).

Thus the perpendicular to an axis of a lead serves as a boundary between the predominantly positive and predominantly negative deflections of a QRS complex in any given lead.

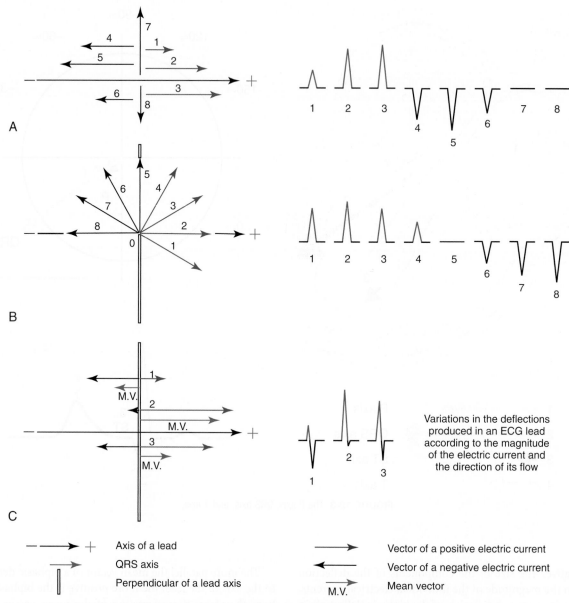

FIGURE 12-4 The axis of a lead, its perpendicular, and the direction of flow of electrical currents.

THE HEXAXIAL REFERENCE FIGURE

The hexaxial reference figure, as noted earlier, is a composite of the two triaxial reference figures, formed by combining the axis of the three standard limb leads (I, II, III) and the three augmented leads (aVR, aVL, aVF) (Figure 12-5, *A*). The primary purpose of the hexaxial reference figure is to aid in the determination of the direction of the QRS axis in the frontal plane with some degree of precision.

Viewed from the front, the six lead axes are arranged like spokes within a wheel through a central point representing the potential "zero" center of the heart. The axis of the leads is positioned within the wheel consistent with their actual direction and polarity in the frontal plane so that their positive and negative poles are spaced 30 degrees apart around the rim of the wheel.

Each positive and negative pole is assigned a degree number ranging from 0° to 180°. The poles around the rim of the upper half of the wheel of the hexaxial reference figure are given negative degree numbers (−30°, −60°, −90°, −120°, −150°, and −180°); those around the lower half of the rim are given positive degree numbers (+30°, +60°, +90°, +120°, +150°, and +180°). The negative and positive degrees should not be confused with the negative and positive poles of the lead axis but are instead merely conventions used for orientation around the hexaxial reference figure.

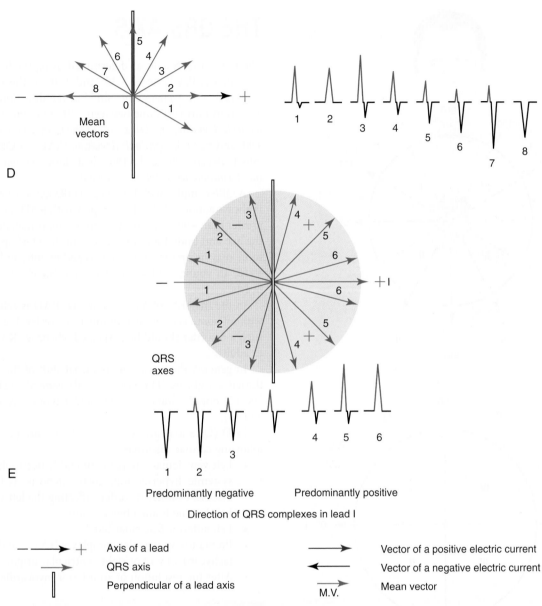

D

Mean vectors

E

QRS axes

Predominantly negative   Predominantly positive

Direction of QRS complexes in lead I

——→ + Axis of a lead	——→ Vector of a positive electric current
—→ QRS axis	←— Vector of a negative electric current
▯ Perpendicular of a lead axis	——→ M.V. Mean vector

FIGURE 12-4, cont'd

The positive and negative poles of the axis of the three standard limb leads and the three augmented leads are assigned the following degree numbers:

Standard leads	−Pole	+Pole
Lead I	±180°	0°
Lead II	−120°	+60°
Lead III	−60°	+120°

Augmented leads	−Pole	+Pole
Lead aVR	+30°	−150°
Lead aVL	+150°	−30°
Lead aVF	−90°	+90°

The hexaxial reference figure is divided into four quadrants by the bisection of lead axis I and aVF (Figure 12-5, *B*). Although there are several different ways to designate the quadrants, the following designation is used in this book:

Degrees	Quadrant
0° to −90°	I
0° to +90°	II
+90° to ±180°	III
−90° to ±180°	IV

The perpendiculars of the lead axis have the same attributes as those of the lead axis with which they coincide (i.e., their

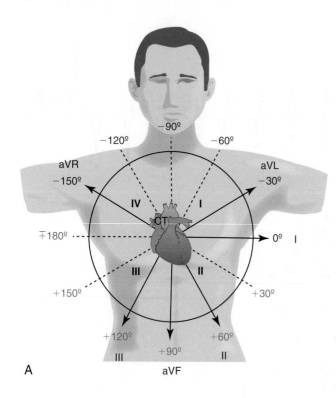

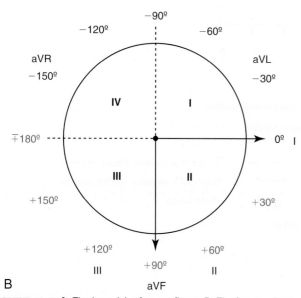

A

B

FIGURE 12-5 A, The hexaxial reference figure. **B,** The four quadrants of the hexaxial reference figure.

THE QRS AXIS

The normal QRS axis, as determined using the hexaxial reference figure, lies between −30° and +90° in the frontal plane (Figure 12-7). A change or "shift" in the direction of the QRS axis from normal to one between −30° and −90° is considered *left axis deviation (LAD)*; a shift of the QRS axis to one between +90° and ±180° is *right axis deviation (RAD)*. A QRS axis rarely falls between −90° and ±180°. If it does, *extreme RAD* or an *indeterminate axis (IND)* is present.

A QRS complex with LAD (i.e., a QRS axis greater than −30°) is always abnormal. A QRS complex with RAD (i.e., a QRS axis greater than +90°) may or may not be abnormal, depending on the age and body build of the patient. RAD of up to +120° or more may be present in newborns and infants, and up to about +110° in young adults with long, narrow chests and vertical hearts.

In the majority of adults, however, RAD is seldom present without some cardiac or pulmonary disorder. For this reason, such a disorder should be suspected whenever RAD is present in adults.

In general, the causes of abnormal shift of the QRS axis to the left or right are (1) ventricular enlargement and hypertrophy and (2) bundle branch and fascicular block (see Chapters 13 and 15).

LAD (QRS axis greater than −30°) occurs in adults in the following cardiac disorders:

- Left ventricular enlargement and hypertrophy caused by systemic hypertension, aortic stenosis, ischemic heart disease, or other disorders affecting the left ventricle
- Left bundle branch block (rare)
- Left anterior fascicular block
- Premature ventricular complexes (PVCs) and ventricular tachycardia (VT) of right ventricular origin
- After the resolution of an inferior myocardial infarction

> LAD in the absence of left ventricular hypertrophy is the single best method of diagnosing a left anterior fascicular block. See Chapter 13.

RAD (QRS axis greater than +90°) occurs in adults with the following cardiac and pulmonary disorders:

- Right ventricular enlargement and hypertrophy secondary to chronic obstructive pulmonary disease (COPD), pulmonary embolism, congenital heart disease, and other disorders that cause severe pulmonary hypertension or cor pulmonale
- Right bundle branch block and left posterior fascicular block
- PVCs and ventricular tachycardia of left ventricular origin
- After the resolution of a lateral myocardial infarction
- Normal variant in the newborn and infants (QRS axis up to +120°) and young adults (QRS axis up to +110°)

coincident leads) (Figure 12-6). For example, the perpendicular to the axis of lead II, which coincides with the axis of lead aVL, has one pole at −30° and the other at +150°.

Table 12-1 summarizes the location of the negative and positive poles of the lead axis and their perpendiculars.

The Lead Axes and Their Perpendiculars

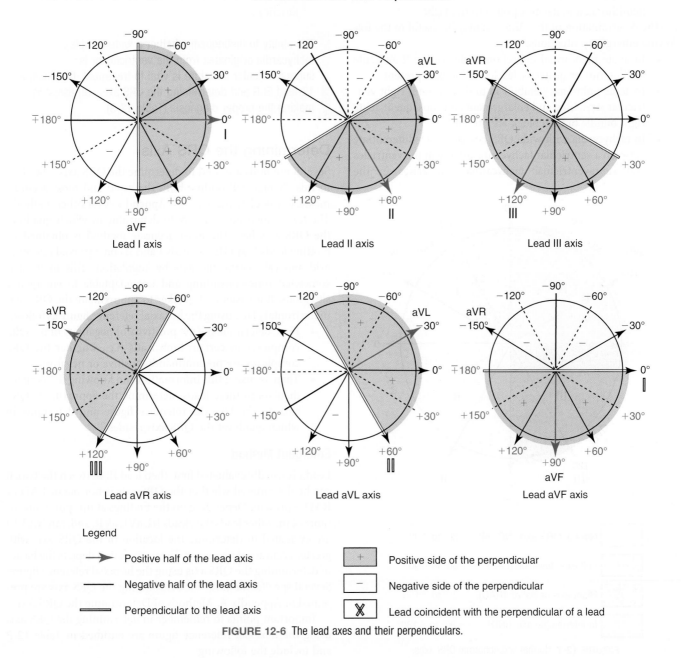

FIGURE 12-6 The lead axes and their perpendiculars.

TABLE 12-1 Negative and Positive Poles of the Lead Axis and Their Perpendiculars

| Lead | Location of Lead Axis Poles | | Location of the Poles of the Perpendicular (and its coincident lead axis) −Pole +Pole |
	−Pole	+Pole	
I	±180°	0°	−90°, +90° (aVF)
II	−120°	+60°	+150°, −30° (aVL)
III	−60°	+120°	+30°, −150° (aVR)
aVR	+30°	−150°	−60°, +120° (III)
aVL	+150°	−30°	−120°, +60° (II)
aVF	−90°	+90°	±180°, 0° (I)

- Dextrocardia, a condition where the heart lies in the right hemithorax and its apex points to the right

The determination of the QRS axis may be useful in the following emergency situations:

- In acute myocardial infarction to determine if an acute left anterior or posterior fascicular block is present
- In acute pulmonary embolism to determine if right ventricular stretching and enlargement and subsequent acute right bundle branch block are present
- In tachycardia with wide QRS complexes to differentiate between a ventricular tachycardia arising in the ventricles and supraventricular tachycardia that arises in the

sinoatrial (SA) node, atria, or atrioventricular (AV) junction.

> The ability to distinguish whether a wide complex tachycardia originates from the ventricles or is supraventricular in nature is vital to treatment. Obtaining a 12-lead ECG and determining the QRS axis can assist in making the proper diagnosis (Table 12-3).

Determining the QRS Axis

Several methods are used to determine the QRS axis. The steps in this chapter will outline both the rapid and most accurate means to calculate the axis. See Appendix A for other methods. The fastest method is simply to determine in which quadrant the QRS axis lies. The most accurate method is obtained by plotting leads I and III (or leads I and II) on a triaxial reference grid and calculating the axis by angulation. This method is somewhat time-consuming and not adaptable to emergency situations. It is easier and quicker to approximate the QRS axis in the frontal plane using the hexaxial reference figure as follows:

- First, determine the net positivity or negativity of the QRS complexes in certain limb leads (i.e., whether the QRS complexes are predominantly positive or negative)
- Then, by using this information and knowing the perpendiculars to these leads, determine the approximate QRS axis on the hexaxial reference figure and determine in which quadrant the QRS axis resides.

Emergent Method

Lead I is usually evaluated first, then lead II. Between the two, it can be determined whether the QRS axis is normal or LAD or RAD is present. Depending on the findings at this point, one or more of the other leads (i.e., leads III, aVF, aVR, and, rarely, aVL) are evaluated to determine the location of the QRS axis with greater accuracy if necessary. The next section depicts the basics of determining the QRS axis using the hexaxial reference figure. Several specific methods for determining the QRS axis are presented in Appendix A, Methods of Determining the QRS Axis.

Important points to remember in determining the QRS axis using the hexaxial reference figure are outlined in Table 12-2 and include the following:

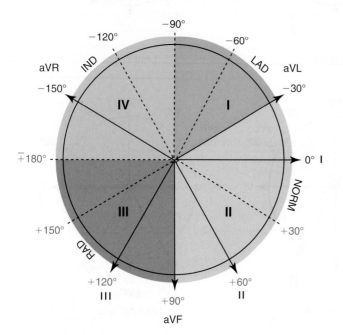

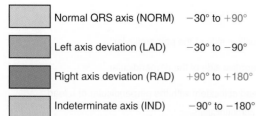

Normal QRS axis (NORM) −30° to +90°

Left axis deviation (LAD) −30° to −90°

Right axis deviation (RAD) +90° to +180°

Indeterminate axis (IND) −90° to −180°

FIGURE 12-7 Normal and abnormal QRS axes.

TABLE 12-2 **Basic Points to Remember in Determining the QRS Axis**

Leads					
I	II	aVF	QRS Axis Range	Quadrant	Axis
Positive	Positive		−30° to +90°		Normal
Positive	Negative		−30° to −90°		LAD
Positive		Positive	0° to +90°	II	Normal
Positive		Negative	0° to −90°	I	LAD, Normal
Negative		Positive	+90° to ±180°	III	RAD
Negative		Negative	−90° to ±180°	IV	IND

TABLE 12-3 QRS Characteristics in Various Leads and Associated QRS Axis

| Leads | | | | | | Equiphasic Leads | | | | | | |
I	II	aVF	III	aVR	Location of QRS Axis	I	II	aVF	III	aVR	aVL	Location of QRS Axis
+	+	+	+		+30° to +90°	±	−	−	−	+		−90
+	+	+	+		0° to +30°	+	−	−	−		±	−60
+	+	−	−		0° to −30°	+	±	−	−	−		−30
+	−	−	−		−30° to −90°	+	+	±	−	−		0
−	+	+	+		±90° to +120°	+	+	+	±	−	±	+30
−	+	+	+	+	+120° to +150°	+	+	+	+	−	±	+60
−	−	−	−		−90° to −150°	±	+	+	+	−		+90
						−	+	+	+	±		+120
						−	±	+	+	+		+150
						−	−	±	+	+		±180
						−	−	−	±	+		−150
						−	−	−	±	±		−120

+, Predominantly positive; −, Predominantly negative; ±, Equiphasic.

1. Lead II in the presence of a predominantly positive QRS complex in lead I helps to determine whether LAD is present (Figure 12-8)
   a. A predominantly positive QRS complex in lead II indicates a normal QRS axis (−30° to +90° = Normal)
   b. A predominantly negative QRS complex in lead II indicates an LAD (−30° to −90° = LAD)
2. Lead aVF, in the presence of a predominantly positive QRS complex in lead I, helps to determine whether the QRS axis lies in quadrant I or II (Figure 12-9)
   a. A predominantly positive QRS complex in lead aVF indicates that the QRS axis is in quadrant II (0° to +90° = Normal)
   b. A predominantly negative QRS complex in lead aVF indicates that the QRS axis is in quadrant I (0° to −90° = partly Normal, partly LAD)
3. Lead aVF, in the presence of a predominantly negative QRS complex in lead I, helps to determine whether the QRS axis lies in quadrant III or IV (Figure 12-10, p. 201)
   a. A predominantly positive QRS complex in lead aVF indicates that the QRS axis is in quadrant III (+90° to ±180° = RAD)
   b. A predominantly negative QRS complex in lead aVF indicates that the QRS axis is in quadrant IV (−90° to +180° = IND)

Other important points to remember include the following:
1. Lead II is the single lead that holds the clue in detecting LAD because its perpendicular coincides with the positive pole of the axis of lead aVL (−30°)
2. A predominantly positive QRS complex in lead I excludes RAD
3. A predominantly negative QRS complex in lead I and a predominantly positive QRS complex in lead aVR indicate a RAD (>+120°)
4. A QRS axis between −90° and ±180° (quadrant IV) indicating IND is rare except in ventricular ectopy

While there are many points to consider in reality the process is simple. Approach the QRS axis determination systematically. First determine whether lead I is positive or negative. Secondly, determine whether lead II is positive or negative and finally do the same with aVF. The information in Table 12-2 shows that the combination of these results places the QRS axis in one of the four quadrants. The only value of examining lead II is to determine whether the QRS axis is normal or there is left axis deviation.

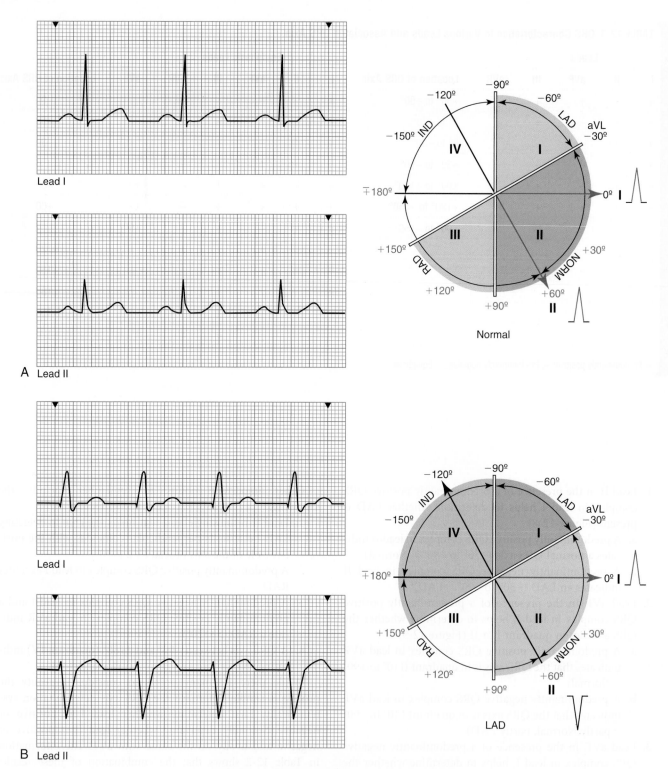

FIGURE 12-8 A, Normal QRS axis. **B,** Left axis deviation.

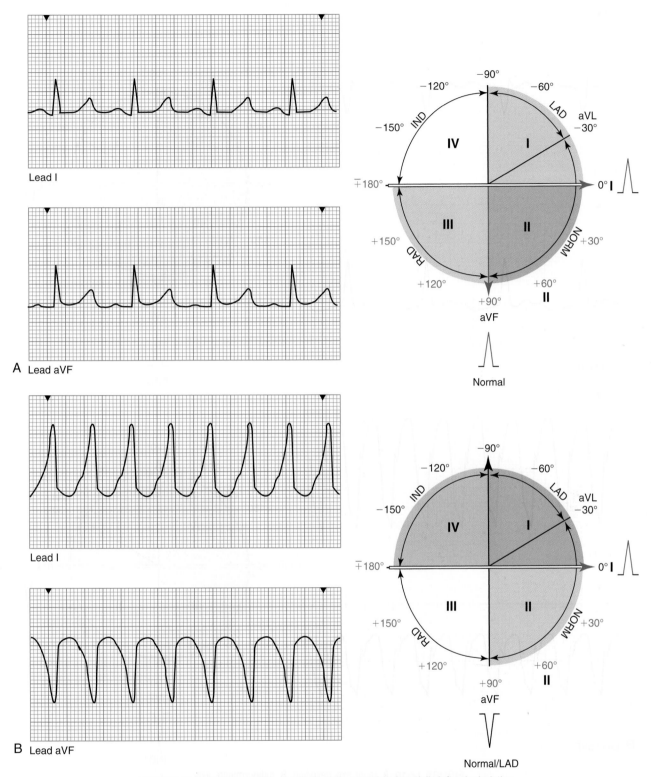

FIGURE 12-9 **A,** Normal QRS axis. **B,** Partially normal and partially left axis deviation.

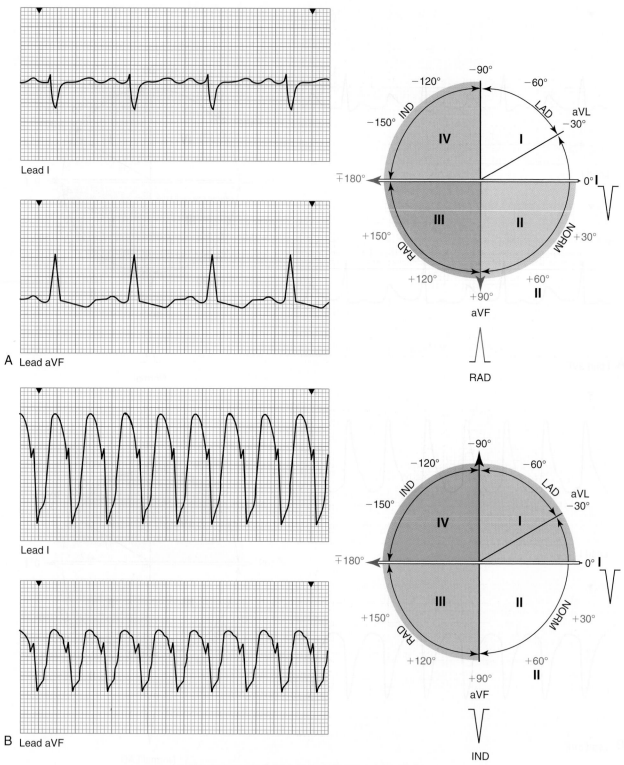

FIGURE 12-10 **A,** Right axis deviation. **B,** Indeterminate axis.

Steps in Determining an Accurate QRS Axis

There are three steps in determining an accurate QRS axis:

- Determine the net positivity or negativity of the QRS complexes in lead I.
  A. If the QRS complexes are predominantly *positive* in lead I, the QRS axis lies between −90° and +90° (i.e., in quadrant I or II). The QRS axis may be between −30° and +90° (normal QRS axis) or between −30° and −90° (LAD).

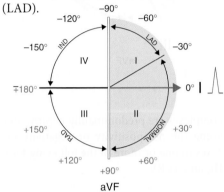

  B. If the QRS complexes are predominantly *negative* in lead I, the QRS axis is greater than +90° (lying between +90° and −90°), indicating right axis deviation. Most likely, the QRS axis lies in quadrant III and, rarely, in quadrant IV.

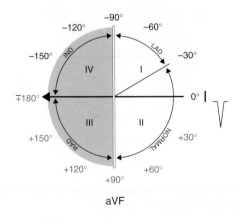

Note: If the QRS complexes are predominately *positive* in lead I, proceed to *Step 2*. If the QRS complexes are predominantly *negative* in lead I, proceed to *Step 3*.

If the QRS complexes are predominantly *positive* in lead I:
- Determine the net positivity or negativity of the QRS complexes in one or more of the following three leads (II, aVF, and III):

Lead II

A. If the QRS complexes are predominantly *positive* in lead II, the QRS axis is between −30° and +90° (normal QRS axis).

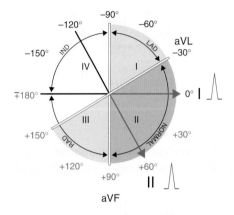

B. If the QRS complexes are predominantly *negative* in lead II, the QRS axis is between −30° and −90° (left axis deviation).

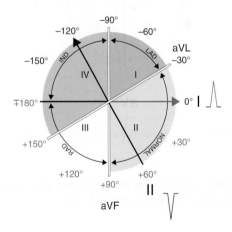

Lead aVF

C. If the QRS complexes are predominantly *positive* in lead aVF, the QRS axis is between 0° and +90° (quadrant II).

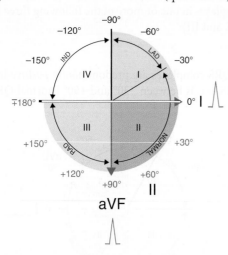

D. If the QRS complexes are predominantly *negative* in lead aVF, the QRS axis is between 0° and −90° (quadrant I).

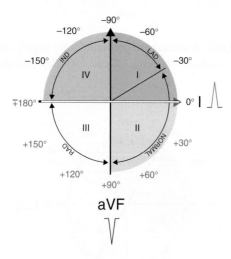

Lead III

E. If the QRS complexes are predominantly *positive* in lead III, the QRS axis is between +30° and +90°.

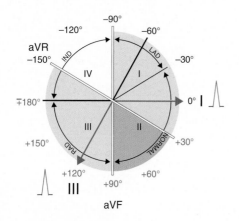

F. If the QRS complexes are predominantly *negative* in lead III, the QRS axis is between +30° and −90°.

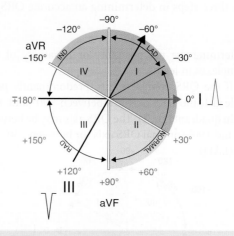

If the QRS complexes are predominantly *negative* in lead I:

- Determine the net positivity or negativity of the QRS complexes in one or more of the following four leads (II, aVF, III, and aVR):

Lead II

A. If the QRS complexes are predominantly *positive* in lead II, the QRS axis is between +90° and +150°.

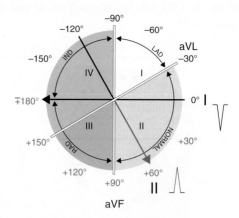

B. If the QRS complexes are predominantly *negative* in lead II, the QRS axis is greater than +150°.

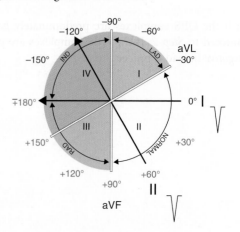

Lead aVF

C. If the QRS complexes are predominantly *positive* in lead aVF, the QRS axis is between +90° and +180° (quadrant III).

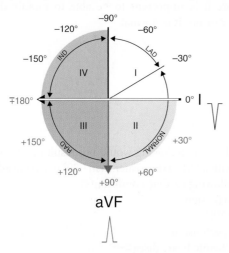

D. If the QRS complexes are predominantly *negative* in lead aVF, the QRS axis is between −90° and −180° (quadrant IV).

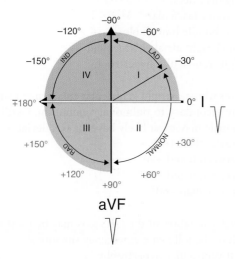

Lead III

E. If the QRS complexes are predominantly *positive* in lead III, the QRS axis is between +90° and −150°.

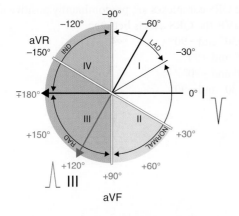

F. If the QRS complexes are predominantly *negative* in lead III, the QRS axis is between −90° and −150°.

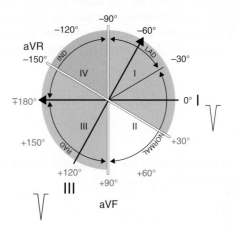

Lead aVR

G. If the QRS complexes are predominantly *positive* in lead aVR, the QRS axis is greater than +120° (severe right axis deviation).

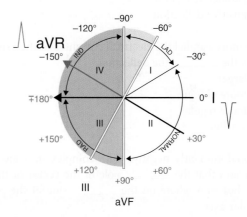

H. If the QRS complexes are predominantly *negative* in lead aVR, the QRS axis is between +90° and +120° (mild to moderate right axis deviation).

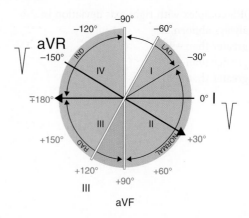

CHAPTER SUMMARY

- The electrical forces of the heart can be described as having both a magnitude and an axis, which we call a vector.
- The ECG records numerous simultaneous vectors and generates results on the screen that represent the cumulative cardiac vectors for the P wave, QRS complex, and T wave.
- The axis, or direction of the QRS complex, can be calculated by using the hexaxial reference figure generated by the limb leads.
- The QRS axis can be affected by multiple conditions and therefore it is important to be able to rapidly determine whether or not it is normal

CHAPTER REVIEW

1. The mean of all vectors generated during the depolarization of the atria is the _____ axis.
   A. P
   B. QRS
   C. ST
   D. T

2. An electrical current flowing toward the positive pole of a lead produces a(n) _____ on the ECG.
   A. elongated deflection
   B. negative deflection
   C. parallel deflection
   D. positive deflection

3. The more parallel the electrical current is to the axis of the lead, the _____ the deflection.
   A. larger
   B. more oblique
   C. more regular
   D. smaller

4. A predominantly negative QRS complex in a given lead indicates that the _____ pole of the vector of the QRS axis lies somewhere on the _____ side of the perpendicular axis.
   A. positive, positive
   B. positive, negative
   C. negative, negative
   D. negative, positive

5. A QRS complex with right axis deviation is:
   A. always abnormal
   B. greater than +90°
   C. greater than −30°
   D. greater than −90°

6. Which of the following would not result in left axis deviation with a QRS axis greater than −30° occurs in adults with the following cardiac condition(s):
   A. aortic stenosis
   B. COPD
   C. hypertension
   D. ischemic heart disease

7. Right axis deviation occurs in adults with which of the following disorders?
   A. anterior fascicular
   B. Left bundle branch block
   C. block right atrial enlargement
   D. right ventricular hypertrophy

8. Patients who have right ventricular enlargement and hypertrophy secondary to pulmonary embolism, COPD, or cor pulmonale may most likely have an axis deviation of:
   A. greater than +90°
   B. between 0 and +90°
   C. between 0 and −60°
   D. greater than −60°

9. The determination of the QRS axis may be most useful in which of the following emergency situations?
   A. left ventricular hypertrophy
   B. premature atrial complexes
   C. pulmonary hypertension
   D. tachycardia with wide QRS complexes

10. If the QRS complexes are predominantly positive in leads I and aVF, the QRS axis is between:
    A. −30° and +90°
    B. 0° and +90°
    C. 0° and −90°
    D. +30° and +90°

13 Bundle Branch and Fascicular Blocks

OBJECTIVES *Upon completion of this chapter, you should be able to complete the following objectives:*

1. Name and identify the atrioventricular (AV) node and the parts of the electrical conduction system within the ventricles on an anatomical drawing.
2. Name the artery or arteries that supply the following structures of the electrical conduction system:
   Interventricular septum
   - Posterior portion
   - Anterior portion
   - Middle portion
   - AV node
   - Bundle of His
   - Proximal part
   - Distal part
   - Right bundle branch
   - Proximal part
   - Distal part
   - Left bundle branch
   - Main stem
   - Left anterior fascicle
   - Left posterior fascicle
3. Describe the anatomical features and the blood supply that make the following structures more or less vulnerable to disruption:
   - Right bundle branch
   - Left bundle branch

- Left anterior fascicle
- Left posterior fascicle

4. Define ventricular activation time (VAT) and intrinsicoid deflection.
5. List five major causes of bundle branch and fascicular blocks.
6. Identify the location of acute myocardial infarctions (AMIs) that may result in the following:
   - Right bundle branch block
   - Left bundle branch block
   - Left anterior fascicular block
   - Left posterior fascicular block
7. Indicate the significance of the following:
   - Bundle branch or fascicular block by itself
   - Bundle branch or fascicular block complicating an acute MI
   - Bundle branch block complicated by a first- or second-degree AV block
   - Right bundle branch block and left posterior fascicular block occurring together
   - Right bundle branch block and left anterior fascicular block occurring together
8. Give the treatment and its rationale for the following:
   - A bundle branch or fascicular block occurring alone
   - A bundle branch block complicated by (1) a fascicular block or (2) a first-degree or second-degree AV block, occurring alone or in the setting of an acute MI
   - A bundle branch block progressing to third-degree AV block in the setting of an acute MI
9. Discuss the pathophysiology, causes, and ECG characteristics in the following bundle branch and fascicular blocks:
   - Right bundle branch block
   - Left bundle branch block
   - Left anterior fascicular block
   - Left posterior fascicular block

ANATOMY AND PHYSIOLOGY OF THE ELECTRICAL CONDUCTION SYSTEM

Anatomy of the Electrical Conduction System

The electrical conduction system located below the atrioventricular (AV) node and within the ventricles—the His-Purkinje system of the ventricles—consists of the bundle of His, the right and left bundle branches, and terminates in the Purkinje network composed of extremely fine Purkinje fibers (Figure 13-1).

The long, thin, round right bundle branch (RBBB) runs down the right side of the interventricular septum to conduct the electrical impulses to the right ventricle. The left bundle branch (LBBB), which consists of a short, thick, flat left common bundle branch and two main divisions—the left anterior and posterior fascicles—conducts the electrical impulses to the left ventricle, including the interventricular septum. The relatively long, thin left anterior fascicle occupies the anterior wall of the interventricular septum. It conducts the electrical impulses from the left bundle branch to the anterior and lateral walls of the left ventricle. The short, broad left posterior fascicle, which runs down the posterior wall of the interventricular septum, conducts the electrical impulses to the posterior wall of the left ventricle.

Blood Supply to the Electrical Conduction System

The anterior two thirds of the interventricular septum is supplied by the left anterior descending (LAD) branch of the left coronary artery; the posterior third of the septum is supplied by the posterior descending coronary artery. The posterior descending coronary artery (PDA) arises from the right coronary artery (RCA) in 85% to 90% of hearts and from the left circumflex coronary artery of the left coronary artery in the other 10% to 15%.

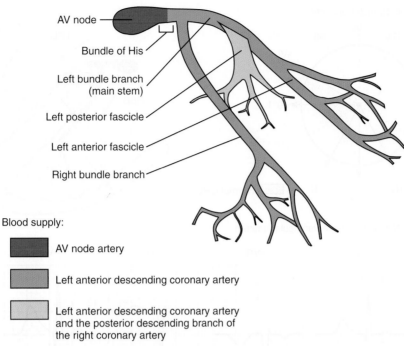

Blood supply:

■ AV node artery

■ Left anterior descending coronary artery

□ Left anterior descending coronary artery
and the posterior descending branch of
the right coronary artery

FIGURE 13-1 The electrical conduction system and its blood supply in most hearts.

The main blood supply of the AV node and proximal part of the bundle of His is the AV node artery (see Figure 13-1), which, like the posterior descending coronary artery, arises from the right coronary artery in 85% to 90% of the hearts and, in the other 10% to 15%, from the left circumflex coronary artery.

In most hearts, the left anterior descending coronary artery, by way of its branches (particularly the septal perforator arteries), is the main blood supply to the distal part of the bundle of His, the entire right bundle branch (including the proximal and distal parts), the main stem of the left bundle branch, and the left anterior fascicle. Occasionally, the posterior descending coronary artery also supplies the distal part of the bundle of His, the proximal part of the right bundle branch, and the main stem of the left bundle branch.

The left posterior fascicle is supplied by both the left anterior descending coronary artery (anteriorly) and the posterior descending coronary artery (posteriorly).

Table 13-1 summarizes the blood supply to the various parts of the electrical conduction system.

Physiology of the Electrical Conduction System

Normally, the electrical impulses progress through the right bundle branch and left bundle branch and its fascicles simultaneously (Figure 13-2), causing first the depolarization of the interventricular septum (1) and then the synchronous depolarization of the right and left ventricles (2). The electrical activity

TABLE 13-1   The Electrical Conduction System and Its Primary and Alternate Blood Supply

Electrical Conduction System	Primary Blood Supply	Alternate Blood Supply
AV node	AV node artery	None
Bundle of His		
Proximal	AV node artery	None
Distal	LAD	PDA
Right bundle branch		
Proximal	LAD	PDA
Distal	LAD	None
Left bundle branch		
Main stem	LAD	PDA
Left anterior fascicle	LAD	None
Left posterior fascicle	LAD and PDA	None

AV, Atrioventricular; *LAD,* left anterior descending artery by way of the septal perforator arteries; *PDA,* posterior descending coronary artery.

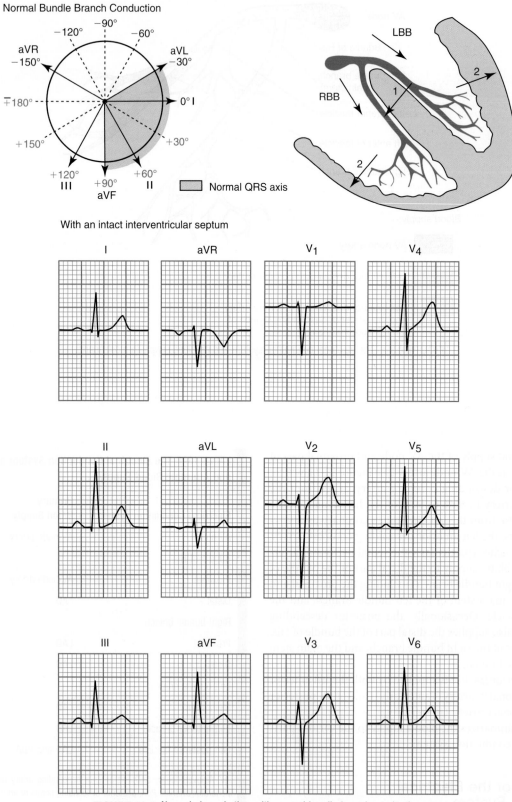

FIGURE 13-2 Normal sinus rhythm with normal bundle branch conduction.

generated by the depolarization of the smaller right ventricle is buried in that generated by the left ventricle.

> An intact, viable interventricular septum is one that is capable of conducting an electrical impulse and depolarizing from left to right, producing an initial small q or r wave in the QRS complex, depending on the lead. An interventricular septum that is not intact or viable because of some form of heart disease, such as an anteroseptal myocardial infarction (MI), is unable to conduct an electrical impulse and depolarize normally. This affects primarily the conduction of the bundle of His and may cause a bundle branch block.

Electrocardiograms (ECGs) typical of normal bundle branch conduction with and without an intact interventricular septum and their QRS axes are shown in Figure 13-2.

The time it takes for depolarization of the interventricular septum and the ventricle under a facing precordial lead, including the endocardial to epicardial depolarization of the ventricular wall, is commonly called the *ventricular activation time* (VAT) (Figure 13-3).

The VAT is measured from the onset of the QRS complex to the peak of the last R wave in the QRS complex. Normally, it is less than 0.035 second in the right precordial leads V_1 and V_2 and less than 0.055 second in the left precordial leads V_5 and V_6. The rest of the QRS complex, from the peak of the R wave to the onset of the ST segment, or the *J point*, represents the final depolarization of the ventricles progressing away from the facing lead.

The down stroke of the R wave, which begins at the peak of the R wave and ends at the J point or tip of the following S wave, is called the *intrinsicoid deflection*. The VAT is prolonged in leads V_1 and V_2 in right bundle branch block (RBBB) and right ventricular hypertrophy and in leads V_5 and V_6 in left bundle branch block (LBBB) and left ventricular hypertrophy.

PATHOPHYSIOLOGY OF BUNDLE BRANCH AND FASCICULAR BLOCKS

Causes of Bundle Branch and Fascicular Blocks

The relatively thin right bundle branch is more vulnerable to disruption than the left bundle branch with its short, thick, wide main stem and widely spread fascicles. A relatively small myocardial lesion can disrupt the right bundle branch and cause a block, whereas a much more widespread lesion is necessary to block the less vulnerable main stem of the left bundle branch.

The left anterior fascicle of the left bundle branch, like the right bundle branch, is also thin and vulnerable to disruption. The left posterior fascicle, on the other hand, because it is short and thick and supplied by both the right coronary artery (via the posterior descending coronary artery) and the left anterior descending coronary artery, is rarely disrupted. Therefore, disruption of perfusion of the coronary artery associated with a given myocardial infarction may result in a particular bundle branch block or fascicular block. The relationship between the area of infarction and the associated bundle branch and fascicular blocks are listed in Table 13-2 and expanded as follows:

- RBBB primarily occurs secondary to an anteroseptal MI and rarely to a right ventricular wall MI.
- LBBB primarily occurs secondary to an anteroseptal and rarely to an inferior wall MI.
- Left anterior fascicle block primarily occurs secondary to an anteroseptal MI.
- Left posterior fascicle block is relatively rare in acute MI because both the left anterior descending coronary artery and the posterior descending coronary artery of the right coronary artery (or less commonly of the left circumflex artery) have to be occluded for left posterior fascicle block to occur, such as in an anteroseptal MI combined with a right ventricular or inferior MI.

Right and left bundle branch block may also be present in a heart with an interventricular septum that is free of coronary artery disease.

Significance of Bundle Branch and Fascicular Blocks

A bundle branch or fascicular block by itself is not significant and requires no treatment. The underlying heart disease that produced the bundle branch or fascicular block usually determines the prognosis.

In general, a bundle branch or fascicular block complicating an acute anteroseptal MI indicates a more serious condition than an acute MI without one, presumably because of greater damage to the myocardium. The incidence of pump failure and life-threatening dysrhythmias, such as sustained ventricular tachycardia and ventricular fibrillation, is much higher in patients with an acute MI complicated by a bundle branch block than in those who do not have such a complication. For this reason, the mortality rate in such patients is several times higher than in those with uncomplicated acute MI.

A bundle branch block may occasionally progress to a third-degree (complete) AV block in the setting of an acute MI, requiring temporary cardiac pacing. This is most likely to happen when a first- or second-degree AV block complicates a right or left bundle branch block occurring during the early stages of the infarction.

The progression of RBBB to complete AV block occurs twice as often as that of LBBB, especially when RBBB is associated with a fascicular block. The occurrence of a complete AV block

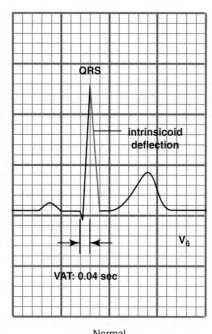

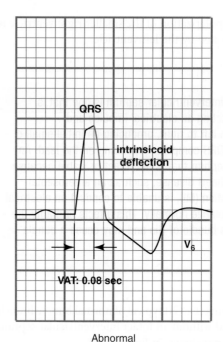

Normal   Abnormal

FIGURE 13-3 The ventricular activation time and intrinsicoid deflection.

TABLE 13-2 The Bundle Branch and Fascicular Blocks and the Acute Myocardial Infarctions That Usually Cause Them

Bundle Branch and Fascicular Block	Acute Myocardial Infarction (Coronary Artery Involved)
Right bundle branch block	Anteroseptal (LAD) OR Right ventricular (RCA) (Rare)
Left bundle branch block	Anteroseptal (LAD) OR Inferior (LCX) (Rare)
Left anterior fascicular block	Anteroseptal (LAD)
Left posterior fascicular block	Anteroseptal (LAD) AND Right ventricular (RCA) OR Inferior (distal RCA or LCX)

LAD, Left anterior descending coronary artery; *LCX,* left circumflex coronary artery; *RCA,* right coronary artery.

in the setting of an acute MI is an ominous sign, indicating the involvement of both the left anterior descending branch of the left coronary artery and the posterior descending branch of either the right coronary artery or left circumflex. Complete AV block, in this instance, is usually transient, however, lasting about 1 to 2 weeks.

Left anterior and posterior fascicular blocks are usually benign and rarely progress to complete LBBB unless they are secondary to an acute MI. A left posterior fascicle

block occurring with an RBBB, although rare, signifies a poor prognosis because occlusion of both the right coronary artery and the left anterior descending coronary artery must occur for this to happen.

Treatment of Bundle Branch and Fascicular Blocks

Specific treatment is usually not indicated for a bundle branch or fascicular block if it is present alone and is not the result of an acute MI.

Temporary cardiac pacing is indicated for the treatment of a right or left bundle branch block under the following conditions:

- If a new right or left bundle branch block or an alternating bundle branch block (one in which an RBBB alternates with an LBBB) results from an acute MI
- If a bundle branch block is complicated by a fascicular block, a first- or second-degree AV block, or both, especially in the setting of an acute MI
- If a bundle branch block progresses to a complete AV block, especially in the setting of an acute MI

RIGHT BUNDLE BRANCH BLOCK

Pathophysiology of Right Bundle Branch Block

In RBBB (Figure 13-4), the electrical impulses are prevented from entering the right ventricle directly because of the

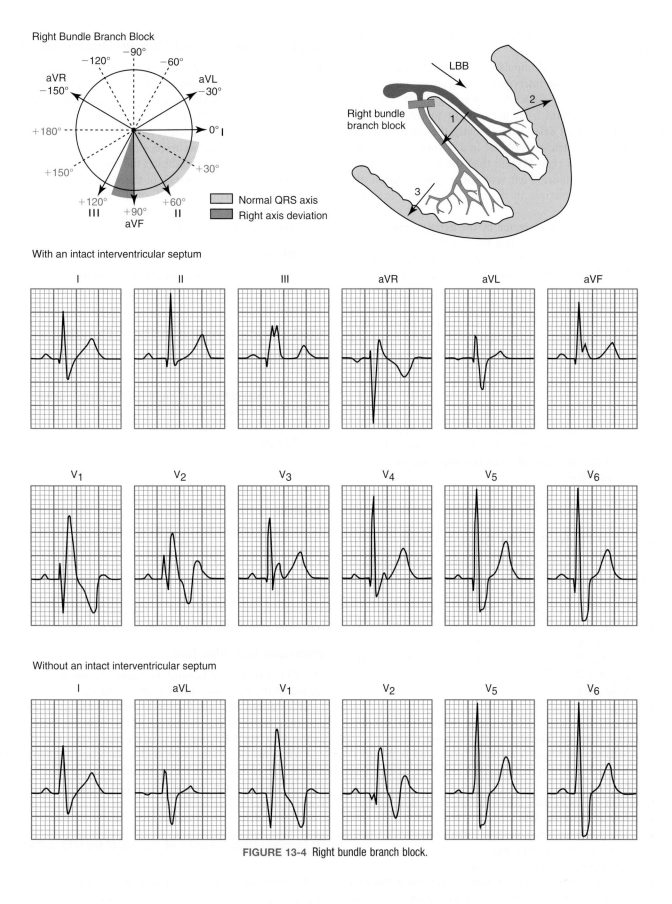

FIGURE 13-4 Right bundle branch block.

disruption of conduction of the electrical impulses through the right bundle branch.

In RBBB, the electrical impulses travel rapidly down the left bundle branch into the interventricular septum and left ventricle, as they normally do, while progressing slowly across the interventricular septum from left to right to enter the right ventricle after a short delay. Consequently, the interventricular septum and left ventricle depolarize in a normal way: first the septum from left to right (1) and then the left ventricle from right to left (2). Following left ventricular depolarization, the right ventricle depolarizes in a normal direction, from left to right (3).

The electrical forces generated by the depolarization of the right ventricle in RBBB occur after those of the interventricular septum and left ventricle and travel in a normal direction (i.e., anteriorly and to the right, toward lead V_1). Because of the delay in the depolarization of the right ventricle, the QRS complex is typically greater than 0.12 second in duration and bizarre in shape and appearance. When it is greater than 0.12 seconds in duration, it is said to be *complete*; between 0.10 and 0.12 second, it is *incomplete*. The term RBBB used alone signifies a complete RBBB.

> Duration of the bundle branch block is only one component of the incomplete RBBB. The axis, VAT, and shape of the QRS must also be considered before interpreting an incomplete RBBB.

Causes of Right Bundle Branch Block

RBBB may be present in otherwise healthy individuals with apparently normal hearts without any apparent cause. Common causes of chronic RBBB include the following:

- Coronary and hypertensive heart disease
- Cardiac tumors
- Cardiomyopathy and myocarditis
- Syphilitic, rheumatic, and congenital heart disease (atrial septal defect)
- Cardiac surgery
- Congenital RBBB
- Idiopathic degenerative disease of the electrical conduction system (i.e., Lenègre and Lev diseases)
- Aberrant ventricular conduction associated with supraventricular premature complexes and tachycardias (see Chapter 6)

Common causes of acute RBBB include the following:

- Acute anteroseptal MI
- Acute pulmonary embolism or infarction
- Acute congestive heart failure
- Acute pericarditis or myocarditis
- After the resolution of these acute causes, the RBBB may or may not persist chronically, depending on the severity of damage inflicted on the right bundle branch.

Significance of Right Bundle Branch Block

The presence of a new RBBB in the context of an acute coronary syndrome is highly suspicious of an anteroseptal myocardial infarction. This will be discussed in greater detail in Chapter 17. The progression of RBBB to complete AV block occurs twice as often as that of LBBB, especially when RBBB is associated with a fascicular block. The occurrence of a complete AV block in the setting of an acute MI indicates the involvement of both the left anterior descending branch of the left coronary artery and the posterior descending branch of the right coronary artery. However, complete AV block, in this instance, is usually transient, lasting about 1 to 2 weeks.

Treatment of Right Bundle Branch Block

Only rarely does RBBB require treatment. In the event of complete AV block, a temporary pacemaker may be utilized until the block resolves.

ECG Characteristics in Right Bundle Branch Block

> **Characteristics of Right Bundle Branch Block**
> QRS greater than 0.12 second
> Slurred S wave in leads I and V_6
> RSR′ pattern in V_1

QRS COMPLEXES (FIGURE 13-5)

Duration

The duration of the QRS complex in RBBB is greater than 0.12 second; in incomplete RBBB, the duration of the QRS complex is 0.10 to 0.12 second.

QRS Axis

The QRS axis may be normal or deviated slightly to the right (i.e., right axis deviation, >+90° but <110°).

Ventricular Activation Time

The VAT is prolonged beyond the upper normal limit of 0.035 second in the right precordial leads V_1 and V_2.

QRS Pattern in Right Bundle Branch Block. In RBBB, the electrical forces of depolarization of the right ventricle occur abnormally late, following those of the interventricular septum and left ventricle. These right ventricular electrical forces are directed anteriorly and to the right and last more than 40 msec (0.04 second), producing the typical late broad, or "terminal," R and S waves in various leads.

> *Terminal* means the last 0.04 seconds of the QRS complex.

The combined electrical forces of the left ventricle and delayed right ventricle depolarization produce the typical wide biphasic QRS complexes of RBBB.

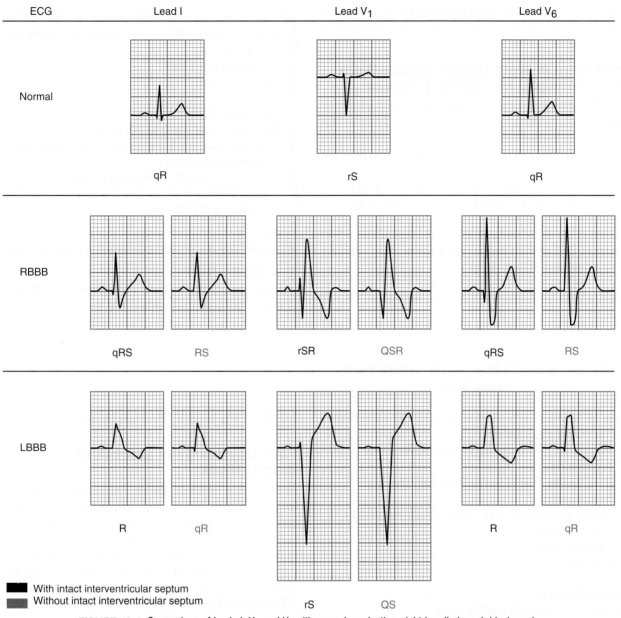

FIGURE 13-5 Comparison of leads I, V$_1$, and V$_6$ with normal conduction, right bundle branch block, and left bundle branch block.

Q waves: Normal small septal q waves may be present in leads I, aVL, and V$_5$-V$_6$, reflecting the normal depolarization of the interventricular septum.

R waves: Small r waves are present in the right precordial leads V$_1$-V$_2$, reflecting the normal depolarization of the interventricular septum. Wide and slurred, tall "terminal" R waves are present in lead aVR and the right precordial leads V$_1$-V$_2$. This produces the classical triphasic rSR′ pattern of RBBB (or the "M" or "rabbit ears" pattern) in leads V$_1$-V$_2$.

S waves: Deep and slurred "terminal" S waves are present in leads I and aVL and the left precordial leads V$_5$-V$_6$. This produces the typical qRS pattern of RBBB in leads V$_5$-V$_6$.

> QRS complexes of RBBB characteristically have a "rabbit ear" appearance with small q waves, rSR′ in V$_1$-V$_2$, and slurring of the terminal S wave in lead I and V$_5$-V$_6$.

ST SEGMENTS

ST-segment depression may be present in leads V$_1$-V$_2$.

T WAVES

T wave inversion may be present in leads V$_1$-V$_2$.

The ST-T waves are, as in LBBB, discordant (deflect in the opposite direction of the QRS) with the QRS complex, so that

T waves are inverted in the right precordial leads (and other leads with a terminal R′ wave) and upright in the left precordial leads and in leads I and aVL.

QRS Pattern in Right Bundle Branch Block with Anteroseptal Myocardial Infarction

An anteroseptal myocardial infarction results in death of the anterior portion of the interventricular septum. RBBB in this context is different than that described above because the initial normal depolarization of the interventricular septum does not occur. The result is the absence of initial small r waves in the precordial leads V_1-V_2 and septal q waves in leads I, aVL, and V_5-V_6. Consequently, the classical triphasic rSR′ pattern of RBBB is replaced by a QSR pattern in V_1-V_2.

However, the QRS complex duration remains prolonged greater than 0.12 seconds and the terminal "slurring" of the S wave is still present in leads I and V_5-V_6.

For a comparison of ECG characteristics of RBBB with and without an intact interventricular septum, see Figure 13-5.

Summary of the ECG Characteristics in Right Bundle Branch Block

Leads V_1-V_2

Wide QRS complex with a classic triphasic rSR′ pattern (the "M" or "rabbit ears" pattern)

- Initial small r wave (normal interventricular septal depolarization)
- Deep, slurred S wave (normal left ventricular depolarization)
- Late (terminal) tall R′ wave (delayed right ventricular depolarization)

ST-segment depression

T wave inversion

Leads I, aVL, V_5-V_6

Wide QRS complex with a qRS pattern

- Initial small q wave (normal interventricular septal depolarization)
- Tall R wave (normal left ventricular depolarization)
- Late (terminal) deep, slurred S wave (delayed right ventricular depolarization)

QRS axis

Normal QRS axis or right axis deviation (+90° to +110°)

Ventricular activation time

Prolonged beyond the upper normal limit of 0.035 second in the right precordial leads V_1 and V_2

RBBB Following Anteroseptal Myocardial Infarction

Leads V_1-V_2

Wide QRS complex with QSR pattern

- Absent initial small r wave (absent interventricular septal depolarization)

- Deep QS wave (normal left ventricular depolarization)
- Late (terminal) tall R wave (delayed right ventricular depolarization)

ST-segment depression

T wave inversion

Leads I, aVL, V_5-V_6

Wide QRS complex with an RS pattern

- Absent initial small q wave (absent interventricular septal depolarization)
- Tall R wave (normal left ventricular depolarization)
- Late (terminal) deep, slurred S wave (delayed right ventricular depolarization)

QRS axis

Normal QRS axis or right axis deviation (+90° to +110°)

Ventricular activation time

Prolonged beyond the upper normal limit of 0.035 second in the right precordial leads V_1 and V_2

LEFT BUNDLE BRANCH BLOCK

Pathophysiology of Left Bundle Branch Block

In LBBB (Figure 13-6), the electrical impulses are prevented from entering the left ventricle directly because of the disruption of conduction of the electrical impulses through the left bundle branch. The presence of LBBB is almost always the result of disease of the interventricular septum. Following an anteroseptal or right ventricular myocardial infarction, the interventricular septum may be injured resulting in a LBBB which differs slightly from the typical LBBB because of the loss of the normal septal depolarization.

In LBBB, the electrical impulses travel rapidly down the right bundle branch into the right ventricle, as they normally do, while progressing slowly across the interventricular septum from right to left into the left ventricle. Consequently, the interventricular septum depolarizes first in an abnormal way, from right to left (1), and either anteriorly or posteriorly. This is followed by the depolarization of the right ventricle in a normal way, left to right (2), and then depolarization of the left ventricle in a normal direction from right to left (3).

The electrical forces generated by the depolarization of the left ventricle in LBBB occur after those of the interventricular septum and right ventricle and travel in a normal leftward direction, away from lead V_1.

Because the electrical impulses enter the left ventricle from the right via the interventricular septum instead of the left bundle branch, the depolarization of the left ventricle occurs slightly behind schedule, but in an essentially normal sequence.

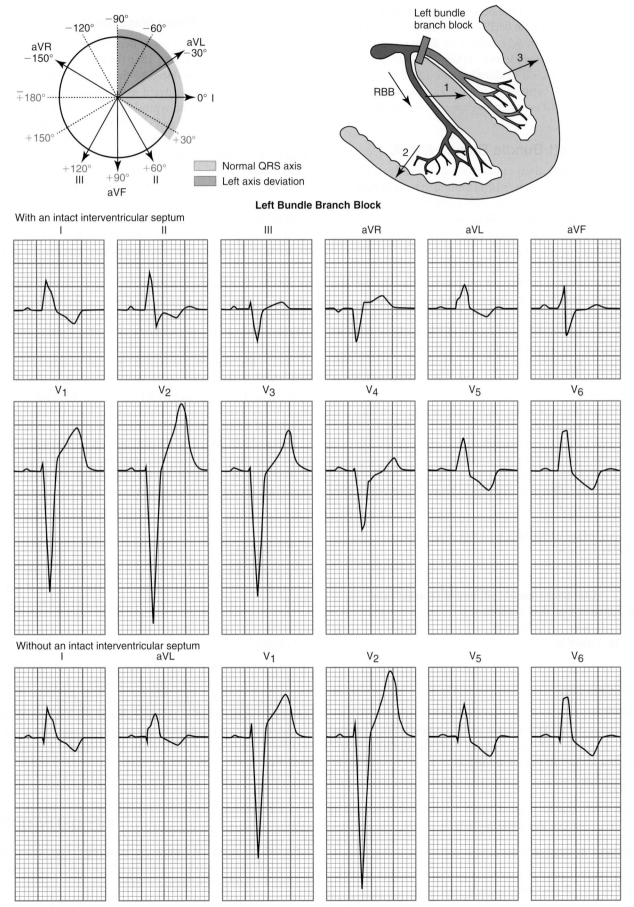

Left Bundle Branch Block

With an intact interventricular septum

I II III aVR aVL aVF

V₁ V₂ V₃ V₄ V₅ V₆

Without an intact interventricular septum

I aVL V₁ V₂ V₅ V₆

FIGURE 13-6 Left bundle branch block.

Because of the delay in the depolarization of the left ventricle, the VAT is greater than 0.055 second and the QRS complex is typically greater than 0.12 second in duration and has an abnormal shape and appearance. When the QRS complex is greater than 0.12 second in duration, the LBBB is said to be *complete;* when it is between 0.10 and 0.12 second, it is *incomplete.* The term *LBBB used alone signifies a complete left bundle branch block.*

Causes of Left Bundle Branch Block

LBBB, unlike RBBB, always indicates a diseased heart because it is a relatively uncommon (<10%) finding in healthy hearts. In general, LBBB is more common than is RBBB. Common causes of chronic LBBB include the following:

- Hypertensive heart disease (the most common cause) and coronary artery disease
- Cardiomyopathy and myocarditis
- Syphilitic, rheumatic, and congenital heart disease and aortic stenosis from whatever cause
- Cardiac tumors
- Idiopathic degenerative disease of the electrical conduction system (i.e., Lenègre and Lev diseases)
- Aberrant ventricular conduction associated with supraventricular premature complexes and tachycardias (see Chapter 6)

Common causes of acute LBBB include the following:

- Acute anteroseptal MI
- Acute congestive heart failure
- Acute pericarditis or myocarditis
- Acute cardiac trauma
- Administration of such drugs as beta-blockers, diltiazem, and verapamil (rare)

ECG Characteristics in Left Bundle Branch Block

> **Characteristics of Left Bundle Branch Block**
> QRS greater than 0.12 seconds
> Broad R wave in Lead I and V_6
> Broad S wave in V_1

QRS COMPLEXES

Duration

The duration of the QRS complex with complete LBBB is greater than 0.12 second; with incomplete LBBB, the duration of the QRS complex is 0.10 to 0.12 second.

QRS Axis

The QRS axis may be normal, but it is commonly deviated to the left (i.e., left axis deviation, >−30°).

Ventricular Activation Time

The VAT is prolonged beyond the upper normal limit of 0.055 second in the left precordial leads V_5 and V_6.

QRS Pattern in Left Bundle Branch Block

In LBBB, the electrical forces of depolarization of the left ventricle occur abnormally late, after those of the right ventricle. The electrical forces produced by the depolarization of the left ventricle are directed leftward and last more than 40 msec (0.04 sec), producing the typical broad R and S waves in the various leads. The combined electrical forces of the right ventricle and delayed left ventricle produce the typical wide monophasic QRS complexes of LBBB.

Q waves: Septal q waves are absent in leads I and aVL and the left precordial leads V_5-V_6, where they normally occur. Their absence results from the depolarization of the interventricular septum in an abnormal direction, from right to left.

R waves: Small to relatively tall, narrow R waves are present in leads V_1-V_3 when the interventricular septum depolarizes from right to left and anteriorly. This occurs in about two thirds of LBBBs. The R waves in leads V_1-V_3 give the typical appearance of a "poor R-wave progression" across the precordial leads. In the other third of LBBBs, where the interventricular septum depolarizes from right to left and posteriorly, R waves are absent in leads V_1-V_3.

Tall, wide, slurred R waves are present in leads I and aVL and the left precordial leads V_5-V_6. These R waves may be notched, particularly near their peaks. The VAT is prolonged up to 0.07 seconds or more, particularly in lead aVL and the left precordial leads V_5-V_6.

S waves: Deep, wide S waves are present in leads V_1-V_3, producing the typical rS or QS complexes. Because of these wide S waves, an anteroseptal MI may be mistakenly diagnosed. S waves are absent in leads I and aVL and the left precordial leads V_5-V_6.

ST SEGMENTS

ST-segment depression is present in leads I and aVL and the left precordial leads V_5-V_6. ST-segment elevation is present in leads V_1-V_3.

T WAVES

T wave inversion is present in leads I and aVL and the left precordial leads V_5-V_6. The T wave is upright in leads V_1-V_3. The T waves are "disconcordant," which means that the QRS complex and the T wave deflect in opposite directions. This is normal for LBBB. If they both deflect in the same direction, the T wave is termed "cordant," which is an indication of underlying ischemia.

KEY DEFINITION

The QRS complexes and T waves are "concordant" when the last part of the QRS complex and the T wave are either both positive or negative. If they are opposite it is called "discordant."

QRS Pattern in Left Bundle Branch Block With Anteroseptal Myocardial Infarction

In LBBB without an intact interventricular septum, the initial depolarization of the septum from right to left does not occur. This leaves the initial electrical forces of right ventricular depolarization (from left to right) unopposed so that significant narrow r waves may be present in leads V_1 and V_2, with small q waves present in leads I and aVL and the left precordial leads V_5-V_6.

For a comparison of ECG characteristics of LBBB with and without an intact interventricular septum, see Figure 13-6.

Summary of the ECG Characteristics in Left Bundle Branch Block

Leads V_1-V_3
- Wide QRS complex with an rS or QS pattern
- Initial small r wave (abnormal interventricular septal depolarization from right to left and anteriorly) OR absent R wave (abnormal septal depolarization from right to left and posteriorly)
- Deep, wide S wave (delayed, essentially normal left ventricular depolarization)

ST-segment elevation
T wave "concordant" with QRS complex

Leads I, aVL, V_5-V_6
Wide QRS complex with an R pattern
- Absent initial small q wave (absent normal interventricular septal depolarization from left to right)
- Tall, wide, slurred R wave with or without notching, and a prolonged VAT (delayed, essentially normal left ventricular depolarization)

ST-segment depression
T wave inversion "concordance"

QRS axis
Normal QRS axis or left axis deviation (−30° to −90°)

Ventricular activation time
Prolonged beyond the upper normal limit of 0.055 second in the left precordial leads V_5 and V_6

Following an Anteroseptal Myocardial Infarction
Leads V_1-V_2
Wide QRS complex with an rS pattern
- Small narrow r wave (unopposed normal right ventricular depolarization)
- Deep, wide S wave (delayed, essentially normal left ventricular depolarization)

ST-segment elevation
T wave "concordant" with QRS complex

Leads I, aVL, V_5-V_6
Wide QRS complex with a qR pattern
- Small q wave (unopposed normal right ventricular depolarization)
- Tall, wide, slurred R wave with or without notching, and a prolonged VAT (delayed, essentially normal left ventricular depolarization)

ST-segment depression
T wave inversion "concordance"

QRS axis
Normal QRS axis or left axis deviation (−30° to −90°)

Ventricular activation time
Prolonged beyond the upper normal limit of 0.055 second in the left precordial leads V_5 and V_6

HEMIBLOCKS

The left bundle branch splits into the anterior and posterior fascicles. A hemiblock exists when there is a conduction block in either fascicle. Thus the name "hemi" referring to "half" of the left bundle branch. Because the conduction block only affects a portion of the left bundle branch, the QRS complex duration does not exceed 0.12 second.

> The QRS duration of a hemiblock is normal.

LEFT ANTERIOR FASCICULAR BLOCK (LEFT ANTERIOR HEMIBLOCK)

Pathophysiology of Left Anterior Fascicular Block

In left anterior fascicular block (LAFB) (Figure 13-7), the electrical impulses are prevented from entering the anterior and lateral walls of the left ventricle directly because of the disruption of conduction of the electrical impulses through the left anterior fascicle of the left bundle branch. The electrical impulses travel rapidly down the left posterior fascicle into the interventricular septum and posterior wall of the left ventricle and then, after a very slight delay, into the anterior and lateral walls of the left ventricle. At the same time, the electrical impulses travel down the right bundle branch into the right ventricle in a normal way.

The interventricular septum depolarizes first in a normal direction, from left to right (1). This is followed by the depolarization of the right ventricle (2) and the posterior wall of the

Left Anterior Fascicular Block

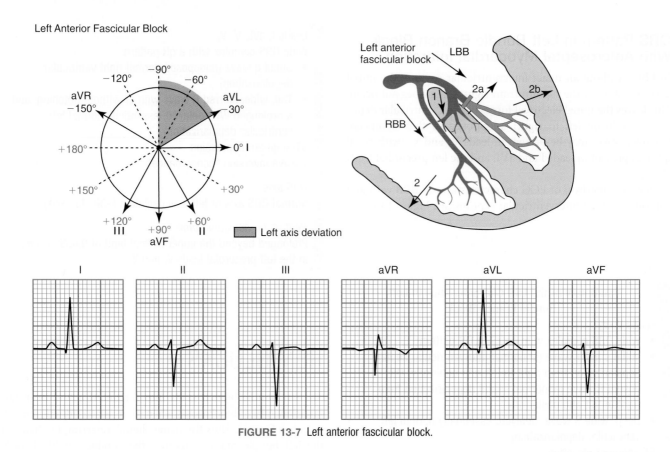

FIGURE 13-7 Left anterior fascicular block.

left ventricle (2a), followed almost instantly by depolarization of the anterior and lateral walls of the left ventricle (2b).

Because there is no appreciable delay between the depolarization of the posterior and anterolateral walls of the left ventricle, the QRS complex is of normal duration. The electrical forces generated by the slightly delayed depolarization of the anterior and lateral walls of the left ventricle travel in an upward and leftward direction, producing a marked left axis deviation.

Causes of Left Anterior Fascicular Block

The most common cause of left anterior fascicular block is acute anteroseptal MI. Left anterior fascicular block can occur alone or in combination with an RBBB.

ECG Characteristics in Left Anterior Fascicular Block

QRS COMPLEXES

Duration

Normal, less than 0.12 second in duration.

QRS Axis

The QRS axis is deviated to the left (i.e., left axis deviation, −30° to −90°).

QRS Pattern

The QRS complexes appear normal without unusual notching or any delay in the VAT. The electrical forces of depolarization of the anterolateral area of the left ventricle, somewhat delayed by 40 msec (0.04 sec), are directed upward and leftward. The presence of an initial small q wave in lead I and an initial small r wave in lead III (q_1r_3 pattern) is an indication of a left anterior fascicular block.

Q waves: Initial small q waves are present in leads I and aVL.

R waves: Initial small r waves are present in leads II, III, and aVF

S waves: The S waves are typically deep and larger than the R waves in leads II, III, and aVF

> The QRS complex of left anterior hemiblock typically has a rS pattern in II, III, and aVF and a qR pattern in lead I. Even in the presence of Q waves the overall deflection will point toward the left axis deviation.

ST SEGMENTS

Normal.

T WAVES

Normal.

LEFT POSTERIOR FASCICULAR BLOCK (LEFT POSTERIOR HEMIBLOCK)

Pathophysiology of Left Posterior Fascicular Block

In left posterior fascicular block (Figure 13-8) the electrical impulses are prevented from entering the interventricular septum and posterior wall of the left ventricle directly because of the disruption of conduction of the electrical impulses through the left posterior fascicle of the left bundle branch. The electrical impulses travel rapidly down the left anterior fascicle into the anterior and lateral walls of the left ventricle and then, after a very slight delay, into the posterior wall of the left ventricle. At the same time, the electrical impulses travel down the right bundle branch into the right ventricle in a normal way and into the interventricular septum.

The interventricular septum depolarizes first in an abnormal direction, from right to left anteriorly and superiorly (1). This is followed by the depolarization of the right ventricle (2) and the anterior and lateral walls of the left ventricle (2a), followed almost instantly by depolarization of the posterior wall of the left ventricle (2b).

Because there is no appreciable delay between the depolarization of the anterolateral and posterior walls of the left ventricle, the QRS complex is of normal duration. The electrical forces generated by the slightly delayed depolarization of the posterior wall of the left ventricle travel in a downward and rightward direction, producing a marked right axis deviation.

Causes of Left Posterior Fascicular Block

Left posterior fascicular block is rare because the fibers of the fascicle are not as organized and discrete as the anterior fascicle and therefore requires a more significant area of the heart to be injured to result in its being blocked. It can occur in an acute anteroseptal MI involving the left anterior descending artery in combination with either an acute right ventricular or inferior MI where the posterior descending artery is also involved. The posterior descending artery most commonly arises from the right coronary artery but can arise occasionally from the left circumflex coronary artery. Left posterior fascicular block can occur alone or in combination with an RBBB.

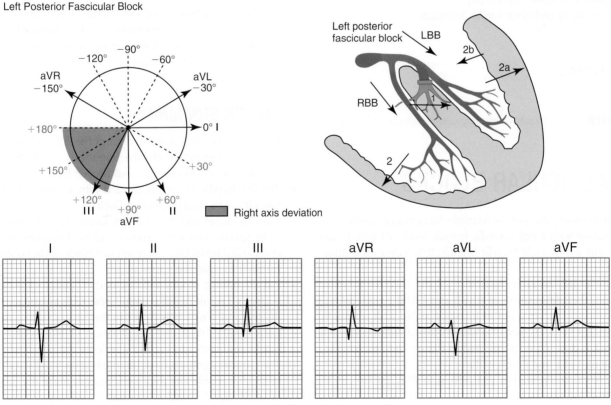

FIGURE 13-8 Left posterior fascicular block.

ECG Characteristics in Left Posterior Fascicular Block

QRS COMPLEXES

Duration

Normal, less than 0.12 second in duration.

QRS Axis

The QRS axis is deviated to the right (i.e., right axis deviation, +90° to +180°).

QRS Pattern

The QRS complexes appear normal without unusual notching or any delay in the VAT. The electrical forces of depolarization of the posterior part of the left ventricle, somewhat delayed by 40 msec (0.04 sec), are directed downward and rightward. The presence of an initial small q wave in lead III and an initial small r wave in lead I (q_3r_1 pattern) is an indication of a left posterior fascicular block.

Q waves: Initial small q waves are present in leads II, III, and aVF and absent in leads I, aVL, and V_5-V_6.

R waves: Initial small r waves are present in leads I and aVL, and tall R waves are present in leads II, III, and aVF.

S waves: Deep S waves are present in leads I and aVL.

> These findings relative to the QRS complexes are significant only in the absence of other causes of right axis deviation, including the following:
> - Right ventricular hypertrophy
> - Pulmonary embolism and/or infarction

ST SEGMENTS

Normal.

T WAVES

Normal.

BIFASCICULAR BLOCKS

As stated before, either of the hemiblocks can occur alone or in combination with a right bundle branch block (RBBB). When they occur with a right bundle branch, this is termed a bifascicular block.

Because left anterior fascicular block (LAFB) is more common, the combination of RBBB and LAFB represents the most common presentation of bifascicular block. It is usually stable except in the context of acute myocardial infarction when the block is new. As demonstrated in Figure 13-9, the characteristics of RBBB and LAFB include:

- Typical configuration of RBBB with RSR′ pattern in V_1 and slurred S in V_6

- QRS complex duration >0.12 second
- Left axis deviation and rS pattern in lead III typical of LAFB

The combination of RBBB and left posterior fascicular block (LPFB) is actually more common than LPFB alone since the ischemia required to injure the posterior fascicle results in injury to the RBBB. This is a very serious condition that can deteriorate into complete heart block particularly in the setting of myocardial infarction. Figure 13-10 shows the characteristic findings of RBBB and LPFB which include;

- Typical configuration of RBBB with RSR′ pattern in V_1 and slurred S in V_6
- QRS complex duration >0.12 seconds
- Right axis deviation with small q wave in lead III

INTRAVENTRICULAR CONDUCTION DELAY

Not all intraventricular conduction delays (IVCDs) will meet the strict criteria presented in this chapter. Some ECGs will exhibit QRS complexes that have the characteristic pattern of a bundle branch block yet only present in one or two leads or their duration will not exceed 0.12 second. These conditions are referred to as nonspecific intraventricular conduction delays.

They may be localized, only seen in one or two leads, or they may be generalized throughout the 12-lead ECG. Localized IVCD is commonly seen in lead III and of no clinical significance. However, a generalized IVCD of greater than 0.12 second, which does not meet the criteria of any of the bundle branch or fascicular blocks, should lead one to consider an electrolyte abnormality such as hyperkalemia.

CHAPTER SUMMARY

- Once the electrical impulse reaches the AV node or the AV node fires independently, the impulse is conducted to the ventricles through the right and the left bundle branches.
- The left bundle branch is divided into a small left anterior fascicle and a larger posterior fascicle.
- Both branches and the fascicles receive their blood supply from specific coronary arteries and its disruption during a myocardial infarction can result in a block of the conduction through the affected pathway.
- Bundle branch blocks and fascicular (hemiblocks) can also occur as a result of other conditions, such as cardiovascular disease and ventricular hypertrophy.
- Each bundle block and combination of blocks and hemiblocks results in specific ECG findings.
- The clinical significance of bundle branch blocks and hemiblocks is variable and their presence can make the detection of an ST elevation MI more difficult.

Bifascicular block: right bundle branch block with left anterior fascicular block

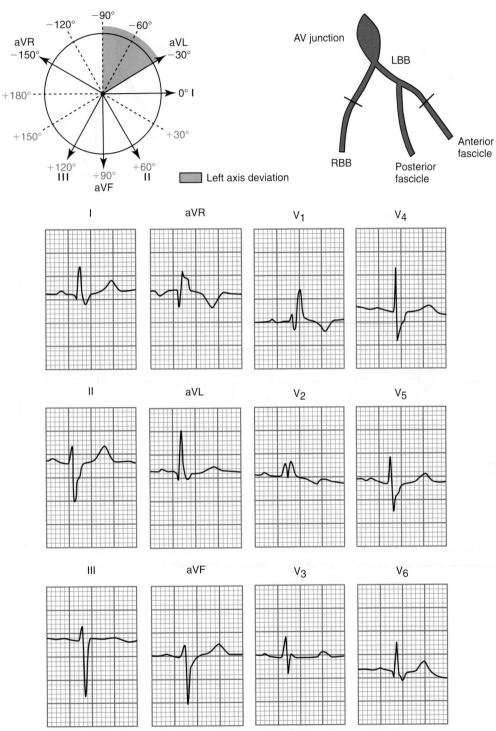

FIGURE 13-9 Bifascicular block, RBBB, and LAHB. (Modified from Goldberger A: *Clinical electrocardiography: a simplified approach*, ed 7, Mosby, St Louis, 2006.)

Bifascicular block: right bundle branch block with left posterior fascicular block

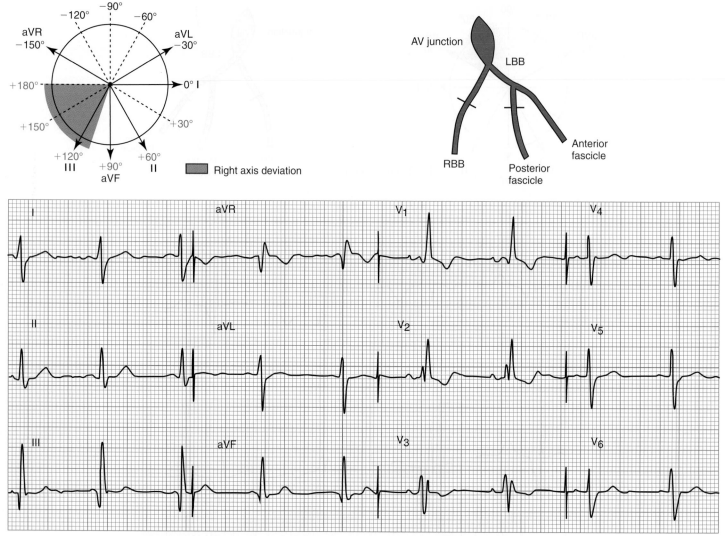

FIGURE 13-10 Bifascicular block, RBBB, and LPHB. (Modified from Goldberger A: *Clinical electrocardiography: a simplified approach*, ed 7, Mosby, St Louis, 2006.)

CHAPTER REVIEW

1. The time from the onset of the QRS complex to the peak of the R wave in the QRS complex is called:
   A. depolarization threshold
   B. interventricular conduction delay
   C. the preintrinsicoid deflection
   D. the ventricular activation time

2. The anterior portion of the septum is supplied with blood from the:
   A. AV nodal artery
   B. left anterior descending coronary artery
   C. posterior descending coronary artery
   D. right coronary artery

3. The main blood supply of the AV node and proximal part of the bundle of His is the AV node artery, which arises from the _____ in the majority of hearts.
   A. circumflex coronary artery
   B. left anterior descending artery
   C. posterior descending coronary artery
   D. right coronary artery

4. A common cause of bundle branch and fascicular blocks is:
   A. electrolyte abnormality, specifically hyperkalemia
   B. ischemic heart disease
   C. severe right ventricular hypertrophy
   D. stroke and seizures

5. In the setting of an acute MI, a right bundle branch block occurs primarily in a(n):
   A. anteroseptal MI
   B. inferior MI
   C. lateral MI
   D. posterior MI

6. In patients with acute MI with a bundle branch block, _____ than in those not complicated by a bundle branch block.
   A. a temporary transcutaneous pacemaker is less frequently indicated
   B. the incidence of pump failure and ventricular dysrhythmias is much higher
   C. the incidence of supraventricular tachycardia is higher
   D. the incidence of ventricular fibrillation is lower

7. Common causes of chronic right bundle branch block include:
   A. congestive heart failure, stroke, and seizures
   B. hyperventilation, acute coronary syndrome, and diabetes
   C. myocarditis, cardiomyopathy, and cardiac surgery
   D. ventricular hypertrophy

8. In a right bundle branch block, the QRS complex in lead V_1 is:
   A. narrow with a QRS pattern
   B. wide with a classic triphasic rSR′ pattern
   C. wide with a tall R wave
   D. wide with deep QS pattern

9. When the electrical impulses are prevented from directly entering the anterior and lateral walls of the left ventricle, the condition is called a:
   A. bifascicular block
   B. left anterior fascicular block
   C. left lateral hemiblock
   D. left posterior fascicular block

10. The most ominous bifascicular block is a RBBB with
    A. left anterior fascicular block
    B. left inferior hemiblock
    C. left posterior fascicular block
    D. right posterior hemiblock

14

Pacemaker and Implantable Defibrillator Rhythms

OBJECTIVES   *Upon completion of this chapter, you should be able to complete the following objectives:*

1. Describe the purpose of pacemakers and list the most common indications for their use.
2. List the components of a pacemaker and compare and contrast a temporary versus a permanent pacemaker.
3. Compare and contrast a fixed-rate versus a demand pacemaker
4. Define the following terms as they relate to pacemakers
   - Lower rate limit
   - Atrioventricular interval
   - Atrial refractory period
   - Ventricular refractory period
5. Be able to determine from the five-letter designation of a pacemaker what type of sensing and pacing function it possesses.
6. Be able to describe the unique features of pacer spikes and their associated QRS complexes
7. List and contrast the following types of pacemaker malfunctions:
   Failure to sense
   Failure to pace
8. Be able by examining an ECG strip to determine whether a pacemaker is failing to sense or pace.
9. Describe the function of an implantable cardiac defibrillator (ICD) and compare and contrast it to a pacemaker.
10. List the types of conditions under which an ICD malfunction may present

PACEMAKERS

A pacemaker is a battery-powered device whose primary purpose is to stimulate the heart electrically. It is indicated for patients with excessively slow heart rhythms. The most common dysrhythmias for which it is indicated include:

- Symptomatic sinus bradycardia
- Atrioventricular block due to
  - Third-degree atrioventricular block associated with symptoms

- Third-degree atrioventricular block with pauses greater than 3 seconds or with an escape rate less than 40 beats/min in awake patients
- Postoperative atrioventricular block that is not expected to resolve
- Second-degree atrioventricular block associated with symptoms
- Chronic bifascicular or trifascicular block with an intermittent third-degree atrioventricular block or type II second-degree atrioventricular block or alternating bundle branch block

- Atrioventricular block associated with myocardial infarction and
  - Second- or third-degree atrioventricular block in the His-Purkinje system
  - Transient second- or third-degree infranodal atrioventricular block and associated bundle branch block
  - Persistent, symptomatic second- or third-degree atrioventricular block
- Sinus node dysfunction
  - Symptomatic sinus bradycardia or sinus pauses
  - Symptomatic sinus arrest
- Carotid sinus syndrome: recurrent syncope or near-syncope as a result of carotid sinus syndrome

A pacemaker has two major components: (1) a controller pack that contains the battery and programmable hardware and (2) wire electrodes that are attached to the heart chamber(s) being stimulated.

Pacemakers are either temporary or permanent (implanted). With temporary pacemakers, the pacing wire is connected to a controller outside the body and the electrode is run through a transvenous catheter into the heart. With long-term implanted pacemakers, the controller is inserted subcutaneously, usually under the chest wall. With both types, the pacemaker wire is threaded through a vein into the right ventricular cavity so that the pacemaker electrode can stimulate the endocardium of the right ventricle (Figure 14-1). Most pacemakers provide the ability to pace the atria as well as the ventricle by placing electrodes in both chambers.

Before obtaining central vascular access, transcutaneous pacing of the heart may be performed using the same self-adhesive pads used for defibrillation. The application and use of transcutaneous pacing is beyond the scope of this text. However, its effects on dysrhythmia interpretation are similar to both temporary and permanent pacemakers.

Regardless of type, all pacemaker leads have the ability to perform two functions. The first function is to sense atrial and/or ventricular electrical activity. The second function is pacing during which the electrode generates an electrical discharge to depolarize the myocardium.

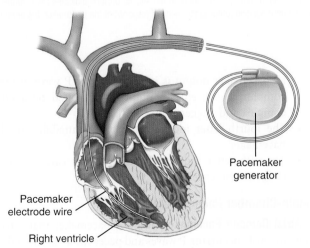

Pacemaker generator

Pacemaker electrode wire

Right ventricle

FIGURE 14-1 Implanted pacemaker.

TYPES OF PACEMAKERS

Fixed-Rate or Demand

There are two basic kinds of pacemakers: *fixed-rate* and *demand.* Fixed-rate pacemakers are designed to fire constantly at a preset rate without regard to the heart's own electrical activity. The first pacemakers on the market were fixed-rate and are uncommon today, although all pacemakers can be placed into a fixed-rate mode. Demand pacemakers have a sensing device that senses the heart's electrical activity and fires at a preset rate only when the heart's electrical activity drops below a predetermined rate. Modern pacemakers are demand pacemakers. A demand pacemaker incorporates two distinct features: (1) a sensing mechanism designed so that the pacemaker is inhibited when the heart rate is adequate, and (2) a pacing mechanism designed to trigger the pacemaker when no intrinsic QRS complexes occur within a predetermined period. By contrast, fixed-rate pacemakers lack a sensing mechanism.

Demand pacemakers can be temporarily converted to fixed-rate mode by placing a special magnet on the chest wall over the battery. This is performed when the pacemaker is firing when it should not. Present-day demand-type pacemakers are also "programmable" by placing a special telemetry device on the chest wall to allow communication with the pacemaker. Besides programming, the device can also interrogate the pacemaker to determine how well it is "sensing" the heart's electrical activity. The demand pacemaker senses the electrical activity of the QRS complex and will not fire. This is vital for the demand pacemaker to function properly.

Each time a demand pacemaker senses a spontaneous QRS complex, formation of a pacemaker pulse is inhibited. Therefore these pacemakers show pacemaker spikes only when the spontaneous heart rate is slower than the preset rate of the pacemaker. The spikes appear before each QRS complex (Figure 14-2).

The timing cycle consists of a defined lower rate limit (LR) and a ventricular refractory period (VRP). The LR is the period of time the pacemaker will wait for an intrinsic electrical discharge from the heart before initiating a pulse. The demand pacemaker also has a ventricular refractory period (VRP) that begins whenever the pacemaker senses a QRS complex or emits a pulse (Figure 14-3). During the refractory period a ventricular demand pacemaker does not sense any electrical activity. When the LR limit is reached, a pacing spike is delivered in the absence of a sensed intrinsic ventricular event. If an intrinsic QRS occurs, the LR time is started from that point. A VRP begins with any sensed or paced ventricular activity.

Single-Chamber and Dual-Chambered

Pacemakers can be either *single-chamber* pacemakers that pace either the ventricles or atria or *dual-chambered* pacemakers that pace both the atria and ventricles. Examples of commonly used pacemakers from each category are described below, with the Intersociety Commission for Heart Disease Resources (ICHD) code noted. While there are five letters in the coding, not all are

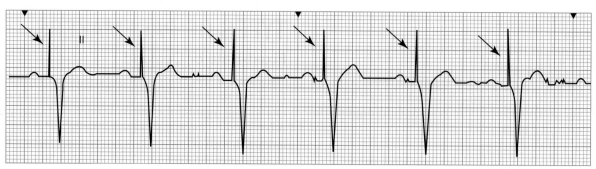

FIGURE 14-2 Pacer spikes in ECG. *Arrows,* pacer spikes.

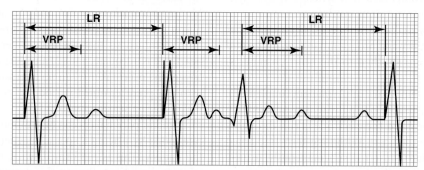

FIGURE 14-3 Lower rate and ventricular refractory period of demand pacemaker. *LR,* Lower rate; *VRP,* ventricular refractory period. (Modified from Libby: *Braunwald's heart disease: a textbook of cardiovascular medicine,* ed 8, Elsevier, Philadelphia, 2007.)

TABLE 14-1 Five Letter Pacemaker Code

Letter 1	Letter 2	Letter 3	Letter 4	Letter 5
Chamber Paced	Chamber Sensed	Sensing Response	Programmability	Antitachycardia Functions
A = atrium	A = atrium	T = triggered[*]	P = simple	P = pacing
V = ventricle	V = ventricle	I = inhibited	M = multiprogrammable	S = shock
D = dual	D = dual	D = dual (A and V inhibited)	R = rate adaptive	D = dual (shock + pace)
0 = none	0 = none	0 = none	C = communicating	
			0 = none	

The letter in the first position indicates the chamber(s) being paced—the *atrium (A), ventricle (V),* or *both (D).* The letter in the second position indicates the chamber(s) where sensing occurs—again the atrium (A), ventricle (V), or both (D). Finally, the letter in the third position refers to the mode of response of the pacemaker-*triggered (T), inhibited (I),* or *dual (D).*

used for every pacemaker. In general, the first three letters provide sufficient information regarding how the pacemaker functions to allow for interpretation of its associated ECG rhythm. Table 14-1 provides a full list of the codes. The codes can be deciphered as follows:

- The first letter of the code indicates which chamber is paced (*A,* atria, *V,* ventricles, *D,* both atria and ventricles)
- The second letter indicates which chamber is sensed (*A,* atria, *V,* ventricles, *D,* both atria and ventricles)
- The third letter indicates the mode of sensing or the response of the pacemaker to a P wave or QRS complex

(*I,* pacemaker output is inhibited by the P wave or QRS complex, *D,* pacemaker output is inhibited by a QRS complex and triggered by a P wave)
- The fourth letter indicates the programmability of the pacemaker
- The fifth letter indicates whether it has cardioversion/defibrillation capability

Single-Chamber Pacemakers

Atrial Demand Pacemaker (AAI). A pacemaker that senses spontaneously occurring P waves and paces the atria when they do not appear (Figure 14-4). The AAI timing cycle consists of

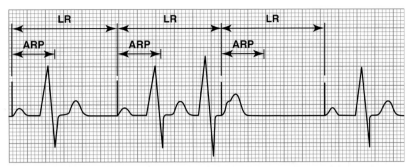

FIGURE 14-4 Single-chamber (AAI) pacemaker. *LR,* Lower rate; *ARP,* Atrial refractory period. (Modified from Libby: *Braunwald's heart disease: a textbook of cardiovascular medicine,* ed 8, Elsevier, Philadelphia, 2007.)

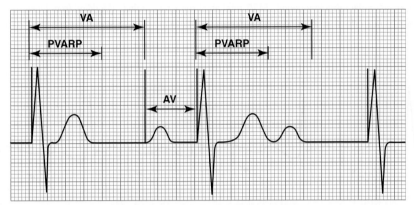

FIGURE 14-5 Dual-chamber (DDI) pacemaker. *VA,* ventricular activation; *AV,* atrioventricular interval; *PVARP,* postventricular atrial refractory period. (Modified from Libby: *Braunwald's heart disease: a textbook of cardiovascular medicine,* ed 8, Elsevier, Philadelphia, 2007.)

a defined lower rate (LR) limit and an atrial refractory period (ARP). During the ARP the pacemaker will not sense any additional atrial electrical activity. When the LR limit is reached, a pacing spike is delivered in the atrium in the absence of a sensed atrial event. If an intrinsic P wave occurs, the LR timer is started from that point. An ARP begins with any sensed or paced atrial activity. The AAI timing cycle should not be affected by events in the ventricle. If a premature ventricular complex (PVC) occurs it is not sensed by the AAI pacemaker, and the atrial pacing spike occurs in the T wave of the PVC. Even though atrial capture presumably would occur, there is no ventricular event after the paced atrial event because the ventricle is still refractory. However, the timing cycle will be reset by anything that is sensed on the atrial sensing circuit.

Ventricular Demand Pacemaker (VVI). A pacemaker that senses spontaneously occurring QRS complexes and paces the ventricles when they do not appear. Figure 14-3 is from a VVI pacemaker.

Dual-Chambered Pacemakers

Atrial Synchronous Ventricular Pacemaker (VDD). A pacemaker that senses spontaneously occurring P waves and QRS complexes and paces the ventricles when QRS complexes fail to appear following spontaneously occurring P waves, as in complete AV block. In this type of pacemaker, the pacing of the ventricles is synchronized with the P waves so that physiologically the ventricular contractions follow the atrial contractions in the normal sequence.

Atrioventricular Sequential Pacemaker (DDI). A pacemaker that senses spontaneously occurring QRS complexes and paces both the atria and ventricles (the atria first, followed by the ventricles following a short delay) when QRS complexes do not appear (Figure 14-5). The timing cycle in DDI pacing consists of a lower rate limit, an atrioventricular (AV) interval, a ventricular refractory period, and an atrial refractory period. The ventricular refractory period is initiated by any sensed or paced ventricular activity, and the atrial refractory period is initiated by any sensed or paced atrial activity. The lower rate limit cannot be violated, even if the sinus rate is occurring at a faster rate. This design allows for a physiologic delay between atrial and ventricular stimulation analogous to the PR interval seen in normal conduction.

Optimal Sequential Pacemaker (DDD). A pacemaker that senses spontaneously occurring P waves and QRS complexes and (1) paces the atria when P waves fail to appear, as in sinus node dysfunction, and (2) paces the ventricles when QRS complexes fail to appear following spontaneously occurring or paced P waves (Figure 14-6). The timing cycle in DDD consists

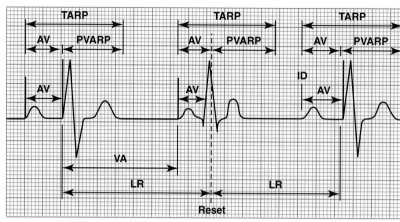

FIGURE 14-6 Dual-chamber (DDD) pacemaker. *LR,* lower rate; *AV,* atrioventricular interval; *PVARP,* postventricular atrial refractory period. *TARP,* total atrial refractory period. (Modified from Libby: *Braunwald's heart disease: a textbook of cardiovascular medicine,* ed 8, Elsevier, Philadelphia, 2007.)

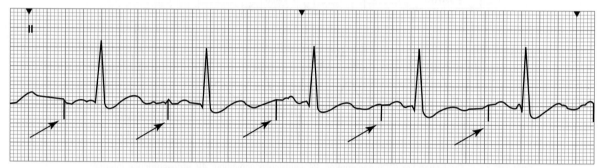

FIGURE 14-7 Atrial pacemaker spikes. *Arrows,* pacemaker spikes.

of a lower rate (LR) limit, an atrioventricular (AV) interval, a postventricular/atrial refractory period (PVARP), and an upper rate limit. The AV interval and PVARP together comprise the total atrial refractory period (TARP). If intrinsic atrial and ventricular activity occur before the LR times out, both channels are inhibited and no pacing occurs. If no intrinsic atrial or ventricular activity occurs, there is AV sequential pacing (first sequence). If no atrial activity is sensed before the ventriculoatrial (VA) interval is completed, an atrial pacing spike is delivered, which initiates the AV interval. If intrinsic ventricular activity occurs before the termination of the AV interval, the ventricular output from the pacemaker is inhibited (i.e., atrial pacing [second sequence]). If a P wave is sensed before the VA interval is completed, output from the atrial channel is inhibited. The AV interval is initiated and, if no ventricular activity is sensed before the AV interval terminates, a ventricular pacing spike is delivered (i.e., P-synchronous pacing [third sequence]).

PACEMAKER RHYTHM

KEY DEFINITION

A pacemaker rhythm consists of the complexes and rhythm produced by a cardiac pacemaker.

Diagnostic Features

Heart rate. The heart rate produced by a permanently implanted cardiac pacemaker is usually between 60 and 70 beats/min, depending on its preset rate of firing. If the pacemaker rate is greater than 90 beats/min, it is probably malfunctioning.

Rhythm. The ventricular rhythm produced by a pacemaker that is pacing constantly is regular. The ventricular rate may be irregular when the pacemaker is pacing on demand (i.e., pacing only when P waves and/or QRS complexes fail to appear).

> It has been noted that in certain cardiac monitors and cardiographs, the pacemaker spikes are difficult to detect. Turning up the gain on the monitor will often times make these spikes more discernable.

P waves. P waves may be present or absent. If present, they may be spontaneously occurring or induced by a pacemaker lead positioned in the atria. When not followed by inherent QRS complexes, spontaneously occurring P waves are usually followed by pacemaker-induced QRS complexes. This indicates that a dual-chamber VDD or DDD pacemaker is present. A narrow, often biphasic spike—the pacemaker spike—precedes pacemaker-induced P waves (Figure 14-7). With the pacemaker

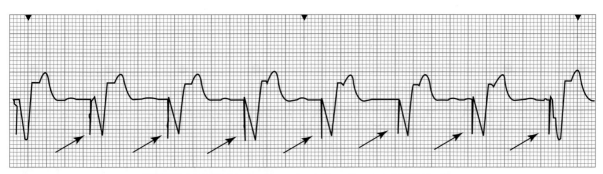

FIGURE 14-8 Ventricular pacemaker spikes. *Arrows,* pacemaker spikes.

electrode placed in the right atrium, a pacemaker spike (A) is seen before each P wave. The QRS complex is normal because the ventricle is not being electronically paced. These P waves may be followed by the inherent QRS complexes or pacemaker-induced QRS complexes, as seen in dual-chamber DDI or DDD pacemakers. A ventricular pacemaker usually does not produce a retrograde, inverted P wave.

PR intervals. The PR intervals of the underlying rhythm may be normal (0.12 to 0.20 second) or abnormal, depending on the dysrhythmia. The PR intervals in atrial synchronous and dual-paced, AV sequential pacemakers are within normal limits.

R-R intervals. The R-R intervals of the pacemaker rhythm are equal. When the pacemaker-induced QRS complexes are interspersed among the patient's normally occurring QRS complexes, the R-R intervals are unequal.

QRS complexes. The QRS complexes of the underlying rhythm may be normal (0.12 second or less in width) or abnormal. Pacemaker-induced QRS complexes are typically greater than 0.12 second in duration (Figure 14-8). The first P-QRS cycle is from a normal sinus beat. It is followed by four pacemaker beats. Notice the pacemaker spike (S) preceding each paced beat.

On the 12-lead ECG, the QRS will have a left bundle branch block pattern because the electrode is in the right ventricle and therefore the conduction moves through the right bundle of His first then leftward to the left bundle. This delay produces the characteristic left bundle branch block pattern. Preceding each pacemaker-induced QRS complex is a narrow deflection, often biphasic—the pacemaker spike—representing the electrical discharge of the pacemaker. If only the atria are being paced, the QRS complexes are those of the underlying rhythm. These are normal unless a preexisting intraventricular conduction disturbance (such as a bundle branch block) or ventricular preexcitation is present.

Pacemaker site. The pacemaker site of a cardiac pacemaker is an electrode usually located in the tip of the pacemaker lead, commonly positioned in the apex of the right ventricular cavity (ventricular pacemaker), in the right atrium (atrial pacemaker), or in both (dual-chamber pacemaker).

Clinical Significance

A pacemaker rhythm indicates that the patient's heart is being electronically paced. Cardiac pacemakers are usually perma-

nently implanted in patients to treat an underlying third-degree AV block or episodes of symptomatic bradycardia, such as second-degree AV block, marked sinus bradycardia or sinus pauses (sick sinus syndrome), slow junctional rhythms, or atrial fibrillation or flutter with an excessively slow ventricular response.

Temporary pacemakers are often employed during cardiac emergencies when an extremely slow heart rate occurs. For example, they may be used immediately after open heart surgery or during cardiac arrest when the ECG shows a slow escape rhythm that does not respond to drug therapy. Occasionally, temporary pacemakers are needed in patients with digitalis or other drug toxicity causing profound bradycardia.

Typically, a $2\frac{1}{2}$- to 3-inch diameter bulge is present, usually in the upper, left anterior chest wall, indicating an implanted cardiac pacemaker.

PACEMAKER MALFUNCTION

The presence of pacemaker spikes followed by a QRS complex indicates that the patient's heart rate is being regulated by a cardiac pacemaker. When a normal or wide and bizarre QRS complex follows every pacemaker spike or every paced P wave (as seen in single-chamber pacing) or every pair of pacemaker spikes (as seen in dual-chamber pacing), the pacemaker is apparently functioning normally even if the patient's own P waves and QRS complexes are interspersed between the pacemaker spikes and associated QRS complexes.

Most problems with pacemakers fall into the following categories: Failure to sense, failure to capture, or both.

- **Failure to sense:** Complete absence of pacemaker spikes in the presence of bradycardia or asystole indicates a failure of the pacemaker to sense the underlying heart rate (Figure 14-9). Notice that after the first two paced complexes, a series of sinus beats with a prolonged PR interval is seen. Failure of the pacemaker unit to sense these intrinsic QRS complexes leads to inappropriate pacemaker spikes (•), which sometimes fall on T waves. Three of these spikes do not capture the ventricle because they occur during the refractory period of the cardiac cycle.

  The two most common causes of failure to sense (without actual battery failure) are dislodgment of the

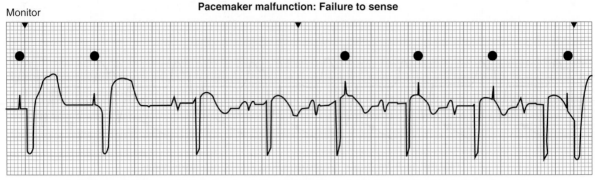

FIGURE 14-9 Failure to sense. *, pacer spike. (Modified from Goldberger A: *Clinical electrocardiography: a simplified approach*, ed 7, Mosby, St Louis, 2006; Adapted from Conover MB: *Understanding electrocardiography*, ed 4, St Louis, Mosby, 1996.)

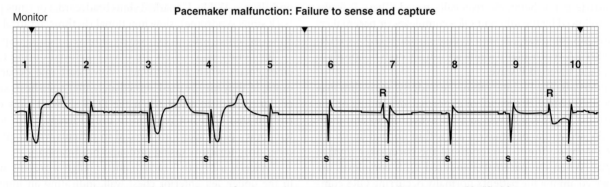

FIGURE 14-10 Failure to capture. *S*, sense and pacer spike. 1, 3, and 4 have capture. (Modified from Goldberger A: *Clinical electrocardiography: a simplified approach*, ed 7, Mosby, St Louis, 2006.)

pacemaker wire and excessive scarring (fibrosis) around the tip of the pacing wire.

- **Failure to capture:** The presence of pacemaker spikes that are not followed by P waves or QRS complexes indicates a malfunctioning pacemaker, one whose electric impulses are unable to stimulate the heart to depolarize; the failure to capture most likely results from the current output from the pacemaker being adjusted too low (Figure 14-10). Notice that beats 1, 3, and 4 show pacemaker spikes (s) and normally paced wide QRS complexes and T waves. The remaining beats show only pacemaker spikes without capture. (R represents the patient's slow spontaneous QRS complexes, which the pacemaker also fails to sense.)

Pacemaker malfunction in patients with temporary pacemakers should always prompt an immediate search for loose connections between the battery and the pacing wire, a faulty battery, or a dislodged wire.

> To determine if the pacemaker is functioning and generating pacer spikes, an insulated circular magnet is placed over the pacemaker generator. This causes the pacemaker to go into the default fixed-rate mode, resulting in pacer spikes at the preset rate. These can then be seen on the ECG strip.

IMPLANTABLE CARDIOVERTER-DEFIBRILLATOR THERAPY

Sudden cardiac arrest, occurring unexpectedly, is most commonly due to the abrupt onset of ventricular fibrillation, often preceded by a run of ventricular tachycardia. Less common causes are asystole and pulseless electrical activity. The goal in modern cardiology is to prevent or interrupt episodes of ventricular dysrhythmias that can lead to sudden cardiac death in these high-risk patients.

The three major approaches to this problem used currently are: (1) antidysrhythmic drug therapy; (2) radiofrequency catheter ablation, designed to destroy areas of the ventricles that generate ectopy; and (3) implantable cardioverter-defibrillators (ICDs).

ICD therapy, as the name implies, involves the internal placement of a device, resembling a pacemaker, capable of delivering electrical shocks to the heart to terminate (cardiovert or defibrillate) a life-threatening run of ventricular tachycardia or ventricular fibrillation. This approach is modeled on conventional external cardioversion/defibrillation devices used in advanced cardiopulmonary resuscitation (CPR), which deliver an electrical shock via paddles placed on the chest wall to treat these types of tachycardias. The clinical indications for an ICD include:

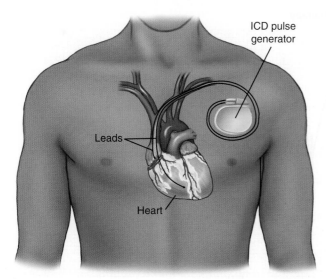

FIGURE 14-11 An implanted cardioverter-defibrillator (ICD). (Modified from Goldberger A: *Clinical electrocardiography: a simplified approach*, ed 7, Mosby, St. Louis, 2006.)

ICD pulse generator

Leads

Heart

- Cardiac arrest resulting from ventricular fibrillation (VF) or ventricular tachycardia (VT) not produced by a transient or reversible cause
- Spontaneous sustained VT in association with structural heart disease
- Syncope of undetermined origin with clinically relevant, hemodynamically significant sustained VT or VF induced during electrophysiological study
- Nonsustained VT in patients with coronary artery disease, prior myocardial infarction, left ventricular dysfunction, and inducible VF or sustained VT during electrophysiological study
- Spontaneous sustained VT in patients who do not have structural heart disease that is not amenable to other treatments.
- Patients with left ventricular ejection fraction of 30% or less, at least 1 month after myocardial infarction and 3 months after coronary artery bypass surgery

ICD devices resemble pacemakers and have two major components: a lead system and a pulse generator (Figure 14-11). The device is very similar to a pacemaker. However, instead of a simple electrode in the right ventricle, there is a special electrode that is touching more surface area of the endocardium. This special electrode delivers the life-saving shock to the heart in the event a lethal ventricular dysrhythmia is detected.

Contemporary ICD devices have many programmable features and have the capacity to deliver *tiered* (staged) therapy when they detect a tachydysrhythmia (Figure 14-12). These devices are capable of automatically delivering staged therapy in treating ventricular tachycardia (VT) or ventricular fibrillation (VF), including antitachycardia pacing (A) and cardioversion shocks (B) for VT, and defibrillation shocks (C) for VF.

For example, the device may be programmed to perform "overdrive" pacing if it detects a presumed episode of ventricular tachycardia. This type of pacing may convert the dysrhythmia without the need for an electrical cardioversion shock. If the dysrhythmia persists or degenerates into ventricular fibrillation, actual shocks are delivered at increasing intensities. Newer ICD models also function as pacemakers in case of bradycardia. The ICD units have data storage capability, allowing cardiac electrophysiologists to interrogate the device periodically and obtain a detailed record of any dysrhythmias sensed and any pacing spikes or shocks delivered.

ICD Malfunction

ICD malfunction occurs for many of the same reasons as those of pacemakers but because of their unique ability to deliver defibrillation, they present with the following list of conditions:

- Increase or abrupt change in shock frequency
  - Increased frequency of VF or VT (consider ischemia, electrolyte disorder, or drug effect)
  - Displacement or break in ventricular lead
  - Recurrent nonsustained VT
  - Sensing and shock of supraventricular tachydysrhythmia
  - Oversensing of T waves
  - Sensing noncardiac signals
- Syncope, near-syncope, dizziness
  - Recurrent VT with low shock strength (lead problem, change in defibrillation threshold)
  - Hemodynamically significant supraventricular tachydysrhythmia
  - Inadequate backup pacing for bradydysrhythmia (spontaneous or drug-induced)
- Cardiac arrest
  - Assume malfunction, but probably due to VF that failed to respond to programmed shock parameters

CHAPTER SUMMARY

- Electronic pacemakers are battery-powered devices used to stimulate the heart electrically, particularly when a patient's own heart rate is excessively slow.
- A temporary pacemaker is a unit with an external battery. Temporary pacing wires can be inserted during cardiac emergencies (e.g., cardiac arrest caused by asystole or myocardial infarction [MI] complicated by high-degree heart block or sinus arrest).
- An implanted permanent pacemaker, in which the battery is inserted subcutaneously (usually in the chest wall) is indicated for patients with symptomatic second- or third-degree AV block or other major bradydysrhythmias (e.g., sinus arrest or slow junctional escape rhythm) leading to inadequate cardiac output.
- Cardiac pacing can be done in a *fixed-rate* or *demand* mode. Demand pacemakers are inhibited when the heart rate is faster than the escape rate of the pacemaker while fixed-rate pacemakers discharge constantly at a preset rate.

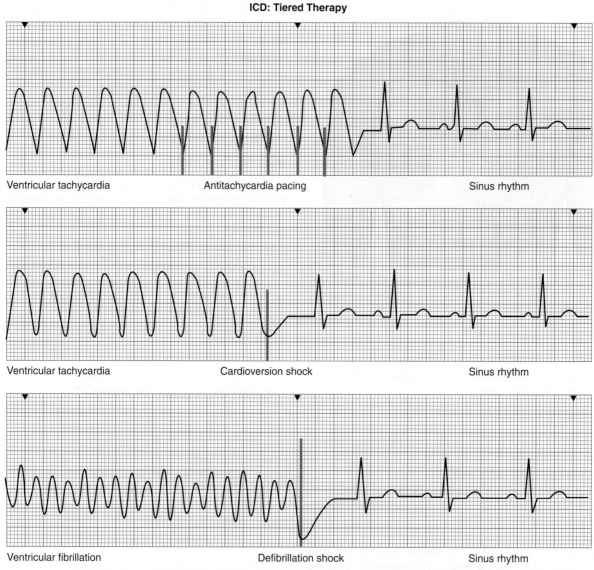

FIGURE 14-12 Tiered dysrhythmia therapy and implanted cardioverter-defibrillators (ICDs). (Modified from Goldberger A: *Clinical electrocardiography: a simplified approach*, ed 7, Mosby, St Louis, 2006.)

- *Dual-chamber* (atrial and ventricular) pacemakers were developed to maintain physiologic timing between atrial and ventricular contractions, thereby increasing cardiac output.
- Pacemaker spikes from an electrode attached to the right ventricular endocardium results in a left bundle branch block pattern because of delayed left ventricular stimulation. Each QRS complex is preceded by a pacemaker spike.

- Failure to sense, capture, or a combination are the most common malfunctions associated with pacemakers and have unique features on the ECG.
- *Implantable cardioverter-defibrillator* (ICD) therapy involves the internal placement of a device capable of delivering electrical shocks to the heart to interrupt a life-threatening run of ventricular tachycardia or ventricular fibrillation and thereby prevent syncope or sudden death.

CHAPTER REVIEW

1. Which of the following is the major indication for a *permanent* pacemaker?
   A. digitalis toxicity
   B. history of multiple prior myocardial infarctions
   C. symptomatic bradydysrhythmia
   D. ventricular bigeminy

2. Fibrosis around the pacemaker electrode primarily affects which of the following?
   A. failure to sense
   B. failure to pace
   C. failure to sense and pace
   D. normal pacemaker function with a ventricular premature beat

3. A pacemaker that fires only when the heart rate falls below a set limit is called:
   A. demand pacemaker
   B. dual-chamber pacemaker
   C. fixed-rate pacemaker
   D. overdrive pacemaker

4. The QRS complex generated by an implanted pacemaker has which of the following characteristics?
   A. duration less than 0.12 seconds
   B. left bundle branch block appearance
   C. normal P wave preceding the QRS complex
   D. right bundle branch block appearance

5. A pacemaker that senses and paces both the atria and ventricles is denoted by what code?
   A. AVI
   B. DDD
   C. DVI
   D. VVI

6. The period following the pacer spike in a VVI pacemaker during which a pacer spike will not discharge is called the:
   A. absolute refractory period
   B. lower set limit
   C. relative refractory period
   D. ventricular refractory period

7. The application of a circular magnet over the controller of an implanted pacemaker will cause it to:
   A. go into demand mode
   B. go into fixed-rate mode
   C. increase power of the discharges to overcome poor capture
   D. stop functioning completely

8. Implantable cardioverter-defibrillator (ICD) is contraindicated for the following condition:
   A. inducible VF or sustained VT during electrophysiological study
   B. spontaneous sustained VT in association with structural heart disease
   C. sustained VT secondary to digitalis toxicity
   D. syncope of undetermined origin with clinically relevant, hemodynamically significant sustained VT

9. Modern pacemakers and ICDs have the following in common:
   A. both can be interrogated by an external controller to determine how well they are functioning
   B. both can cardiovert ventricular tachycardia
   C. both can provide overdrive pacing when needed
   D. both have the same type of electrode attached to the endocardium

10. A patient presents complaining that he can feel his ICD firing in his chest:
    A. He is obviously mistaken since he is awake and not in cardiac arrest.
    B. He most likely has a severe bradycardia.
    C. He should be immediately placed on a cardiac monitor.
    D. The most common cause is a dead battery.

15

Other Assorted ECG Findings

OBJECTIVES *Upon completion of this chapter, you should be able to complete the following objectives:*

1. Discuss the pathophysiology of atrial and ventricular dilatation and hypertrophy and list four examples of atrial and ventricular dilatation and four examples of atrial and ventricular hypertrophy or enlargement.

2. Discuss the pathophysiology of enlargement or hypertrophy of the following heart chambers and list the electrocardiogram (ECG) abnormalities characteristic of each:
   - Right atrial enlargement
   - Left atrial enlargement
   - Right ventricular hypertrophy
   - Left ventricular hypertrophy

3. Discuss the effect each of the following conditions has on the heart and list the ECG changes characteristic of each:
   - Pericarditis
   - Cor pulmonale
   - Pulmonary embolism

4. List the characteristic ECG changes in the following serum electrolyte imbalances according to the serum levels where applicable:
   - Hyperkalemia
   - Hypokalemia
   - Hypercalcemia
   - Hypocalcemia

5. List the excitatory and inhibitory effects of the following drugs on the heart and its electrical conduction system and the characteristic ECG changes that occur with each:
   - Digitalis
   - Procainamide
   - Quinidine
6. Describe the ECG abnormalities characteristic of early repolarization and discuss the implications of diagnosing certain cardiac disorders when it is present.
7. Describe the ECG changes in hypothermia and when they occur.
8. Discuss the anatomical features and pathophysiology of the accessory conduction pathways, the ECG abnormalities characteristic of each, and the potential for misinterpretation of such ECG abnormalities.
9. Define Brugada syndrome and describe its clinical manifestations and unique ECG characteristics.

CHAMBER ENLARGEMENT

Pathophysiology

Enlargement of the atria and ventricles often occurs when heart disease forces them to accommodate greater pressure and/or volume than they normally do. The term *enlargement* includes *dilatation* and *hypertrophy*.

Dilatation

Dilatation is the distention of an individual heart chamber; it may be acute or chronic. Acute dilatation is usually not associated with hypertrophy of the chamber wall, whereas chronic dilatation commonly is. Examples of acute chamber dilatation include the following:
- Left atrial dilatation in acute left heart failure
- Right atrial and ventricular dilatation in acute pulmonary edema and acute pulmonary embolism

Examples of chronic chamber dilatation include the following:
- Left ventricular dilatation in severe aortic valve stenosis or insufficiency
- Left atrial dilatation in severe mitral valve stenosis or insufficiency

Hypertrophy

Hypertrophy is a chronic condition of the heart characterized by an increase in the thickness of a chamber's myocardial wall secondary to the increase in the size of the muscle fibers. This is the usual response of the myocardium to an increase in its workload over time. Examples of chamber hypertrophy include the following:
- Left ventricular hypertrophy in aortic valve stenosis or insufficiency and systemic hypertension
- Right ventricular hypertrophy in pulmonary valve stenosis and chronic obstructive pulmonary disease (COPD)
- Left atrial enlargement in mitral valve stenosis and insufficiency and left ventricular hypertrophy from any cause
- Right atrial enlargement in tricuspid valve stenosis and insufficiency and right ventricular hypertrophy from any cause

Dilatation and hypertrophy affect the ECG differently. Dilatation results in stretching of the walls of the myocardium, resulting in a change in the normal pathway of conduction. This is similar to a bundle branch block and its effects are most noticeable in the atria resulting in prolongation of the P wave duration. Hypertrophy, because of greater muscle mass, results in a QRS complex of larger amplitude. Since the walls of the atria contain less muscle mass to begin with, dilatation is the predominant result of any pathology. Increased workload on the ventricles results primarily in hypertrophy.

RIGHT ATRIAL ENLARGEMENT

Pathophysiology

Right atrial enlargement (generally more dilatation than hypertrophy) is usually caused by increased pressure and/or volume in the right atrium—*right atrial overload*. It occurs in the following conditions:
- Pulmonary valve stenosis
- Tricuspid valve stenosis and insufficiency (relatively rare)
- Pulmonary hypertension from various causes, such as the following:
  - COPD
  - Status asthmaticus
  - Pulmonary embolism
  - Pulmonary edema
  - Mitral valve stenosis or insufficiency
  - Congenital heart disease

The result of right atrial enlargement is, typically, a tall, symmetrically peaked P wave—the *P pulmonale*.

ECG Characteristics (Figure 15-1)
P Waves

Duration. The duration of the P waves is usually normal (0.10 second or less).

Shape. P waves characteristic of right atrial enlargement include the following:

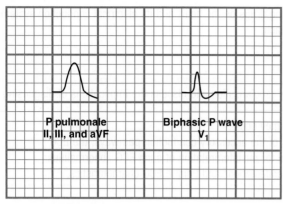

Right atrial enlargement

FIGURE 15-1 Right atrial enlargement.

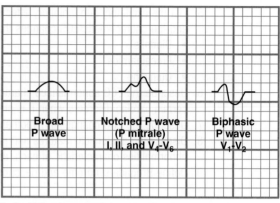

Left atrial enlargement

FIGURE 15-2 Left atrial enlargement.

- Typically tall and symmetrically peaked P wave—the P pulmonale present in leads II, III, and aVF
- Sharply peaked biphasic P wave in leads V_1 and V_2

Direction. The direction of the P waves are positive (upright) in leads II, III, and aVF and biphasic in V_1 and V_2, with the initial deflection greater than the terminal deflection.

Amplitude. The amplitude of the P waves is 2.5 mm or greater in leads II, III, and aVF.

KEY DEFINITION

P pulmonale refers to tall, symmetrically peaked P waves characteristic of right atrial enlargement.

LEFT ATRIAL ENLARGEMENT

Pathophysiology

Left atrial enlargement (generally more dilatation than hypertrophy) is usually caused by increased pressure and/or volume in the left atrium—*left atrial overload.* It occurs in the following conditions:

- Mitral valve stenosis and insufficiency
- Acute myocardial infarction (MI)
- Left heart failure
- Left ventricular hypertrophy from various causes, such as the following:
  - Aortic stenosis or insufficiency
  - Systemic hypertension
  - Hypertrophic cardiomyopathy

The result of left atrial enlargement is typically a wide notched P wave—the *P mitrale.* Such P waves may also result from a delay or block of the progression of the electrical impulses through the interatrial conduction tract (Bachmann's bundle) between the right and left atria.

ECG Characteristics (Figure 15-2)

P Waves

Duration. The duration of the P waves is usually greater than 0.10 second.

Shape. P waves characteristic of left atrial enlargement include the following:

- A broad positive (upright) P wave, 0.10 second or greater in duration, in any lead.
- A wide notched P wave with two "humps" 0.04 second or more apart—the P mitrale. The first hump represents the depolarization of the right atrium; the second hump represents the depolarization of the enlarged left atrium. The P mitrale is usually present in leads I, II, and V_4-V_6.
- A biphasic P wave, greater than 0.10 second in total duration, with the terminal, negative component 1 mm (0.1 mV) or more deep and 1 mm (0.04 second) or more in duration (i.e., 1 small square or greater). The initial, positive (upright) component of the P wave represents the depolarization of the right atrium; the terminal, negative component represents the depolarization of the enlarged left atrium. Such biphasic P waves are commonly present in leads V_1-V_2.

Direction. The direction of the P waves is positive (upright) in leads I, II, and V_4-V_6 and biphasic in leads V_1-V_2. The P wave may be negative in leads III and aVF.

Amplitude. The amplitude of the P waves is usually normal (0.5 to 2.5 mm).

RIGHT VENTRICULAR HYPERTROPHY

Pathophysiology

Right ventricular hypertrophy is usually caused by increased pressure and/or volume in the right ventricle—*right ventricular overload.* It occurs in the following conditions:

- Pulmonary valve stenosis and other congenital heart defects (e.g., atrial and ventricular septal defects)
- Tricuspid valve insufficiency (relatively rare)
- Pulmonary hypertension from various causes, such as the following:
  - COPD
  - Status asthmaticus
  - Pulmonary embolism
  - Pulmonary edema
  - Mitral valve stenosis or insufficiency

Right ventricular hypertrophy produces abnormally large rightward electrical forces that travel toward lead V_1 and away from the left precordial leads V_5-V_6. The sequence of depolarization of the ventricles, however, remains normal.

ECG Characteristics (Figure 15-3)

P Waves

Changes indicative of right atrial enlargement are present (i.e., tall, symmetrically peaked P waves [P pulmonale] in leads II, III, and aVF and sharply peaked biphasic P waves in leads V_1 and V_2).

QRS Complexes

Duration. The duration of the QRS complexes is 0.12 second or less.

QRS Axis. A right axis deviation of +90° or more is usually present: +110° in adults and +120° in the young.

Ventricular Activation Time. The ventricular activation time (VAT) is prolonged beyond the upper normal limit of 0.035 second in the right precordial leads V_1 and V_2.

QRS Pattern.
- **R waves:** Tall R waves are present in leads II, III, and V_1. The R waves are usually 7 mm or more (0.7 mV) in height in lead V_1. They are equal to or greater than the S waves in depth in this lead. Relatively tall R waves are also present in the adjacent precordial leads V_2-V_3.
- **S waves:** Relatively deeper than normal S waves are present in lead I and the left precordial leads V_4-V_5. In lead V_6, the depth of the S waves may be greater than the height of the R waves.

> Tall R waves equal to or greater than the S waves in lead V_1 may also be present in acute posterior wall MI.

ST Segments

"Downsloping" ST-segment depression of 1 mm or more may be present in leads II, III, aVF, and V_1 and sometimes in leads V_2 and V_3.

T Waves

T wave inversion is often present in leads II, III, aVF, and V_1 and sometimes in leads V_2 and V_3.

> The downsloping ST-segment depression and the T wave inversion together form the "strain" pattern characteristic of long-standing right or left ventricular hypertrophy. This pattern gives the so-called "hockey stick" appearance to the QRS-T complex.

LEFT VENTRICULAR HYPERTROPHY

Pathophysiology

Left ventricular hypertrophy is usually caused by increased pressure and/or volume in the left ventricle-*left ventricular overload.* It occurs in the following conditions:
- Mitral insufficiency
- Aortic stenosis or insufficiency
- Systemic hypertension
- Acute MI
- Hypertrophic cardiomyopathy

Left ventricular hypertrophy produces abnormally large leftward electrical forces that travel toward the left precordial leads V_5-V_6 and away from lead V_1. The sequence of depolarization of the ventricles, however, remains normal.

ECG Characteristics (Figure 15-4)

P Waves

Changes indicative of left atrial enlargement are present (i.e., wide, notched P waves [P mitrale] in leads I, II, and V_4 and V_6 and biphasic P waves in leads V_1 and V_2).

QRS Complexes

Duration. The duration of the QRS complexes is 0.12 second or less.

QRS axis. The QRS axis is usually normal, but it may be deviated to the left (i.e., left axis deviation of > −30°).

Ventricular Activation Time. The VAT is prolonged beyond the upper normal limit of 0.04 to 0.05 second or more in the left precordial leads V_5 and V_6.

QRS Pattern.
- **R waves:** Tall R waves are present in leads I and aVL and the left precordial leads V_5-V_6. The following criteria concerning the amplitude (or voltage) of the R wave in various leads are often used to diagnose left ventricular hypertrophy:
  - An R wave of 20 mm (2.0 mV)* or more in lead I
  - An R wave of 11 mm (1.1 mV) or more in lead aVL
  - An R wave of 30 mm (3.0 mV) or more in lead V_5 or V_6
- **S waves:** Deep S waves are present in lead III and the right precordial leads V_1 and V_2. The following criteria concerning the depth (or voltage) of the S wave in various leads are often used to diagnose left ventricular hypertrophy:
  - An S wave of 20 mm (2.0 mV) or more in lead III
  - An S wave of 30 mm (3.0 mV) or more in lead V_1 or V_2

---

*10 mm = 1.0 mV.

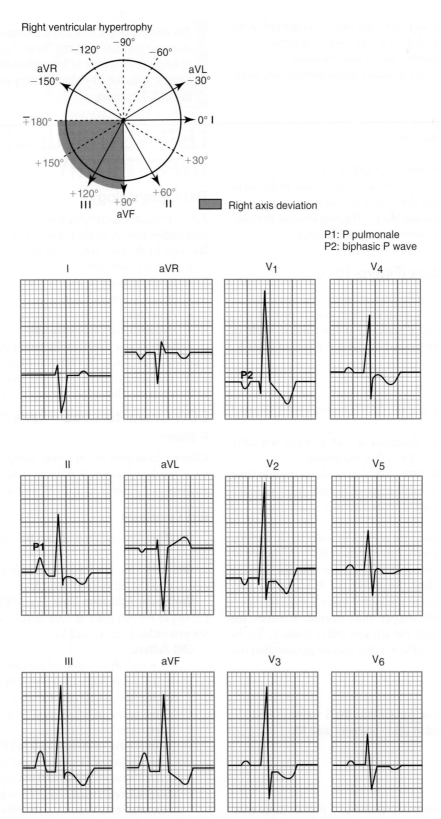

FIGURE 15-3 Right ventricular hypertrophy with right atrial enlargement.

P1: broad P wave
P2: wide notched P wave (P mitrale)
P3: biphasic P wave

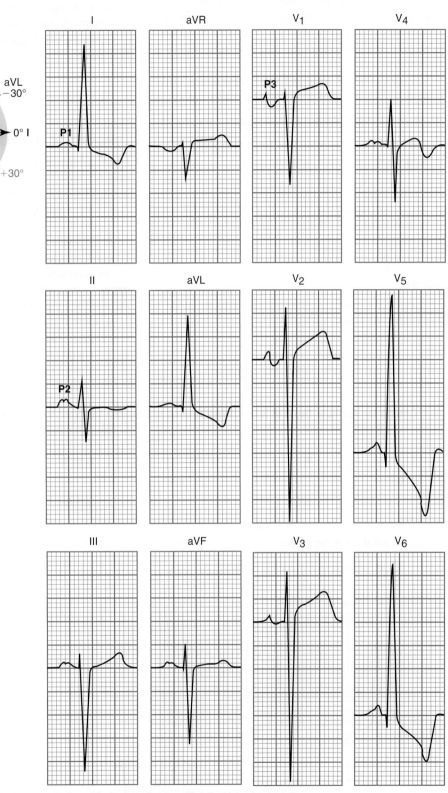

FIGURE 15-4 Left ventricular hypertrophy with left atrial enlargement.

- **Sum of R and S waves:** The sum of the height of the R waves and the depth of the S waves (in mm or mV) in the leads in which these two waves are most prominent is often used to determine the presence of left ventricular hypertrophy. Left ventricular hypertrophy is considered to be present if any one of the following summations is exceeded:
  - The sum of any R wave and any S wave in any of the limb leads I, II, or III is 20 mm (2.0 mV) or more

R (I, II, or III) + S (I, II, or III) ≥ 20 mm (= 2.0 mV)

  - The sum of the R wave in lead I and the S wave in lead III is 25 mm (2.5 mV) or more

R I + S III ≥ 25 mm (= 2.5 mV)

  - The sum of the S wave in lead V_1 or V_2 and the R wave in lead V_5 or V_6 is 35 mm (3.5 mV) or more

S V_1 (or S V_2) + R V_5 (or R V_6) ≥ 35 mm (= 3.5 mV)

ST Segments

"Downsloping" ST-segment depression of 1 mm or more is present in leads I, aVL, and V_5-V_6.

T Waves

T wave inversion is present in leads I, aVL, and V_5-V_6.

> The downsloping ST-segment depression and T wave inversion seen with ventricular hypertrophy is referred to as a "strain pattern" because the myocardial hypertrophy requires greater deopolarization and subsequently greater repolarization. Repolarization affects the ST segment and T waves.

DIAGNOSIS OF LEFT VENTRICULAR HYPERTROPHY

Many criteria for the diagnosis of left ventricular hypertrophy may be caused by other conditions, yet all are based on three major ECG characteristics:
- Increased amplitude or depth of the R and S waves in specific limb and precordial leads
- QRS axis greater than −15° (left axis deviation)
- ST-segment depression

An acceptable set of criteria for diagnosing left ventricular hypertrophy, which would differentiate from other causes, include the following:
- Increased amplitude or depth of the R and S waves in any appropriate lead(s) satisfying the amplitude (or voltage) criteria of left ventricular hypertrophy, expressed in mm or mV (Table 15-1):

TABLE 15-1 Criteria for Height or Depth of R and S Waves Used to Diagnose Left Ventricular Hypertrophy

Wave	I	III	aVL	V_1 or V_2	V_5 or V_6
R Wave	≥20 mm		≥11 mm		≥30 mm
S Wave		≥20 mm		≥30 mm	
Summation	R (I, II, or III) + S (I, II, or III) = ≥20 mm (≥20 mV)				
	R I + S III = ≥25 (≥2.5 mV)				
	S V_1 or V_2 + R V_5 or V_6 = ≥mm (≥3.5 mV)				
R-wave	I		aVL	V_5-V_6	

TABLE 15-1 Criteria for Height or Depth of R and S Waves Used to Diagnose Left Ventricular Hypertrophy—cont'd

			Lead		
Wave	**I**	**III**	**aVL**	**V₁ or V₂**	**V₅ or V₆**
S-wave	III	V₁-V₂			

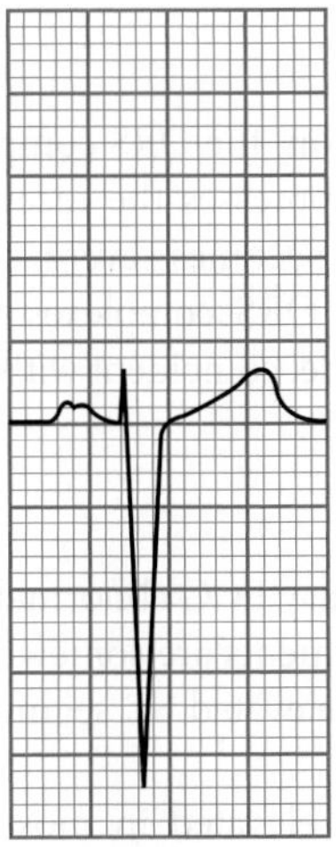

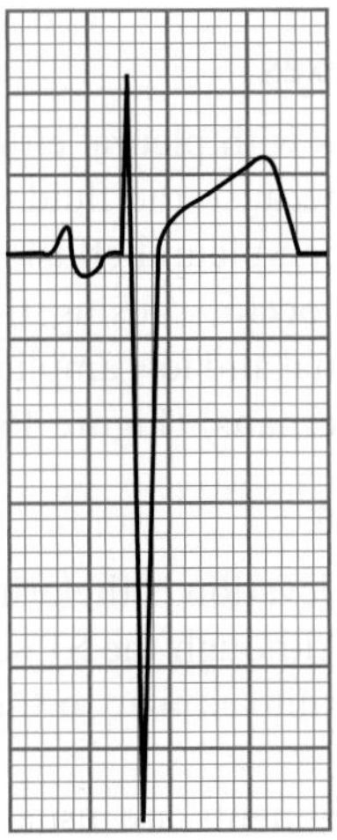

Summation	R (I, II, III)	S (I, II, III)	RI	S III	SV₁/V₂	R V₅/V₆

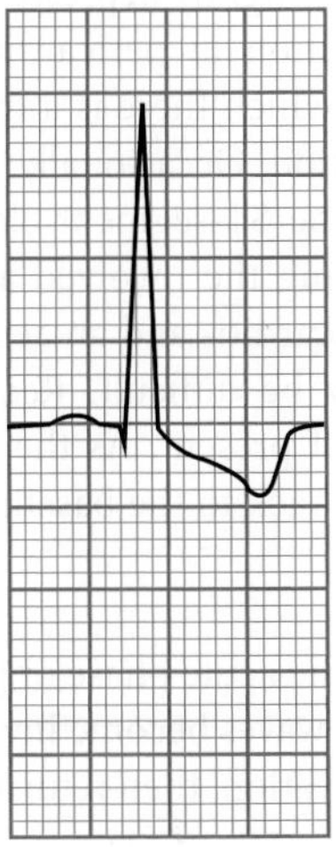

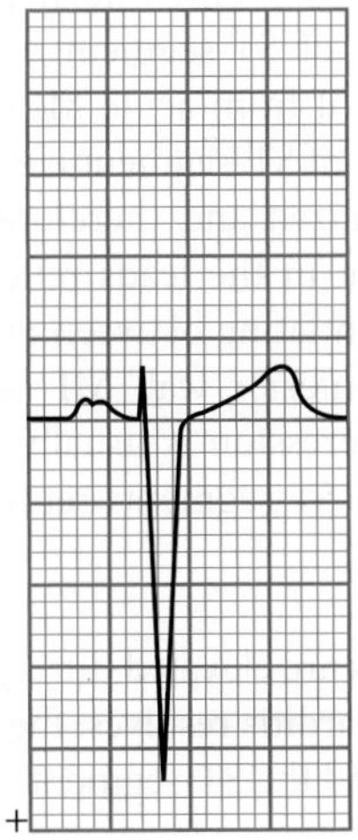

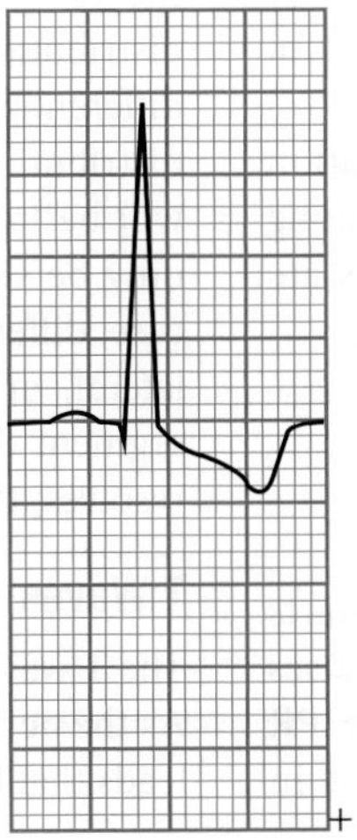

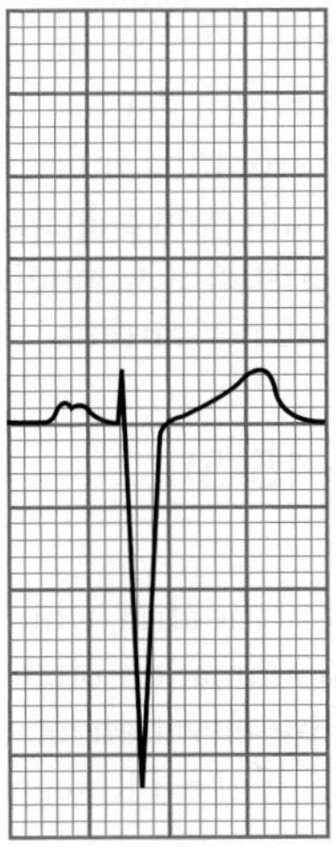

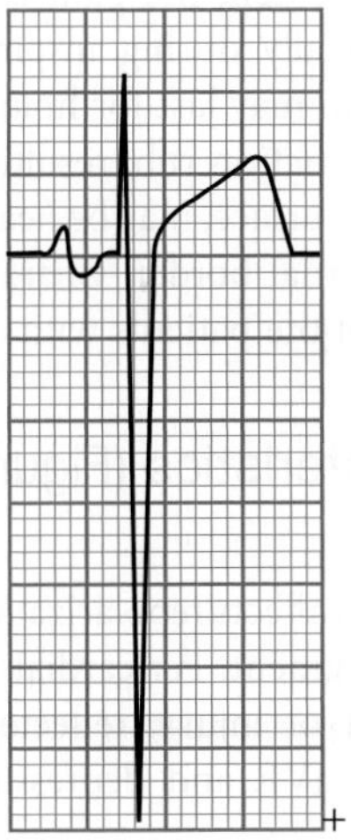

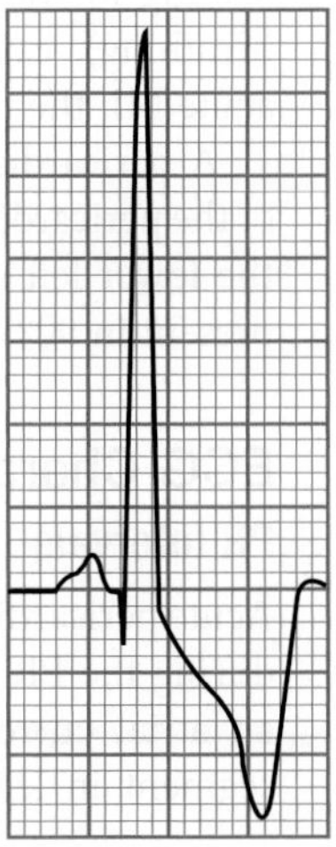

R+S = ≥20 mm   R+S = ≥25 mm   S+R = ≥35 mm

1. The amplitude of the R wave in lead I or the depth of the S wave in lead III of 20 mm (2.0 mV) or greater

OR

2. The sum of the S wave in lead V₁ or V₂ and the R wave in V₅ or V₆ of greater than 35 mm (3.5 mV)

AND one of the following:

1. QRS axis between −15° and −30° or greater than −30° (left axis deviation)

OR

2. ST segment depression of 1 mm in leads with an R wave having the amplitude (or voltage) criteria of left ventricular hypertrophy

PERICARDITIS

PATHOPHYSIOLOGY

Pericarditis is an inflammatory disease of the pericardium, directly involving the epicardium with deposition of inflammatory cells and a variable amount of serous, fibrous, purulent, or hemorrhagic exudate within the pericardial sac. Depending on the nature of the exudate, acute fibrinous pericarditis, pericardial effusion, cardiac tamponade, or constrictive pericarditis may develop. A variety of agents and conditions can cause acute pericarditis, including the following:

- Infectious agents (bacteria, viruses, tuberculosis, and mycotic [fungus] agents)
- Acute MI
- Trauma
- Connective tissue disorders
- Allergic and hypersensitivity diseases
- Metabolic disorders

Unlike acute coronary syndromes, which pericarditis may mimic, pericarditis usually occurs in younger patients without cardiac risk factors who are not suspected of having coronary artery disease. The signs and symptoms of acute pericarditis include the following:

- Chest pain
- Dyspnea
- Tachycardia
- Fever
- Malaise
- Weakness
- Chills

The chest pain, which can mimic that of acute MI, is sharp and severe, with radiation to the neck, back, left shoulder, and, rarely, to the arm. Characteristically, it is present along the sternum, made worse by lying flat, and relieved by sitting up or leaning forward. Often, the pain is pleuritic (made worse by breathing), especially during inspiration. Unlike the pain of acute MI, the pain may last for hours or even days.

A pericardial friction rub, resulting from the inflammation of the pericardial surface, may be heard and even palpated along the lower left sternal border. Characteristic ECG findings are present in 90% of the patients with acute pericarditis.

ECG Characteristics (Figure 15-5)
PR Intervals

Acute pericarditis affects repolarization of the atria, which starts during the PR-segment. Pericardial inflammation often causes an atrial current of injury, reflected by elevation of the PR segment in lead aVR and depression of the PR segment in other limb leads and the left chest leads (V₅ and V₆). The PR and ST segments typically point in opposite directions, with the PR segment being elevated (often by only 1 mm, or so) in lead aVR and the ST segment usually being slightly depressed in that lead. Other leads may show PR-segment depression and ST-segment elevation.

QRS Complexes

In pericarditis with pleural effusion, the QRS complexes are of low voltage because the fluid suppresses the reception of the impulses. When pleural effusion becomes severe, cardiac tamponade may occur, causing the QRS complexes to alternate between normal and low amplitude, coincident with respiration (electrical alternans) (Figure 15-6).

ST Segments

ST-segment elevation is the primary ECG abnormality in acute pericarditis. Although the ST segments are somewhat concave, they appear quite similar to the elevated ST segments present in acute MI.

The ST segments are usually elevated in most, if not all, leads—except leads aVR and V₁—because pericarditis usually affects the entire myocardial surface of the heart. In lead aVR, the ST segment is either normal or slightly depressed. This wide distribution of ST-segment elevation in pericarditis helps to differentiate it from acute MI in which there is a more limited distribution of ST-segment elevation. Occasionally, pericarditis will be localized and therefore the ST-segment elevation will only be seen in the leads reflecting the involved area. In this case, differentiating between pericarditis and an acute anterior, lateral, or inferior wall MI may be difficult. Reciprocal ST-segment depression is usually not present. As the pericarditis resolves, the ST segments return back to the baseline.

T Waves

The T waves are elevated during the acute phase of pericarditis. As the pericarditis resolves, the T waves become inverted in the leads that had the ST-segment elevation, then return to normal.

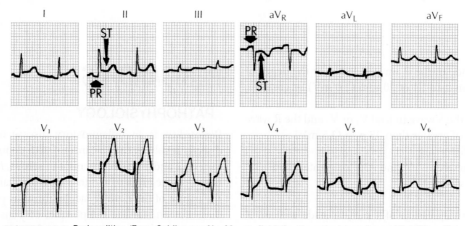

FIGURE 15-5 Pericarditis. (From Goldberger AL: *Myocardial infarction: electrocardiographic differential diagnosis*, ed 4, St Louis, Mosby, 1991.)

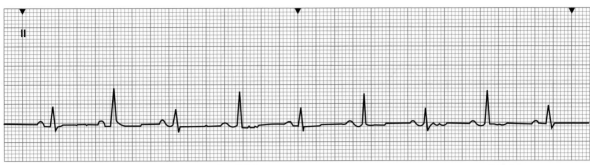

FIGURE 15-6 Electrical alternans. (Modified from Goldberger A: *Clinical electrocardiography: a simplified approach*, ed 7, Mosby, St Louis, 2006.)

ELECTROLYTE IMBALANCE

HYPERKALEMIA

Pathophysiology

Hyperkalemia is the excess of serum potassium above the normal range of 3.5 to 5.0 milliequivalents per liter (mEq/L). The most common causes of hyperkalemia are kidney failure and certain diuretics (e.g., triamterene) that cause the body to retain potassium. Characteristic ECG changes occur at various levels of hyperkalemia. The first changes occur to repolarization and are therefore seen in the T wave and ST segments. As the levels continue to rise, depolarization abnormalities occur resulting in changes to the QRS complex. Sinus arrest may occur when the serum potassium level reaches about 7.5 mEq/L, and asystole or ventricular fibrillation may occur at about 10 to 12 mEq/L. Recognition of the early "peaking" of the T wave in hyperkalemia described below may be life-saving.

ECG Characteristics (Figure 15-7)

P Waves

The P waves begin to flatten out and become wider when the serum potassium level reaches about 6.5 mEq/L, and they disappear at 7 to 9 mEq/L.

PR Intervals

The PR intervals may be normal or prolonged, greater than 0.20 second. The PR interval is absent when the P waves disappear.

QRS Complexes

The QRS complexes begin to widen when the serum potassium level reaches about 6 to 6.5 mEq/L. The QRS pattern qualifies as an interventricular conduction delay because V_1 resembles a left bundle branch block with the typical rS pattern and leads I and V_6 look like a right bundle branch block with deep slurred S waves. As the potassium level approaches 10 mEq/L the QRS complex becomes markedly slurred and abnormally widened

beyond 0.12 second. The QRS complexes may widen to the point that they "merge" with the following T waves, resulting in a "sine wave" QRS-T pattern.

> The presence of an interventricular conduction delay with LBBB *and* RBBB characteristics is highly suspicious for hyperkalemia.

ST Segments

The ST segments disappear when the serum potassium level reaches about 6 mEq/L.

T Waves

The T waves become typically narrow, tall, and peaked when the serum potassium level reaches about 5.5 to 6.5 mEq/L. These T waves, described as tentlike, reach a height of at least 50% of the total height of the QRS complex. The earliest T wave changes are best seen in leads II, III, and V_2-V_4 in most cases.

QT Interval

The QT interval is not affected by hyperkalemia. However, since renal failure is one of the most common causes of hyperkalemia, the ECG may demonstrate QT interval prolongation secondary to associated hypocalcemia.

HYPOKALEMIA

Pathophysiology

Hypokalemia is the deficiency of serum potassium below the normal levels of 3.5 to 5 mEq/L. The most common cause of hypokalemia is loss of potassium in body fluids through vomiting, gastric suction, and excessive use of diuretics. Hypokalemia may also result from low serum magnesium levels (hypomagnesemia). Incidentally, the ECG characteristics of hypomagnesemia resemble those of hypokalemia.

Symptoms of hypokalemia are polyuria in mild cases and muscle weakness in more severely affected patients. Digitalis in the presence of hypokalemia may precipitate serious ventricular dysrhythmias, including the torsades de pointes form of ventricular tachycardia. The diagnosis of hypokalemia is often

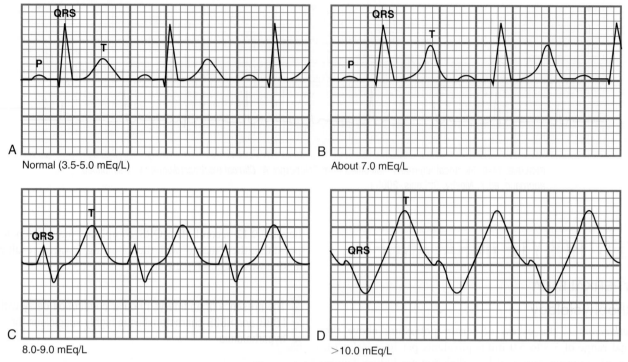

FIGURE 15-7 Changes in lead II caused by hyperkalemia.

made by its characteristic ECG changes. These characteristic ECG changes occur at various levels of hypokalemia.

ECG Characteristics (Figure 15-8)

P Waves

The P waves become typically tall and symmetrically peaked with an amplitude of 2.5 mm or greater in leads II, III, and aVF in severe hypokalemia of about 2 mEq/L or less. Because these P waves resemble P pulmonale, they are called "pseudo P pulmonale."

QRS Complexes

The QRS complexes begin to widen when the serum potassium level drops to about 3 mEq/L.

ST-Segments

The ST-segments may become depressed by 1 mm or more.

T Waves

The T waves begin to flatten when the serum potassium level drops to about 3 mEq/L and continue to become smaller as the U waves increase in size. The T waves may either merge with the U waves or become inverted.

U Waves

The U waves begin to increase in size, becoming as tall as the T waves, when the serum potassium level drops to about 3 mEq/L; they become taller than the T waves at about 2 mEq/L.

The U wave is considered to be "prominent" when it is equal to or taller than the T wave in the same lead. The U waves reach "giant" size and fuse with the T waves at 1 mEq/L.

QT Intervals

The QT intervals may appear to be prolonged when the U waves become prominent and fuse with the T waves.

HYPERCALCEMIA

Pathophysiology

Hypercalcemia is the excess of serum calcium above the normal levels of 2.1 to 2.6 mEq/L (or 4.25 to 5.25 mg/100 mL). Common causes of hypercalcemia include the following:

- Adrenal insufficiency
- Hyperparathyroidism
- Immobilization
- Kidney failure
- Malignancy
- Sarcoidosis
- Thyrotoxicosis
- Vitamin A and D intoxication

Severe hypercalcemia is life threatening. Digitalis in the presence of hypercalcemia may precipitate serious dysrhythmias.

ECG Characteristics (Figure 15-9, *B*)

QT Intervals

The QT intervals are shorter than normal for the heart rate.

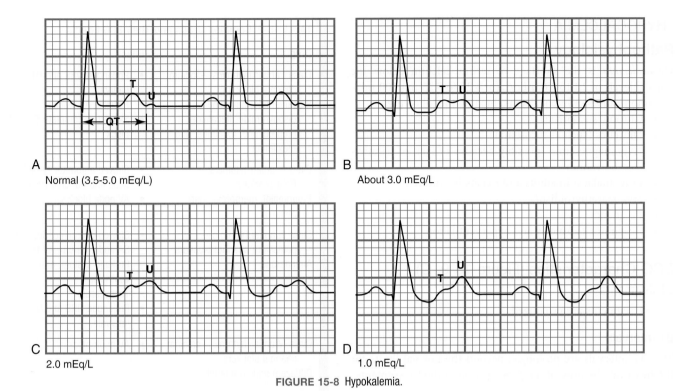

FIGURE 15-8 Hypokalemia.

A
Normal (3.5-5.0 mEq/L)

B
About 3.0 mEq/L

C
2.0 mEq/L

D
1.0 mEq/L

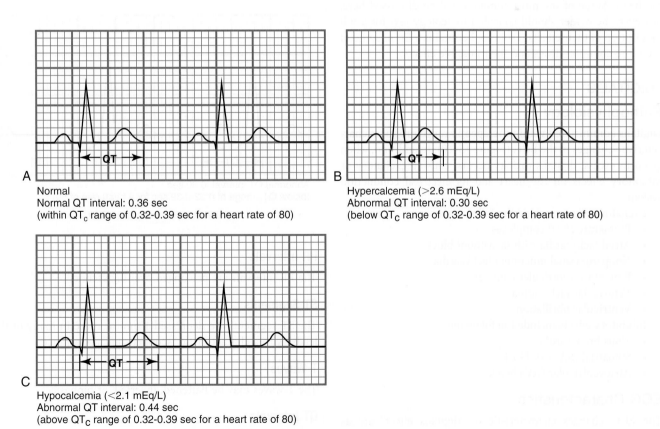

A
Normal
Normal QT interval: 0.36 sec
(within QT$_c$ range of 0.32-0.39 sec for a heart rate of 80)

B
Hypercalcemia (>2.6 mEq/L)
Abnormal QT interval: 0.30 sec
(below QT$_c$ range of 0.32-0.39 sec for a heart rate of 80)

C
Hypocalcemia (<2.1 mEq/L)
Abnormal QT interval: 0.44 sec
(above QT$_c$ range of 0.32-0.39 sec for a heart rate of 80)

FIGURE 15-9 Hypercalcemia and hypocalcemia.

HYPOCALCEMIA

Pathophysiology

Hypocalcemia is the shortage of serum calcium below the normal levels of 2.1 to 2.6 mEq/L (or 4.25 to 5.25 mg/100 mL). Common causes of hypocalcemia include the following:

- Chronic steatorrhea
- Diuretics (such as furosemide)
- Hypomagnesemia (possibly because of lack of parathyroid hormone)
- Osteomalacia in adults and rickets in children
- Hypoparathyroidism
- Pregnancy
- Respiratory alkalosis and hyperventilation

ECG Characteristics (Figure 15-9, *C*)

ST Segments

The ST segments are prolonged.

QT Intervals

The QT intervals are prolonged beyond the normal limits for the heart rate because of the prolongation of the ST segments.

DRUG EFFECTS

Many pharmaceutical agents have electrophysiologic effects on the heart. Some of the most common will be discussed here; however, the reader should consult a toxicology text for a full description of their effects. Table 15-2 contains a list of some of the more common drugs and their possible effects.

DIGITALIS

Pathophysiology

Digitalis administered within therapeutic range produces characteristic changes in the ECG (Figure 15-10). In addition, when given in excess, digitalis toxicity occurs, causing excitatory or inhibitory effects on the heart and its electrical conduction system.

Excitatory effects include the following:

- Premature atrial complexes
- Atrial tachycardia with or without block
- Nonparoxysmal junctional tachycardia
- Premature ventricular complexes
- Ventricular tachycardia
- Ventricular fibrillation

Inhibitory effects include the following:

- Sinus bradycardia
- Sinoatrial (SA) exit block
- Atrioventricular (AV) block

ECG Characteristics

The ECG changes characteristic of "digitalis effect" are as follows.

TABLE 15-2 Common Drugs and Their ECG Effects

Drug	Effect
Class I antiarrhythmics—sodium channel blockers: Procainamide, quinidine, disopyramide, flecainide, propafenone, tocainide, and mexiletine	• Prolonged QRS and QT intervals • Possible AV blocks • Slowed or complete SA nodal block
Class II antiarrhythmics— Beta-blockers Propranolol, metoprolol, and atenolol	• Slowed automaticity of SA node and Purkinje system • AV node block
Class III antiarrhythmic— potassium channel blockers Amiodarone	• Slowed overall conduction: SA node, atrium, AV node, Purkinje system, and ventricles • Tachycardia • Prolonged QRS and QT intervals
Class IV antiarrhythmic—calcium channel blockers Diltiazem and verapamil	• AV node block
Other agents Phenothiazines and tricyclic antidepressants	• QRS prolongations • T wave changes

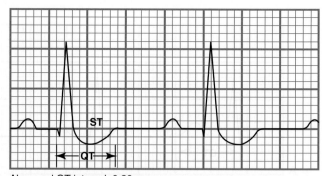

Abnormal QT interval: 0.30 sec
(below QT_c range of 0.32-0.39 sec for a heart rate of 80)

FIGURE 15-10 Digitalis effect.

PR Intervals

The PR intervals are prolonged over 0.2 second.

ST Segments

The ST segments are depressed 1 mm or more in many of the leads, with a characteristic "scooped-out" appearance.

T Waves

The T waves may be flattened, inverted, or biphasic.

QT Intervals

The QT intervals are shorter than normal for the heart rate.

PROCAINAMIDE

Pathophysiology

Procainamide administered within therapeutic range produces characteristic changes in the ECG (Figure 15-11). In addition, when given in excess, procainamide toxicity occurs, causing excitatory or inhibitory effects on the heart and its electrical conduction system.

Excitatory effects include the following:

- Premature ventricular complexes
- Ventricular tachycardia in the form of torsades de pointes (occurrence less common than in quinidine administration)
- Ventricular fibrillation

Inhibitory effects include the following:

- Depression of myocardial contractility, which may cause hypotension and congestive heart failure
- AV block
- Asystole

ECG Characteristics

QRS Complexes

The duration of the QRS complexes may be increased beyond 0.12 second. QRS complex widening is a sign of toxicity. The R waves may be decreased in amplitude.

T Waves

The T waves may be decreased in amplitude. Occasionally the T waves may be widened and notched because of the appearance of a U wave.

PR Intervals

The PR intervals may be prolonged.

ST Segments

The ST segments may be depressed 1 mm or more.

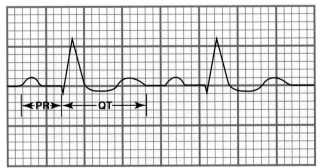

PR interval: >0.20 sec
QT interval: Prolonged, 0.45 sec
(above QT$_C$ range of 0.32-0.39 sec for a heart rate of 80)
QRS complex: Widened, >0.12 sec

FIGURE 15-11 Procainamide and quinidine toxicity.

QT Intervals

The QT intervals may occasionally be prolonged beyond the normal limits for the heart rate. Prolongation of the QT intervals is a sign of procainamide toxicity.

QUINIDINE

Pathophysiology

Quinidine administered within therapeutic range produces characteristic changes in the ECG (see Figure 15-11). In addition, when given in excess, quinidine toxicity occurs, causing excitatory or inhibitory effects on the heart and its electrical conduction system.

Excitatory effects include the following:

- Premature ventricular complexes
- Ventricular tachycardia in the form of torsades de pointes (occurrence more common than in procainamide administration)
- Ventricular fibrillation

Inhibitory effects include the following:

- Depression of myocardial contractility, which may cause hypotension and congestive heart failure
- SA exit block
- AV block
- Asystole

ECG Characteristics

P Waves

The P waves may be wide, often notched.

QRS Complexes

The duration of the QRS complexes may be increased beyond 0.12 second. QRS complex widening is a sign of toxicity.

T Waves

The T waves may be decreased in amplitude, wide, and notched, or they may be inverted. The notching is caused by the appearance of a U wave as the T wave widens.

PR Intervals

The PR intervals may be prolonged beyond normal.

ST Segments

The ST segments may be depressed 1 mm or more.

QT Intervals

The QT intervals may be prolonged beyond the normal limits for the heart rate. Prolongation of the QT intervals is a sign of quinidine toxicity.

ACUTE PULMONARY EMBOLISM

Pathophysiology

Pulmonary embolism (Figure 15-12) occurs when a blood clot (thromboembolus) or other foreign matter (solid, liquid, or gaseous) lodges in a pulmonary artery and causes obstruction (occlusion) of blood flow to the lung segment supplied by the artery. The thromboemboli originate most commonly in the deep leg veins or the pelvic veins and infrequently in the veins of the upper extremities or in the right heart.

If the area of the pulmonary circulation affected by pulmonary embolization is small, the symptoms, if any, are minimal, such as sinus tachycardia and dyspnea. If pulmonary embolization shuts off a large part of the pulmonary circulation, it is considered a massive pulmonary embolism. This results in hypoxemia and the following signs and symptoms.

Symptoms

- Sudden severe dyspnea
- Anxiety, restlessness, and apprehension
- Chilliness, dizziness, and mental confusion
- Nausea, vomiting, and abdominal pain (acute congestion of the liver caused by right-sided congestive heart failure)
- Precordial or substernal chest pain similar to that of acute MI

Signs

- Sinus tachycardia
- Tachypnea, cough, and wheezing
- Cyanosis
- Distended neck veins (right-sided congestive heart failure)
- Forceful pulsation, seen and palpated, in the second left intercostal space with a systolic pulmonic murmur (dilated pulmonary artery)
- Hypotension, shock, and, rarely, cardiac arrest

Because of the increased pressure in the pulmonary artery (pulmonary hypertension) caused by the major obstruction of blood flow through the pulmonary circulation, the right ventricle and atrium become distended, unable to function properly, leading to right heart failure. This condition is called *acute cor pulmonale*.

In minimally to moderately significant pulmonary emboli, the ECG may be normal. However, in massive acute pulmonary embolization (acute cor pulmonale), the ECG shows a "P pulmonale" and a characteristic $S_1Q_3T_3$ pattern described below.

ECG Characteristics

P Waves

Changes indicative of right atrial enlargement are present (i.e., tall, symmetrically peaked P waves [P pulmonale] in leads II, III, and aVF and sharply peaked biphasic P waves in leads V_1 and V_2).

QRS Complexes

An S wave in lead I, a Q wave in lead III, and an inverted T wave in lead III (the $S_1Q_3T_3$ pattern) may occur acutely. In addition, a right bundle branch block may also occur.

QRS Axis

The QRS axis is greater than +90°.

ST Segments/T Waves

A right ventricular "strain" pattern may be present (inverted T waves in leads V_1-V_3).

CHRONIC COR PULMONALE

Pathophysiology

Chronic cor pulmonale (Figure 15-13) is the enlargement of the right ventricle (dilatation and/or hypertrophy) commonly accompanied by right heart failure. It is usually the end stage result of prolonged pulmonary hypertension that occurs with

Pulmonary Embolism (Acute)

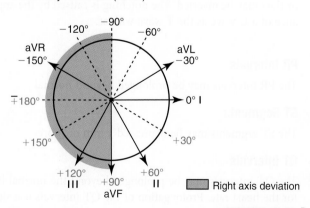

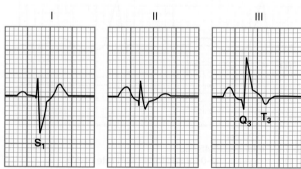

FIGURE 15-12 Pulmonary embolism.

Cor pulmonale

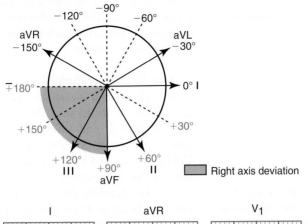

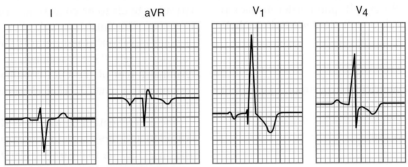

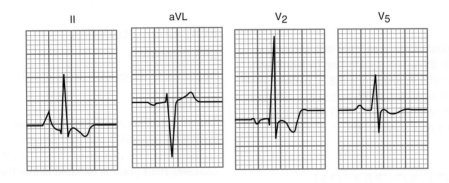

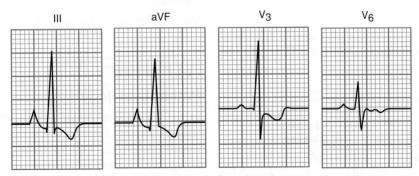

FIGURE 15-13 Cor pulmonale.

many diseases of the lung, including COPD and recurrent pulmonary embolization.

Chronic cor pulmonale is often associated with atrial dysrhythmias, including the following:

- Premature atrial complexes
- Wandering atrial pacemaker
- Multifocal atrial tachycardia
- Atrial flutter
- Atrial fibrillation

ECG Characteristics

P Waves

Changes indicative of right atrial enlargement are present (i.e., tall, symmetrically peaked P waves [P pulmonale] in leads II, III, and aVF and sharply peaked biphasic P waves in leads V_1 and V_2).

QRS Complexes

Changes indicative of right ventricular hypertrophy are present.

QRS Axis

The QRS axis is greater than +90°.

ST Segments/T Waves

A right ventricular "strain" pattern is present (inverted T waves in leads V_1-V_3).

> The ECG in a small percentage of patients with chronic cor pulmonale, especially those with severe lung hyperinflation, shows S waves in leads I, II, and III (the $S_1S_2S_3$ pattern) along with a "P pulmonale" and a QRS axis in the −90° to −150° range. Patients with this type of ECG pattern have been shown to have a poor survival rate.

EARLY REPOLARIZATION

Pathophysiology

Early repolarization (Figure 15-14) is a term used to describe a form of myocardial repolarization in which the ST segment is

elevated or depressed 1 to 3 mm above or below the baseline, respectively. The ST elevations are most commonly seen in leads I, II, and aVF and the precordial leads V_2-V_6. ST depression may be present in lead aVR. Early repolarization can occur in normal healthy people, commonly in young persons and sometimes in the elderly. The ST elevations can mimic the ECG pattern seen in acute MI and pericarditis.

The ST-segment elevations present in early repolarization are similar to those seen during the early phase of acute anterior, lateral, and inferior MIs. However, there are no typical reciprocal ST depressions in the opposite leads. Unlike the elevated ST segments in early acute coronary syndromes that later return to the baseline, these ST elevations persist. Another difference is that the ST segment of early repolarization tends to be concave in shape while that of ischemia is convex. One final hallmark of early repolarization is called "J point elevation." The J point is the point at which the QRS complex meets the ST segment. In early repolarization, the terminal forces of the QRS complex will be slightly positive resulting in a small J point elevation before the ST-segment elevation.

The differentiation between the ST elevations of early repolarization and those seen in acute pericarditis is often difficult. The only clues are that early repolarization ST segments do not return to the baseline and that the T waves do not invert as they do over time in resolving pericarditis.

ECG Characteristics

QRS Complexes

Abnormal Q waves are usually absent.

ST Segments

The ST segments are elevated by about 1 to 3 mm or more in leads I, II, and aVF and the precordial leads V_2-V_6. The ST segment may be depressed in lead aVR. The ST segment is concave. The J point is elevated before the ST segment.

T Waves

The T waves are usually normal.

HYPOTHERMIA

Pathophysiology

In the majority of hypothermic patients with a core body temperature of 89°F, a distinctive narrow, positive wave (Figure 15-15), the Osborn wave (also referred to as "the J wave," "the J deflection," or "the camel's hump"), occurs at the junction of the QRS complex and the ST segment. Associated ECG changes include prolonged PR and QT intervals and widening of the QRS complex.

Sinus bradycardia and junctional and ventricular dysrhythmias also occur in hypothermia. The abnormal ECG changes and dysrhythmias noted here are reversed after normalization of the body's temperature.

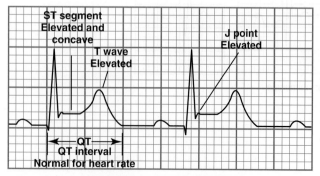

FIGURE 15-14 Early repolarization.

ECG Characteristics

PR Intervals

The PR intervals may occasionally be greater than 0.20 second.

QRS Complexes

The QRS complexes may occasionally be abnormally wide, greater than 0.12 second.

QT Interval

The corrected QT interval (QTc interval) may occasionally be prolonged.

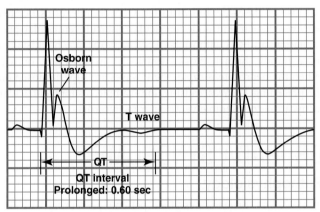

FIGURE 15-15 Hypothermia.

Osborn Wave

An Osborn wave is present, typically in the leads facing the left ventricle. It is a narrow positive deflection that is closely attached to the end of the R or S wave of the QRS complex at the point where the QRS complex joins the ST segment—the J point.

PREEXCITATION SYNDROMES

Pathophysiology

Preexcitation syndromes (Figure 15-16) occur when electrical impulses travel from the atria or AV junction into the ventricles through accessory conduction pathways, causing the ventricles to depolarize earlier than they normally would. Accessory conduction pathways are abnormal strands of myocardial fibers that conduct electrical impulses (1) from the atria to the ventricles or AV junction or (2) from the AV junction to the ventricles, bypassing various parts of the normal electrical conduction system (see Chapter 1). These pathways cannot only conduct electrical impulses forward (antegrade), but most of them can also conduct the impulses backward (retrograde) as well, a potential set-up for reentry tachydysrhythmias, such as paroxysmal supraventricular tachycardias (PSVT).

The following are the three major accessory conduction pathways:

- **Accessory AV pathways (bundles of Kent).** These accessory tracts, located between the atria and ventricles, are

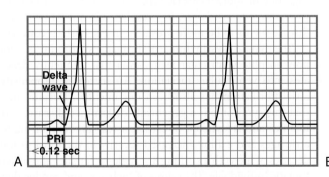

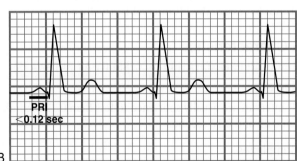

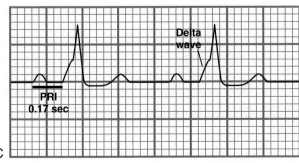

A. Ventricular preexcitation
B. Atrio-His preexcitation
C. Nodoventricular/fasciculoventricular preexcitation

FIGURE 15-16 Preexcitation syndromes.

responsible for accessory AV pathway conduction, also known as the *Wolff-Parkinson-White (WPW) conduction.* These pathways conduct electrical impulses from the atria to the ventricles, bypassing the AV junction, producing premature depolarization of the ventricles-*ventricular preexcitation.* This results in a slurring of the onset of the QRS complex, the *delta wave.* When accessory AV pathway conduction is associated with episodes of PSVT, it is called the *Wolff-Parkinson-White (WPW) syndrome.* During the tachycardia, the changes in the QRS complex characteristic of ventricular preexcitation described below disappear and the QRS complexes appear normal.

- **Atrio-His fibers (James fibers).** This accessory conduction pathway connects the atria with the lowermost part of the AV node, bypassing the slower conducting AV node. This results in *atrio-His preexcitation,* typified by an abnormally short PR interval. This is called *Lown-Ganong-Levine (LGL) syndrome.* Because this type of accessory AV conduction does not conduct the electrical impulse directly into the ventricles, a delta wave is not produced.
- **Nodoventricular/fasciculoventricular fibers (Mahaim fibers).** These rarely occurring accessory conduction pathways provide bypass channels between the lower part of the AV node and the ventricles (the nodoventricular fibers) and between the bundle of His and the ventricles (the fasciculoventricular fibers), resulting in *nodoventricular* and *fasciculoventricular preexcitation.* Like ventricular preexcitation, this form of preexcitation also involves the conduction of the electrical impulse directly into the ventricles with premature depolarization of the ventricles, producing a delta wave. Because the AV node is not bypassed, the PR interval is usually normal.

ECG Characteristics

VENTRICULAR PREEXCITATION (ACCESSORY AV PATHWAYS)
PR Intervals

The PR intervals are usually shortened to less than 0.12 second, between 0.09 and 0.12 second.

QRS Complexes

The duration of the QRS complexes are greater than 0.12 second and abnormally shaped, with a delta wave (the slurring of the onset of the QRS complex).

ATRIO-HIS PREEXCITATION (ATRIO-HIS FIBERS)
PR Intervals

The PR intervals are usually shortened to less than 0.12 second.

QRS Complexes

The duration of the QRS complexes is normal: 0.12 second or less in adults and 0.08 second or less in children. A delta wave is not present.

NODOVENTRICULAR/FASCICULOVENTRICULAR PREEXCITATION (NODOVENTRICULAR/FASCICULOVENTRICULAR FIBERS)
PR Intervals

The PR intervals are usually normal, 0.12 second or greater.

QRS Complexes

The duration of the QRS complexes are greater than 0.12 second and abnormally shaped, with a delta wave (the slurring of the onset of the QRS complex) in both of these preexcitation syndromes.

CLINICAL SIGNIFICANCE

Because of the wide and distorted QRS complexes associated with ventricular and nodoventricular/fasciculoventricular preexcitation, an ECG with such QRS complexes may be mistaken for a bundle branch block, ventricular hypertrophy, or MI. When the heart rate is rapid, the P waves are superimposed on the preceding T waves, causing, for example, a supraventricular tachycardia to resemble ventricular tachycardia.

BRUGADA SYNDROME
Pathophysiology

In 1992, Drs. Brugada described patients presenting with ST-segment elevation in the right precordial leads (V_1 to V_3) (in the absence of acute coronary syndrome), right bundle branch block, susceptibility to ventricular tachydysrhythmias, and structurally normal hearts. These individuals had a significantly high rate of sudden cardiac arrest. This disease is now referred to as *Brugada syndrome.* Its prevalence is not known, but the disease seems to be more prevalent in Far Eastern countries.

The typical dysrhythmia of Brugada syndrome is a rapid polymorphic ventricular tachycardia that frequently degenerates into ventricular fibrillation. An increased propensity to atrial fibrillation has also been documented. Despite the fact that this syndrome is a genetically determined disease, clinical manifestations (syncope or cardiac arrest) are rare during pediatric ages and exhibit increased severity in the third to fourth decades of life with a striking 8 : 1 male-to-female ratio in symptomatic individuals. The causes of such age- and gender-dependent risk are not yet understood. Cardiac events occur during sleep or at rest. Fever, tricyclic antidepressant usage, and cocaine consumption have been identified as specific triggers for events in some patients.

The incidence of premature sudden cardiac arrest is estimated to be as high as 30 percent for those with Brugada syndrome. They are often diagnosed only after suffering a syncopal episode. Conservative treatment consists of an implantable defibrillator.

ECG Characteristics (Figure 15-17)
QRS Complexes

The QRS complexes in V_1-V_3 resemble a right bundle branch block without the typical RSR' pattern.

Brugada Pattern

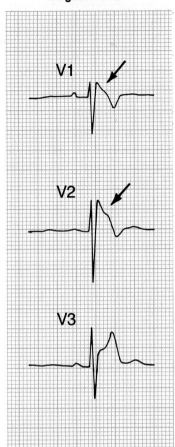

FIGURE 15-17 Brugada syndrome. Arrows denote nonischemic downsloping ST-segment elevation. (From Goldberger A: *Clinical electrocardiography: a simplified approach*, ed 7, Mosby, St Louis, 2006.)

ST Segments

The ST segments associated with the abnormal QRS complexes in the precordial leads have a nonischemic elevation pattern (no reciprocal changes).

CHAPTER SUMMARY

- The two physiologic changes to the myocardium that effect conduction are dilatation and hypertrophy.
- Significantly elevated or depressed levels of physiologic electrolytes, potassium and calcium in particular, result in characteristic ECG changes. Potassium is associated with T wave changes while calcium is associated with changes in the QT interval.
- Left atrial enlargement results in P mitrale while right atrial enlargement results in P pulmonale.
- Certain drugs, particularly those used to treat cardiac rhythm disturbances, can cause significant cardiac conduction changes.
- Accessory conduction pathways predispose the heart to tachydysrhythmias such as PSVT of which there are several types depending on the particular pathway involved.
- An assortment of physiologic conditions such as hypothermia, inflammation, and medical conditions can result in characteristic ECG changes.

CHAPTER REVIEW

1. A chronic condition of the heart characterized by an increase in the thickness of a chamber's myocardial wall secondary to the increase in the size of the muscle fibers is called:
   A. atrophy
   B. dilatation
   C. hypertrophy
   D. stenosis

2. A patient who has mitral valve insufficiency or left heart failure may have:
   A. left atrial and ventricular enlargement
   B. left ventricular enlargement alone
   C. right atrial and ventricular enlargement
   D. right ventricular enlargement alone

3. Left ventricular hypertrophy, a condition usually caused by increased pressure or volume in the left ventricle, is often found in:
   A. COPD
   B. pulmonary hypertension
   C. systemic hypertension and acute MI
   D. ventricular septal defect

4. An inflammatory disease directly involving the epicardium with deposition of inflammatory cells and a variable amount of serous, fibrous, purulent, or hemorrhagic exudate within the sac surrounding the heart is called:
   A. cardiac tamponade
   B. electrical alternans
   C. myocarditis
   D. pericarditis

5. In a diffuse pericarditis (i.e., one that is not localized), the ST-segments are elevated in:
   A. all leads except aVR and V_1
   B. leads aVR, aVL, and aVF
   C. the bipolar leads only
   D. the precordial leads V_1 through V_4

6. An excess serum potassium above the normal levels of 3.5 to 5.0 mEq/L is called:
   A. hypercalcemia
   B. hypercarbia
   C. hyperkalemia
   D. hypernatremia

7. The ECG changes that occur at various levels of excess serum potassium are:
   A. appearance of U waves
   B. prolonged QT interval
   C. shortened PR interval
   D. the QRS complexes widen and the T waves become tall

8. A medication normally prescribed to heart patients, which when taken in excess causes depression of myocardial contractility, AV block, ventricular asystole, and PVCs, is:
   A. digitalis
   B. furosemide
   C. procainamide
   D. verapamil

9. The ECG changes in acute pulmonary embolism include:
   A. a QRS axis of greater than +90°
   B. a right ventricular "strain" pattern in leads V_5 and V_6
   C. an $S_3Q_1T_3$ pattern in leads I and III
   D. left axis deviation

10. The Osborn wave is a sign of:
    A. hyperthermia
    B. hypothermia
    C. pericarditis
    D. ventricular preexcitation

OBJECTIVES *Upon completion of this chapter, you should be able to complete the following objectives:*

1. Name and identify the right and left coronary arteries and their branches on an anatomical drawing of the coronary circulation.
2. Given a list of the arteries of the coronary circulation and a list of the regions of the heart, match the arteries with the regions of the heart they supply.
3. List the major risk factors for coronary heart disease.
4. Describe the sequence of pathologic changes in the evolution of coronary atherosclerosis and the formation of a thrombus.
5. List the causes of myocardial ischemia, injury, and infarction.
6. Define *myocardial ischemia, myocardial injury*, and *myocardial infarction* and indicate which are reversible and which are not.
7. List and define the three coronary syndromes.
8. Define the following terms:
   - Thrombolysis
   - Transmural infarction
   - Subendocardial infarction
9. On a drawing of an acute myocardial infarction, identify the zones of ischemia, injury, and infarction (necrosis).
10. Identify nine anatomic locations in the heart where acute myocardial infarctions occur and list the coronary arteries that supply these areas.
11. Describe the sequence of changes in the myocardium that occurs during the four phases of evolution of a transmural myocardial infarction, including the timing and duration of each phase and sequence.
12. Define "facing," "reciprocal," and "contiguous" ECG leads.
13. Describe the changes in the Q, R, T waves and ST segments in facing and reciprocal ECG leads in myocardial ischemia, injury, and necrosis and when they appear following the onset of an acute myocardial infarction.

14. Give the explanations for the following changes in the T waves associated with an acute myocardial infarction:
    - Inverted T waves over ischemic tissue
    - Tall and peaked T waves over ischemic tissue
    - Inverted T waves over necrotic tissue
15. Describe the T wave changes in a typical transmural myocardial infarction and those in a subendocardial myocardial infarction.
16. Give the measurement characteristic of an elevated or depressed ST segment associated with acute coronary syndromes.
17. Explain the theory behind ST-segment elevation in acute myocardial infarction, namely, the current of injury.
18. Name three cardiac conditions, other than acute myocardial infarction, in which ST-segment elevation occurs.
19. List the three kinds of sloping of the ST segment found in ST depression associated with myocardial ischemia.
20. Name three cardiac conditions, other than myocardial ischemia, in which ST-segment depression occurs.
21. Define "septal" q and r waves, and indicate in which leads they normally appear.
22. Define and discuss the criteria of physiologic Q waves
23. Discuss the following with regard to pathologic Q waves:
    - Diagnostic characteristics
    - Significance of appearance in the ECG
    - Q wave and non–Q wave myocardial infarctions
    - Time of appearance following the onset of an acute myocardial infarction
    - "Window" theory
24. Describe the following:
    - Q wave
    - QS wave; QS complex
    - QR complex; Qr complex
25. Discuss the significance of pathologic Q waves appearing in the following leads:
    - aVR
    - aVL
    - aVF
    - III
    - V₁
26. Discuss the significance of pathologic Q waves when they occur in the presence of the following conditions:
    - ST-segment elevation and T wave inversion
    - Left or right bundle branch block
    - Left anterior or left posterior fascicular block
    - Left ventricular hypertrophy
27. Explain why a Q wave myocardial infarction cannot be classified solely as a transmural myocardial infarction and why a non–Q wave myocardial infarction cannot be classified solely as a nontransmural myocardial infarction.
28. Describe the typical changes in the Q, R, and T waves and ST segments in relation to each of the four phases in the evolution of the following:
    - Q wave "transmural" infarction
    - Non–Q wave "nontransmural" infarction
29. Review the pathophysiologic changes in the ventricular wall with respect to the associated ECG changes that occur during each of the four phases of a transmural myocardial infarction.
30. Name the facing and reciprocal ECG leads used in the diagnosis of the following acute myocardial infarctions:
    - Septal MI
    - Anterior MI
    - Anteroseptal MI
    - Lateral MI
    - Anterolateral MI
    - Inferior MI
    - Posterior MI
    - Right ventricular MI

31. Name the potential complications of acute myocardial infarctions that involve the following regions of the heart:
    - Septum
    - Anterior left ventricular wall
    - Lateral left ventricular wall
    - Inferior left ventricular wall
    - Posterior left ventricular wall
    - Right ventricular and inferior left ventricular wall

CORONARY CIRCULATION

The coronary circulation (Table 16-1 and Figure 16-1) consists of the *left* and *right coronary arteries*. The left coronary artery arises from the base of the aorta just above the left coronary cusp of the aortic valve. The right coronary artery arises from the aorta just above the right aortic coronary cusp.

Left Coronary Artery

The left coronary artery consists of the *left main coronary artery*, a short main stem of about 2 to 10 mm in length that usually divides into two equal major branches, the *left anterior descending coronary artery* (LAD) and the *left circumflex coronary artery* (LCx). Sometimes, a third major branch, the *diagonal (or intermediate) coronary artery*, arises from the left main coronary artery instead of from the left anterior descending coronary artery.

> **AUTHOR'S NOTE** The term *artery(ies)* is used interchangeably with the term *branch(es)* in this chapter as it relates to the coronary circulation.

The left anterior descending coronary artery travels anteriorly and downward within the interventricular groove over the interventricular septum and circles the apex of the heart to end behind it. The left anterior descending coronary artery gives rise to at least one and often up to six diagonal branches, three to five septal perforator branches, and, sometimes, one or more right ventricular branches.

The diagonal arteries, the first of which may originate from the left main coronary artery or from the left circumflex coronary artery course over the anterior and lateral surface of the left ventricle between the left anterior descending coronary artery and the anterolateral marginal branch of the left circumflex coronary artery. The diagonal arteries give rise to the septal perforator arteries at a right angle from the left anterior descending coronary artery and run directly into the interventricular

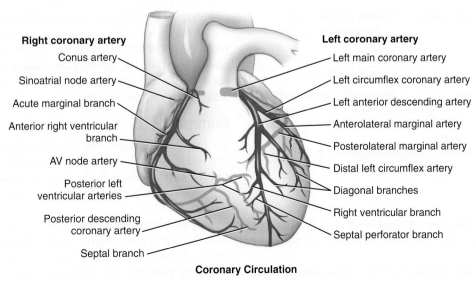

Coronary Circulation

FIGURE 16-1 The coronary circulation.

TABLE 16-1 The Coronary Circulation and the Regions of the Heart it Supplies

Coronary Artery	Region Supplied
Left Coronary Artery	
Left anterior descending	
Diagonal	Anterolateral wall of the left ventricle
Septal perforator	Anterior two thirds of the interventricular septum
Right ventricular	Anterior wall of the right ventricle
Left circumflex	
SA node (40%-60%)*	SA node
Left atrial circumflex	Left atrium
Anterolateral marginal	Anterolateral wall of the left ventricle
Posterolateral marginal	Posterolateral wall of the left ventricle
Distal left circumflex	Posterior wall of the left ventricle
Posterior descending (10%-15%)	Posterior one third of the interventricular septum
AV node (10%-15%)	AV node
	Proximal bundle of His
Posterior left ventricular (10%-15%)	Inferior wall of the left ventricle
Right Coronary Artery	
Conus	Upper anterior wall of the right ventricle
SA node (50%-60%)	SA node
Anterior right ventricular	Anterolateral wall of the right ventricle
Right atrial	Right atrium
Acute marginal	Lateral wall of the right ventricle
Posterior descending (85%-90%)	Posterior one third of the interventricular septum
AV node (85%-90%)	AV node
	Proximal bundle of His
Posterior left ventricular (85%-90%)	Inferior wall of the left ventricle

AV, Atrioventricular; *SA*, sinoatrial.
*The percentage figures indicate in what percentage of hearts the indicated coronary artery is present.

septum. The right ventricular arteries branch off of the diagonal arteries and course over the anterior surface of the right ventricle.

The left circumflex coronary artery arises from the left main coronary artery at an obtuse angle (between 90 and 180 degrees) and runs posteriorly along the left atrioventricular (AV) groove to end as the distal circumflex coronary artery supplying the posterior wall of the left ventricle in about 85% to 90% of hearts. In the remaining 10% to 15%, the left circumflex coronary artery continues along the AV groove to become the posterior left ventricular arteries, where it supplies the inferior wall of the left ventricle. When this occurs, the left circumflex coronary artery usually continues further to enter the posterior interventricular groove to become the posterior descending coronary artery where it gives rise to the AV node artery. A left coronary artery with a circumflex coronary artery that gives rise to both the posterior left ventricular arteries and the posterior descending coronary artery is considered to be a "dominant" left coronary artery because it supplies a dominant proportion of the myocardium and AV conduction.

The left circumflex coronary artery gives rise to the sinoatrial (SA) node artery in 40% to 50% of the hearts, one or two left atrial circumflex branches, the left obtuse marginal branches (the large anterolateral marginal artery and one or more smaller posterolateral marginal arteries), and the distal left circumflex artery.

The anterolateral marginal artery runs over the anterolateral surface of the left ventricular wall toward the apex, lateral to the diagonal branches of the left anterior descending coronary artery. The posterolateral marginal arteries run down the posterolateral wall of the left ventricle, and the distal left circumflex artery runs down the left AV groove.

Right Coronary Artery

The right coronary artery travels downward and then posteriorly in the right AV groove, giving rise to the conus artery, the sino-atrial (SA) node artery in 50% to 60% of hearts, several anterior right ventricular branches, the right atrial branch, and the acute marginal branch.

In 85% to 90% of hearts, it also gives rise to the atrioventricular (AV) node artery and the posterior descending coronary artery (with its septal branches), which runs down the posterior interventricular groove, and, then, continuing into the left AV groove, the right coronary artery terminates as the posterior left ventricular arteries. A right coronary artery that gives rise to both the posterior descending coronary artery and the posterior left ventricular arteries is considered to be a "dominant" right coronary artery.

Summary

The left anterior descending coronary artery supplies the anterior two thirds of the interventricular septum, most of the right and left bundle branches, the anterior (apical) and lateral wall of the left ventricle, and sometimes the anterior wall of the right ventricle.

The left circumflex coronary artery supplies the left atrial wall, the lateral and posterior wall of the left ventricle, and, in 40% to 50% of hearts, the SA node. In 10% to 15% of hearts, when the posterior left ventricular, AV node, and posterior descending coronary arteries arise from the left circumflex artery, the left circumflex artery also supplies the inferior wall of the left ventricle, the AV node, the proximal bundle of His, and the posterior (inferior) one third of the interventricular septum. When this occurs, the entire interventricular septum is supplied by the left coronary artery.

The right coronary artery supplies the right atrial and ventricular wall; the AV node, the proximal bundle of His, the posterior one third of the interventricular septum, and the inferior wall of the left ventricle in 85% to 90% of hearts; and the SA node in 50% to 60% of hearts.

CORONARY HEART DISEASE

Cardiovascular disease is the leading cause of death in the United States. It comprises coronary heart disease, stroke, heart failure, hypertension, and atherosclerosis. Coronary heart disease (CHD) previously referred to as coronary artery disease represents over half the deaths from cardiovascular disease annually. The name change reflects a better understanding of the pathophysiology of the disease recognizing that while the primary site of pathology rests in the arteries, the entire cardiovascular system is affected.

The prevalence of CHD in adults over 20 in the United States as of 2005 is estimated to be 16 million (8.7 million men and 7.3 million women). It is estimated that in 2008, 770,000 Americans suffered their first acute coronary syndrome and 430,000 had a recurrent attack. There are 600,000 new heart attacks and 320,000 recurrent ones annually. The average age of a person having their first heart attack is 64.5 for men and 70.4 for women. In 2004, congestive heart failure caused one of every five deaths in the United States and an acute coronary syndrome occurred every 26 seconds resulting in one death every minute.

While the death rate from CHD remains high it has continued to decline over the past 2 decades primarily due to increased awareness of the signs and symptoms and aggressive treatment of modifiable risk factors. The major modifiable risk factors for CHD include the following:

- Cigarette smoking
- Diabetes mellitus
- Hypertension
- Elevated lipid blood levels
- Abdominal obesity
- Lack of exercise
- Stress
- Illicit drug (stimulant) use

Coronary atherosclerosis, a form of arteriosclerosis (hardening of the arteries), is the primary disease process involved in CHD. It is responsible for the formation of atheromatous plaques in large and medium-sized coronary arteries, often followed by plaque disruption, thrombosis, and coronary artery occlusion. The consequence of coronary atherosclerosis is a group of clinical syndromes, the "acute coronary syndromes," that include *unstable angina, non–ST-segment elevation myocardial infarction (NSTEMI)*, and *ST-segment elevation myocardial infarction (STEMI)*.

> As the name implies, a syndrome is a collection of signs and symptoms associated with a particular condition. Unstable angina, NSTEMI, and STEMI are all acute coronary syndromes and the patient experiencing chest pain/discomfort may be suffering from any of the three and may progress from one to the other depending on the underlying cause.

Pathophysiology of Coronary Atherosclerosis and Thrombosis

The first phase in the evolution of coronary atherosclerosis is the appearance of *atherosclerotic plaques* within the inner layer of the coronary arteries (Figure 16-2, stage 1) after damage to the endothelium. Inflammation-mediated response by myocytes (Figure 16-2, stage 2) results deposition of low-density lipoproteins (LDL) from the plasma into the intima, where they evolve into small clumps of lipid-filled foam cells seen as yellow dots or streaks on the intimal (internal) surface of the artery. These progress over time to large plaques (Figure 16-2, stage 3) consisting of a soft gruel-like lipid and cholesterol rich atheromatous core and an external fibrous cap (Figure 16-2, stage 4) composed primarily of smooth muscle cells and collagen. The volume and composition of the atheromatous core and the thickness of the fibrous cap vary from plaque to plaque, even in the same coronary artery. Atherosclerotic plaques may remain stable for years without causing any symptoms.

Stable, Vulnerable, and Unstable Plaques

Any atherosclerotic plaque can rupture, resulting in a total occlusion of the coronary artery. Atherosclerotic plaques are categorized as "stable" if they are less prone to rupture. A "stable" intracoronary plaque (Figure 16-3) has a lipid core separated from the arterial lumen by a thick fibrous cap. They develop slowly and result in a narrowing of the arterial lumen due to the fact that the lipid core does not stretch the arterial wall but instead intrudes into lumen of the artery. Over time they may narrow the lumen to the point that anginal symptoms occur with exertion because they limit the amount of blood flow to the myocardium. They rarely result in an acute myocardial infarction.

"Vulnerable" (Figure 16-3) plaques are intracoronary lesions that have a thin fibrous cap. They are lipid-rich and result in a compensatory enlargement of the artery and are therefore referred to as nonstenotic lesions. They are often located at branch points or bends in the coronary arteries. Owing to the thinness of the fibrous cap, these plaques are susceptible to erosion and rupture, which can lead to thrombus formation and an acute coronary syndrome. The leading edge of the vulnerable plaque is impacted by coronary blood flow and can become inflamed. This inflammation further weakens the plaque making it more prone to rupture. As the inflammation increases, so does the risk of rupture. At this point the plaque is referred to as "unstable."

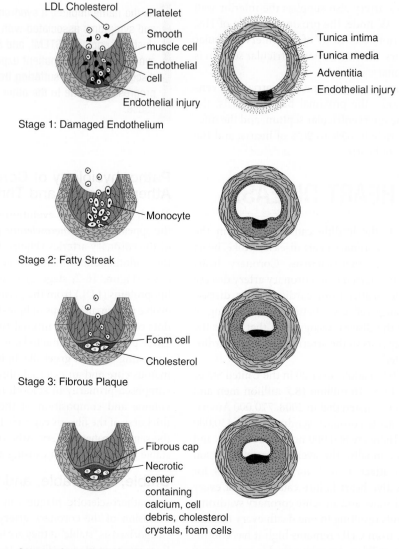

LDL Cholesterol — Platelet
Smooth muscle cell
Endothelial cell
Endothelial injury

Tunica intima
Tunica media
Adventitia
Endothelial injury

Stage 1: Damaged Endothelium

Monocyte

Stage 2: Fatty Streak

Foam cell
Cholesterol

Stage 3: Fibrous Plaque

Fibrous cap
Necrotic center containing calcium, cell debris, cholesterol crystals, foam cells

Stage 4: Complicated Lesion

FIGURE 16-2 Plaque formation. (From Libby P: The vascular biology of atherosclerosis. In Zipes DP, Libby P, Bonow RO, et al, eds, *Braunwald's heart disease: A textbook of cardiovascular medicine*, ed 7, Philadelphia, 2005, Saunders.)

Plaque Erosion and Rupture

A *thrombus* (blood clot) forms on the surface of the plaque after its erosion or in the plaque itself after rupture of the fibrous cap, often with an extension of the thrombus into the arterial lumen. Generally, a plaque does not rupture until its core becomes highly saturated with lipids. The rupture of the fibrous cap is at least three times more common than is erosion of the plaque surface.

Erosion occurs when the endothelial layer covering the plaque is torn away, exposing the plaque itself. A platelet-rich thrombus immediately forms on the exposed surface of the plaque, increasing the size of the plaque.

Rupture (disruption) of the fibrous cap is most likely to occur at its leading edge, the area of the cap where it connects with the normal arterial wall. The cause of the rupture may be one or more of the following:

- Progressive weakening and/or thinning of the fibrous wall at one point
- Sudden surges in blood pressure, heart rate, or blood flow (as seen with emotional stress, heavy physical exertion in otherwise sedentary people, or the process of getting up in the morning)
- Vasospasm of the coronary artery at the site of the plaque
- Repetitive flexion of the artery at the site of the plaque

After rupture of the fibrous cap, blood enters the plaque mixing with the atheromatous lipid rich gruel, which appears to greatly enhance thrombus formation, and immediately produces a thrombus rich in platelets and fibrin. Initially the thrombus may not extend beyond the plaques, causing no

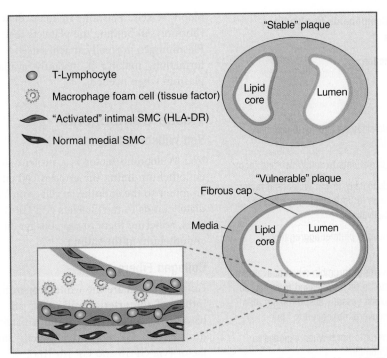

FIGURE 16-3 Stable and vulnerable plaques. (From Aehlert B: *ACLS study guide,* ed 3, St Louis, 2007, Mosby.)

further occlusion. However, as it often does, the thrombus continues to grow, extending beyond the fibrous cap into the arterial lumen, partially or completely occluding it. As the thrombus grows into the lumen, it becomes rich in fibrin. Sometimes clumps of platelets break off the distal end of the main thrombus and flow downstream, resulting in microemboli and resulting in additional obstruction of smaller terminal coronary arteries.

Once the thrombus is formed, it may partially or completely disintegrate spontaneously, (spontaneous thrombolysis), undergo further rethrombosis and enlarge, or undergo organization by connective tissue into a fibrotic lesion (scar).

THROMBUS FORMATION AND LYSIS

To understand the rationale for the treatment of acute coronary syndromes, one must understand the components of thrombus formation in the presence of damage to an atherosclerotic plaque within a coronary artery wall and of the eventual lysis (breakdown) of the thrombus. Of the numerous factors necessary for thrombus formation and lysis normally present in the blood and connective tissue of the blood vessel wall, the following are considered the principal components (Table 16-2).

Blood Components

Platelets

Platelets contain adhesive glycoproteins (GP) receptors that bind with various components of connective tissue and blood to form thrombi. The major GP receptors and their function include the following:

- GP Ia binds the platelets directly to collagen fibers present in connective tissue
- GP Ib binds the platelets to von Willebrand factor (a tissue component)
- GP IIb/IIIa binds the platelets to von Willebrand factor and, after the platelets are activated, to fibrinogen

Platelets also contain several substances that, when released after platelet activation, promote thrombus formation by stimulating platelet aggregation. These substances include the following:

- Adenosine diphosphate (ADP)
- Serotonin
- Thromboxane A_2 (TxA_2)

Prothrombin

Prothrombin is a plasma protein that when activated by exposure of the blood to tissue factor released from the damaged arterial wall is converted to thrombin. Thrombin in turn converts fibrinogen to fibrin.

TABLE 16-2 **Blood and Tissue Components Involved in Thrombus Formation and Lysis**

Component	Function
Thrombus Formation	
Blood	
Platelets	
GP Ia	Binds platelets directly to collagen fibers
GP Ib	Binds platelets to von Willebrand factor
GP IIb/IIIa	Binds initially to von Willebrand factor, then to fibrinogen after platelet activation
Adenosine (ADP), serotonin, thromboxane A$_2$ (TxA$_2$)	Stimulates platelet aggregation
Prothrombin	Converts to thrombin when activated by tissue factor released from injured blood vessel walls; thrombin then converts fibrinogen to fibrin
Fibrinogen	Converts to fibrin when exposed to thrombin
Tissue	
von Willebrand factor	Binds to platelets' GP Ib and GP IIb/IIIa and to collagen fibers
Collagen fibers	Bind directly to platelets' GP Ia and to GP Ib and GP IIb/IIIa via von Willebrand factor
Tissue factor	Initiates the conversion of prothrombin to thrombin
Thrombolysis	
Blood	
Plasminogen	Converts to plasmin when activated by tissue plasminogen activator (tPA); plasmin then dissolves the fibrin (fibrinolysis), causing the thrombus to break apart (thrombolysis)
Tissue	
Tissue plasminogen activator (tPA)	Activates plasminogen to convert to plasmin

Fibrinogen

Fibrinogen is a plasma protein that converts to fibrin, an elastic, threadlike filament, when exposed to thrombin.

Plasminogen

Plasminogen is a plasma glycoprotein that converts to an enzyme—plasmin—when activated by tissue plasminogen activator (tPA) normally present in the endothelium lining the blood vessels. Plasmin, in turn, dissolves the fibrin strands (fibrinolysis) binding the platelets together within a thrombus. Plasminogen normally attaches itself to fibrin during thrombus formation, making it instantly available for conversion to plasmin when needed.

Tissue Components

Von Willebrand Factor

Von Willebrand factor is a protein stored in the cells of the endothelium lining the arteries. When exposed to blood after an injury to the endothelial cells, von Willebrand factor immediately binds to the platelets (via GP Ib and GP IIb/IIIa receptors), adhering them to the collagen fibers located beneath the endothelium in the intima.

Collagen Fibers

Collagen fibers are the white protein fibers present within the intima of the arterial wall. After an injury and exposure to blood, the collagen fibers immediately bind to the platelets directly (via GP Ia) and indirectly through von Willebrand factor (via GP Ib and GP IIb/IIIa).

Tissue Factor

Tissue factor is a substance present in tissue, platelets, and leukocytes that, when released after injury, initiates the conversion of prothrombin to thrombin.

Tissue Plasminogen Activator

Tissue plasminogen factor (tPA) is a glycoprotein present primarily in the vascular endothelium that when released into the plasma activates plasminogen to convert to plasmin. Plasmin in turn dissolves fibrinogen and fibrin.

Phases of Thrombus Formation

Formation of a coronary artery thrombus consists of five phases: (1) Subendoethelial exposure (2) platelet adhesion, (3) platelet activation, (4) platelet aggregation, and (5) thrombus formation (Figure 16-4).

Phase 1: Subendothelial Exposure

At the moment an atherosclerotic plaque becomes denuded or ruptures, the platelets are exposed to collagen fibers and von Willebrand factor present within the cap of the atherosclerotic plaques. Platelets begin to fill the gap and natural vasoconstriction occurs in an attempt to lessen the size of the rupture. This is mediated by thromboxane A$_2$.

Phase 2: Platelet Adhesion

The platelets' GP Ia receptors bind with the collagen fibers directly, and the GP Ib and GP IIb/IIIa receptors bind with von Willebrand factor, which in turn also binds with the collagen fibers. The result is the adhesion of platelets to the collagen fibers within the plaque, forming a layer of platelets overlying the damaged plaque.

A VASOCONSTRICTION

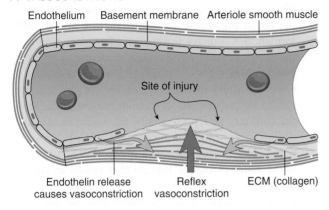

B PRIMARY HEMOSTASIS

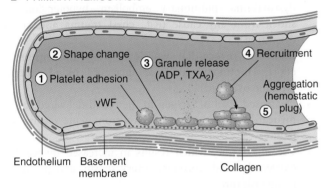

C SECONDARY HEMOSTASIS

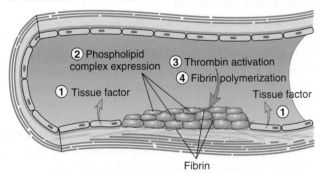

D THROMBUS AND ANTITHROMBOTIC EVENTS

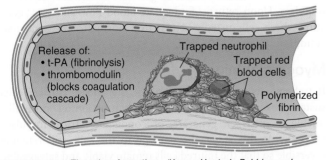

FIGURE 16-4 Thrombus formation. (Kumar V, et al: *Robbins and Cotran's pathologic basis for disease*, ed 7, Philadelphia, 2005, Saunders.)

Phase 3: Platelet Activation

Upon being bound to the collagen fibers, the platelets become activated. The platelets change their shape from smooth ovals to tiny spheres while releasing adenosine diphosphate (ADP), serotonin, and thromboxane A_2 (TxA_2), substances that stimulate platelet aggregation. Platelet activation is also stimulated by the lipid-rich gruel within the atherosclerotic plaque. At the same time, the GP IIb/IIIa receptors are turned on to bind with fibrinogen. While this is going on, tissue factor is being released from the tissue and platelets.

Phase 4: Platelet Aggregation

Once activated, the platelets bind to each other by means of fibrinogen, a cordlike structure that binds to the platelets' GP IIb/IIIa receptors. One fibrinogen can bind to two platelets, one at each end. Stimulated by ADP and TxA_2, the binding of fibrinogen to the GP IIb/IIIa receptors is greatly enhanced, resulting in a rapid growth of the platelet plug. By this time, the prothrombin in the vicinity of the damaged plaque has been converted to thrombin by the tissue factor.

Phase 5: Thrombus Formation

At first, the platelet plug is rather unstable but becomes firmer as the fibrinogen between the platelets is replaced by stronger strands of fibrin. This occurs after prothrombin is converted to thrombin by tissue factor. Thrombin in turn converts fibrinogen to fibrin threads. Plasminogen usually becomes attached to the fibrin during its formation. As the thrombus grows, red cells and leukocytes (white cells) become entrapped in the platelet-fibrin mesh.

Phases of Thrombolysis

Normally, the breakdown of a thrombus—*thrombolysis*—occurs when the thrombus is no longer needed to maintain the integrity of the blood vessel wall. Thrombolysis can also be initiated by the intravenous injection of thrombolytic agents such as alteplase, reteplase, and tenecteplase. Natural thrombolysis consists of three phases: (1) activation of intrinsic and extrinsic pathways, (2) plasmin formation, and (3) fibrinolysis (Figure 16-5).

Phase 1: Activation of Intrinsic and Extrinsic Pathways

The central reaction is the conversion of plasminogen to the enzyme plasmin. Activation of plasminogen is achieved by the extrinsic pathway (Figure 16-5 blue) initiated by the release of tissue plasminogen activator (tPA) released from the endothelial cells and by the intrinsic pathway (Figure 16-5 gold) from factor XIIa and urokinase.

Phase 2: Plasmin Formation

tPA, factor XIIa, or urokinase activate plasminogen resulting in its conversion to plasmin.

Phase 3: Fibrinolysis

Plasmin breaks down the fibrin into soluble fragments, causing the platelets to separate from each other and the thrombus breaks apart (thrombolysis).

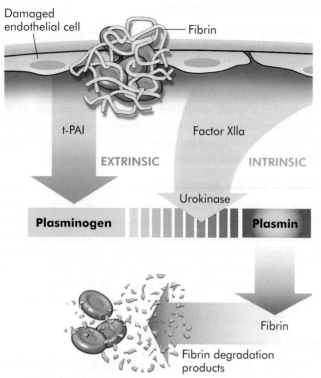

FIGURE 16-5 Thrombolysis. (Huether S: *Understanding pathophysiology*, ed 4, St Louis, 2008, Mosby.)

There are multiple points in the process of thrombus formation that can be inhibited by the administration of pharmaceutical agents to augment the body's natural mechanisms. Additionally, thrombolysis can be augmented by the administration of fibrinolytic agents to enhance thrombolysis. Together these constitute the mainstay of noninvasive revascularization for acute myocardial infarction.

MYOCARDIAL ISCHEMIA, INJURY, AND INFARCTION

Myocardial ischemia, injury, and infarction result from the failure of local coronary arteries to supply sufficient oxygenated blood to the myocardial tissue they supply to meet the tissue's need for oxygen. This can result from a variety of causes (Figure 16-6), including the following:

- Occlusion (or obstruction) of a severely narrowed atherosclerotic coronary artery by a coronary thrombus after rupture of an atherosclerotic plaque with hemorrhage within the plaque extending into the arterial lumen. Acute increase in arterial pressure or heart rate such as that associated with physical exertion or emotional stress

commonly precedes the rupture of an atherosclerotic plaque. Coronary artery spasm and hypercoagulability of the blood predispose to plaque rupture and thrombus formation. Coronary thrombosis after plaque rupture is the most common cause of MI, occurring in about 90% of acute MIs.

- Coronary artery spasm, in the absence of plaque rupture, caused by constriction of smooth muscle in the wall of the coronary artery. Generally, the spasm occurs at the site of narrowing from coronary atherosclerosis. As noted above, coronary artery spasm may accompany or is the cause of plaque rupture that results in coronary thrombosis.
- Decreased coronary arterial blood flow for any reason other than coronary artery occlusion or spasm, such as a dysrhythmia, pulmonary embolism, hypotension, or shock from any cause (e.g., chest trauma and aortic dissection).
- Increased myocardial workload from unaccustomed effort, emotional stress, or increased blood volume (volume overload).
- Decreased level of oxygen in the blood delivered to the myocardium because of hypoxia from acute respiratory failure.
- Use of cocaine, which results in increased myocardial oxygen demand, coronary artery spasm, and promotes plaque rupture.

Myocardial Ischemia

Myocardial ischemia is present the moment the supply of oxygen to the myocardium is insufficient to meet the demands of cellular metabolism. This results in a lack of oxygen (anoxia) within the cardiac cells. For a short time after the onset of anoxia, certain reversible ischemic changes occur in the internal structure of the affected cells. These ischemic changes cause a delay in the depolarization and repolarization of the cells. Mild to moderate anoxia can be tolerated for a short period of time by the cardiac cells without greatly affecting their function. During this period there may be some loss in the ability of the myocardial cells to contract and of the specialized cells of the electrical conduction system to generate or conduct electrical impulses. Upon return of adequate blood flow and reoxygenation, these cells usually return to a normal or near normal condition.

Myocardial Injury

If ischemia is severe or prolonged, the anoxic cardiac cells sustain *myocardial injury* and stop functioning normally, unable to contract, generate, or conduct electrical impulses properly. At this stage, the damage to the cells still remains reversible so that the injured cells remain viable and salvageable for some time. As in ischemic cells, injured cells may also return to normal or near normal after the return of adequate blood flow and reoxygenation. The degree to which they can withstand injury and the extent to which they will return to normal depends on the length and severity of the ischemia they

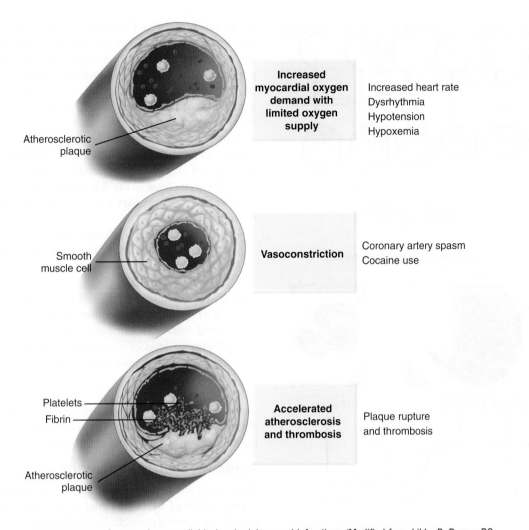

FIGURE 16-6 Causes of myocardial ischemia, injury, and infarction. (Modified from Libby P, Bonow RO, Mann DL, et al: *Braunwald's heart disease*, ed 8, Philadelphia, 2008, Saunders.)

suffered and their preexisting health before the period of ischemia.

Myocardial Infarction

If severe myocardial ischemia continues because of a persistent absence of blood supply, the anoxic cardiac cells eventually sustain irreversible injury and die, becoming electrically inert. At the moment of cellular death, necrosis, the process of scarring begins and *myocardial infarction* is said to have occurred. Necrotic cells *do not* return to normal upon revascularization or reoxygenation.

> Myocardial ischemia and injury is reversible. Myocardial infarction is not. The goal of therapy is to minimize the amount of myocardium infarcted.

ACUTE CORONARY SYNDROMES

The *acute coronary syndromes* (Figure 16-7) include unstable angina, non–ST-segment elevation myocardial infarction (NSTEMI), and ST-segment elevation myocardial infarction (STEMI). Sudden cardiac death can occur in any of these conditions.

Angina

Angina is the discomfort associated with an acute coronary syndrome. We will discuss the signs and symptoms of angina in Chapter 18.

Stable Angina

Exertion-induced angina (Canadian Cardiovascular Society Angina Classification [CCSC] class II or III) (Table 16-3), that characteristically remains unchanged from episode to episode

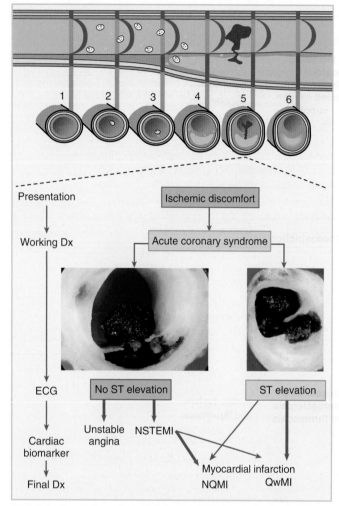

FIGURE 16-7 Acute coronary syndromes. (From Libby P, Bonow RO, Mann DL, et al: *Braunwald's heart disease: A textbook of cardiovascular medicine*, ed 8, Philadelphia, 2008, Saunders.)

after the same amount of exertion and is relieved promptly with rest is considered *stable angina*. It is the result of a stable atherosclerotic plaque causing significant coronary artery stenosis. The ECG usually shows ST-segment depression with or without T wave inversion during angina, indicating subendocardial ischemia.

Unstable Angina

Unstable angina is considered to be present if one or more of the following occurs:

- A new onset of exertional angina of CCSC class III or IV
- Preexisting angina that has become more frequent, longer in duration, or lower in threshold (i.e., increased by one or more CCSC classes to at least class III severity)
- The appearance of angina at rest (usually prolonged for 20 minutes or longer)

The most common cause of unstable angina is disruption of an atherosclerotic plaque secondary to inflammation. This is followed by plaque expansion, erosion or rupture, and thrombus formation. Then spontaneous thrombolysis occurs and

blood flow is restored. First-time partial occlusion of the coronary artery results in a new onset of exertional angina, worsening of an existing stenosis results in an increase in the pre-existing anginal pattern, and temporary total obstruction results in angina at rest. The ECG usually shows ST-segment depression with or without T wave inversion, indicating subendocardial ischemia and injury.

It must be noted that unstable angina may also occur under certain circumstances in which an imbalance between oxygen demand and supply suddenly arises without being necessarily caused by an increase in the degree of the stenotic lesion within an atherosclerotic coronary artery. These circumstances include the following:

- Tachycardia from any cause, such as tachydysrhythmias, congestive heart failure, anemia, fever, hypoxia, hypotension, or shock
- Bradydysrhythmia
- Increased myocardial workload from unaccustomed effort, emotional stress, unrelieved fatigue, or increased blood volume (volume overload)
- Decreased level of oxygen in the blood delivered to the myocardium because of hypoxia from acute respiratory failure
- Use of cocaine

The ECG under these circumstances also usually shows ST-segment depression with or without T wave inversion, indicating subendocardial ischemia and injury.

Acute Myocardial Infarction

Acute myocardial infarction (AMI) is the result of a plaque rupture followed by the formation of a large thrombus that partially or completely occludes the lumen of a coronary artery, resulting in myocardial ischemia, injury, and necrosis of myocytes. This necrosis results in the release of cardiac enzymes—"cardiac markers"—which will be discussed in Chapter 18, and is diagnostic of acute myocardial infarction. As was described earlier in this text, the ST segment is generally elevated when myocardial infarction occurs. However, this does not always occur. An AMI without ST segment elevation is called a non–ST-segment elevation MI, "non-STEMI," or "NSTEMI," while one with ST-segment elevation is called an ST-segment elevation MI or "STEMI." Both result in release of cardiac markers and both are acute coronary syndromes.

> The presence of elevated cardiac enzymes is diagnostic of myocardial infarction. They are not elevated in myocardial ischemia and injury.

ACUTE MYOCARDIAL INFARCTION

Myocardial infarction usually follows the occlusion of an atherosclerotic pericardial coronary artery by a thrombus—

TABLE 16-3 **Canadian Cardiovascular Society Functional Classification of Angina Pectoris**

Class	Activity Evoking Angina	Specific Activity Scale
I	Ordinary physical activity, such as walking and climbing stairs, does not cause angina. Angina with strenuous or rapid or prolonged exertion at work or recreation.	Patients can perform to completion any activity requiring >7 metabolic equivalents (e.g., can carry 24 lb up eight steps; carry objects that weigh 80 lb; do outdoor work [shovel snow, spade soil]; do recreational activities [skiing, basketball, squash, handball, jog/walk 5 mph]).
II	Slight limitation of ordinary activity. Walking or climbing stairs rapidly, walking uphill, walking or stair climbing after meals, in cold, in wind, or when under emotional stress, or only during the few hours after awakening. Walking more than two blocks on the level and climbing more than one flight of ordinary stairs at a normal pace and in normal conditions.	Patients can perform to completion any activity requiring >5 metabolic equivalents (e.g., have sexual intercourse without stopping, garden, rake, weed, roller skate, dance fox trot, walk at 4 mph on level ground), but cannot and do not perform to completion activities requiring ≥7 metabolic equivalents.
III	Marked limitation of ordinary physical activity. Walking one to two blocks on the level and climbing more than one flight in normal conditions.	Patients can perform to completion any activity requiring >2 metabolic equivalents (e.g., shower without stopping, strip and make bed, clean windows, walk 2.5 mph, bowl, play golf, dress without stopping), but cannot and do not perform to completion any activities requiring ≥5 metabolic equivalents.
IV	Inability to carry on any physical activity without discomfort—anginal syndrome *may be* present at rest.	Patients cannot or do not perform to completion activities requiring ≥2 metabolic equivalents. *Cannot* carry out activities listed above (Specific Activity Scale, Class III).

coronary thrombosis. This process, as described earlier, involves an intricate interaction between the rupture of an atherosclerotic plaque lining the coronary artery (often accompanied by vasospasm of the coronary artery smooth muscle), platelet activation, and formation of an occluding thrombus.

Angiographic studies of the coronary arteries performed within the first few hours after the onset of symptoms of a STEMI show that approximately 90% of coronary artery occlusions are the result of thrombi, while only 35% to 75% of NSTEMI show evidence of thrombi formation.

After the occlusion of a coronary artery, the myocardium evolves through various stages of impairment severity, beginning with myocardial ischemia, then progressing to myocardial injury, both of which are reversible, and ending with myocardial infarction, the stage of tissue necrosis, an irreversible condition. Along the way, characteristic changes in the ECG reflect the changes in the myocardium, which will be described later.

Typically, an MI at its height consists of a central area of dead, necrotic tissue—the *zone of infarction (or necrosis)* surrounded by a layer of injured myocardial tissue—*the zone of injury*, and then by an outer layer of ischemic tissue—*the zone of ischemia* (Figure 16-8).

An acute MI may be either transmural or nontransmural. A *transmural infarction* is one in which the zone of infarction involves the entire or almost entire thickness of the ventricular wall, including both the subendocardial and subepicardial areas of the myocardium. A *nontransmural infarction*, on the other hand, is one in which the zone of infarction only involves a part of the ventricular wall, usually the inner, subendocardial area of the myocardium (Figure 16-9).

Anatomic Locations of Myocardial Infarctions

The site of the MI depends on which coronary artery is occluded (Figure 16-10). Table 16-4 lists the locations of the MI and the coronary artery or arteries most likely occluded to produce them. Because the distribution of the coronary arteries varies from person to person, the arteries occluded in any specific MI may differ from the ones listed in the table.

The Four Phases of a Transmural Myocardial Infarction

The evolution and resolution of a typical transmural MI can be divided into four phases, depending on the stage and severity of involvement of the myocardium. The transmural MI usually begins in the subendocardium, presumably because this area has the highest myocardial oxygen demand and the least supply of blood. The infarct then progresses outward in a wave front until it involves the entire myocardium. While the necrosis is progressing from the endocardium to the epicardium, the acute MI is said to be *"evolving."*

Phase 1

Within the first 2 hours after coronary artery occlusion, the following sequence of changes occurs in the myocardium supplied by the occluded artery (Figure 16-11, *A* p. 273):

1. Within seconds of the coronary artery occlusion, extensive myocardial ischemia occurs.
2. During the first 20 to 40 minutes (average, 30 minutes) after the onset of the MI, reversible myocardial injury appears in the subendocardium.

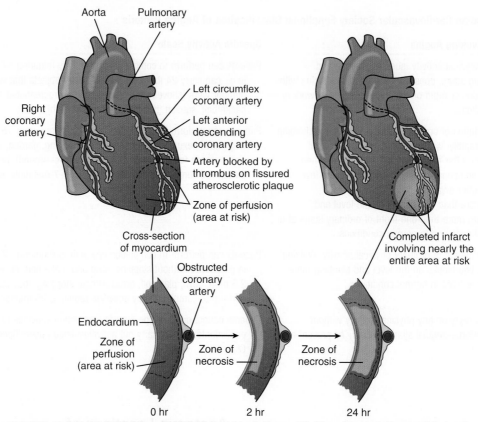

FIGURE 16-8 Zone of infarction. (Modified from Libby P, Bonow RO, Mann DL, et al: *Braunwald's heart disease*, ed 8, Philadelphia, 2008, Saunders.)

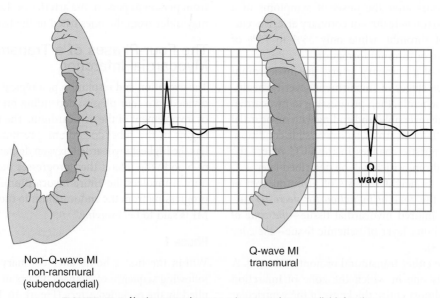

FIGURE 16-9 Nontransmural versus a transmural myocardial infarction.

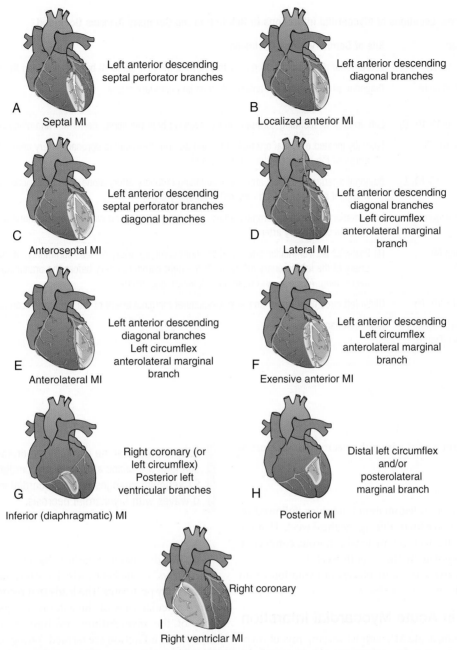

A   Left anterior descending
septal perforator branches
Septal MI

B   Left anterior descending
diagonal branches
Localized anterior MI

C   Left anterior descending
septal perforator branches
diagonal branches
Anteroseptal MI

D   Left anterior descending
diagonal branches
Left circumflex
anterolateral marginal
branch
Lateral MI

E   Left anterior descending
diagonal branches
Left circumflex
anterolateral marginal
branch
Anterolateral MI

F   Left anterior descending
Left circumflex
anterolateral marginal
branch
Exensive anterior MI

G   Right coronary (or
left circumflex)
Posterior left
ventricular branches
Inferior (diaphragmatic) MI

H   Distal left circumflex
and/or
posterolateral
marginal branch
Posterior MI

I   Right coronary
Right ventriclar MI

FIGURE 16-10 Location of myocardial infarction in relation to the coronary arteries occluded.

3. About 30 minutes after the interruption of blood flow, irreversible myocardial necrosis (infarction) occurs in the subendocardium as myocardial injury begins to spread toward the epicardium.
4. By 1 hour after the onset, myocardial necrosis has spread through over one third of the myocardium.
5. By 2 hours after the onset, myocardial necrosis has spread through about half of the myocardium.

Phase 2

Between the second and twenty-fourth hour after the occlusion, the evolution of the MI is completed in the following sequence (Figure 16-11, *B*):

1. By 3 hours, about two thirds of the myocardial cells within the affected myocardium become necrotic.
2. By 6 hours, only a small percentage of the cells remain viable. For all practical purposes, the evolution of the transmural MI is complete.
3. By 24 hours, the progression of myocardial necrosis to the epicardium is usually complete.

Phase 3

After the first day, during the next 24 to 72 hours, little or no ischemic or injured myocardial cells remain because all cells have either died or recovered. Acute inflammation with edema

TABLE 16-4 Anatomic Locations of Myocardial Infarctions in Relation to the Coronary Arteries Occluded

Location of Infarction	Site of Coronary Artery Occlusion
Septal MI (Figure 16-10, *A*)	Left anterior descending coronary artery beyond the first diagonal branch, involving the septal perforator arteries
Anterior (localized) MI (Figure 16-10, *B*)	Diagonal arteries of the left anterior descending coronary artery
Anteroseptal MI (Figure 16-10, *C*)	Left anterior descending coronary artery involving both the septal perforator and diagonal arteries
Lateral MI (Figure 16-10, *D*)	Laterally located diagonal arteries of the left anterior descending coronary artery and/or the anterolateral marginal artery of the left circumflex coronary artery
Anterolateral MI (Figure 16-10, *E*)	Diagonal arteries of the left anterior descending coronary artery alone or in conjunction with the anterolateral marginal artery of the left circumflex coronary artery
Extensive anterior MI (Figure 16-10, *F*)	Left anterior descending coronary artery alone or in conjunction with the anterolateral marginal artery of the left circumflex coronary artery
Inferior (diaphragmatic) MI (Figure 16-10, *G*)	(1) Posterior left ventricular arteries of the right coronary artery or, less commonly, of the left circumflex coronary artery of the left coronary artery or (2) the right coronary artery before the branching of the posterior descending, AV node, and posterior left ventricular arteries
Posterior MI (Figure 16-10, *H*)	Distal left circumflex artery and/or posterolateral marginal artery of the circumflex coronary artery
Right ventricular MI with inferior (diaphragmatic) MI (Figure 16-10, *I*)	Right coronary artery

MI, Myocardial infarction.

and cellular infiltration begins within the necrotic tissue during this phase.

Phase 4

During the second week, inflammation continues, followed by proliferation of connective tissue during the third week. Healing with replacement of the necrotic tissue with fibrous connective tissue is generally complete by the seventh week.

Table 16-5 summarizes the four phases of evolution of an acute transmural MI.

ECG Changes in Acute Myocardial Infarction

The ECG in an evolving acute MI, with its varying mix of myocardial ischemia, injury, and necrosis, is characterized by changes in three components of the ECG—the T wave, ST segment, and Q wave. The changes in the ECG ascribed to myocardial ischemia, injury, and necrosis include the following:

- *Myocardial ischemia:* Ischemic T waves and ST-segment elevation or depression
- *Myocardial injury:* ST-segment elevation or depression
- *Myocardial necrosis:* Pathologic Q waves

The nature of these ECG changes and the leads in which they appear will depend on (1) the anatomical location of the acute MI in the ventricles (anterior, posterior, inferior, or right ventricular) and (2) the extent of the involvement of the myocardial wall (transmural or nontransmural). The changes that acute MIs produce in the T waves, ST segments, and Q waves are summarized in Table 16-6 and described in detail in the following sections.

> As it relates to acute coronary syndromes, T waves changes are associated with myocardial ischemia, ST segment changes with myocardial injury, and pathologic Q waves with myocardial necrosis.

As was discussed in earlier chapters, certain leads have specific "views" of the heart, which correspond to anatomical areas of coronary perfusion. The leads that record the electrical forces in a particular view of the exterior or epicardial surface of the area of the myocardium involved by myocardial ischemia, injury, and infarction are termed *"facing"* leads in this book. The leads that record the electrical forces that view the epicardial surface of the uninvolved myocardium directly opposite the area of ischemia, injury, or infarction are termed *"reciprocal"* leads. The ECG findings in the reciprocal lead are referred to as "reciprocal changes." ECG leads that examine the same area of the heart are referred to as "contiguous." For example, the precordial leads V_1 and V_2 both face the anterior wall of the left ventricle and therefore are contiguous. Finding abnormal changes in contiguous leads enhances their accuracy.

> Facing leads view the area of ischemia, injury, or infarction while reciprocal leads view the area from the opposite direction. Adjacent or leads facing the same area of the heart are referred to as "contiguous."

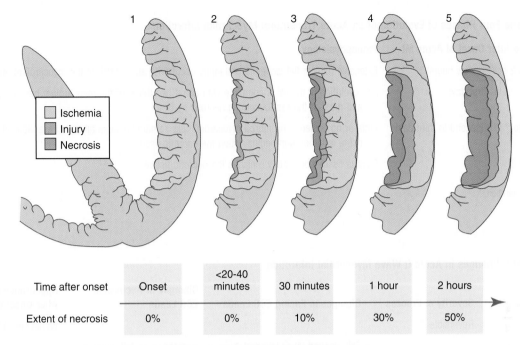

Time after onset	Onset	<20-40 minutes	30 minutes	1 hour	2 hours
Extent of necrosis	0%	0%	10%	30%	50%

A   Phase 1: Transmural MI (0-2 hours)

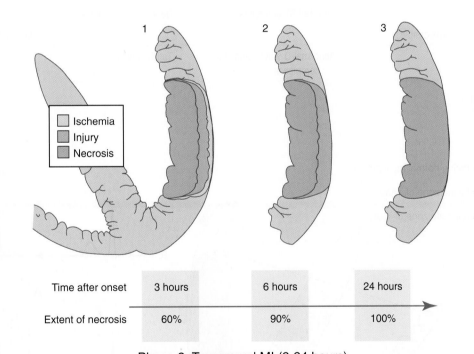

Time after onset	3 hours	6 hours	24 hours
Extent of necrosis	60%	90%	100%

B   Phase 2: Transmural MI (2-24 hours)

FIGURE 16-11 The first two early phases of an acute myocardial infarction. **A,** Phase 1. **B,** Phase 2.

ISCHEMIC T WAVES

Changes to the T waves indicating myocardial ischemia usually appear within seconds of the onset of an acute MI. These ischemic T waves, which appear over the zone of ischemia in the facing leads, are primarily caused by a delay or change in direction in repolarization of the myocardium because of hypoxia (Figure 16-12). They may be abnormally tall and peaked or deeply inverted. In addition, the QT intervals associated with the ischemic T waves are usually prolonged.

Whether the ischemic T waves are upright or inverted depends on whether the ischemia is subendocardial or subepicardial, respectively. In normal hearts, repolarization begins at

TABLE 16-5 **The Four Phases of Evolution of an Acute Transmural Myocardial Infarction**

Phase	Time After Onset of Acute MI	Pathophysiology
1	0 to 2 hr (first few hours)	Extensive myocardial ischemia and injury occur with about 50% of the myocardium becoming necrotic
2	2 to 24 hr (first day)	The evolution of the MI is complete with about two thirds of the myocardium becoming necrotic by 3 hr and most of the rest becoming necrotic by 6 hr
3	24 to 72 hr (second to third day)	Little or no ischemic or injured myocardial cells remain because all cells have either died or recovered; acute inflammation begins within the necrotic tissue
4	2 to 8 wk	Fibrous tissue completely replaces the necrotic tissue

MI, Myocardial infarction.

TABLE 16-6 **ECG Changes in Acute Q Wave Myocardial Infarction**

Stage of Acute MI	Severity of Process	Changes in Facing ECG Leads	Changes in Reciprocal ECG Leads	Appearance of ECG Changes After Onset of Acute MI
Ischemia	Reversible			Within seconds of onset
		Tall, peaked (a) or inverted (b) T waves	Inverted (a) or tall, peaked (b) T waves	
Ischemia, injury	Reversible			Within minutes of onset
		Elevated ST segments	Depressed ST segments	
Necrosis	Irreversible			In about 2 hr after onset
		Abnormal Q waves and QS complexes	Tall R waves	

MI, Myocardial infarction.

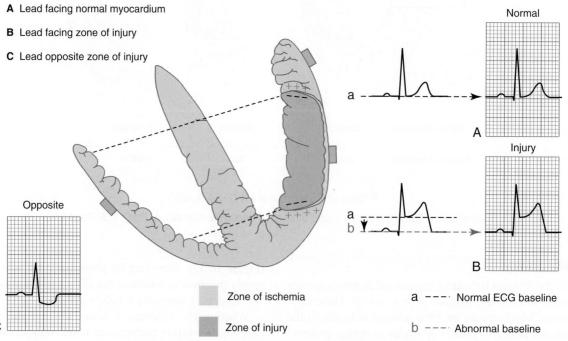

A Lead facing normal myocardium

B Lead facing zone of injury

C Lead opposite zone of injury

Normal

Injury

Opposite

Zone of ischemia

Zone of injury

a - - - Normal ECG baseline

b - - - Abnormal baseline

FIGURE 16-12 The mechanism of formation of abnormal T waves.

the epicardium and progresses toward the endocardium, producing a positive T wave.

In subendocardial ischemia, there is a delay in repolarization of the subendocardial cardiac cells. Repolarization progresses in the normal direction from the epicardium to the endocardium but is slowed when it reaches the ischemic subendocardial area. This produces a prolonged QT interval and a symmetrically positive, tall, and peaked T wave.

In subepicardial ischemia, on the other hand, there is a delay in the repolarization in the subepicardial cardiac cells. Because of this, repolarization begins at the endocardium and progresses in a reverse direction, from the endocardium to the epicardium, slowing when it reaches the ischemic subepicardial area. This produces a prolonged QT interval and a symmetrically negative and deep T wave.

Ischemic T waves are often associated with depression or elevation of the ST segment, another manifestation of myocardial ischemia. Ischemic T waves and associated ST segment changes revert to normal quickly after an anginal attack. Those present in acute MI secondary to myocardial ischemia may disappear more gradually or not at all as healing proceeds.

Deeply inverted T waves also appear in association with pathologic Q waves over the zone of necrosis in the later phases of acute MI. These T waves are deeply inverted, mirror images of the upright T waves normally generated in the opposite ventricular wall, being produced the same way as pathologic Q waves (the window theory), which will be described later.

In a typical transmural MI (Table 16-7), the leads that normally (in the absence of an MI) show positive T waves, ischemic T waves are initially prolonged, abnormally tall, symmetrical, and peaked. Occasionally, the ischemic T waves become extremely tall—the so-called *hyperacute T waves*—appearing for only a short time at the onset. Almost immediately after the onset of ischemia, the ST segments become elevated, resulting in the typical ST-T complex elevation seen during the early ischemic phase of a typical transmural infarction. This ST-T complex pattern continues through the injury phase into the

necrosis phase, at which time pathologic Q waves begin to appear. As the infarction evolves, the T waves revert to normal and then become deeply inverted in about 24 hours. Such an MI with Q waves is referred to as a *Q wave MI*.

In a typical subendocardial MI (Table 16-8), the T waves that follow the onset of infarction appear isoelectric, biphasic, or inverted. They are usually associated with depressed ST segments resembling those seen with angina pectoris. Unlike the ST-T complexes associated with angina, which quickly revert to normal after an anginal attack, these abnormal ST-T complexes return to normal more gradually, if at all, as healing proceeds. Q waves usually do not appear in subendocardial MI. An MI in which Q waves are absent is called a *non-Q wave MI*.

ST SEGMENT CHANGES

ST segment changes occur in myocardial infarction, indicating myocardial ischemia and injury, and in noninfarction-related myocardial ischemia from any cause. The ST segments may be elevated or depressed.

ST-Segment Elevation

ST-segment elevation is an ECG sign of severe, extensive, usually transmural, myocardial ischemia and injury in the evolution of an acute Q wave MI. It may also be seen less frequently in the evolution of an acute non-Q wave MI. An ST segment is considered to be elevated when it is 1 mm (0.1 mV) above the baseline, measured 0.04 second (1 small square) after the J point of the QRS complex.

ST elevation usually appears within minutes after the onset of infarction, initially indicating extensive myocardial ischemia and foreshadowing a progression first to myocardial injury within 20 to 40 minutes (average, 30 minutes) and then to significant myocardial necrosis in about 2 hours. Such ST segments are elevated in the leads facing the zone of ischemia and injury and depressed in the reciprocal leads (Figure 16-13). ST-segment elevation is often accompanied by an increase in the size of the R wave.

TABLE 16-7 Changes in the Facing ECG Leads During the Four Phases of a Transmural, Q Wave Myocardial Infarction

Phase of Infarction	Q Waves	R Waves	ST Segments	T Waves
Phase 1 (0 to 2 hr) Onset of extensive ischemia occurs immediately, subendocardial injury occurs within 20 to 40 min, and subendocardial necrosis occurs in about 30 min; necrosis extends to about half of the myocardial wall by 2 hr	Unchanged	Unchanged or abnormally tall	Onset of elevation	Amplitude increases; peaking may occur
Phase 2 (2 to 24 hr) Transmural infarction is considered complete by 6 hr as necrosis involves about 90% of the myocardial wall; the rest of the necrosis occurs by the end of phase 2	Width and depth begin to increase	Amplitude begins to decrease	Maximum elevation	Amplitude and peaking lessen; T waves still positive
Phase 3 (24 to 72 hr) Little or no ischemia or injury remains as healing begins	Reach maximum size	Absent	Return to baseline	Become maximally inverted
Phase 4 (2 to 8 wk) Replacement of the necrotic tissue by fibrous tissue	Q waves persist	May return partially	Usually normal	Slight inversion

TABLE 16-8 Changes in the Facing ECG Leads During the Four Phases of a Subendocardial Non-Q Wave Myocardial Infarction

Phase of Infarction	Q Waves	R Waves	ST Segments	T Waves
Phase 1 (0 to 2 hr) Onset of localized ischemia occurs immediately, subendocardial injury occurs within 20 to 40 min, and subendocardial necrosis occurs in about 30 min	Unchanged	Unchanged	Onset of depression	Amplitude may or may not increase slightly
Phase 2 (2 to 24 hr) Subendocardial infarction is considered complete by 6 hr; generally, the necrosis involves only the inner parts of the myocardium, usually the subendocardial area, without extending to the epicardial surface	Unchanged	Amplitude may begin to decrease somewhat	May or may not return to normal	Inversion may occur
Phase 3 (24 to 72 hr) Little or no ischemia or injury remains as healing begins	Unchanged	Unchanged	May or may not return to normal	Inversion may occur
Phase 4 (2 to 8 wk) Replacement of the infarcted tissue by fibrous tissue	Unchanged	Unchanged	May or may not return to normal	May or may not return to normal

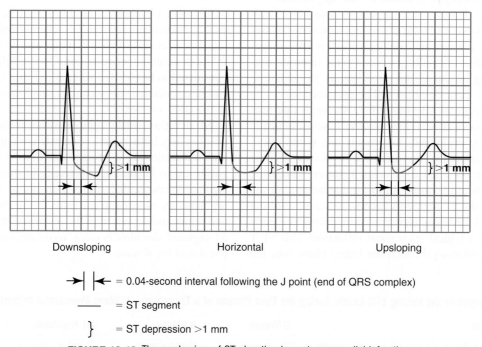

Downsloping   Horizontal   Upsloping

$\rightarrow| |\leftarrow$ = 0.04-second interval following the J point (end of QRS complex)

—— = ST segment

} = ST depression >1 mm

FIGURE 16-13 The mechanism of ST elevation in acute myocardial infarction.

The cause of ST-segment elevation in acute MI is the "current of injury," an electrical manifestation of the inability of cardiac cells "injured" by severe ischemia to maintain a normal resting membrane potential during diastole.

Following the ischemic and injury phases, as the MI progresses, the injured myocardial tissue turns necrotic and the current of injury disappears as the tissue becomes electrically inert. The ST segments become less elevated in the facing leads and finally return to the baseline. As this is occurring, the R waves begin to become smaller and disappear and significant Q waves and T wave inversion begin to appear in the facing leads.

ST-segment elevation can be caused by other processes and can be confused with that of acute MI. They include:

- **Coronary vasospasm.** Intense transmural myocardial ischemia brought on by vasospasm of a major coronary artery, termed Prinzmetal angina, may mimic an acute MI electrocardiographically. Clinically, patients with Prinzmetal angina have recurrent chest pain not related to exercise or other precipitating factors, often several times a day or night, and sometimes associated with significant dysrhythmias.

- **Acute pericarditis.** The pain of acute pericarditis may mimic that of acute MI, but the younger age of the patient, who usually lacks the coronary risk factors, makes the diagnosis of acute MI unlikely. The pain of pericarditis is often pleuritic in nature, made worse on inspiration, and relieved by the patient sitting upright and leaning forward. The pleuritic pain, the presence of a pericardial friction rub, and the appearance of ST-segment elevations in practically all of the ECG leads support the diagnosis of pericarditis. (See the Pericarditis section, p. 243)
- **Hyperkalemia** (see Hyperkalemia section, p. 245)
- **Early repolarization** (see Early Repolarization section, p. 252)

ST-Segment Depression

ST-segment depression is an ECG sign of subendocardial ischemia and injury. Similar to the criteria for ST elevation, an ST segment is considered to be depressed when it is 1 mm (0.1 mV) below the baseline, measured 0.04 second (1 small square) after the J point of the QRS complex.

ST depression usually appears within minutes after the onset of subendocardial non–Q wave MI, during an anginal attack or after exercise. ST depression may also be seen, but less frequently, in Q wave MI. The ST segments are depressed in the leads facing the ischemic tissue and elevated in the reciprocal leads. Such abnormal ST segments are due to altered repolarization of the myocardium because of anoxia.

The ST-segment depressions of subendocardial ischemia and injury have been classified as to the nature of the sloping of the segment (i.e., downsloping, horizontal, and upsloping) (Figure 16-14). The downsloping of an ST-segment is most specific for subendocardial ischemia and injury, as present in subendocardial infarction; horizontal sloping is of intermediate specificity; and upsloping is the least specific. However, regardless of the slope, an ST segment that is depressed 1 mm 0.04 second after the end of the QRS complex is significant. ST-segment depression is often associated with ischemic biphasic or inverted T waves, another manifestation of myocardial ischemia.

ST-segment depression quickly reverts to normal after an anginal attack or after exertion as myocardial ischemia is relieved or corrected. When associated with myocardial injury from an acute MI, the ST depression may disappear more gradually or not at all resulting in a permanent ST depression on the ECG.

Although ST-segment depression is commonly associated with subendocardial ischemia and injury, other common causes include the following:

- Left and right ventricular hypertrophy
- Left and right bundle branch blocks
- Digitalis in therapeutic and toxic doses

PATHOLOGIC Q WAVES

The Q wave is the first negative deflection of the QRS complex. It may be normal (physiologic) or abnormal (pathologic) (Figure 16-15).

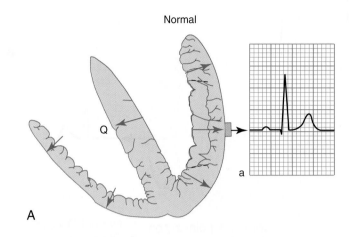

Normal

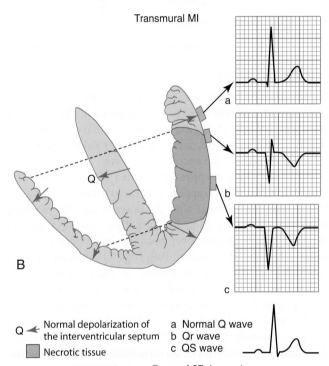

Transmural MI

Q ← Normal depolarization of the interventricular septum

▢ Necrotic tissue

a Normal Q wave
b Qr wave
c QS wave

FIGURE 16-14 Types of ST depression.

Physiologic Q Waves

Physiologic Q waves result from the normal depolarization of the interventricular septum from left to right. These relatively small electrical forces are the first step in the depolarization of the ventricles. The electrical forces responsible for the normal Q wave are negative because they travel away from the leads in which they appear, being opposite in direction to the positive electrical forces producing the R wave. Because the interventricular septum is thin, the electrical forces are small and of short duration—within 0.04 second and of low amplitude. The resultant "septal" q wave is less than 0.04 second wide and of a depth of less than 25% of the height of the succeeding R wave. Such small normal q waves are commonly present in the QRS complexes in leads I, II, III, aVL, aVF, V_5, and V_6.

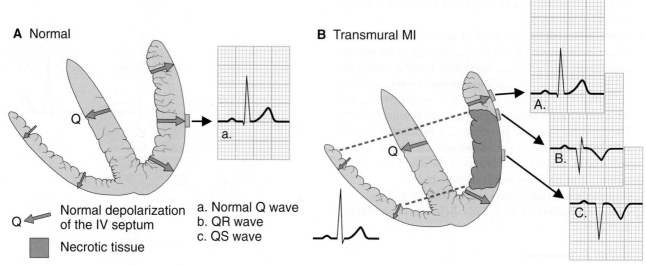

A Normal

Q

Normal depolarization of the IV septum

Q

Necrotic tissue

a. Normal Q wave
b. QR wave
c. QS wave

a.

B Transmural MI

Q

A.

B.

C.

FIGURE 16-15 The mechanism of formation of Q waves and QS waves in acute myocardial infarction.

Pathologic Q Waves

A pathologic or "significant" Q wave is usually considered an ECG sign of irreversible myocardial necrosis in the evolution of an acute MI, specifically a Q wave MI. A Q wave is considered significant if it is 0.04 second wide and has a depth of at least 25% of the height of the succeeding R wave.

Pathologic Q waves appear in less than 50% of patients with acute MI. When they do appear, they do so within 8 to 12 hours (but as early as 2 hours) after the onset of the MI, reaching maximum size within 24 to 48 hours. They typically appear in the facing leads directly over necrotic, infarcted myocardial tissue—the zone of infarction. Pathologic Q waves may persist indefinitely or disappear in months or years. As mentioned earlier, an acute MI with pathologic Q waves is called a *Q-wave MI*; one in which they are absent is a *non–Q-wave MI*.

The cause of pathologic Q waves differs from that of normal Q waves. A popular theory is referred to as the "window" theory. It reasons that because infarcted myocardium does not depolarize or repolarize, no electrical forces are generated, resulting in an electrically inert area. This electrically inert area can be considered a "window" through which the facing leads actually view, electrocardiographically speaking, the endocardium of the opposite noninfarcted ventricular wall. Because depolarization progresses from the endocardium outward, the electrical forces generated by the wall opposite the infarct will be traveling away from the leads facing the infarct. Therefore these leads will detect the negative electrical forces generated by the opposite, noninfarcted ventricular wall as large negative Q waves. These Q waves are actually mirror images of the R waves produced by the opposite ventricular wall.

The presence and size of pathologic Q waves and the number of leads in which they occur depend on the size of the infarct, both as to its depth (thickness) and width. The larger the infarct (i.e., the larger the "window"), the larger the Q waves are and the greater the number of contiguous leads in which they appear. A large pathologic Q wave with or without a succeeding R wave is often called a *QS wave.*

> In general, the greater the depth of the infarct, the deeper the Q waves; the wider the infarct; therefore, the more contiguous leads they appear in.

In contrast, the smaller the infarct, the smaller the Q waves both in width and depth and the fewer the facing leads with Q waves. If the infarct is relatively small and nontransmural, such as a subendocardial MI, pathologic Q waves may be completely absent, resulting in a non–Q-wave MI. Even transmural MIs, if small enough will not result in pathologic Q waves. The QS waves that occur in the right precordial leads V_1-V_2 within the first few hours of the onset of an acute anterior wall MI involving the interventricular septum result from the severe ischemia of the septum. The "septal" r waves normally produced by the left-to-right depolarization of the interventricular septum fail to occur, changing the normal rS pattern of the QRS complex in the right precordial leads to a QS complex.

Pathologic Q waves are *not* present in the 12-lead ECG of a posterior wall MI because there are no leads facing the infarct.

Q waves may be present in certain leads without being considered significant. A Q wave is commonly ignored in the following leads, especially if it occurs under certain circumstances. Box 16-1 lists the leads and conditions in which such a Q wave may be considered clinically nonrelevant.

Other considerations in determining the significance of Q waves include the following:

- Q waves accompanied by ST-segment elevation and T wave inversion are more significant and more reliable in making a diagnosis of acute MI than when they occur alone.
- Q waves in the presence of left bundle branch block and left anterior and posterior fascicular blocks are usually not considered significant.

BOX 16-1 Leads and Conditions in Which a Q Wave May Be Considered Clinically Non-Relevant

- Lead aVR. A Q wave in lead aVR is usually ignored because the QRS complex in this lead normally consists of a large S wave.
- Lead aVL. A QS or a QR wave in lead aVL alone in which the QRS axis is greater than + 60° (i.e., an electrically vertical heart) is usually ignored.
- Lead aVF. A QS or a QR wave in lead aVF alone is considered insignificant unless it is accompanied by significant Q waves, ST-segment elevation, and abnormal T wave changes in one or both of the other inferior leads—leads II and III.
- Lead III. A Q wave in this lead by itself is considered insignificant unless (1) it is accompanied by significant Q waves, ST-segment elevation, and abnormal T wave changes in the other inferior leads (lead II or aVF or both) and (2) the Q wave in lead III is wider and deeper than those in leads II and aVF.
- Lead V_1. A Q wave in this lead by itself is considered insignificant unless it is accompanied by significant Q waves, ST-segment elevation, and abnormal T wave changes in the other precordial leads-leads V_2-V_6.
- **Other considerations**
  - Q waves in the presence of left bundle branch block and left anterior and posterior fascicular blocks are usually not considered significant.
  - The presence of right bundle branch block does not affect the significance of Q waves.
  - Left ventricular hypertrophy may or may not affect the significance of Q waves.

- The presence of right bundle branch block does not affect the significance of Q waves.
- Left ventricular hypertrophy may or may not affect the significance of Q waves.

Determining the Site of a Myocardial Infarction

The location of an acute Q-wave MI relates to the leads in which ST-segment elevation and subsequent pathologic Q waves appear (i.e., the facing leads) (Table 16-9 and Figure 16-16). It is generally held that the ECG changes must be present in 2 or more contiguous leads. That is, two more leads that face or view the same area of the heart. For example, if ST-segment elevation and pathologic Q waves appear in any leads I, aVL, and V_1-V_6, the MI is "anterior." If ST-segment elevation and pathologic Q waves appear in leads II, III, and aVF, the MI is "inferior." If, in an inferior infarction, the ST segment in V_{4R} also becomes elevated, a "right ventricular" MI is present. Because there are no facing leads in a posterior MI, there are no diagnostic ST-segment elevations or pathologic Q waves present in the ECG leads. A posterior MI is diagnosed if reciprocal ECG changes of ST-segment depression and tall R waves are present in leads V_1-V_4. This topic will be discussed in greater detail in the next chapter.

TABLE 16-9 The Facing and Reciprocal Leads Relative to the Various Sites of Acute Q Wave Myocardial Infarction

Site of Infarction	Facing Leads	Reciprocal Leads
Anterior wall		
Septal	V_1-V_2	None
Anterior (localized)	V_3-V_4	None
Anteroseptal	V_1-V_4	None
Lateral	I, aVL, and V_5 or V_6	II, III, and aVF
Anterolateral	I, aVL, and V_3-V_6	II, III, and aVF
Extensive anterior	I, aVL, and V_1-V_6	II, III, and aVF
Inferior wall	II, III, and aVF	I and aVL
Posterior wall	None	V_1-V_4
Right ventricular	II, III, aVF, and V_{4R}	I and aVL

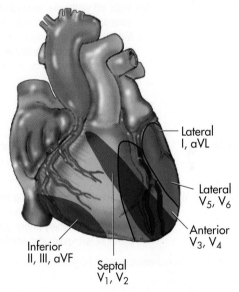

FIGURE 16-16 Site of infarction and associated ECG leads. (From Sanders MJ: *Mosby's paramedic textbook-revised reprint*, ed 3, St Louis, Mosby, 2007.)

> To localize the site of ischemia, injury, or infarction, ECG abnormalities must be present in at least 2 leads that view the same area of the heart. These are referred to as contiguous leads.

Complications of Acute Myocardial Infarction

The two major complications of acute MI are (1) myocardial dysfunction secondary to myocardial damage, resulting in right or left ventricular failure, and (2) the disruption of the electrical conduction system, resulting in various dysrhythmias, AV

TABLE 16-10 Coronary Arteries Involved, Diagnostic ECG Leads, and Associated Potential Complications of Specific Myocardial Infarctions

Infarction	Coronary Arteries Involved	Facing ECG Leads	Potential Complications
Septal MI	Septal perforator arteries of the left anterior descending coronary artery	V_1-V_2 (ST↑)	*AV blocks:* Second-degree, type II AV block* Second-degree, 2:1 and advanced AV block* Third-degree AV block* *Bundle branch blocks:* RBBB LBBB LAFB LPFB‡
Anterior (localized) MI	Diagonal arteries of the left anterior descending coronary artery	V_3-V_4 (ST↑)	*LV dysfunction:* CHF Cardiogenic shock
Lateral MI	Diagonal arteries of the left anterior descending coronary artery and/or the anterolateral marginal artery of the left circumflex coronary artery	I, aVL, V_5-V_6 (ST↑)	*LV dysfunction:* CHF (moderate)
Inferior MI	Posterior left ventricular arteries of the right coronary artery or, less commonly, of the left circumflex coronary artery, the posterior descending coronary artery and the AV node artery may also be involved	II, III, aVF (ST↑)	*LV dysfunction:* CHF (mild, if any) *AV blocks:* First-degree AV block† Second-degree, type I AV block† Second-degree, 2:1 and advanced AV block† Third-degree AV block† *Bundle branch blocks:* LPFB§
Posterior MI	Distal left circumflex artery and/or posterolateral marginal artery of the circumflex coronary artery	None Opposite leads: V_1-V_4 (ST↓)	*LV dysfunction:* CHF (mild, if any)
Right ventricular MI	Right coronary artery, including the SA node and AV node arteries, the posterior descending coronary artery, and the posterior left ventricular arteries	II, III, aVF, V_{4R} (ST↑)	*RV dysfunction:* Right heart failure *Dysrhythmias:* Sinus arrest Sinus bradycardia Atrial premature beats Atrial flutter Atrial fibrillation *AV blocks:* First-degree AV block† Second-degree type I AV block† Second-degree, 2:1 and advanced AV block† Third-degree AV block† *Bundle branch blocks:* LPFB§

CHF, Congestive heart failure; *LAFB*, left anterior fascicular block; *LBBB*, left bundle branch block; *LPFB*, left posterior fascicular block; *LV*, left ventricular; *RBBB*, right bundle branch block; *RV*, right ventricular.

*With abnormally wide QRS complexes.
†With normal QRS complexes.
‡In conjunction with a right ventricular or inferior infarction.
§In conjunction with a septal infarction.

blocks, or fascicular blocks. Which ventricle becomes dysfunctional and what types of dysrhythmias or disruptions of the electrical conduction system may develop depends on which coronary artery and related area of the heart is involved in the infarction. Table 16-10 details the relationship between the location of the infarction, the coronary arteries occluded, the ECG leads affected, and the complications that may be incurred. Because the distribution of the coronary arteries varies from person to person, and the location and degree of coronary artery occlusion varies from infarct to infarct, the type and extent of the complications will also vary from infarct to infarct. We will address the treatment of these complications in Chapter 19.

CHAPTER SUMMARY

- The myocardium is perfused by the left and right coronary arteries, which branch and feed specific areas of the heart with oxygen. Interruption of blood supply to specific coronary arteries results in myocardial ischemia and infarction of predictable areas of the heart.
- Atheromatous plaques form in the coronary arteries as a result of coronary artery disease and by a combination of erosion and/or disruption can result in occlusion of the coronary artery.
- When coronary artery perfusion is diminished from any cause, it can result in an acute coronary syndrome. The three recognized syndromes include unstable angina, non–ST-segment elevation myocardial infarction (NSTEMI), and ST-segment elevation myocardial infarction (STEMI).
- Once a plaque ruptures thrombosis begins. The phases of thrombosis involve multiple blood and tissue components, the action of which may be inhibited by the administration of pharmacologic agents.
- Likewise, thrombolysis involves multiple steps and may be augmented by drug therapy.
- The specific ECG changes associated with acute coronary syndromes include ischemic T waves, ST-segment elevation and depression, and pathologic Q waves.

CHAPTER REVIEW

1. The artery that arises from the left main coronary artery at an obtuse angle and runs posteriorly along the left atrioventricular groove to end in back of the left ventricle is called the:
   A. left anterior descending coronary artery
   B. left circumflex coronary artery
   C. right ventricular artery
   D. septal perforator artery

2. The SA node may be supplied with blood from:
   A. the conus artery
   B. the left anterior descending coronary artery
   C. the left circumflex coronary
   D. the right coronary artery

3. The most common cause of myocardial ischemia or infarction is caused by:
   A. cocaine toxicity
   B. coronary artery spasm
   C. increased myocardial workload
   D. occlusion of an atherosclerotic coronary artery

4. An increase in existing angina from a CCSC class II to a class III indicates the following:
   A. a decrease in the coronary artery stenosis
   B. the appearance of angina at rest
   C. the occurrence of an acute MI
   D. the onset of unstable angina

5. The most common cause of acute MI is a (n):
   A. air embolism
   B. coronary artery spasm
   C. coronary thrombosis
   D. hypertension

6. Upon revascularization or reoxygenation, necrotic cells:
   A. do not return to normal function
   B. return to normal or near normal function
   C. revert to a previous state of injury
   D. usually take 24 hours to return to normal function

7. An MI in which the zone of infarction involves the entire full thickness of the ventricular wall, from the endocardium to the epicardial surface, is called a:
   A. necrotic infarction
   B. nontransmural infarction
   C. subendocardial infarction
   D. transmural infarction

8. The "window" theory best describes the mechanism for the presence of which of the following:
   A. inverted T waves
   B. pathologic Q wave
   C. ST-segment elevation
   D. ST-segment depression

9. Inverted or tall peaked T waves in a facing lead during the early phase of an acute MI are an indication of:
   A. infarct
   B. injury
   C. ischemia
   D. necrosis

10. The most likely cause of an inferior MI is an occlusion of the:
    A. anterolateral marginal artery
    B. left anterior descending artery
    C. posterior descending artery
    D. right coronary artery

17

Diagnostic ECG Changes in Specific Myocardial Infarctions

OBJECTIVES *Upon completion of all or part of this chapter, you should be able to complete the following objectives:*

1. Name the coronary artery or arteries occluded and the region of the heart involved in the following acute myocardial infarctions (MIs):
   - Septal MI
   - Anterior (localized) MI
   - Anteroseptal MI
   - Lateral MI
   - Anterolateral MI
   - Inferior MI
   - Posterior MI
   - Right ventricular MI

2. List the diagnostic changes in the Q waves, R waves, ST segments, and T waves in the facing and reciprocal ECG leads (where applicable) during the early and late phases of the following acute MIs:
   - Septal MI
   - Anterior (localized) MI
   - Anteroseptal MI
   - Lateral MI
   - Anterolateral MI
   - Inferior MI
   - Posterior MI
   - Right ventricular MI

4. Identify the facing and opposite ECG leads that show the ST segment and T wave changes of early transmural Q wave MIs in the following:
   - Septal MI
   - Anterior (localized) MI
   - Anteroseptal MI
   - Lateral MI
   - Anterolateral MI
   - Extensive anterior MI
   - Inferior MI
   - Posterior MI
   - Right ventricular MI

INTRODUCTION

It should be noted that if the ECG being analyzed has changes consistent with both an anterolateral and an inferior MI, for example, then the patient has both an inferior and an anterolateral MI. This would also be true of an anterolateral and a posterior MI, an inferior and a posterior MI, and so forth.

The changes in the ECG presented for each specific MI are based on typical first-time infarcts and may not represent actual changes in a particular patient's ECG. The reasons for this include individual variations in the size, position in the chest, and rotation of the heart and in the distribution of the coronary artery circulation; the presence of bundle branch blocks, ventricular hypertrophy, and previous MIs; and coexisting drug- and electrolyte-related ECG changes.

SEPTAL MYOCARDIAL INFARCTION

Coronary Arteries Involved and Site of Occlusion

The major coronary artery involved is the left coronary artery, specifically the following branches:

- The left anterior descending coronary artery beyond the first diagonal branch, involving the septal perforator arteries (Figure 17-1).

Location of Infarct

The septal MI involves (1) the anterior wall of the left ventricle overlying the interventricular septum and (2) the anterior two thirds of the interventricular septum.

ECG Changes (Table 17-1)

In facing leads V_1-V_2:
    Early: Absence of normal "septal" r waves in the right precordial leads V_1-V_2, resulting in QS waves in these leads.
    Absence of normal "septal" q waves where normally present (i.e., in leads I, II, III, aVF, and V_4-V_6).
    ST-segment elevation with tall T waves in leads V_1-V_2.
    Late: QS complexes with T wave inversion in leads V_1-V_2.
In reciprocal leads II, III, and aVF:
    Early: No significant ECG changes.
    Late: No significant ECG changes.

TABLE 17-1 ECG Changes in Septal MI

	Q Waves (Abnormal Q Waves and QS Complexes)	R Waves (Abnormally Tall or Small)	ST Segments (Elevated or Depressed)	T Waves (Abnormally Tall or Inverted)
Early				
Phase 1				
First few hours (0 to 2 hr)	Absent "septal" q waves in I, II, III, aVF, and V_4-V_6 QS waves in V_1-V_2	Absent "septal" r waves in V_1-V_2	Elevated in V_1-V_2	Sometimes abnormally tall with peaking in V_2-V_2
Phase 2				
First day (2 to 24 hr)	Same as in phase 1	Same as in phase 1	Maximally elevated in V_1-V_2	Less tall, but generally still positive, in V_1-V_2
Late				
Phase 3				
Second and third day (24 to 72 hr)	QS complexes in V_1-V_2	Same as in phase 1	Return of the ST segments to the baseline throughout	T wave inversion in V_1-V_2

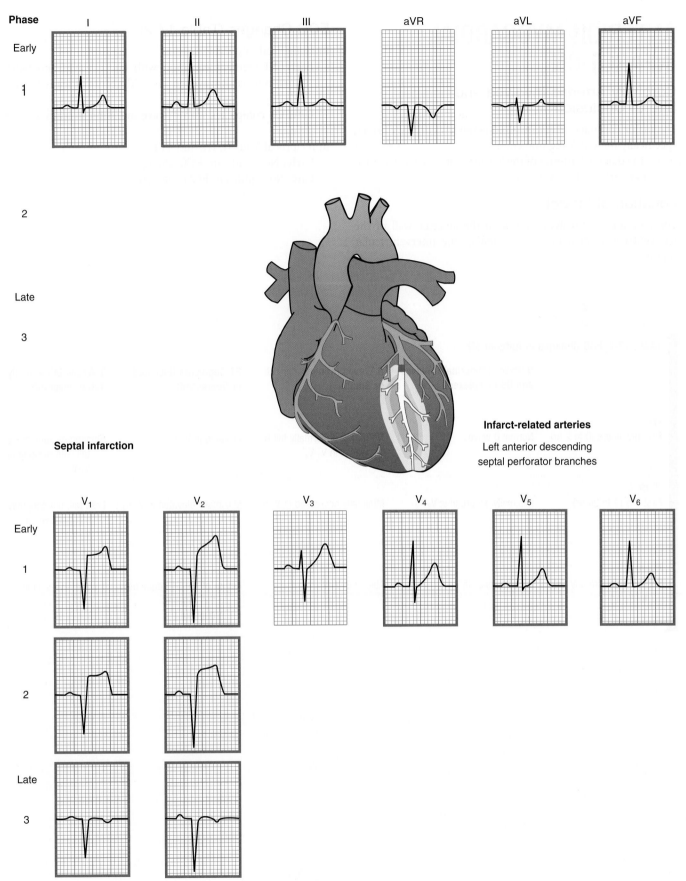

FIGURE 17-1 Septal MI.

ANTERIOR MYOCARDIAL INFARCTION

Coronary Arteries Involved and Site of Occlusion

The major coronary artery involved is the left coronary artery, specifically the following branches:

- The diagonal arteries of the left anterior descending coronary artery (Figure 17-2).

Location of Infarct

The anterior MI involves an area of the anterior wall of the left ventricle immediately to the left of the interventricular septum.

ECG Changes (Table 17-2)

In facing leads V_3-V_4:

Early: ST-segment elevation with tall T waves and taller than normal R waves in the midprecordial leads V_3 and V_4.

Late: QS complexes with T wave inversion in leads V_3 and V_4.

In reciprocal leads II, III, and aVF:

Early: No significant ECG changes.

Late: No significant ECG changes.

TABLE 17-2 ECG Changes in Anterior MI

	Q Waves (Abnormal Q Waves and QS Complexes)	R Waves (Abnormally Tall or Small)	ST-Segments (Elevated or Depressed)	T Waves (Abnormally Tall or Inverted)
Early *Phase 1* First few hours (0 to 2 hr)	Normal Q waves	Normal or abnormally tall R waves in V_3-V_4	Elevated in V_3-V_4	Sometimes abnormally tall with peaking in V_3-V_4
Phase 2 First day (2 to 24 hr)	Minimally abnormal in V_3-V_4	Minimally decreased in V_3-V_4	Maximally elevated in V_3-V_4	Less tall, but generally still positive, in V_3-V_4
Late *Phase 3* Second and third day (24 to 72 hr)	QS complexes in V_3-V_4	Absent in V_3-V_4	Return of the ST segments to the baseline throughout	T wave inversion in V_3-V_4

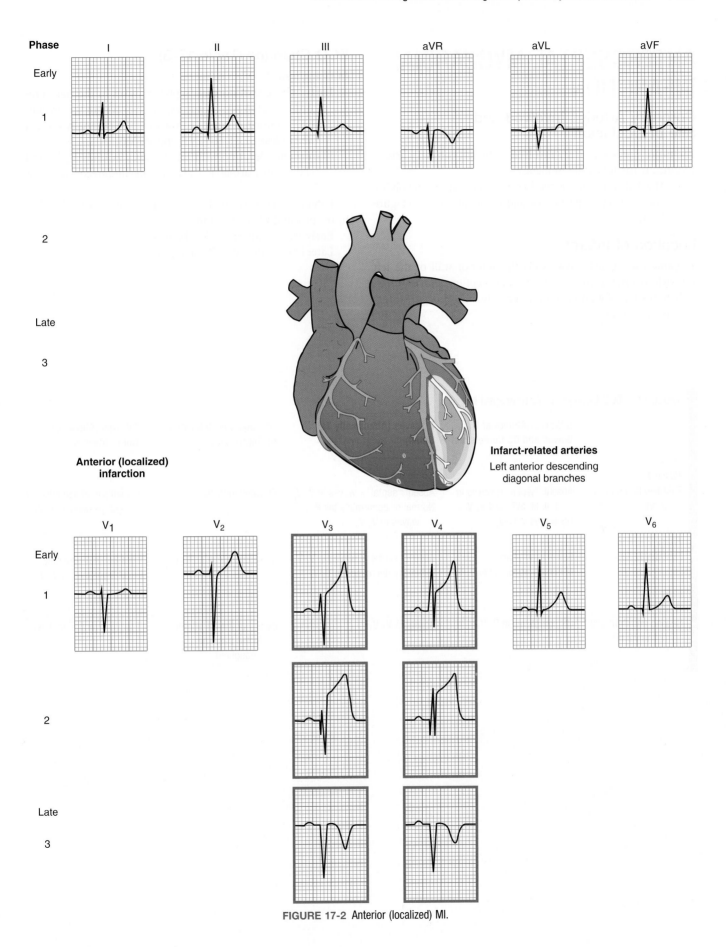

FIGURE 17-2 Anterior (localized) MI.

ANTEROSEPTAL MYOCARDIAL INFARCTION

Coronary Arteries Involved and Site of Occlusion

The major coronary artery involved is the left coronary artery, specifically the following branches:

- The left anterior descending coronary artery involving both the septal perforator and diagonal arteries (Figure 17-3).

Location of Infarct

The anteroseptal MI involves (1) the anterior wall of the left ventricle overlying the interventricular septum and immediately to the left of it and (2) the anterior two thirds of the interventricular septum.

ECG Changes (Table 17-3)

In facing leads V_1-V_4:

Early: Absence of normal "septal" r waves in the right precordial leads V_1-V_2, resulting in QS waves in these leads. Absence of normal "septal" q waves where normally present (i.e., in leads I, II, III, aVF, and V_4-V_6).

ST-segment elevation with tall T waves in leads V_1-V_4 and taller than normal R waves in the midprecordial leads V_3-V_4.

Late: QS complexes with T wave inversion in leads V_1-V_4.

In reciprocal leads II, III, and aVF:

Early: No significant ECG changes.

Late: No significant ECG changes.

TABLE 17-3 ECG Changes in Anteroseptal MI

	Q Waves (Abnormal Q Waves and QS Complexes)	R Waves (Abnormally Tall or Small)	ST Segments (Elevated or Depressed)	T Waves (Abnormally Tall or Inverted)
Early *Phase 1* First few hours (0 to 2 hr)	Absent "septal" q waves in I, II, III, aVF, and V_4-V_6 QS waves in V_1-V_2	Absent "septal" r waves in V_1-V_2 Normal or abnormally tall R waves in V_3-V_4	Elevated in V_1-V_4	Sometimes abnormally tall with peaking in V_1-V_4
Phase 2 First day (2 to 24 hr)	Same as in phase 1 Minimally abnormal in V_3-V_4	Absent "septal" r waves in V_1-V_2 Minimally decreased in V_3-V_4	Maximally elevated in V_1-V_4	Less tall, but generally still positive, in V_1-V_4
Late *Phase 3* Second and third day (24 to 72 hr)	QS complexes in V_1-V_4	Absent in V_1-V_4	Return of the ST segments to the baseline throughout	T wave inversion in V_1-V_4

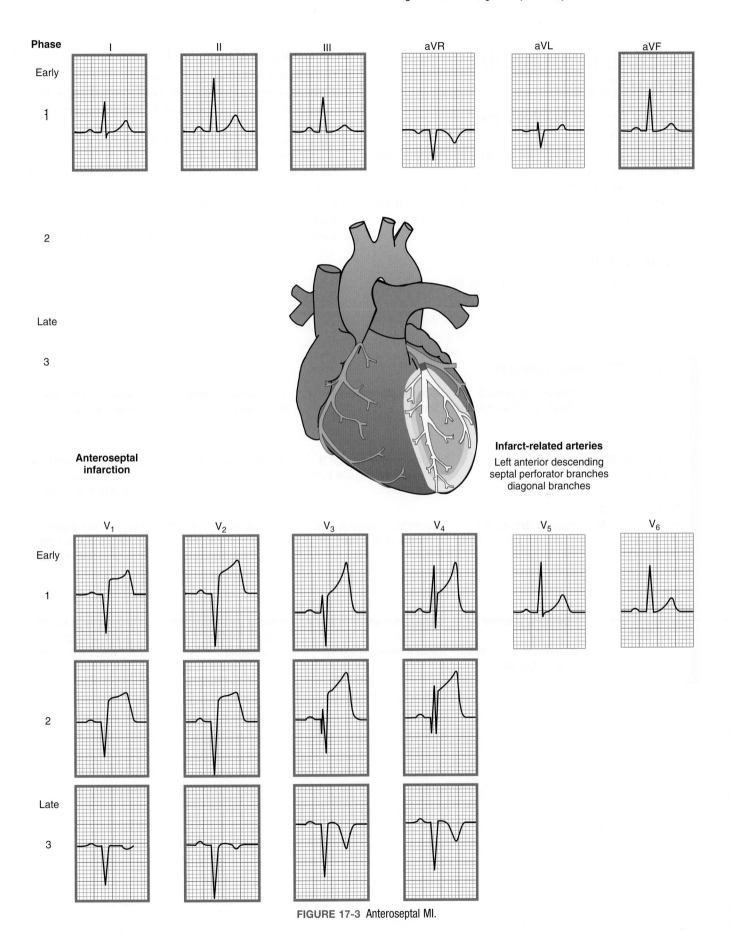

Phase

Infarct-related arteries
Left anterior descending
septal perforator branches
diagonal branches

Anteroseptal infarction

FIGURE 17-3 Anteroseptal MI.

LATERAL MYOCARDIAL INFARCTION

Coronary Arteries Involved and Site of Occlusion

The major artery involved is the left coronary artery, specifically the following branches:

- The laterally located diagonal arteries of the left anterior descending coronary artery and/or the anterolateral marginal artery of the left circumflex coronary artery (Figure 17-4).

Location of Infarct

The lateral MI involves the lateral wall of the left ventricle.

ECG Changes (Table 17-4)

In facing leads I, aVL, and V_5 or V_6, or both:

Early: ST-segment elevation with tall T waves and taller than normal R waves in leads I, aVL, and the left precordial lead V_5 or V_6 or both.

Late: Abnormal Q waves and small R waves with T wave inversion in leads I and aVL.

QS waves or complexes with T wave inversion in lead V_5 or V_6 or both.

In reciprocal leads II, III, and aVF:

Early: ST-segment depression in leads II, III, and aVF.

Late: Abnormally tall T waves in leads II, III, and aVF.

TABLE 17-4 ECG Changes in Lateral MI

	Q Waves (Abnormal Q Waves and QS Complexes)	R Waves (Abnormally Tall or Small)	ST Segments (Elevated or Depressed)	T Waves (Abnormally Tall or Inverted)
Early *Phase 1* First few hours (0 to 2 hr)	Normal Q waves	Normal or abnormally tall R waves in I, aVL, and V_5 or V_6 or both	Elevated in I, aVL, and V_5 or V_6 or both Depressed in II, III, and aVF	Sometimes abnormally tall with peaking in I, aVL, and V_5 or V_6 or both
Phase 2 First day (2 to 24 hr)	Minimally abnormal in I, aVL, and V_5 or V_6 or both	Minimally decreased in I, aVL, and V_5 or V_6 or both	Maximally elevated in I, aVL, and V_5 or V_6 or both Maximally depressed in II, III, and aVF	Less tall, but generally still positive, in I, aVL, and V_5 or V_6 or both
Late *Phase 3* Second and third day (24 to 72 hr)	Significantly abnormal in I and aVL QS waves or complexes in V_5 or V_6 or both	Decreased or absent in V_5 or V_6 or both Small R waves in I and aVL	Return of the ST segments to the baseline throughout	T wave inversion in I, aVL, and V_5 or V_6 or both Tall T waves in II, III, and aVF

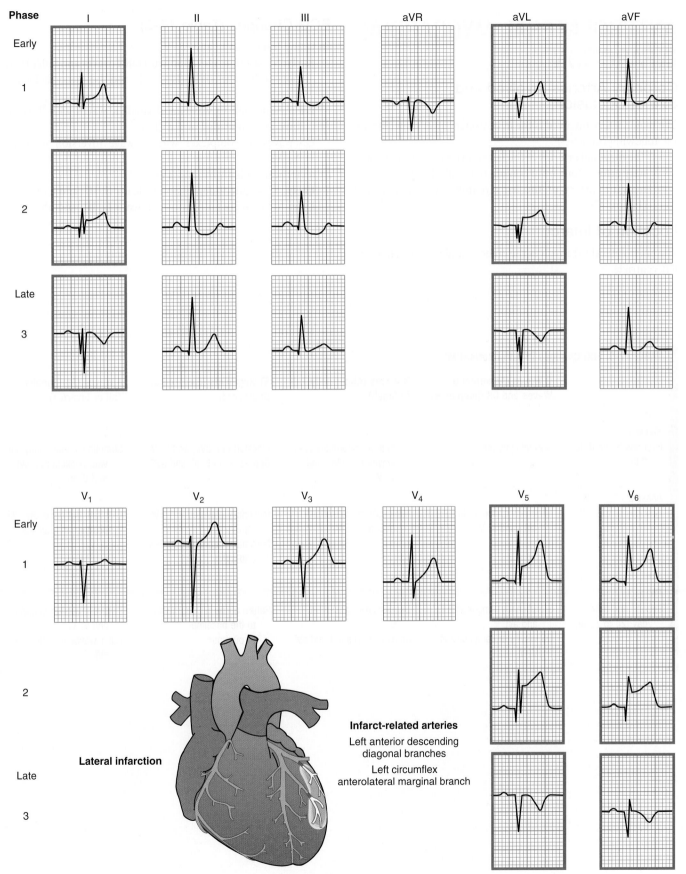

FIGURE 17-4 Lateral MI.

ANTEROLATERAL MYOCARDIAL INFARCTION

Coronary Arteries Involved and Site of Occlusion

The major artery involved is the left coronary artery, specifically the following branches:

- The diagonal arteries of the left anterior descending coronary artery alone or in conjunction with the anterolateral marginal artery of the left circumflex coronary artery (Figure 17-5).

Location of Infarct

The anterolateral MI involves the anterior and lateral wall of the left ventricle.

ECG Changes (Table 17-5)

In facing leads I, aVL, and V_3-V_6:

Early: ST-segment elevation with tall T waves and taller than normal R waves in leads I, aVL, and the precordial leads V_3-V_6.

Late: Abnormal Q waves and small R waves with T wave inversion in leads I and aVL.

QS waves or complexes with T wave inversion in leads V_3-V_6.

In reciprocal leads II, III, and aVF:

Early: ST-segment depression in leads II, III, and aVF.

Late: Abnormally tall T waves in leads II, III, and aVF.

TABLE 17-5 ECG Changes in Anterolateral MI

	Q Waves (Abnormal Q Waves and QS Complexes)	R Waves (Abnormally Tall or Small)	ST Segments (Elevated or Depressed)	T Waves (Abnormally Tall or Inverted)
Early *Phase 1* First few hours (0 to 2 hr)	Normal Q waves	Normal or abnormally tall R waves in I, aVL, and V_3-V_6	Elevated in I, aVL, and V_3-V_6 Depressed in II, III, and aVF	Sometimes abnormally tall with peaking in I, aVL, and V_3-V_6
Phase 2 First day (2 to 24 hr)	Minimally abnormal in I, aVL, and V_3-V_5	Minimally decreased in I, aVL, and V_3-V_6	Maximally elevated in I, aVL, and V_3-V_6 Maximally depressed in II, III, and aVF	Less tall, but generally still positive, in I, aVL, and V_3-V_6
Late *Phase 3* Second and third day (24 to 72 hr)	Significantly abnormal in I and aVL QS waves or complexes in V_3-V_6	Decreased or absent in V_3-V_6 Small R waves in I and aVL	Return of the ST segments to the baseline throughout	T wave inversion in I, aVL, and V_3-V_6 Tall T waves in II, III, and aVF

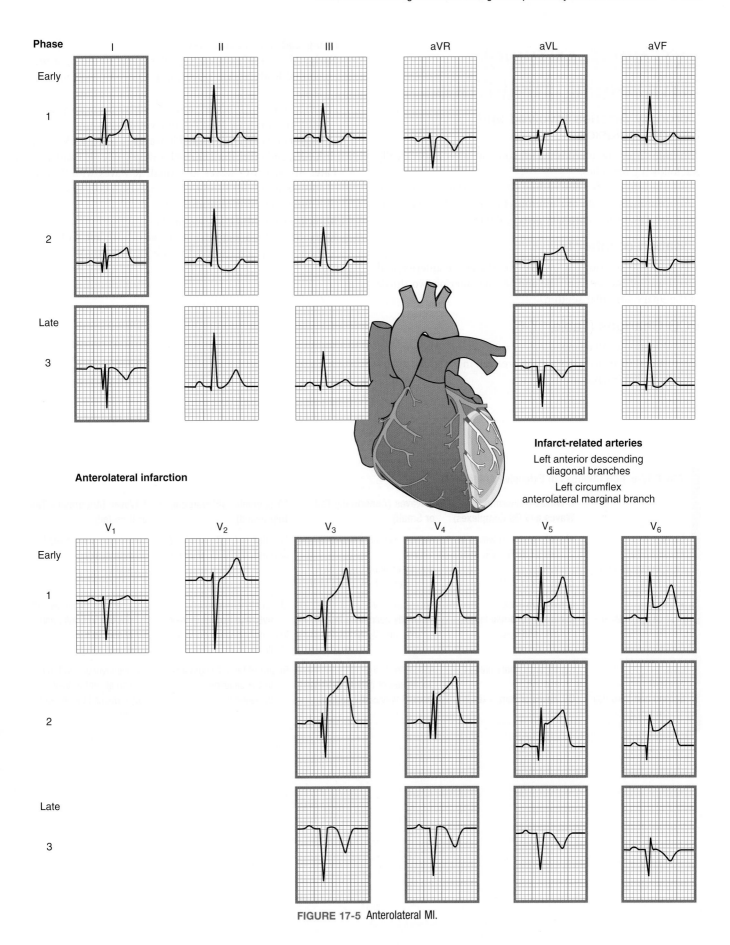

Anterolateral infarction

Infarct-related arteries

Left anterior descending
diagonal branches

Left circumflex
anterolateral marginal branch

FIGURE 17-5 Anterolateral MI.

EXTENSIVE ANTERIOR MYOCARDIAL INFARCTION

Coronary Arteries Involved and Site of Occlusion

The major artery involved is the left coronary artery, specifically the following branches:

- The left anterior descending coronary artery alone or in conjunction with the anterolateral marginal artery of the left circumflex coronary artery (Figure 17-6).

Location of Infarct

The extensive anterior MI involves (1) the entire anterior and lateral wall of the left ventricle and (2) the anterior two thirds of the interventricular septum.

ECG Changes (Table 17-6)

A combination of all changes seen in anteroseptal, anterior, and anterolateral myocardial infarction are seen in extensive anterior myocardial intarction.

In facing leads I, aVL, and V_1-V_6:

Early: Absence of normal "septal" r waves in the right precordial leads V_1-V_2, resulting in QS complexes in these leads.

Absence of normal "septal" q waves where normally present (i.e., in leads I, II, III, aVF, and V_4-V_6).

ST-segment elevation with tall T waves in leads I, aVL, and V_1-V_6, and taller than normal R waves in leads I and aVL.

Late: Abnormal Q waves and small R waves with T wave inversion in leads I and aVL. QS waves or complexes with T wave inversion in leads V_1-V_6.

In reciprocal leads II, III, and aVF:

Early: ST-segment depression in leads II, III, and aVF. Late: Abnormally tall T waves in leads II, III, and aVF.

TABLE 17-6 ECG Changes in Extensive Anterior MI

	Q Waves (Abnormal Q Waves and QS Complexes)	R Waves (Abnormally Tall or Small)	ST segments (Elevated or Depressed)	T Waves (Abnormally Tall or Inverted)
Early *Phase 1* First few hours (0 to 2 hr)	Absent "septal" q waves in leads I, II, III, aVR, and V_4-V_6 QS waves in V_1-V_2	Absent "septal" r waves in V_1-V_2 Normal or abnormally tall R waves in I, aVL, and V_3-V_6	Elevated in I, aVL, and V_1-V_6 Depressed in II, III, and aVF	Sometimes abnormally tall with peaking in I, aVL, and V_1-V_6
Phase 2 First day (2 to 24 hr)	Same as in Phase 1 Minimally abnormal in I, aVL, and V_3-V_6	Absent in V_1-V_2 Minimally decreased in I, aVL, and V_3-V_6	Maximally elevated in I, aVL, and absent in V_1-V_6 Maximally depressed in II, III, and aVF	Less tall, but generally still positive in I, aVL, and absent in V_1-V_6
Late *Phase 3* Second and third day (24 to 72 hr)	Significantly abnormal in I and aVL QS waves or complexes in V_1-V_6	Absent in V_1-V_2 Decreased or absent in V_3-V_6 Small R waves in I and aVL	Return of the ST segments to the baseline throughout	T wave inversion in I, aVL, and absent in V_1-V_6 Tall T waves in II, III, and aVF

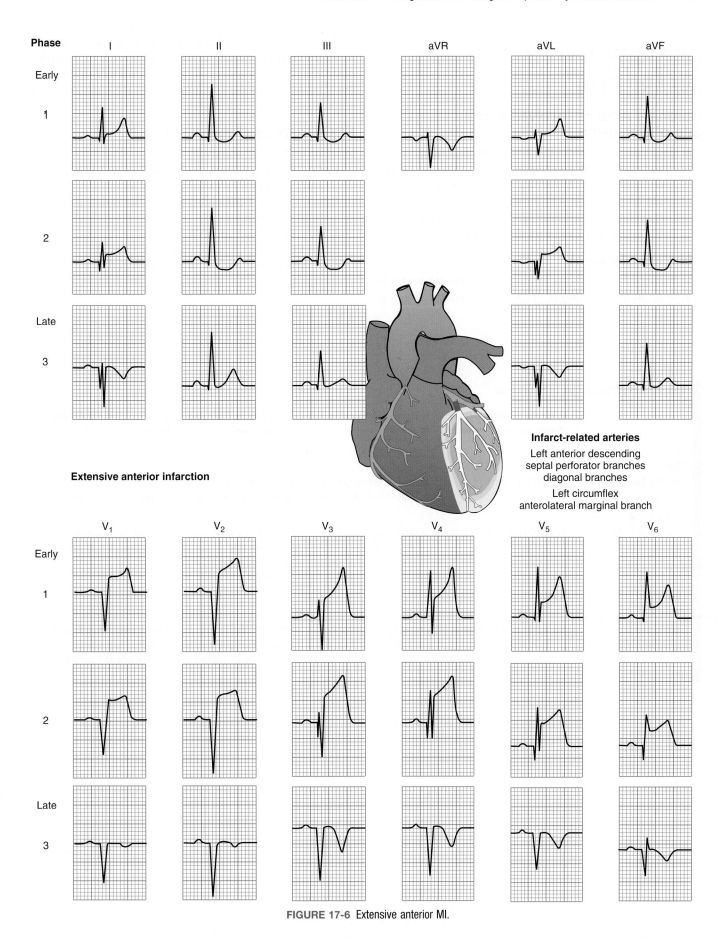

Phase

I   II   III   aVR   aVL   aVF

Early

1

2

Late

3

Extensive anterior infarction

Infarct-related arteries

Left anterior descending
septal perforator branches
diagonal branches

Left circumflex
anterolateral marginal branch

V_1 V_2 V_3 V_4 V_5 V_6

Early

1

2

Late

3

FIGURE 17-6 Extensive anterior MI.

INFERIOR MYOCARDIAL INFARCTION

Coronary Arteries Involved and Site of Occlusion

The major coronary arteries involved are the following:

- The posterior left ventricular arteries of the right coronary artery or, less commonly, of the left circumflex coronary artery of the left coronary artery. The posterior descending coronary artery and the atrioventricular (AV) node artery may also be involved (Figure 17-7).

Location of Infarct

The inferior MI involves the inferior wall of the left ventricle that rests on the diaphragm. If the left circumflex artery is occluded, the infarction extends somewhat into the lateral wall of the left ventricle, causing an inferolateral MI. If the posterior descending coronary artery and the AV node artery are involved, the MI extends into the posterior third of the interventricular septum and the AV node as well.

ECG Changes (Table 17-7)

In facing leads II, III, and aVF:

Early: ST-segment elevation with tall T waves and taller than normal R waves in leads II, III, and aVF.

Late: QS waves or complexes with T wave inversion in leads II, III, and aVF.

In reciprocal leads I and aVL:

Early: ST-segment depression in leads I and aVL.

Late: Abnormally tall T waves in leads I and aVL.

TABLE 17-7 ECG Changes in Inferior MI

	Q Waves (Abnormal Q Waves and QS Complexes)	R Waves (Abnormally Tall or Small)	ST Segments (Elevated or Depressed)	T Waves (Abnormally Tall or Inverted)
Early				
Phase 1				
First few hours (0 to 2 hr)	Normal Q waves	Normal or abnormally tall R waves in II, III, and aVF	Elevated in II, III, and aVF Depressed in I and aVL	Sometimes, abnormally tall with peaking in II, III, and aVF
Phase 2				
First day (2 to 24 hr)	Minimally abnormal in II, III, and aVF	Minimally decreased in II, III, and aVF	Maximally elevated in II, III, and aVF Maximally depressed in I and aVL	Less tall, but generally still positive, in II, III, and aVF
Late				
Phase 3				
Second and third day (24 to 72 hr)	QS waves or complexes in II, III, and aVF	Decreased or absent in II, III, and aVF	Return of the ST segments to the baseline throughout	T wave inversion in II, III, and aVF Tall T waves in I and aVL

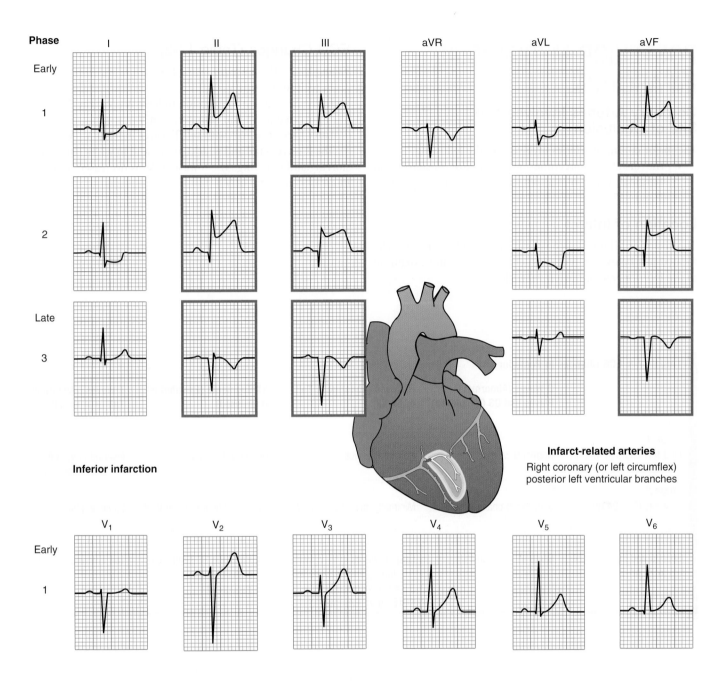

FIGURE 17-7 Inferior MI.

POSTERIOR MYOCARDIAL INFARCTION

Coronary Arteries Involved and Site of Occlusion

The major coronary arteries involved are the following:

- The distal left circumflex artery and/or posterolateral marginal artery of the left circumflex coronary artery (Figure 17-8).

Location of Infarct

The posterior MI involves the posterior wall of the left ventricle, located just below the posterior left AV groove and extending to the inferior wall of the left ventricle.

ECG Changes (Table 17-8)

Facing leads: There are no facing leads.

In reciprocal leads V_1-V_4:

Early: ST-segment depression in leads V_1-V_4. The T wave is inverted in V_1 and sometimes in V_2.

Late: Large R waves with tall T waves in leads V_1-V_4.

The R wave is tall and wide (0.04 second in width) in V_1 with slurring and notching. The S wave in V_1 is decreased, resulting in an R/S ratio of 1 in V_1.

TABLE 17-8 ECG Changes in Posterior MI

	Q Waves (Abnormal Q Waves and QS Complexes)	R Waves (Abnormally Tall or Small)	ST Segments (Elevated or Depressed)	T Waves (Abnormally Tall or Inverted)
Early *Phase 1* First few hours (0 to 2 hr)	Normal Q waves	Normal R waves	Depressed in V_1-V_4	Inverted in V_1 and sometimes in V_2
Phase 2 First day (2 to 24 hr)	Same as in phase 1	Minimally increased in V_1-V_4	Maximally depressed in V_1-V_4	Same as phase 1
Late *Phase 3* Second and third day (24 to 72 hr)	Same as in phase 1	Large R waves in V_1-V_4 with slurring and notching in V_1 S waves decreased in V_1 NOTE: In V_1, R/S ratio ≥ 1	Return of the ST segments to the baseline throughout	Tall T waves in V_1-V_4

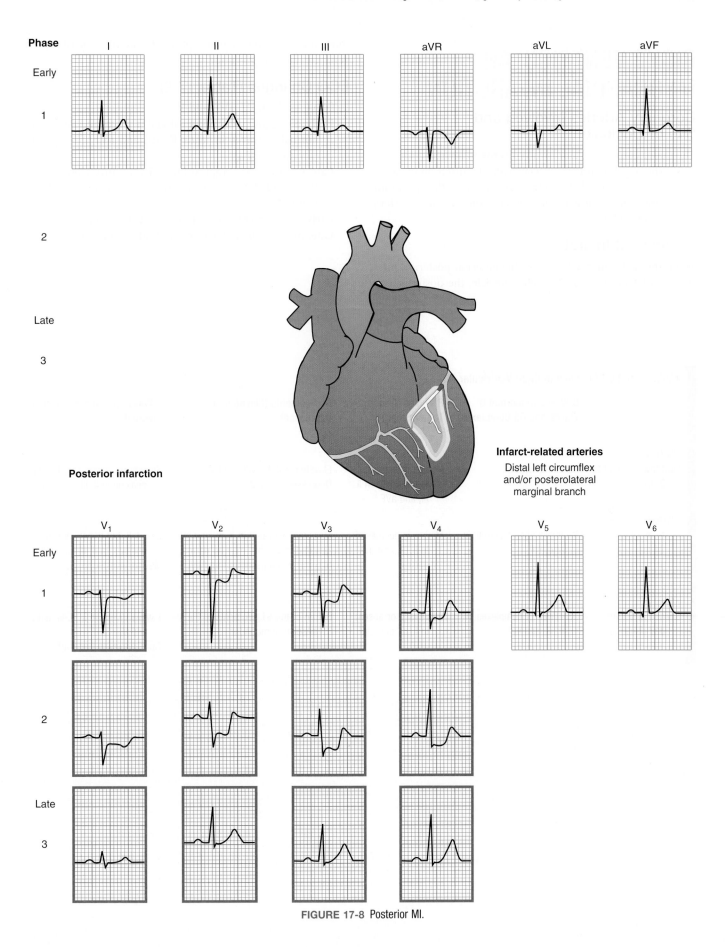

FIGURE 17-8 Posterior MI.

RIGHT VENTRICULAR MYOCARDIAL INFARCTION

Coronary Arteries Involved and Site of Occlusion

The major coronary artery involved is the following:

- The right coronary artery with its distal branches—the posterior left ventricular arteries, the posterior descending coronary artery, and the AV node artery (Figure 17-9).

Location of Infarct

The right ventricular MI involves the anterior, posterior, inferior, and lateral walls of the right ventricle, the posterior one third of the interventricular septum, the inferior wall of the left ventricle, and the AV node.

ECG Changes (Table 17-9)

In facing leads II, III, aVF, and V_{4R}.

Early: ST-segment elevation with tall T waves and taller than normal R waves in leads II, III, and aVF. ST-segment elevation in V_{4R}.

Late: QS waves or complexes with T wave inversion in leads II, III, and aVF. T wave inversion in V_{4R}. In opposite leads I and aVL:

Early: ST-segment depression in leads I and aVL.

Late: Abnormally tall T waves in leads I and aVL.

TABLE 17-9 **ECG Changes in Right Ventricular MI**

	Q Waves (Abnormal Q Waves and QS Complexes)	R Waves (Abnormally Tall or Small)	ST Segments (Elevated or Depressed)	T Waves (Abnormally Tall or Inverted)
Early				
Phase 1				
First few hours (0 to 2 hr)	Normal Q waves	Normal or abnormally tall R waves in II, III, and aVF	Elevated in II, III, aVF, and V_{4R} Depressed in I and aVL	Sometimes abnormally tall with peaking in II, III, and aVF
Phase 2				
First day (2 to 24 hr)	Minimally abnormal in II, III, and aVF	Minimally decreased in II, III, and aVF	Maximally elevated in II, III, and aVF Elevated in V_{4R}, but may be normal Maximally depressed in I and aVL	Less tall, but generally still positive, in II, III, and aVF May be inverted in V_{4R}
Late				
Phase 3				
Second and third day (24 to 72 hr)	QS waves or complexes in II, III, and aVF	Decreased or absent in II, III, and aVF	Return of the ST segments to the baseline throughout	T wave inversion in II, III, aVF, and V_{4R} Tall T waves in I and aVL

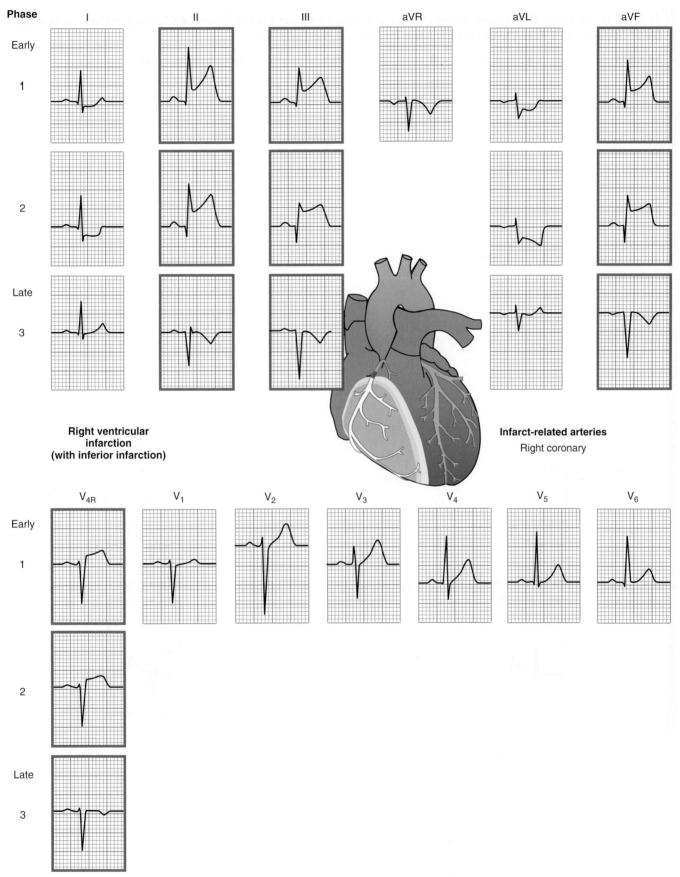

FIGURE 17-9 Right ventricular MI.

TABLE 17-10 The Facing ECG Leads of Anterior, Inferior, and Right Ventricular MIs and Reciprocal ECG Leads of Posterior MI Showing the ST-Segment and T Wave Changes in Early Acute Transmural Q Wave Infarction

Infarction	I	II	III	aVR	aVL
Septal MI					
Anterior MI					
Anteroseptal MI					
Lateral MI					
Anterolateral MI					

V_{4R}	V₁	V₂	V₃	V₄	V₅	V₆

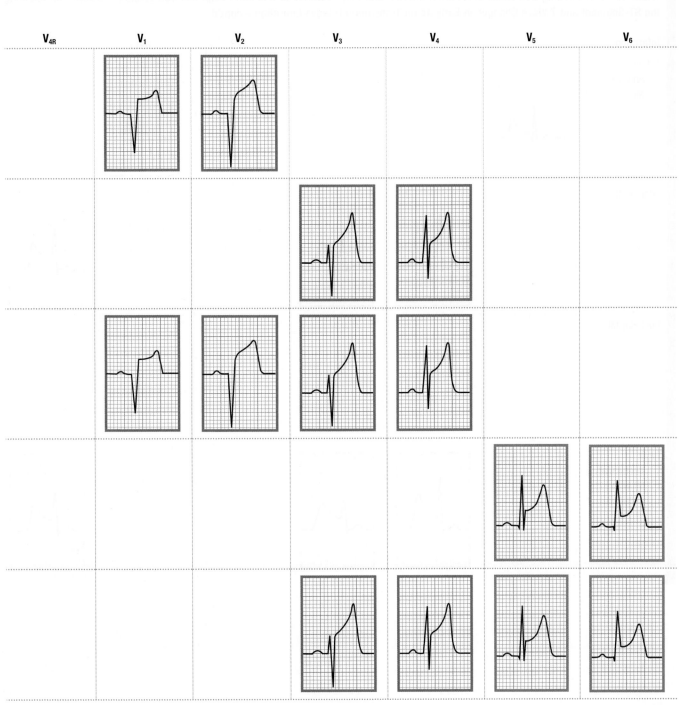

Continued

TABLE 17-10 The Facing ECG Leads of Anterior, Inferior, and Right Ventricular MIs and Reciprocal ECG Leads of Posterior MI Showing the ST-Segment and T Wave Changes in Early Acute Transmural Q Wave Infarction—cont'd

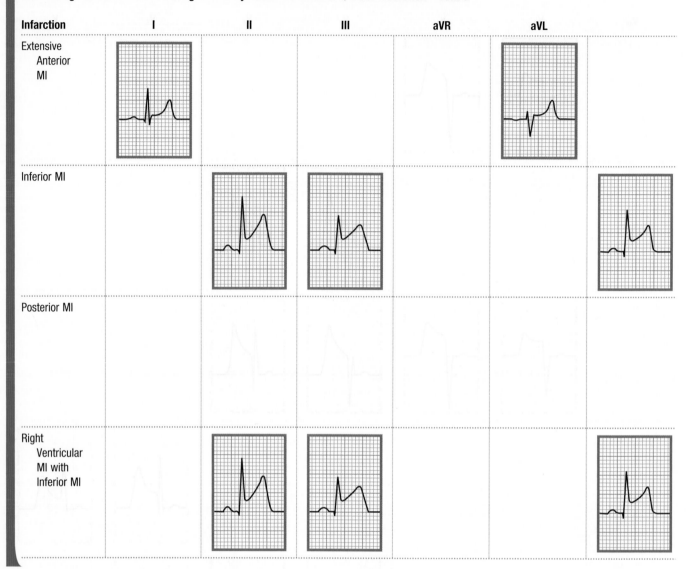

Infarction	I	II	III	aVR	aVL
Extensive Anterior MI					
Inferior MI					
Posterior MI					
Right Ventricular MI with Inferior MI					

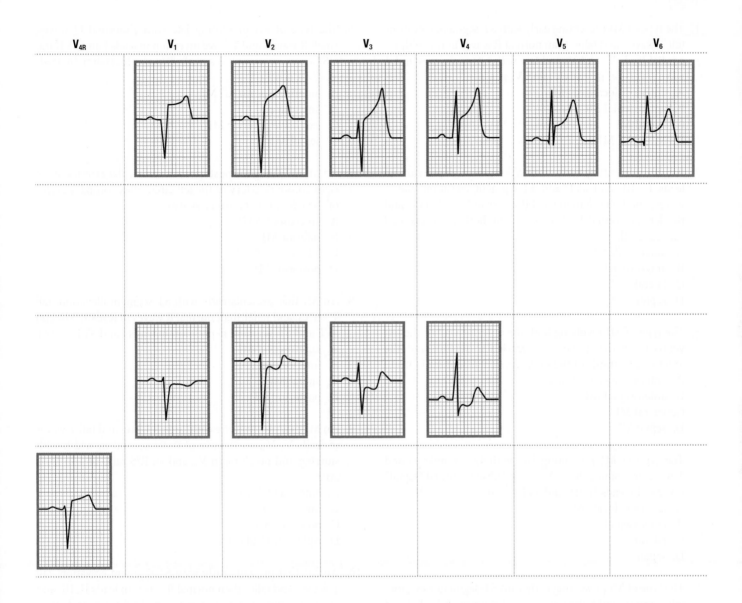

CHAPTER REVIEW

1. The type of MI presenting early with ST-segment elevation, tall T waves, and taller than normal R waves in the midprecordial leads V_3 and V_4 and late with QS complexes and T wave inversion in leads V_3 and V_4 is a(n):
   A. anterior (localized) MI
   B. anteroseptal MI
   C. lateral MI
   D. MI septal MI

2. An MI presenting early with ST-segment depression in leads II, III, and aVF and ST-segment elevation, tall T waves, and taller than normal R waves in leads I, aVL, and the left precordial lead V_5 or V_6 or both indicates a(n) _____ MI.
   A. anterior (localized)
   B. anteroseptal
   C. lateral
   D. septal

3. The type of MI involving both the anterior wall of the left ventricle overlying the interventricular septum and the anterior two thirds of the interventricular septum is a(n):
   A. anterior (localized) MI
   B. anteroseptal MI
   C. lateral MI
   D. septal MI

4. The type of MI presenting late with QS complexes and T wave inversion in leads V_1-V_2 and absent normal "septal" q waves in leads II, III, and aVF is a(n) _____ MI.
   A. anterior (localized)
   B. anteroseptal
   C. lateral
   D. septal

5. The type of MI presenting early with ST-segment elevation, tall T waves, and taller than normal R waves in leads I and aVL and the precordial leads V_3-V_6 and ST segment depression in leads II, III, and aVF is a(n):
   A. anterior (localized) MI
   B. anterolateral MI
   C. lateral MI
   D. septal MI

6. The type of MI presenting late with abnormal Q waves, small R waves, and T wave inversion in leads I and aVL and QS waves or complexes with T wave inversion in leads V_1-V_6 is a(n):
   A. anterior (localized) MI
   B. anterolateral MI
   C. extensive anterior MI
   D. septal MI

7. An MI involving the posterior left ventricular arteries of the right coronary artery or the left circumflex coronary artery of the left coronary artery is a(n):
   A. anteroseptal MI
   B. inferior MI
   C. left ventricular MI
   D. posterior MI

8. An MI that presents early with ST-segment elevation, tall T waves, and taller than normal R waves in leads II, III, and aVF and ST-segment depression in leads I and aVL is a(n):
   A. anteroseptal MI
   B. inferior MI
   C. lateral MI
   D. posterior MI

9. An MI that presents late with large R waves and tall T waves in leads V_1-V_4, an R wave of 0. 04 second in width with slurring and notching in V_1, and an R/S ratio of 1 in V_1 is a(n):
   A. anteroseptal MI
   B. inferior MI
   C. posterior MI
   D. right ventricular MI

10. An MI that presents early with ST-segment elevation, tall T waves, and taller than normal R waves in leads II, III, and aVF; ST-segment elevation in V_{4R}; and ST segment depression in leads I and aVL is a(n):
    A. anteroseptal MI
    B. inferior MI
    C. posterior MI
    D. right ventricular MI with inferior myocardial infarction

18 Signs, Symptoms, and Diagnosis of Acute Coronary Syndromes

OBJECTIVES *Upon completion of this chapter, you should be able to complete the following:*

1. Discuss the importance of recognizing signs and symptoms and taking a thorough history to making the diagnosis of an acute coronary syndrome (ACS).
2. Define the following:
   - Chief complaint
   - History of present illness
   - Past medical history
3. List the specific questions to be asked during the history taking of a patient with a suspected acute coronary syndrome
4. List the specific symptoms commonly experienced by the patient during an acute coronary syndrome and their causes under the following categories:
   - General and neurologic symptoms
   - Cardiovascular symptoms
   - Respiratory symptoms
   - Gastrointestinal symptoms
5. Discuss the characteristics of the pain encountered in an acute MI according to:
   - Frequency of occurrence
   - Location and radiation
   - Quality, intensity, and duration
   - Relation to body movement
   - Associated emotional and psychological manifestations
   - Responsiveness to rest and/or nitroglycerin
6. List other conditions that can mimic the pain of acute coronary syndromes (ACS) and be able to differentiate them.
7. List the specific signs commonly found on physical examination of the patient experiencing an acute coronary syndrome and their causes under the following categories:
   - The general appearance and neurologic signs of a patient with ACS.
   - The vital signs in ACS, both normal and abnormal:
   - Pulse: rate, rhythm, and force
   - Respirations: rate, rhythm, depth, and character
   - Blood pressure: systolic blood pressure, diastolic blood pressure
   - The physical appearance of the following as they might appear in the ACS, both normally or abnormally:
     - Skin
     - Veins
   - The cardiovascular and respiratory signs that may be found in ACS: abnormal heart and lung sounds

8. Be able to, based on the history and physical examination of a patient to estimate their risk of having an acute coronary syndrome.
9. Appreciate the role of ECG changes in the process of categorizing type of acute coronary syndrome.
10. List and describe the various cardiac markers released and measured during a myocardial infarction and relate their value in making the diagnosis of an acute coronary syndrome.

INTRODUCTION

The acute coronary syndromes (ACS) are so named because they are a constellation of signs and symptoms along with ECG findings and cardiac markers in the context of a patient having risk factors for coronary heart disease. Making the diagnosis accurately and efficiently requires the clinician to recognize these signs and symptoms, perform a rapid risk assessment of the patient, and obtain the diagnostic aids of an ECG and proper lab tests and consultations.

In the prehospital arena, it is vital to quickly determine if the patient is suffering a ST segment elevation myocardial infarction (STEMI) and rapidly deliver them to a facility capable of reperfusion therapy.

Therefore, to promote proficiency, the clinician should develop a standard strategy or approach to the patient having chest pain. This should include a detailed history and physical examination, paying particular attention to the signs and symptoms of acute coronary syndromes.

Obtaining an accurate history remains crucial to making the diagnosis of an acute coronary syndrome. Without it the clinician will have an insufficient index of suspicion to pursue further testing. Failure to obtain an accurate history and subsequently misinterpreting the diagnostic ECG is a leading cause of malpractice suits from patients with unrecognized myocardial infarctions.

> Failing to maintain a high index of suspicion for ACS when examining patients with chest pain is a leading cause of unrecognized myocardial infarctions.

Two groups of patients who are at risk for unrecognized myocardial infarction include women and diabetics.

Sex- and age-related differences in presentation. It has been noted in studies that women have STEMI at an older age than men. There must be an elevated index of suspicion during the evaluation of women for STEMI. Although some variation exists, when large databases of MI patients are examined, symptom profiles for STEMI by sex generally appear more similar than different between men and women. Elderly patients with STEMI are significantly less likely than younger patients to complain of chest discomfort. However, elderly patients with STEMI are more likely to complain of shortness of breath and other atypical symptoms, such as syncope, generalized weakness, or unexplained nausea.

Diabetes mellitus. Diabetics may have impaired pain (angina) recognition, especially in the presence of autonomic neuropathy. A diabetic may misinterpret dyspnea, nausea, vomiting, fatigue, and diaphoresis as disturbance of diabetic control. Up to 50% of diabetic individuals with type 2 diabetes for longer than 10 years will have autonomic nervous system dysfunction manifested by impaired heart rate variability. Diabetics with STEMI should be evaluated for renal dysfunction.

A patient's history includes information about his or her symptoms and any previous illness. It includes the chief complaint, history of present illness, and past medical history. The *chief complaint* is a short statement of the patient's major symptom(s) requiring emergency medical care. The history of present illness is a more detailed description of the patient's chief complaint and includes the symptoms, onset, severity, duration, and relationship to precipitating causes, such as exercise, emotion, body position, and so forth.

Past cardiac history is a brief review of previous cardiovascular diseases and their treatment. This includes any history of previous MIs, angina, congestive heart failure (CHF), dysrhythmias, syncope, hypertension, and so forth; previous hospitalizations; medications currently being taken; and any known allergies.

Once an appropriate history is obtained or even while questioning the patient, a physical examination is performed to determine whether the patient's physical signs, including the vital signs, are consistent with an acute coronary syndrome. These signs, in conjunction with the patient's history and the presence of abnormal ECG changes (ST segment elevation or depression and T wave changes) will help to determine the correct diagnosis and appropriate management.

Acute coronary syndromes manifest themselves by significant signs and symptoms. The symptoms and signs in ACS vary, depending on the location and extent of the heart damage and degree of autonomic nervous system activity (sympathetic or parasympathetic) present.

A *symptom* is defined as an abnormal feeling of distress or an awareness of disturbances in bodily function experienced by the patient. Symptoms are "subjective" expressions of what the patient is experiencing. The symptoms are obtained during the taking of the patient's history. Examples of symptoms of ACS are marked apprehension, chest pain, dyspnea, palpitations, and nausea.

Signs are abnormalities of the patient's body structure and function that are detected by initial inspection of the patient and by the physical examination. Signs are "objective" findings, which can be physically seen or monitored. Some examples of signs of ACS include tachycardia, distention of the neck veins, edema, and cyanosis.

HISTORY TAKING IN SUSPECTED ACUTE CORONARY SYNDROMES

The three primary questions to be addressed when assessing the patient suspected of acute coronary syndrome include: (1) Are their signs and symptoms consistent with ACS? (2) Do they have risk factors for ACS? (3) If STEMI is present on the ECG, are they a candidate for reperfusion? Therefore, taking the history of a patient suspected of having an acute coronary syndrome must be done in a methodical manner that covers the all areas with sufficient detail yet be concise enough not to delay the implementation of reperfusion therapy if the patient is a suitable candidate. It is important to be cognizant of the factors that cause some patients to delay seeking medical care. Box 18-1 lists some of them. Taking them into consideration will improve the quality of the clinician-patient interaction.

Chief Complaint

In an attempt to expedite the interview, ask the patient to describe in their own words their primary concern. This should generally be the only open-ended question you ask during this interview when you want to limit the length of the interview to a minimum. Be prepared to keep the patient's answers focused on the primary concern, which is whether or not they have an ACS. However, this question must be open ended because it allows the patient to express things in ways you might not be able to elicit otherwise. Start by asking the patient "What seems to be bothering you the most currently?" While you may want to hone in on chest pain, the patient may answer with their difficulty breathing or their fear of dying. Address those

> **BOX 18-1 Reasons Patients Delay Seeking Medical Attention for Symptoms of ACS**
>
> - They expected a more dramatic presentation
> - Thought symptoms were not serious or would go away
> - Tried "self-treatment," antacids, their own nitroglycerin, aspirin, etc.
> - Attributed symptoms to chronic conditions such as arthritis, muscle spasm, etc.
> - Lacked awareness of benefits of reperfusion treatments or importance of 9-1-1
> - Fear of embarrassment if "false alarm," thought they needed "permission" to come to office
> - Did not perceive themselves at risk
>   - Young and healthy (especially men)
>   - Women
>   - Under a doctor's care or making lifestyle changes for risk factors
>
> *Based on findings from Finnegan et al. Preventive Med 2000; 31:205-13 (114)

concerns then proceed with the following set of generally accepted questions.

- Do you have any chest pain or discomfort?
  - If so, when did it start?
  - Can you rate it on a scale of 0 to 10 with 10 being the worst pain you've experienced and 0 being no pain at all?
  - Is it sharp or dull?
  - Does it radiate?
  - Does anything make it better or worse?
  - Have you taken anything for it? Did it help?
- Are you having any difficulty breathing or are you feeling fatigued?
- Are you nauseated or have any other symptoms I should be aware of?

Chest discomfort. The severity of discomfort varies and is typically graded on a scale of 0 to 10, with 10 being the most severe pain and 0 being pain-free. It is important to keep in mind that many patients will not admit having chest "pain" but will acknowledge the presence of chest "discomfort," "pressure," or "heaviness." Chest discomfort is often described as a crushing, vicelike constriction, a feeling equivalent to an "elephant sitting on the chest," or heartburn. Usually the discomfort is substernal but may originate in or radiate to areas such as the neck, jaw, interscapular area, upper extremities, and epigastrium. The duration of the discomfort, which typically lasts longer than 30 minutes, may wax and wane and may be remitting. It may be described as "indigestion in the chest" and occasionally may be relieved with belching.

The possibility of precipitation of STEMI by use of illicit drugs such as cocaine should be considered.

> Asking only about chest "pain" and not including "discomfort" may result in failing to obtain an accurate history.

The clinician should ask when did the discomfort begin, how long did it last, what seemed to precipitate it, and did anything make it better or worse? For the patient with a history of stable angina, does the current discomfort represent a change in its pattern or severity? If the patient took their own nitroglycerin before your examination, it is important to determine its effect and consider whether their medication may have been outdated or simply ineffective.

Despite the quality or severity of the discomfort the most important feature to determine is the time of its onset. Determining the role and value of reperfusion therapy is dependent upon knowing the onset of ischemia as accurately as possible.

It is important to ask about associated symptoms, such as shortness of breath or fatigue. Other symptoms to be aware of when taking a patient's history include nausea and vomiting. Diaphoresis associated with a pale complexion may also appear, as well as weakness or profound fatigue. Dizziness, lightheadedness, syncope, and paresthesia may occur because of pain and hyperventilation. The presence of these associated symptoms in the absence of typical angina are referred to as *anginal equivalents* and are often seen in patients with unstable angina and non–ST-segment elevation myocardial infarction (NSTEMI).

Past medical history. The past medical history of patients with suspected ACS should focus on cardiac related issues. Ascertain whether the patient has had prior episodes of myocardial ischemia, such as stable or unstable angina, MI, coronary bypass surgery, or primary cardiac intervention (angioplasty), hypertension, diabetes mellitus, possibility of aortic dissection, risk of bleeding, and clinical cerebrovascular disease (amaurosis fugax, face/limb weakness or clumsiness, face/limb numbness or sensory loss, ataxia, or vertigo).

Hypertension. Hypertension should be assessed, because chronic, severe, poorly controlled hypertension or severe uncontrolled hypertension on presentation is a relative contra-indication to fibrinolytic therapy.

Possibility of aortic dissection. Severe tearing pain radiating directly to the back associated with dyspnea or syncope and without ECG changes indicative of STEMI should raise the suspicion for aortic dissection, and appropriate studies should be undertaken. Clinicians should have a heightened index of suspicion for aortic dissection in elderly hypertensive patients. In addition, it must be kept in mind that the dissection may extend to the pericardial sac and produce cardiac tamponade or disrupt the origin of a coronary artery.

Risk of bleeding. Patients should be questioned about previous bleeding problems (e.g., during surgery or dental procedures, history of ulcer disease, cerebral vascular accidents, unexplained anemia, or melena). The use of antiplatelet, anti-thrombin, and fibrinolytic agents as part of the treatment for STEMI will exacerbate any underlying bleeding risks.

Clinical cerebrovascular disease. The patient with STEMI frequently has medical conditions that are risk factors for both MI and stroke. Evidence for prior episodes suggestive of clinical cerebrovascular disease should be sought. For example, the patient should be asked whether he/she has ever had symptoms of transient retinal or cerebral ischemia, such as amaurosis fugax, face/limb weakness or clumsiness, face/limb numbness or sensory loss, ataxia, or vertigo. Transient ischemic attacks (TIAs) typically last less than 30 minutes, whereas symptoms that last more than 60 to 90 minutes are more likely to indicate the presence of a stroke. In addition, the patient should be asked whether he/she has ever had an ischemic stroke, intracerebral hemorrhage (ICH), or subarachnoid hemorrhage. Finally, a history regarding recent head and facial trauma should be obtained.

SIGNS AND SYMPTOMS OF ACUTE CORONARY SYNDROMES

The signs and symptoms of ACS generally reflect the extent of myocardial ischemia, injury, infarction, and the severity of the complications that may be present (i.e., dysrhythmia, heart failure, or shock). Although pain is the most common symptom in ACS, it is important to note that many of the following signs and symptoms may be present even in the absence of pain. This is referred to as "anginal equivalents." The symptoms of ACS most often involve the following areas:

- General well-being and neurologic
- Cardiovascular
- Respiratory
- Gastrointestinal

The signs of ACS include the following areas:

- General appearance and neurologic signs
- Vital signs (pulse, respirations, blood pressure)
- Appearance of the skin
- Appearance of the veins
- Cardiovascular signs
- Respiratory signs
- Appearance of body tissues
- Appearance of the abdomen

Symptoms of Acute Coronary Syndromes

Early recognition of symptoms of ACS by a patient or their friends and family is the first and most important step that must occur for the patient to seek medical attention. Despite public awareness of the signs and symptoms of MIs such as chest pain, many are unaware of other common associated symptoms such as arm, shoulder, neck, and jaw pain, or less common symptoms such as shortness of breath and diaphoresis (Box 18-2).

The typical patient waits on average 2 hours before seeking medical attention, often thinking the symptoms are self-limited. The reason for these delays include fear that they may in fact be having a heart attack, denial of the severity of the symptoms, or misinterpretation of the symptoms as being caused by something else such as indigestion.

GENERAL AND NEUROLOGIC SYMPTOMS

General and neurologic symptoms of ACS include the following in varying degrees:

- Anxiety and apprehension
- Restlessness and agitation with a fear of impending death (or a sense of impending doom)
- Extreme fatigue and weakness

> **BOX 18-2 Characteristics Typical of ACS Chest Pain**
>
> - Location of the pain—substernal, diffuse, poorly localized
> - Description of the pain—crushing, pressure, squeezing, heaviness
> - Radiation of the pain—shoulder(s), left arm/elbow/wrist, neck, jaw, teeth
> - Relationship to body movement—not positional, not reproducible with palpation
> - Duration of the pain—usually greater than 20 minutes or longer
> - Associated emotional and psychological manifestations
> - Unresponsiveness to rest and/or nitroglycerin

- Light-headedness
- Confusion, disorientation, or drowsiness
- Fainting or loss of consciousness (syncope)

When first seen, the patient with an acute coronary syndrome may appear fully alert and oriented. If the supply of oxygen to the brain becomes inadequate at any time because of (1) decreased cardiac output resulting from heart failure, myocardial rupture, or a dysrhythmia resulting in shock or (2) hypoxia from CHF, symptoms of cerebral hypoperfusion (lowered blood flow) rapidly appear. Commonly, these symptoms of cerebral anoxia are marked anxiety and apprehension, restlessness, and agitation, with a fear of impending death (or a sense of impending doom, as some would describe it) while the patient is still alert and oriented. Extreme fatigue or weakness and light-headedness are usually also present if the cardiac output is inadequate.

These vague symptoms of weakness are more common in patients with less typical presentations of acute coronary syndromes. This is particularly true of the elderly, the diabetic patient, and women. Additionally, heart transplant patients, who have surgically lost their vagal nerve attachments to the heart may be pain free and only present with complaints of weakness, fatigue, and shortness of breath.

CARDIOVASCULAR SYMPTOMS

Cardiovascular symptoms of ACS include the following:
- Chest pain
- Palpitations (or "skipping of the heart")

Pain

Pain is the most conspicuous symptom of an ACS. It appears in the majority (70% to 80%) of the patients with acute MI as a substernal (or retrosternal) constriction or crushing sensation. In the remaining 20% to 30% of patients, who may be experiencing their first attack, are elderly, diabetic, and women, the pain of acute MI may be atypical or absent. When pain is absent, as it is in about 8% to 10% of the patients with acute MI, the MI is called *silent*. Even though pain may be atypical or absent in acute MI, other signs and symptoms are usually present to lead one to suspect an acute MI.

The pain of ACS results from the same factors that are responsible for angina (i.e., lack of oxygen to the myocardium and the accumulation of carbon dioxide and lactic acid). It is important to recognize that this anginal pain is produced by the ischemic myocardium and not by that which is already infarcted. Infarcted myocardium is dead and therefore produces no pain. The zone of ischemia surrounding the infarct is responsible for the pain, therefore as long as the patient has pain there is ongoing ischemia and the potential for further infarction.

Although the pain of stable angina and the pain of ACS often have similar characteristics, they can be differentiated from each other by an accurate and detailed history. Unlike the pain of stable angina, which usually occurs after a certain amount of physical activity, the onset of pain in over half of those experiencing ACS appears during rest. A smaller percentage of persons experience pain during activity, and a few are awakened from sleep by the pain, usually during the early morning hours. Often, many of the patients suffering their first acute MI (about 50%) have experienced recurrent warning attacks of anginal pain (preinfarction or prodromal angina) hours or days before the attack.

The pain of acute MI usually occurs in the middle or upper substernal area, the same as stable angina except that it is generally more intense and lasts longer. The pain may radiate over the anterior chest and frequently to either of the shoulders and arms (usually the left), often extending down the medial aspect of the arm as far as the elbow, forearm, wrist, and, in some cases, the ring and little fingers. Less commonly, the pain radiates to the neck, jaw, and upper teeth; upper back, particularly between the scapulae; or the upper part of the abdomen in the midline (epigastrium). The pain may occasionally appear in these areas without first presenting substernally. About a third of patients have substernal pain without radiation.

The pain of ACS is typically terrifying for its victims, who describe it as constricting, compressing, crushing, bursting, oppressive, heavy, tight, squeezing, burning, aching, or a pressure or fullness. The pain varies in intensity, often being severe and sometimes intolerable. At other times it may be mild in intensity, described as a dull substernal discomfort and easily ignored. If the pain radiates to the epigastrium, it may resemble that of indigestion. Rarely does the patient describe the chest pain as sharp, stabbing, or throbbing.

The pain is usually continuous after its crescendo-like appearance, varying sometimes in intensity. It does not move, nor does coughing, breathing, or changes in body position alter or alleviate it. In localizing the pain, the patient may place a clenched fist against his or her sternum. This is referred to as the Levine sign after Dr. Samuel Levine.

Although the pain of ACS sometimes lasts only a few minutes and disappears spontaneously, it generally lasts longer than 30 minutes, commonly for an hour or longer. In most cases it can only be relieved by medication, such as morphine sulfate. Nitroglycerin may ease the pain of ACS but this is neither diagnostic nor does it mean that no further workup is needed. For example, if the pain of ACS is associated with exertion, it can be confused with stable angina. If the pain is unresponsive to rest or three nitroglycerin tablets during the first 15 minutes after its onset, it is more likely due to an acute MI. However, if the pain is relieved yet not completely resolved after one nitroglycerin tablet the patient should seek medical attention immediately as they may have a partially obstructed lesion causing ischemia and infarction. A patient with chest pain having one or more of the characteristics listed in Table 18-1 should, until proven otherwise, be considered as having an ACS and managed accordingly, regardless of age.

There are several conditions that present with pain that mimics that of ACS (Box 18-3 and Box 18-4). Acute myocarditis and pericarditis tends to be more sharp and stabbing, and is worsened when the patient leans forward. The pain lasts seconds to minutes and the condition is associated with other signs and symptoms not consistent with ACS. The pain of aortic dissection is considered to be excruciating and often referred to as

TABLE 18-1 Likelihood of Signs and Symptoms Representing Acute Coronary Syndrome

Feature	High Likelihood Any of the following:	Intermediate Likelihood Absence of high-likelihood and presence of any of the following:	Low Likelihood Absence of high or intermediate likelihood features but may have:
History	• Chest or left arm pain or discomfort as chief symptom reproducing prior documented angina • Known history of CHD, including MI	• Chest or left arm pain or discomfort as chief symptom • Age greater than 70 years • Male • Diabetes	• Probable ischemic symptoms in absence of any of the intermediate likelihood characteristics
Examination	• Transient mitral regurgitation murmur, hypotension, diaphoresis, pulmonary edema, or rales	• Extracardiac vascular disease	• Chest discomfort reproduced by palpation
ECG	• New, or presumably new, transient ST-segment elevation (1 mm or greater) or T wave inversion in multiple precordial leads	• Fixed Q waves • ST depression 0.5-1 mm or T wave inversion >1 mm	• T wave flattening or inversion less than 1 mm in leads with dominant R waves • Normal ECG
Cardiac markers	• Elevated cardiac TnI, TnT, or CK-MB	• Normal	• Normal

Modified from Braunwald: Unstable angina: diagnosis and management. U.S. Dept of Health and Human Services 1994 publication no. 94-0602 (124)

BOX 18-3 Characteristics of non-ACS Chest Pain

• Location of the pain—"pin-point," well localized
• Description of the pain—sharp, stabbing
• Radiation of the pain—lower abdomen, pelvis
• Relationship to body movement—pleuritic, painful to touch
• Duration of the pain—seconds to less than a few minutes
• Physical activity alleviates pain

BOX 18-4 Chest Pain Which Can Mimic That of ACS

• Myocarditis
• Pericarditis
• Aortic Dissection
• Spontaneous Pneumothorax
• Pulmonary Embolus

"tearing" with referral to the back. It is associated with a loss of one or more major pulses. Spontaneous pneumothorax occurs when the parietal and visceral pleura of the lung separate leading to a collapse of the affected lung. The pain associated with a spontaneous pneumothorax is usually pleuritic, being worsened with inspiration. It is generally well localized. A pulmonary embolism occurs when thrombi lodge in distal pulmonary arteries leading to infarction of the affected lung tissue. Pain from pulmonary embolism tends to be well localized and is generally located in the lateral chest wall with little if any radiation.

Palpitations

A regular heart beat interrupted by one or more extra beats (premature contractions) is a very common cardiac irregularity present in the majority of patients with acute MI. Such irregularities in the heart beat are also commonly experienced by most people under stress. This sensation occurs under the left breast or substernally and is described as palpitations, or "skipping of the heart." It is difficult to assess the significance of the palpitations in asymptomatic people. In persons with symptoms consistent with ACS, however, palpitations may indicate the presence of a potentially life-threatening ventricular dysrhythmia that could lead to impending cardiac arrest. The most common cause of grossly irregular pulses is atrial fibrillation, which is often chronic. Other causes include premature atrial and ventricular contractions. The presence of the latter, particularly if multiform and frequent in number is consistent with myocardial ischemia.

RESPIRATORY SYMPTOMS

Respiratory symptoms of ACS include the following:
• Shortness of breath (dyspnea), with or without a sensation of suffocation; a tight, constricted feeling in the chest
• Wheezing
• Spasmodic coughing, productive of copious, frothy sputum that is frequently pink- or blood-tinged (hemoptysis)

Dyspnea

Dyspnea, described as shortness of breath or difficulty breathing, is commonly seen in ACS, appearing gradually or suddenly. It is the primary symptom of left ventricular failure and is characterized by rapid, shallow, and labored respirations. Dyspnea is always accompanied by an awareness of discomfort and, when it is severe, by extreme apprehension and agitation. A sensation of suffocation and a tight, constricting sensation in the chest and possibly pain on breathing may accompany dyspnea. Dyspnea occurs in pulmonary congestion and edema during exertion and even at rest. It may assume several forms, including dyspnea on exertion, orthopnea, and paroxysmal nocturnal dyspnea.

- *Dyspnea on exertion (DOE)* is usually the first noticeable symptom of left heart failure. It first appears after an exercise or effort, such as climbing a flight of stairs or walking a distance that previously did not produce shortness of breath.
- *Orthopnea* is severe dyspnea that is relieved only by the patient assuming a sitting or semireclining position or standing up.
- *Paroxysmal nocturnal dyspnea (PND)* is characterized by sudden attacks of dyspnea, occurring at night, in a patient who may be asymptomatic during the day. It is caused by the gradual redistribution of the blood and body fluids from the lower extremities into the lungs after the patient has been lying in bed for several hours. Because the left heart cannot cope with the increased volume of fluid presented to it, left heart failure and pulmonary congestion and edema result, forcing the patient to sit up in bed or use extra pillows to breathe.

Cough

Cough accompanied by sputum, or a *productive cough*, is a symptom in patients with pulmonary edema secondary to left heart failure. It is caused by excessive bronchial secretions arising from congested mucous membranes. The cough can be spasmodic and productive of copious, frothy sputum. Frequently the sputum is pink- or blood-tinged (hemoptysis), the result of hemorrhaging from congested bronchial mucosa.

Wheezing

Wheezing may accompany the cough. This is particularly true in patients with a coexisting history of COPD/emphysema. Even in the absence of lung disease, the presence of the aforementioned bronchial secretions can cause the patient to wheeze and worsen their sense of dyspnea.

GASTROINTESTINAL SYMPTOMS

Gastrointestinal symptoms of ACS include the following:
- Loss of appetite (anorexia)
- Nausea
- Vomiting
- Thirst

Loss of appetite (anorexia) and nausea with or without vomiting are common in ACS. The patient may misinterpret these gastrointestinal symptoms as being caused by "indigestion" and ignore them, especially if the pain radiates from the chest into the epigastric region. Patients with inferior wall myocardial infarctions are more likely to have nausea and other GI symptoms than other infarctions owing to what has been termed the Bezold-Jarisch reflex from increased parasympathetic stimulation.

The patient with an ACS generally has increased sympathetic tone due to the combination of pain and fear. This leads to such typical symptoms as dry mouth and thirst.

Signs of Acute Coronary Syndromes

GENERAL APPEARANCE AND NEUROLOGIC SIGNS

General appearance and neurologic signs of ACS include the following:
- Fright
- Anxiety and apprehension
- Restlessness and agitation
- Disorientation and drowsiness
- Unconsciousness

The patient with acute MI may be alert and oriented, but frightened, anxious, and apprehensive, appearing restless, agitated, and in pain. If hypotension or shock occurs, the patient becomes confused and disoriented, then drowsy and unresponsive, and finally unconscious.

A patient who has severe pulmonary congestion and edema is typically sitting up, struggling to breathe.

VITAL SIGNS

The patient's vital signs, which include the pulse, respirations, and blood pressure vary, depending on the site and extent of the myocardial damage and on the degree of imbalance of the autonomic nervous system.

Pulse

Rate. The pulse rate is usually rapid (>100 beats/min [tachycardia]) because of the predominance of sympathetic nervous system activity. It may, however, be normal (60 to 100 beats/min) or even slow (<60 beats/min [bradycardia]) if the parasympathetic nervous system activity predominates or a slow dysrhythmia is present. Patients with an acute inferior wall myocardial infarction are more prone to be bradycardic owing to increased vagal stimulation and/or the appearance of atrioventricular (AV) block.

Rhythm. The rhythm of the pulse may be regular or irregular. An irregular pulse caused by numerous premature ventricular contractions (PVCs) or ventricular bigeminy may indicate a potentially life-threatening dysrhythmia and impending cardiac arrest in a small percentage of patients.

The most common cause of gross pulse irregularity is chaotic beating of the atria (atrial fibrillation). This dysrhythmia is characterized by variations in the force of contractions and pulsations in addition to a grossly irregular rhythm.

KEY DEFINITION

Note that PVCs in the context of the physical examination are called premature ventricular "contractions" because they are generating a pulse. In contrast PVCs on the ECG are referred to as "complexes" because they may or may not be resulting in a mechanical *contraction* of the heart.

When any irregular heart rhythm is present, it is not uncommon to find that the radial pulse is slower than the pulse obtained over the cardiac apex. This discrepancy occurs because some of the cardiac contractions are weak and cannot produce a strong enough pulse wave to reach the radial artery. This is called a *pulse deficit*.

Force. The force of the pulse is related to the stroke volume and the pulse pressure (the difference between the systolic and diastolic pressures in mm Hg). The exceptionally strong and full (bounding) pulse present during states of anxiety and emotional stress (increased sympathetic nervous system activity), strenuous exercise, and fever indicates a large stroke volume and a wide pulse pressure. The weak, thready (varying strength) pulse present in hypotension and shock, on the other hand, indicates a low stroke volume and a narrow pulse pressure.

In early phases of CHF, the pulse is initially bounding and strong due to hypertension; then as the heart failure worsens and cardiogenic shock ensues, it becomes weak and thready.

Respirations

The respirations in ACS may vary depending on the presence or absence of anxiety, CHF, hypoxia, hypotension, and shock. The rate of respirations may be normal, 16 to 20 per minute at rest (eupnea); slow, less than 16 per minute; or rapid, greater than 20 per minute (tachypnea). The rhythm of breathing may be regular or irregular. The depth of respirations may be normal, shallow, or deep. The respirations may appear quiet, labored and noisy, or gasping. Usually, the respirations are greater than 20 per minute (tachypnea) and shallow. In CHF, the respirations are typically rapid and shallow, often labored and noisy. In addition, use of the accessory muscles of respiration may be prominent during labored breathing.

Blood Pressure

The blood pressure is usually elevated (greater than 160/90) initially in ACS because of increased sympathetic nervous system activity. Additionally, many of these patients have pre-existing hypertension, which further manifests itself during the attack. Later the blood pressure often returns to normal (about 120/80) or slightly below normal (<120/80 but >90/60) unless hypotension or shock occurs, in which case the systolic blood pressure is less than 90 mm Hg. Initially, if excessive parasympathetic nervous activity is present initially or if the cardiac output is decreased because of significant heart failure or a dysrhythmia, the blood pressure will be low.

APPEARANCE OF THE SKIN

The skin in ACS may be:
- Pale, cold, sweaty, and clammy
- Cyanotic
- Mottled bluish-red

The skin is usually pale, cold, and clammy in acute coronary syndromes because of increased sympathetic nervous system activity or because of hypotension and shock. Both result in the vasoconstriction of superficial blood vessels and stimulation of the sweat glands. The vasoconstriction causes the skin to feel cool to the touch and the sweating gives it a clammy feel. The stimulation of sweat glands can lead to profuse sweating that can be so severe as to make it difficult to keep the ECG electrodes attached to the skin by their adhesive pads.

If cyanosis (the result of decreased oxygenation of arterial blood) of the skin, fingernail beds, and mucous membranes is present, pulmonary congestion and edema may be present causing hypoxemia. In the presence of both severe shock and cyanosis, the skin assumes a mottled bluish-red appearance. The lips may be normal, pale, or cyanotic.

While medical devices can measure the oxygen saturation to determine oxygen levels in the blood, the primary concern for the clinician is the quality of tissue perfusion. This can be loosely monitored by assessing capillary refill. This is performed by compressing the nailbed and counting the number of seconds for the color to return. Normal perfusion should return color to the nailbeds in less than 2 seconds. Any prolongation indicates decreased perfusion and should lead the clinician to have a higher index of suspicion for the presence of shock.

APPEARANCE OF THE VEINS

The veins in ACS may be:
- Normal
- Distended and pulsating
- Collapsed

The veins of the neck may be normal, distended, and/or pulsating, or collapsed. Generally, the patient's neck veins are assessed with the patient in a supine, semireclining position, propped up at a 45-degree angle. Normally, when laying flat the jugular neck veins are moderately distended but flat when sitting up. Coughing or grunting while sitting or reclining will usually distend the jugular veins in the patient without evidence of CHF. Distention of the neck veins typically occurs in right heart failure when the venous pressure is significantly increased. The degree of distention depends on the severity of right-sided failure. In mild right heart failure, the neck veins are only slightly to moderately distended. When the failure is severe, the jugular veins become markedly distended and pulsate even when the patient is sitting upright. The neck veins may also be slightly distended in left heart failure because of the increased pressure in the right ventricle and atrium reflecting the increased pressure in the left atrium by way of the pulmonary circulation.

In hypotension and shock, by contrast, the neck veins are usually collapsed when the patient is sitting or propped up at a 45-degree angle. If right heart failure is also present in hypotension and shock, however, the neck veins may be distended and pulsating.

CARDIOVASCULAR SIGNS

Cardiovascular signs in ACS may include:
- Distant heart sounds
- A third heart sound (S_3) early in diastole
- A fourth heart sound (S_4) late in diastole
- A pericardial friction rub

Heart Sounds

The heart sounds, particularly the first sound (S_1), which correlates to closure of the atrioventricular valves, are frequently muffled and occasionally inaudible during the early phases of a myocardial infarction, and their intensity returns to normal during recovery. A soft first heart sound may also reflect prolongation of the PR interval. Patients with marked ventricular dysfunction and/or left bundle branch block may have paradoxical splitting of the second heart (S_2) sound caused by the aortic valve closing prematurely before the pulmonary valve.

A third heart sound (S_3) in patients with STEMI usually reflects severe left ventricular dysfunction with elevated ventricular filling pressure. It is caused by rapid deceleration of blood flowing across the mitral valve impacting a poorly functioning left ventricular wall. This is particularly true in patients with large infarctions. This sound is detected best at the apex, with the patient in the left lateral recumbent position. A third heart sound may be caused not only by left ventricular failure but also by increased inflow into the left ventricle, as occurs when a mitral regurgitation or ventricular septal defect complicates ST segment elevation myocardial infarction (STEMI).

A fourth heart sound (S_4) is almost universally present in patients in sinus rhythm with STEMI but has limited diagnostic value because it is commonly audible in most patients with chronic ischemic heart disease and is recordable, although not often audible, in many normal subjects older than 45 years. Third and fourth heart sounds emanating from the left ventricle are heard best at the apex; in patients with right ventricular infarcts, these sounds can be heard along the left sternal border and increase on inspiration.

A pericardial friction rub is the sound of the myocardium rubbing against the pericardial sac. This occurs due to the inflammation of the affected epicardium. Pericardial friction rubs may be heard in patients with STEMI, especially those sustaining large transmural infarctions. Rubs are probably more common than reported. Although friction rubs can be heard within 24 hours or as late as 2 weeks after the onset of infarction, most commonly they are noted on the second or third day. Occasionally, in patients with extensive infarction, a loud rub can be heard for many days. Patients with STEMI and a pericardial friction rub may have a pericardial effusion, a collection of fluid within the pericardial sac, which can be detected by an echocardiogram but only rarely does it cause the classic ECG changes of pericarditis. Delayed onset of the rub and the associated discomfort of pericarditis (as late as 3 months postinfarction) are characteristic of the now rare postmyocardial infarction (Dressler) syndrome. Pericardial friction rubs are most readily audible along the left sternal border or just inside the point of maximal impulse at the apex of the heart. Loud rubs may be audible over the entire precordium and even over the back.

RESPIRATORY SIGNS

Respiratory signs in ACS may include:

- Rales
- Rhonchi
- Wheezing
- Dullness to percussion over both lungs, particularly at the bases, posteriorly

Breath Sounds

The breath sounds produced by the flow of air through the pulmonary air passages may be normal, labored and noisy, decreased, or absent. In pulmonary congestion and edema the breath sounds on auscultation are usually slightly diminished or even absent at one or both bases of the lungs posteriorly. This results from the decrease or absence of flow of air through partially or completely obstructed air passages in the congested and edematous parts of the lungs.

Rales, Rhonchi, and Wheezes

The passage of air through bronchi and bronchioles narrowed by edema and spasm and filled with fluid and foam produces abnormal respiratory sounds called *rales*, *rhonchi*, and *wheezes*. They vary in sound texture and intensity, depending on the size of the air passages involved and the degree of fluid accumulation. Rales may be "fine" or "course" according to their site of origin. They are very fine ("crepitant," "crackling," or "bubbling") when originating in the very small air passages, such as the alveoli and terminal bronchioles, and coarse ("gurgling") when originating in larger bronchioles. Rales have a "moist" sound to them. The most common source of rales is from fluid collecting in the alveoli. Rales are the most common sign in pulmonary edema due to left heart failure. They are worse in the lower lung fields where pulmonary congestion occurs first and progresses upwards as heart failure worsens.

Rhonchi are rougher sounds that are generally louder and courser than rales. They usually originate in the larger air passages (i.e., the trachea and larger bronchi), most often because of increased secretion from mucous membranes. Rhonchi may occur in pulmonary edema, but are more common in bronchitis and pneumonia. Dry, coarse rattling in the throat may also be present. Rhonchi clear with coughing and then return over a period of time as the secretions accumulate while rales do not.

Spasmodic coughing with expectoration of frothy sputum, often pink- or blood-tinged (hemoptysis), and choking may be present. This occurs in fulminate cases of heart failure when the amount of fluid that has transited the pulmonary vasculature into the bronchial tree is excessive. Wheezing occurs when there is narrowing of the bronchi and bronchioles. This is often associated with asthma and emphysema but can be heard with heart failure. Patients with emphysema and CHF may present with both wheezes and rales as the fluid precipitates narrowing of the terminal bronchioles. This has been termed "cardiac asthma" but unlike the typical exacerbation of emphysema, the underlying cause is congestive heart failure rather than the collapse or spasm of terminal bronchial. Rales, rhonchi, and wheezes are heard best by auscultation, although if they are loud enough they can be heard without a stethoscope. In patients with early left heart failure, fine, crepitant rales and wheezes are frequently heard at both bases of the lungs posteriorly and sometimes as high up as the scapulae. These sounds may be present at one or both bases of the lungs only or up to the scapulae posteriorly or throughout the lungs and anteriorly as well. Rales can be elicited by having the patient breathe deeply and forcefully through a wide-open mouth. They are best heard during inspiration, especially toward the end of deep breaths. Rhonchi can be heard during both exhalation and late inspiration over the bronchi and trachea.

Consolidation and Pleural Effusion

When a segment of the lung becomes completely filled with fluid, preventing air from entering, consolidation is present. Breath sounds and rales that were once there initially disappear. The breath sounds may also be markedly decreased and even absent over one or both bases of the lungs posteriorly because of fluid in the pleural space (pleural effusion) caused by right heart failure. This results primarily because of compression of the lungs by the effusion. The areas of the lungs where the breath sounds decrease or disappears because of consolidation or pleural effusion lose their resonance and become dull to percussion. Thus dullness to percussion may be present over one or both lungs, particularly at the bases of the lungs posteriorly.

APPEARANCE OF BODY TISSUES

The tissues of the body in ACS may show the following:

- Pitting edema in front of the tibia (pretibial edema), over the lower part of the back over the spine (presacral edema), in the abdominal wall, and over the entire body (anasarca)

Edema

Edema is the accumulation of serous fluid in body tissue. It may be confined to one or more areas or exist throughout the body. When generalized, it is known as *anasarca*.

Some degree of edema is always present in right heart failure. Early in the course of fluid retention, weight gain is the only sign indicating the presence of increased body fluid. As failure increases, however, further fluid accumulates, producing noticeable swelling of the legs, especially the anterior lower leg in front of the tibia (pretibial edema) and feet and ankles (pedal edema), the lower part of the back over the spine (presacral edema), and abdominal wall. The skin usually becomes taut and shiny over the edematous tissue. When pressure is applied with a finger, a dent appears in the edematous tissue that does not disappear immediately upon withdrawal of pressure. This sign of peripheral edema is called *pitting edema.* This is in contrast to *nonpitting edema,* which results from tissue swelling caused by trauma or inflammation.

RISK STRATIFICATION

Once the history and physical examination is completed, the clinician should be able with a fair degree of accuracy determine the likelihood that the patient's symptoms are consistent with an acute coronary syndrome. It is important to perform this risk assessment at this point before relying solely on the ECG and cardiac enzymes for the following reason; (1) the ECG may be nondiagnostic and/or (2) the cardiac enzymes may not be available or the patient may need to be transferred to definitive care. Table 18-1 provides a method of assessing the likelihood that the pain is consistent with ACS. At this point a diagnostic 12-lead ECG should be performed and the indications of STEMI and non-STEMI assessed.

THE 12-LEAD ECG

The 12-lead ECG is critical to proceeding with the workup of the suspected ACS patient. If the ECG shows diagnostic ST elevation in contiguous leads as discussed in Chapter 17, then the diagnosis of STEMI is made. If the ST depression and T wave inversion is present then non-STEMI is more likely; however; a posterior wall MI must be considered. In the absence of ST-segment changes, the working diagnosis is unstable angina. Until the levels of the cardiac markers are known, the patient is now in the unstable angina/NSTEMI category. However, recognizing the limitations of the 12-lead ECG will provide the astute clinician more confidence in the diagnosis of acute coronary syndromes.

The diagnosis of myocardial infarction is confirmed with cardiac markers in more than 90% of patients with ST-segment elevation. Up to 25% of patients with NSTEMI and elevated CK-MB develop Q wave myocardial infarctions while the remaining 75% have non-Q wave MIs. Somewhere between 1% and 6% of patients with a completely normal ECG and chest pain are eventually diagnosed with NSTEMI and at least 4% will have unstable angina.

In the event the initial ECG is nondiagnostic, obtaining serial 12-lead ECGs or monitoring the patient with continuous ST-segment deviation monitoring allows the clinician to detect subtle changes in the ECG, which can confirm the diagnosis and appropriately alter the therapy. Obtaining 12-lead ECGs when the patient is symptomatic is significantly more accurate in detecting ST changes if the pain is secondary to an acute coronary syndrome.

ECG Changes

Not all patients with chest pain are suffering a heart attack. In fact, less than 10% of patients with typical signs and symptoms of an ACS are ultimately determined to have an ACS. As has been discussed in earlier chapters, the 12-lead ECG is extremely useful as a diagnostic aid in detecting the presence of myocardial ischemia and injury during the first half hour or so of an acute MI. Diagnostic ECG changes include the appearance of T wave changes (myocardial ischemia) and ST-segment elevation or depression (myocardial ischemia and injury).

Serial ECGs obtained during the next few hours of an acute MI show the evolution of T wave changes and ST-segment elevation or depression. ST elevation, the prime sign of myocardial injury, has been shown to appear in less than 50% of the patients suffering an acute MI. Q waves denoting myocardial necrosis, however, do not begin to appear until several hours or more into the acute MI, becoming fully developed 24 to 72 hours after the onset. Thus the clinical evaluation and the ST-segment and T wave changes in the ECG are usually the only available data on which to base the diagnosis of an acute MI during the prehospital phase and the early minutes after admission to the emergency department (ED). It should be noted that in a very small number of acute MIs, the only change is the sudden appearance of a complete left bundle branch block (LBBB). This can only be confirmed by having previous 12-lead ECGs with which to compare.

The ST-segment and T wave changes in the early phase of acute MI are described in Chapters 16 and 17. These changes and the leads in which they appear are summarized below for the most common MIs.

ST-Segment Elevation MI

In the majority of STEMI, the following ST-segment and T wave changes are present:

- ST-segment elevation of 0.1 mV or greater, measured 0.04 second (1 small square) after the J point, and abnormally tall peaked T waves in two or more contiguous facing leads:
  - Anterior wall infarction: leads I, aVL, and V_1-V_6
  - Inferior wall infarction: leads II, III, and aVF

Non–ST-Segment Elevation MI

In the majority of NSTEMI, the following ST-segment and T wave changes are present:

- ST-segment depression of 0.1 mV or greater and isoelectric, biphasic, or inverted T waves in two or more contiguous facing leads:
  - Anterior wall infarction: leads I, aVL, and V_1-V_6
  - Inferior wall infarction: leads II, III, and aVF

CARDIAC MARKERS

Upon admission to the ED, blood studies are routinely performed to determine whether certain proteins and enzymes (*cardiac markers*) released from damaged or necrotic myocardial tissue are abnormally elevated. Another reason to obtain the cardiac markers is that almost 50% of patients with chest pain suspicious of ACS have a nondiagnostic ECG and are later found to have had an MI. This can only be confirmed by measuring cardiac markers. Among patients admitted to the hospital with a chest pain syndrome, less than 20% are subsequently diagnosed as having had an MI. In the majority of patients, therefore, clinicians must obtain serum cardiac marker measurements at periodic intervals to either establish or exclude the diagnosis of MI.

These cardiac markers include the following:

- *Myoglobin.* Increase in myoglobin occurs with damage to both skeletal and cardiac muscle. Despite the fact that it peaks 4 to 6 hours before other enzymes, its lack of cardiac specificity makes it a poor solitary test for the diagnosis of myocardial infarction. Myoglobin is rarely used now for the diagnosis of ACS due to its poor specificity (not particularly unique to the heart).
- *CK-MB (creatinine kinase MB isoenzyme).* CK-MB, unlike myoglobin, is more specific, increasing primarily after myocardial necrosis. Three isoenzymes of CK exist (MM, BB, and MB). Brain and kidney tissue contain predominantly the BB isoenzyme; skeletal muscle contains principally MM but does contain some MB (1% to 3%); and cardiac muscle contains both MM and MB isoenzymes. Strenuous exercise, particularly in trained long-distance runners or professional athletes, can cause elevation of both total CK and CK-MB. Although small quantities of CK-MB isoenzyme occur in tissues other than the heart, elevated levels of CK-MB may be considered, for practical purposes, to be the result of MI (except in the case of trauma or surgery on the aforementioned organs). Accurate CK-MB levels, especially in patients presenting within 4 hours of the onset of STEMI, may be used to diagnose a myocardial infarction.
- However, after 4 hours significant damage has occurred to the heart and it is therefore recommended that CK-MB levels not be relied upon as the primary cardiac marker for the diagnosis of acute myocardial infarction when reperfusion therapy is being considered. One notable exception is reinfarction within a matter of days following an acute MI. Because troponins remain elevated for upwards of 5 to 14 days, a sudden rise in CK-MB levels may be the only usable cardiac marker to indicate reinfarction.
- *Troponin T and I (cTnT, cTnI).* The troponins, like CK-MB, are also myocardium specific, but they increase not only after myocardial necrosis but also after myocardial injury. The troponin complex consists of three subunits that regulate the calcium-mediated contractile process of striated muscle. These include troponin C, which binds Ca^{2+}; troponin I (TnI), which binds to actin and inhibits actin-myosin interactions; and troponin T (TnT), which binds to tropomyosin, thereby attaching the troponin complex to the thin filament.
- Because cardiac-specific troponins I and T (cTnI and cTnT) accurately distinguish skeletal from cardiac muscle damage, the troponins are now considered the preferred cardiac marker for diagnosing myocardial infarction.

As shown in Figure 18-1, myoglobin is the first serum marker to become elevated after an acute MI, followed by the troponins and CK-MB. Each clinical laboratory will have a predetermined diagnostic level for ACS based on the type of testing performed. Therefore the clinician must be familiar with the test being used and the diagnostic value set by the laboratory performing the test when interpreting the results. Because diagnostic levels of these serum enzymes do not appear immediately in the blood after an acute MI and their determination may take more than 20 minutes, these markers may not be helpful during the early phase of acute MI to help in its diagnosis. However, the proliferation of bedside "point of care" testing for cardiac markers continues to improve in both speed and accuracy.

> The diagnostic level of each cardiac marker is determined by the clinical laboratory performing the test and therefore there is no "standard" value for any of the cardiac markers.

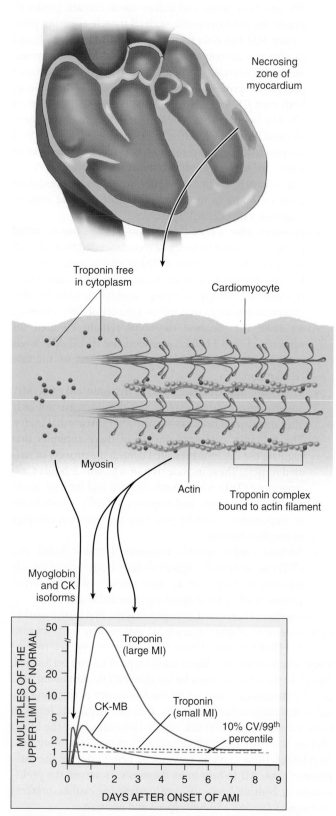

FIGURE 18-1 Time of appearance and degree of elevation of serum markers after the onset of acute myocardial infarction. *(Modified from Antman EM: Decision making with cardiac troponin tests. N Engl J Med 346:2079, 2002 and Jaffe AS, Babiun L, Apple FS: Biomarkers in acute cardiac disease: The present and the future. J Am Coll Cardiol 48:1, 2006.)*

MAKING THE DIAGNOSIS

At this point the clinician has all the information necessary to make the diagnosis. Again referring to Table 18-1, the clinician can further hone the previous risk stratification and more accurately categorize the patient.

If the 12-lead ECG was diagnostic, then the patient has STEMI. If the 12-lead ECG is nondiagnostic, the patient has unstable angina or NSTEMI and the diagnosis hinges on the cardiac markers. If the cardiac markers are elevated, the diagnosis is NSTEMI and if normal the patient is treated for unstable angina.

CHAPTER SUMMARY

The patient presenting with chest pain represents a significant clinical challenge. Using a methodical approach to obtaining the history and performing the physical examination while recognizing the signs and symptoms of acute coronary syndromes is fundamental to avoid missing the diagnosis. Table 18-2 summarizes these signs and symptoms.

Understanding the role and limitation of the 12-lead ECG and the timing of cardiac marker release from the myocardium improves the ability to accurately stratify the patient's risk for an acute coronary syndrome.

TABLE 18-2 Symptoms and Signs of Acute Coronary Syndrome

	Symptom	Sign
General and neurologic	• Anxiety • Apprehension • Extreme fatigue and weakness • Restlessness, and agitation, with a fear of impending death (or a sense of impending doom) are common.	• Alert and oriented • Restless • Anxious • Apprehensive
Cardiovascular	• Chest pain • Palpitations or "skipping of the heart" are frequent	• Distant heart sounds • A third heart sound (S_3) early in diastole (left ventricular dysfunction) • A fourth heart sound (S_4) late in diastole (nondiagnostic) • A pericardial friction rub
Respiratory	• Dyspnea • Chocking • Cough	• Normal or labored • Rapid and shallow • Rales (fluid in alveoli) • Rhonchi (secretions in bronchials) • Wheezing "cardiac asthma" • Dullness to percussion (pleural effusion)
Gastrointestinal	• Nausea • Loss of appetite (anorexia)	• Vomiting

Vital signs		• **Pulse**
		  • Usually rapid, >100/min (tachycardia), but may be 60 to 100/min (normal) or <60/min (bradycardia).
		  • The rhythm may be regular or irregular.
		  • The force of the pulse may be normal, strong, and full, or if hypotension or shock is present, it may be weak and thready.
		• **Respirations**
		  • Typically >20/min (tachypnea) and shallow, but may be 16 to 20/min (normal, eupnea) or less
		  • May be regular or irregular
		  • Depth may be normal, shallow, or deep
		  • Labored and noisy or gasping.
		  • Accessory muscles use may be prominent if severe pulmonary congestion and edema are present.
		• **Blood pressure**
		  • May be normal, elevated (>140 mm Hg), or low (<90 mm Hg) if hypotension or shock is present

Skin		• Pale • Clammy • Sweating (diaphoresis) • Cyanosis • Delayed capillary refill
Veins		• Normal • Moderately distended (in left heart failure and mild right heart failure) • Markedly distended and pulsating (in severe right heart failure) • Collapsed (in hypotension or shock)
Body tissue		• Pitting edema tibia (pretibial edema) • Lower part of the back over the spine (presacral edema) • Abdominal wall • Entire body (anasarca)

CHAPTER REVIEW

1. Which of the following plays the greatest role in avoiding unrecognized myocardial infarctions?
   A. accurate interpretation of the ECG
   B. early administration of nitroglycerin
   C. rapid availability of cardiac markers
   D. recognizing the signs and symptoms of ACS

2. The ACS patient who presents without chest pain but has other signs and symptoms consistent with ACS has:
   A. anginal equivalents
   B. a silent MI
   C. not had a heart attack
   D. unstable angina

3. The primary cause of the signs and symptoms of ACS are a result of:
   A. elevated cardiac markers
   B. hypoxia
   C. increased sympathetic discharge
   D. shock

4. The chest pain of ACS is most often described as:
   A. a heavy pressure
   B. lasting less than a minute
   C. painful to the touch
   D. worse with breathing

5. The first noticeable symptom of left heart failure is usually:
   A. chest pain
   B. cough
   C. dyspnea on exertion (DOE)
   D. orthopnea

6. A patient suffering from an ACS usually presents with skin that is:
   A. cyanotic, diaphoretic, and dry
   B. cyanotic, warm, and moist
   C. pale, cool, and clammy
   D. pale, warm, and dry

7. If left ventricular dysfunction occurs with an acute MI, which of the following heart sounds will most likely be present?
   A. friction rub
   B. split S_1
   C. S_3 early in diastole
   D. S_4 late in diastole

8. Generalized edema over the entire body is called:
   A. anasarca
   B. predominate edema
   C. presacral edema
   D. pretibial edema

9. An agitated patient presents with dyspnea on exertion, wheezing, and a cough productive of blood-tinged sputum. The vital signs are as follows: the pulse is 104 and regular, the respirations are 24 and shallow, and the blood pressure is 160/90 mm Hg. The neck veins are distended, and a S_3 heart murmur is noted. This patient is most likely suffering from:
   A. cardiogenic shock
   B. left heart failure
   C. right heart failure
   D. uncomplicated acute MI

10. In NSTEMI the 12-lead ECG is nondiagnostic and the diagnosis is based on:
    A. cardiac markers
    B. serial ECG changes
    C. the history
    D. the history in combination with elevated cardiac marker

19 Management of Acute Coronary Syndromes

OBJECTIVES *Upon completion of this chapter, you should be able to complete the following objectives:*

1. List and describe the primary goals in the management of acute coronary syndromes.
2. List and describe the time-critical goals in the management of acute myocardial infarction.
3. List and describe the roles EMS and the Emergency Department play in meeting the time-critical goal of limiting myocardial ischemic time.
4. List and describe the two primary goals in the treatment of ST elevation myocardial infarction.
5. Identify the antithrombus drugs used in the management of acute myocardial infarction (MI), the drug category in which they belong, and their action.
6. List and describe the various techniques of interventional coronary revascularization.
7. Compare and contrast the risks and benefits of fibrinolytic therapy with percutaneous coronary intervention for reperfusion therapy in ST elevation myocardial infarction.
8. Describe and discuss the following protocols in the management of acute MI:
   - Initial assessment and management of a patient with chest pain
   - Initial management of ACS
   - Reperfusion therapy: STEMI Protocol
   - Management of congestive heart failure (CHF)
   - Management of cardiogenic shock
9. Discuss the rationale of using a checklist to determine a patient's eligibility for thrombolytic therapy.
10. Identify the absolute contraindications for the use of fibrinolytic agents.

GOALS IN THE MANAGMENT OF ACUTE CORONARY SYNDOMES

Once the clinician suspects the patient is suffering an acute coronary syndrome, diagnosis and management occur simultaneously because time is of the essence. The primary diagnostic goal is to determine whether the patient is suffering a STEMI or an unstable angina/non-STEMI event. Regardless of the final diagnosis, the primary goal of management is to correct the ischemia and stop the progression or at least limit the damage of infarction through reperfusion if it is indicated (Figure 19-1). Each of these goals is time-critical because with each passing minute more myocardial damage occurs and the potential benefit of the various management strategies diminishes. Therefore, time-dependent goals have been set for systems to maximally benefit the needs of the patient suffering an acute coronary syndrome (Figure 19-2). The goal is to limit the *total ischemic time to less than 120 minutes*. Other, more specific goals include:

Medical System: EMS Transport

- Use of prehospital, 12-lead on-scene for the detection of STEMI
- Consider the use of prehospital fibrinolytics
- EMS identified STEMI patients should be transported to percutaneous coronary intervention (PCI) capable hospitals if EMS *transport to balloon time within 90 minutes*

- EMS identified STEMI patients should be transported to non-PCI capable hospitals if *door-to-needle (time to fibrinolytic administration) time within 30 minutes*

Patient Self-Transport
- If a patient arrives at a non-PCI capable hospital, the *door-to-needle time should be within 30 minutes*
- If the patient arrives at a PCI capable hospital, the *door-to-balloon time should be within 90 minutes*
- If the patient arrives at a non-PCI capable hospital, it is appropriate to consider emergency transfer of the patient to a PCI capable hospital if:
  ○ There is a contraindication to fibrinolysis
  ○ PCI can be initiated within 90 minutes of the time the patient comes to the initial hospital
  ○ Fibrinolysis is administered and is unsuccessful (i.e., "rescue PCI")

Role of EMS to Meet Goal
Prehospital ECG

The earlier the STEMI patient is identified, the earlier management can be instituted. The 12-lead ECG is critical to making this diagnosis and therefore it is reasonable to attempt to acquire it as soon as possible. Current ECG monitor/defibrillators have the capability to perform 12-lead ECG and built-in algorithms to detect ST changes indicative of myocardial ischemia and injury. Research has shown that paramedics can accurately interpret them and appropriately triage patients to PCI facilities based on prehospital 12-leads. Combining these capabilities with cellular technology allows EMS to transmit the ECG to the receiving hospital for interpretation and

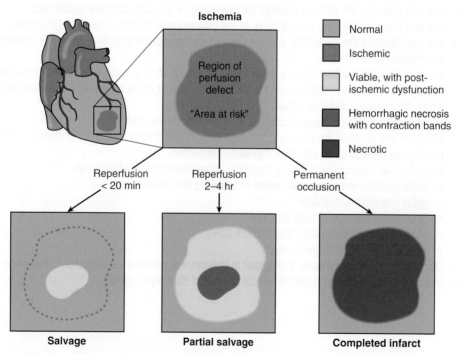

FIGURE 19-1 Myocardial salvage from reperfusion. *(From Libby P, Bonow RO, Mann DL, et al: Braunwald's heart disease, ed 8, Philadelphia, Saunders, 2008.)*

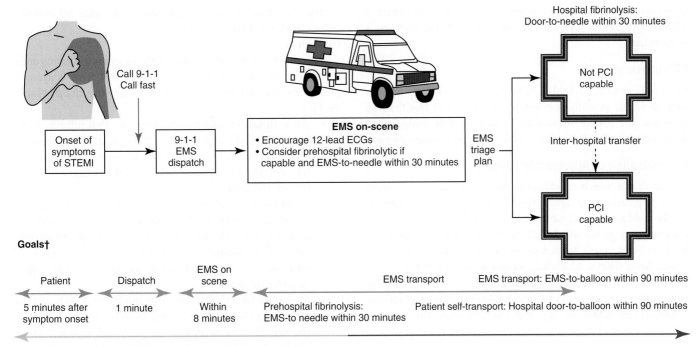

FIGURE 19-2 Reperfusion treatment goals. *(Antnam, et al: 2007 Focused Update of the ACC/AHA 2004 Guidelines for the Management of Patients with ST Elevation Myocardial Infarction. Circulation 2008;117;296-329.)*

verification. Typical prehospital STEMI programs function in the following manner:

- Acquire ECG and apply the following criteria (systems may use either criteria A or B)
- Criteria A: 1 mm or more ST elevation in the inferior leads, or 1 mm or more ST elevation in the precordial leads
- Criteria B: 1 mm or more ST elevation in the inferior leads, or 2 mm or more ST elevation in the precordial leads
- If criteria met, then transport patient to the nearest appropriate facility (PCI capable facility preferred)
  a. If facility is PCI capable, notify facility as soon as possible to mobilize catheterization team and interventional cardiologist
  b. If facility is non-PCI capable, notify facility as soon as possible to ensure that ED is prepared to receive patient and begin fibrinolytic therapy quickly.

> Criteria A is more sensitive than criteria B because as it would result in activating the STEMI system with less ST elevation in the precordial leads. However, there is evidence that 1 mm of ST elevation in the precordial leads may be due to other conditions besides STEMI and therefore using this criteria would result in an higher rate of false-positive activations (patients with actual myocardial infarction). Regardless, with proper quality improvement and oversight, either criteria may be used in a prehospital STEMI program.

Prehospital Fibrinolytic Administration

For the patient with STEMI, the goal is early reperfusion. With the goal of door-to-needle time of 30 minutes or less, it has been proposed that the clock should start at the time the first diagnostic ECG is acquired. This would be particularly applicable when the time to transport the patient to the nearest non-PCI capable facility is greater than 30 minutes or the time to transfer the patient to a PCI capable facility is greater than 90 minutes. In these instances, research has shown value in having EMS administer the initial dose of the fibrinolytic.

STEMI System Design

It can be daunting to design a STEMI system that takes into account all the variables previously discussed combined with the time-critical goals of management and reperfusion whereby the patient is delivered as rapidly as possible to definitive care. Such systems combine the ability of EMS providers to recognize the potential STEMI patient, acquire an ECG, interpret and/or transmit it for interpretation and confirmation and then begin appropriate management while transporting the patient to the closest most appropriate hospital. In many instances this may not be the closest hospital but instead one further away, which has been predesignated as the preferred receiving facility.

Role of Emergency Department to Meet Goal

Triage

Patients with complaints suggestive of acute coronary syndrome should receive priority attention and be taken immediately into an examining room for evaluation. The goal is to obtain a 12-lead ECG within 10 minutes of arrival at the emergency department.

ECG Interpretation

Once obtained the 12-lead ECG should be evaluated by a qualified physician as soon as possible with a goal of less than 10 minutes. The patient must then be immediately evaluated to determine whether they are a candidate for reperfusion therapy.

Determination of Appropriate Therapy

The choice of which reperfusion therapy to use will, in most cases, be based on the capability of the facility but should generally be predetermined by existing policies developed by a multidisciplinary group of physicians and hospital policymakers. Such policies result in preapproved orders and procedures, which limit delays. Multidisciplinary review of STEMI cases provides continuous quality improvement of the process to ensure that management practices are kept current and address issues preventing the facility from meeting time-critical goals.

GOALS IN THE MANAGEMENT OF ST-ELEVATION MYOCARDIAL INFARCTION

The primary goals in the management of acute MI are (1) to stop the formation of the thrombus, (2) to dissolve or lyse the thrombus already formed, or (3) to recanalize the occluded coronary artery. As stated before, the first two goals, the arrest of the formation of the thrombus and the beginning of its dissolution (fibrinolytic therapy), should be initiated within 30 minutes after admission to the emergency department. The third goal, the recanalization of the coronary artery, is performed through percutaneous transluminal coronary angioplasty (PTCA) and/or coronary artery stenting, both being referred to as percutaneous coronary intervention (PCI), as soon as possible after admission to the emergency department (ED), ideally within 90 minutes.

The three goals in the management of an acute MI and the means to attain them are as follows:

Goal One:

Prevent the further expansion of the original thrombus and/or prevent the formation of a new thrombus. This is accomplished by the administration of the following drugs (Table 19-1):

- An **antiplatelet agent**, such as aspirin, that inhibits TxA_2 formation and its release from the platelets, thus partially impeding platelet aggregation. It does not, however, interfere with the adhesion of platelets to the collagen fibers in the arterial wall.
- An **anticoagulant**, such as enoxaparin (Lovenox®), a low-molecular-weight (LMW) heparin, or unfractionated heparin, blocks the conversion of prothrombin to thrombin, and, in addition, inhibits the action of thrombin on fibrinogen, thus preventing the conversion of fibrinogen to fibrin threads.
- A **platelet GP IIb/IIIa receptor inhibitor (GPI)**, such as abciximab (ReoPro®) or eptifibatide (Integrilin®), blocks the GP IIb/IIIa receptors on activated platelets from binding to fibrinogen, thus inhibiting platelet adhesion and aggregation and further thrombus formation.
- A thienopyridine such as Clopidogrel that reduces platelet aggregation through a mechanism different from aspirin.

Goal Two:

Dissolve or lyse the existing thrombus using a fibrinolytic agent, such as alteplase (t-PA), reteplase (r-PA), or tenecteplase (TNK-tPA), which converts plasminogen, normally present in the blood, to plasmin, an enzyme that dissolves fibrin (fibrinolysis) within the thrombus, helping to break the thrombus apart (thrombolysis).

OR

Enlarge the lumen of the occluded section of the affected coronary artery mechanically by means of one or more of the following catheter-based percutaneous coronary interventions (PCI).

- **Percutaneous transluminal coronary angioplasty (PTCA).** (Figure 19-3) The insertion of a balloon-tipped

TABLE 19-1 Antithrombus Drugs Used in the Management of Acute Myocardial Infarction

Drug Category	Action	Drug
Antiplatelet agent	Inhibits thromboxane A_2 (TxA_2) formation and release from platelets, thereby inhibiting platelet aggregation	Aspirin Clopidogrel (Plavix)
Anticoagulant	Blocks conversion of fibrinogen to fibrin by inhibiting the action of thrombin on fibrinogen	Low-molecular-weight heparin such as enoxaparin (Lovenox) Unfractionated heparin
GP IIb/IIIa receptor inhibitor	Inhibits platelet adhesion and aggregation by blocking the platelets' GP IIb/IIIa receptors	Abciximab (ReoPro) Eptifibatide (Integrilin)
Thrombolytic agent	Converts plasminogen to plasmin, which in turn dissolves the fibrin binding the platelets together	Alteplase (Activase) (tPA) Reteplase (Retavase) (rPA) Tenecteplase (TNKase) (TNK-tPA)
Thienopyridines	Inhibits ATP receptor on platelets, resulting in reduction in platelet aggregation	Clopidogrel (Plavix)

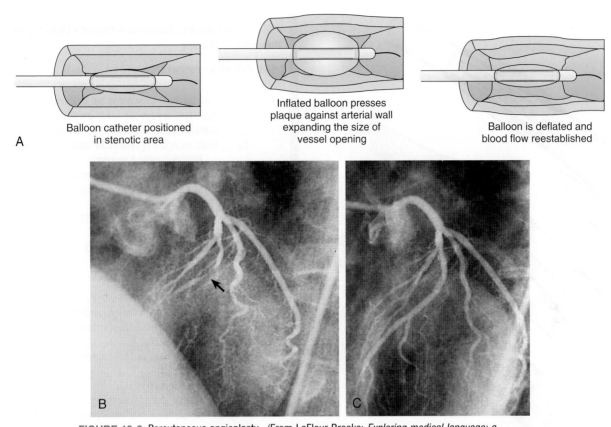

Balloon catheter positioned
in stenotic area

Inflated balloon presses
plaque against arterial wall
expanding the size of
vessel opening

Balloon is deflated and
blood flow reestablished

A

B

C

FIGURE 19-3 Percutaneous angioplasty. (From LaFleur Brooks: *Exploring medical language: a student-directed approach*, ed 7, St Louis, Mosby, 2009.)

catheter into the occluded or narrowed coronary artery followed by the inflation of the balloon, thus fracturing the atherosclerotic plaque and dilating the arterial lumen. This procedure, also referred to as *balloon angioplasty,* is the most commonly performed invasive treatment for coronary artery occlusion. It is often followed by insertion of a coronary artery stent.

- **Coronary artery stenting.** (Figure 19-4) The insertion of a cylindrical wire sheath into the occluded or narrowed coronary artery, followed by the expansion of the sheath to fit snugly within the dilated lumen of the coronary artery. Stents may be used alone as a primary procedure or after balloon angioplasty. Often these stents coated with agents to prevent re-stenosis (drug eluting stents).
- **Directional coronary atherectomy (DCA).** The mechanical removal of a noncalcified thrombus through a catheter inserted in the occluded or narrowed coronary artery.
- **Rotational atherectomy.** The use of a rotational, drill-like device to remove a calcified thrombus.

Emergency coronary artery bypass grafting (CABG) should be considered under the following conditions if still within 4 to 6 hours of the onset of symptoms of acute MI:

- Reperfusion of the occluded coronary artery fails using the above percutaneous coronary interventions and the patient is hemodynamically unstable (i.e., in cardiogenic shock) or continues to have persistent chest pain

- The percutaneous coronary interventions listed above are contraindicated
- Multivessel coronary artery disease is present

REPERFUSION THERAPY: PCI VERSUS FIBRINOLYTICS

Once the patient has been diagnosed as being a candidate for reperfusion therapy through either fibrinolytic or interventional therapy, the patient must be moved to definitive care as quickly as possible. From the onset of pain the clock begins to tick. The decision as to which reperfusion therapy is most appropriate will depend on local and regional resources. The following steps should be taken to make the determination.

STEP 1: Assess Time and Risk

- Time since onset of symptoms
- Degree of certainty of STEMI
- Determine if patient is eligible for fibrinolytic therapy (Box 19-1)
- Time required to transport patient to skilled PCI facility

STEP 2: Determine if fibrinolysis or PCI is preferred

Primary percutaneous coronary interventional therapy is generally preferred if:

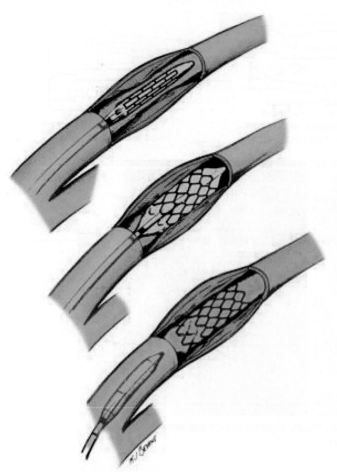

FIGURE 19-4 Stent placement. (From Bevans M, McLimore E: Intracoronary stents: a new approach to coronary artery dilatation. *J Cardiovasc Nurs* 7(1):34–49, 1992.)

- Skilled PCI facility available*
- High-risk STEMI
  - Cardiogenic shock
- Contraindication for fibrinolytic therapy including increased bleeding risk and intracerebral hemorrhage
- Late presentations
  - Symptom onset greater than 3 hours
- Diagnosis of STEMI in doubt

Fibrinolysis is generally preferred if:

- Catheterization lab occupied or not available
- Vascular access difficult
- Lack of access to a skilled PCI facility†

---

*The management of acute MI presented in this section is based on the 2007 focused Update of the ACC/AHA 2004 Guidelines for the Management of Patients With ST-Elevation Myocardial Infarction: A Report of the American college of Cardiology/American Heart Association task Force on Practice Guidelines *Circulation* 2008;117;296-329.

†Skilled PCI facility is defined as one that performs more than 200 cases per year and the procedures are performed by interventional cardiologists who perform more than 75 PCI cases per year.

- Time to transport to skilled PCI facility would result in a medical contact balloon time greater than 90 minutes

MANAGEMENT OF ACUTE ST-ELEVATION MYOCARDIAL INFARCTION*

A suspected acute MI must be regarded as an extreme emergency and be provided emergency medical care immediately, even before a full history is obtained and a physical examination is performed. The immediate management of an acute MI includes the following:

1. Oxygen if indicated
2. Termination of dysrhythmias

3. Relief of chest pain (nitroglycerin, morphine sulfate), apprehension and anxiety (diazepam, lorazepam), and nausea and vomiting (promethazine hydrochloride, ondansetron)

4. Increase coronary perfusion through maximal vasodilation of the coronary arteries (nitroglycerin)

5. Prevention of any further thrombus formation by the administration of the following:

   An antiplatelet agent (aspirin)

   An anticoagulant (LMW heparin or unfractionated heparin)

   A GP IIb/IIIa receptor inhibitor (abciximab or eptifibatide)

6. Reperfusion therapy

MANAGEMENT OF NON–ST-ELEVATION MYOCARDIAL INFARCTION

The absence of ST elevation does not preclude the possibility of an acute myocardial infarction as has been discussed in previous chapters. The patient may have a non-STEMI or in the case of ST depression they be have a posterior myocardial infarction. in addition, the initial 12-lead may be normal or nondiagnostic. The workup for all these outcomes can be extremely complex and is outlined briefly in the accompanying treatment algorithms. Clinicians should work collaboratively with cardiologists to develop policies and protocols for their institutions to address ACS patients who do not meet STEMI criteria. It is highly recommended that in the emergency department setting that cardiology consultation be sought early.

Generally, the approach to the non-STEMI patient involves cardiology consultation, appropriate hospitalization of at-risk-patients, and series of tests consisting of serial cardiac markers, repeat 12-lead ECGs, and additional cardiac imaging such as echocardiography, catheterization, and cardiac stress testing.

> **AUTHOR'S NOTE** The breadth and scope of the possible strategies for the management of non-STEMI patients after initial stabilization is beyond the scope of this text.

ACUTE CORONARY SYNDROME MANAGEMENT STRATEGIES

The following management strategies are based on the current literature and endorsed by the author. However, state, regional, and local protocol may vary. Therefore, all management strategies should be modified based on applicable scope of practice, medical control approval, and in consultation with medical specialists and professional organizations.

Additionally, while protocols and strategies may be presented in a linear format, it is reasonable to assume that several steps will occur simultaneously and therefore the particular sequence of a protocol is a general outline and should not necessarily be interpreted as a step-by-step process.

A. Initial Assessment and Management of Patient with Chest Pain

Prehospital/Emergency Department

1. Administer oxygen 4 L/min nasal cannula or 100% NRB if signs of respiratory distress or oxygen saturation <94%.

2. Quickly assess the patient's circulatory status while obtaining the vital signs, including level of consciousness, and repeat as the situation requires and circumstances permit.

3. Start monitoring the electrocardiogram (ECG) for significant dysrhythmias.

4. Start an intravenous (IV) line with either normal saline (NS) or 5% dextrose in water (D5W) to keep the vein open (TKO) to administer medications.

5. While performing the above, obtain a brief history and physical examination to determine the cause of the chest pain.

6. Obtain a 12-lead ECG (plus lead V_{4R}, if indicated), using an ECG monitor with or without computerized ECG interpretation, and, if appropriate, transmit the 12-lead ECG and/or the computerized ECG interpretation to the base hospital for physician interpretation.

   - Determine if
     - Normal ECG
     - Nondiagnostic ECG
     - ST depression
     - ST elevation MI (Criteria A)

   Evaluate the ECG. If any of the following ECG changes are present, the ECG is diagnostic of an acute MI:

     - ST segment elevation greater than or equal to 1 mm in two or more contiguous leads (indicative of an acute anterior, lateral, inferior, or right ventricular MI)
     - ST segment depression of greater than or equal to 1 mm in two or more contiguous precordial leads (indicative of an acute posterior MI)
     - New or presumably new LBBB; the ECG is diagnostic of an acute MI

B. Management of Suspected Acute Coronary Syndrome

1. Administer a chewable aspirin 162 to 325 mg.

2. If chest pain is present:

   - Administer nitroglycerin 0.4 mg by sublingual tablet or lingual aerosol if the patient's systolic blood pressure is 100 mm Hg or greater. Administer with the patient sitting or lying down. If hypotension does not occur, repeat approximately every 5 minutes as necessary, for a total dose of three tablets or three lingual aerosol applications.

AND

If nitroglycerin is not effective after the third dose or the pain is severe:

- Administer morphine sulfate 2 to 4 mg IV slowly over 3 to 5 minutes and repeat in 5 to 10 minutes as necessary, up to a total dose of 10 to 20 mg.
3. Start an IV infusion of nitroglycerin at a rate of 5 µg/min and increase the rate of infusion by 5 µg/min every 5 to 10 minutes until one of the following occurs, at which time stop increasing the infusion rate and continue it at its current rate:
    - The chest pain is relieved
    - The mean arterial blood pressure drops by 10% in a normotensive patient
    - The mean arterial blood pressure drops by 30% in a hypertensive patient

AND

If the mean arterial blood pressure drops below 80 mm Hg or the systolic blood pressure drops below 90 mm Hg at any time:
    - Slow or temporarily stop the IV infusion of nitroglycerin

> Nitroglycerin infusion should be administered using infusion pumps to ensure properly controlled dosing and avoidance of accidental overdose resulting in hypotension.

4. If the patient is apprehensive and anxious but has little or no pain consider an anxiolytic:
    - Administer diazepam 2.5 to 5 mg IV slowly, or lorazepam 0.5 to 1 mg IV slowly.
5. If nausea or vomiting is present:
    - Administer ondansetron 4 mg IV or promethazine hydrochloride 12.5 to 25 mg IV.
6. If STEMI is confirmed:
    - Proceed immediately to section B, Reperfusion Therapy: STEMI Protocol
7. If dysrhythmias, CHF, or cardiogenic shock are present initially or at any time:
    - Chapter 10, Clinical Significance and Treatment of Dysrhythmias.
    - Section C, Management of Congestive Heart Failure
    - Section D, Management of Cardiogenic Shock

C. Reperfusion Therapy: STEMI Protocol

1. Once the 12-lead ECG is obtained and meets STEMI criteria a decision must be made as to the most appropriate reperfusion therapy.
2. If PCI can be accomplished within 90 minutes proceed to Primary PCI

PRIMARY PCI

Emergency Department

1. Administer an anticoagulant such as LMW heparin (enoxaparin) or unfractionated heparin.
    - Administer enoxaparin 30 mg IV followed in 15 minutes by 1 mg/kg enoxaparin subcutaneously.

OR

Administer a 60 units/kg bolus of unfractionated heparin IV (maximum 4000 U bolus for patients ≥70 kg) followed by a 12 U/kg/hr unfractionated heparin IV infusion (maximum 1000 U/hr for patients >70 kg) to maintain an aPTT of 50 to 70 seconds.

2. Consider the administration of a GP IIb/IIIa receptor inhibitor for patients younger than 75 with extensive anterior MIs and minimal risk of bleeding.
    - Administer abciximab 0.25 mg/kg IV.
    AND
    Start an abciximab infusion at 0.125 µg/kg/min.
    OR
    Administer eptifibatide 180 µg/kg IV
    AND
    Start an eptifibatide infusion at 2 µg/kg/min.
3. Move rapidly to catheterization lab

If PCI cannot be performed within 90 minutes:

1. Determine patients eligibility for fibrinolytic therapy (see Box 19-1)
2. Determine if any absolute contraindications for fibrinolytic therapy exist (Box 19-2)
3. Proceed to fibrinolytic administration

> **BOX 19-2** **Contraindications and Cautions for the Use of Fibrinolytic Agents in Acute Myocardial Infarction**
>
> **Absolute Contraindications**
> - Active internal bleeding (e.g., gastrointestinal or genitourinary); excluding menses
> - Any prior intracerebral hemorrhage
> - Significant closed-head or facial trauma within 3 months
> - Ischemic stroke within 3 months
> - Recent intracranial or intraspinal surgery or trauma
> - Known intracranial neoplasm, arteriovenous malformation, or cerebral aneurysm
> - Suspected aortic dissection
>
> **Relative Contraindications**
> - Recent puncture of noncompressible blood vessels
> - Known bleeding diathesis
> - For streptokinase/anistreplase: prior exposure (more than 5 days ago) or prior allergic reaction to these agents
> - Traumatic or prolonged (>10 minutes) CPR
> - Major surgery (<3 weeks)
> - Current use of oral anticoagulants (e.g., warfarin sodium) with INR ≥2-3
> - History of recent (within 2-4 weeks) gastrointestinal, genitourinary, or other internal bleeding
> - Active peptic ulcer
> - History of chronic, severe, poorly controlled hypertension
> - Severe uncontrolled hypertension on presentation (SBP >180 mm Hg or DBP >110 mm Hg)
> - History of prior ischemic cerebrovascular accident >3 months, dementia, or known intracranial pathology not covered in contraindications
> - Pregnancy

FIBRINOLYTICS

Emergency Department

If acute MI is confirmed and no contraindications to fibrinolytic therapy are present:

1. Administer a fibrinolytic agent.
- Administer reteplase 10 units IV over 2 minutes and repeat in 30 minutes.

OR

- Administer tenecteplase 30 to 50 mg IV over 5 seconds based on the patient's weight as indicated in Table 19-2.
2. Administer an anticoagulant such as LMW heparin (enoxaparin) or unfractionated heparin.
- Administer a 30-mg bolus of enoxaparin IV followed in 15 minutes by 1 mg/kg enoxaparin subcutaneously.

OR

- Administer a 60 units/kg bolus of unfractionated heparin IV (maximum 4000 units bolus for patients greater than or equal to 70 kg) followed by 12 units/kg/hr unfractionated heparin IV infusion (maximum 1000 units/hr for patients >70 kg) to maintain an aPTT of 50 to 70 seconds.
3. Consider the administration of a GP IIb/IIIa receptor inhibitor (GPI) for patients younger than 75 with extensive anterior MIs and minimal risk of bleeding.
- Administer abciximab 0.25 mg/kg IV

AND

- Start an abciximab infusion at 0.125 µg/kg/min IV

OR

- Administer eptifibatide 180 µg/kg IV

AND

- Start an eptifibatide infusion at 2 µg/kg/min IV

> **AUTHOR'S NOTE** If a GP IIb/IIa receptor inhibitor is administered in combination with a fibrolytic agent, the dosage of the fibrinolytic agent should be reduced to approximately half of that indicated above (e.g., 5 units bolus of reteplase IV initially; 15 to 25 mg bolus of tenecteplase IV).

> **CAUTION** After the administration of any of the above, closely monitor the patient for bleeding.

D. Management of Congestive Heart Failure

Prehospital/Emergency Department

If the patient has signs and symptoms of CHF secondary to left heart failure:

1. Place the patient in a semireclining or full upright position, if possible, while reassuring the patient and loosening any tight clothing.
2. Secure the airway and administer high-concentration oxygen to maintain oxygen saturation 94–98%.
3. Reassess the patient's vital signs, including the respiratory and circulatory status.
4. Administer a vasodilator, if the patient's systolic blood pressure is 100 mm Hg or greater, to reduce pulmonary congestion and edema.
- Administer nitroglycerin 0.4 mg by sublingual tablet or lingual aerosol, and repeat every 5 to 10 minutes as needed

AND/OR

Start an IV infusion of nitroglycerin at a rate of 10 to 20 µg/min and increase the rate of infusion by 5 to 10 µg/min every 5 to 10 minutes until signs and symptoms of congestive heart failure improve or maximum dose of 400 µg/min is reached.

If the mean arterial blood pressure drops below 80 mm Hg or the systolic blood pressure drops below 90 mm Hg at any time:

Slow or temporarily stop the IV infusion of nitroglycerin

> Nitroglycerin infusions should be administered using infusion pumps to ensure properly controlled dosing and avoidance of accidental overdose resulting in hypertension.

5. Institute continuous positive airway pressure (CPAP) ventilation (Box 19-3)
6. Consider the administration of an angiotensin-converting enzyme inhibitor (ACE);
- Administer captopril 6.25 to 12.5 mg sublingually.
7. Consider the administration of a rapidly acting diuretic to reduce pulmonary edema if there are signs of volume overload such as significant peripheral edema.
- Administer furosemide 20 to 40 mg (0.25 to 0.50 mg/kg) IV slowly over 4 to 5 minutes

> The role of diuretics in the treatment of acute CHF is controversial and should be guided by a determination of the patient's volume status in combination with renal function and the level of critical electrolytes such as sodium and potassium.

TABLE 19-2 Tenecteplase Dosage Table

Patient Weight	<60 kg	60-<70 kg	70-<80 kg	80-<90 kg	≥90 kg
TNK-tPA (mg)	30 mg	35 mg	40 mg	45 mg	50 mg
Volume (mL)	(6 mL)	(7 mL)	(8 mL)	(9 mL)	(10 mL)

BOX 19-3 Sample Protocol for CPAP Administration

Continuous positive airway pressure (CPAP) has been shown to rapidly improve vital signs, gas exchange, the work of breathing, decrease the sense of dyspnea, and decrease the need for endotracheal intubation in patients who suffer from shortness of breath from asthma, COPD, pulmonary edema, CHF, and pneumonia. In patients with CHF, CPAP improves hemodynamics by reducing preload and afterload.

Indications:

Any patient who is complaining of shortness of breath for reasons other than trauma and:

a. Is awake and able to follow commands

b. Is more than 12 years old and is able to fit the CPAP mask

c. Has the ability to maintain an open airway (GCS >10)

d. Has a systolic blood pressure >90 mm Hg

e. Signs and symptoms consistent with asthma, COPD, pulmonary edema, CHF, or pneumonia

Contraindications:

1. Patient is in respiratory arrest

2. Patient is suspected of having a pneumothorax

3. Patient has a tracheostomy

4. Patient is vomiting

Precautions:

Use care if patient:

Has failed at past attempts at noninvasive ventilation

a. Complains of nausea or vomiting

b. Has inadequate respiratory effort

Procedure:

1. Explain the procedure to the patient

2. Ensure adequate oxygen supply to ventilation device

3. Place the patient on continuous pulse oximetry and cardiac monitoring

4. Place the delivery device over the mouth and nose and use 5 cm H_2O PEEP initially and titrate as needed. Do not exceed 20 cm H_2O pressure

5. Check for air leaks

7. Monitor vital signs at least every 5 minutes. CPAP can cause BP to drop. Level of consciousness is the most sensitive indicator of degree of respiratory distress

8. If respiratory status deteriorates, remove device and consider positive pressure ventilation with BVM or proceed to endotracheal intubation.

Removal procedure:

1. CPAP therapy should be continuous and should not be removed unless the patient cannot tolerate the mask or experiences respiratory failure.

Special notes:

1. For EMS do not remove CPAP until hospital device is ready to be placed on patient.

2. Most patients will improve in 5 to 10 minutes. If no improvement within this time, consider intermittent positive pressure ventilation.

3. Watch patient for gastric distention. Have patient breath through nose to prevent swallowing air.

4. Use nitroglycerin infusion rather than spray to prevent dispersal on rescuers. If nitroglycerin tablets used, attempt to minimize interruptions of CPAP.

5. May be the treatment of choice in a patient with a DNR/DNI order.

6. Consider the administration of lorazepam for anxiety associated with CPAP use bearing in mind that lorazepam may result in respiratory suppression.

E. Management of Cardiogenic Shock

Prehospital/Emergency Department

1. Assess the patient's circulatory status and vital signs, including the level of consciousness, and repeat as the situation requires and circumstances permit.

2. Administer a vasoconstrictive agent (norepinephrine) or an inotropic/vasoconstrictive agent (dopamine) as follows:

If the systolic blood pressure is less than 70 mm Hg:

- Start an IV infusion of norepinephrine at an initial rate of 0.5 to 1.0 µg/min, and adjust the rate of infusion up to 30 µg/min to increase the systolic blood pressure to 70 to 100 mm Hg.

Note: The infusion of norepinephrine may be replaced by an infusion of dopamine at this point.

Systolic blood pressure 70 to 100 mm Hg and signs/symptoms of shock

- Start an IV infusion of dopamine at an initial rate of 2.5 to 5.0 µg/kg/min and adjust the rate of infusion up to 20 µg/kg/min to increase the cardiac output and to elevate and maintain the systolic blood pressure within normal limits.

Systolic blood pressure 70 to 100 mm Hg and no signs/symptoms of shock

- Start an IV infusion of dobutamine at an initial rate of 2 to 5 µg/kg/min and adjust the rate of infusion up to 20 µg/kg/min to maintain systolic blood pressure within normal limits.

AUTHOR'S NOTE When administering vasoconstrictive agents, the systolic blood pressure must be monitored frequently so that the systolic blood pressure stays within a certain range. The rate of administration of such agents is decreased if the systolic blood pressure rises above 100 mm Hg and increased if the systolic blood pressure drops below 90 mm Hg.

Emergency Department

If cardiogenic shock continues despite maximal therapy, the use of a mechanical device such as an intraaortic balloon pump to augment the vascular circulation should be considered.

ACUTE CORONARAY SYNDROME MANAGEMENT ALGORITHMS

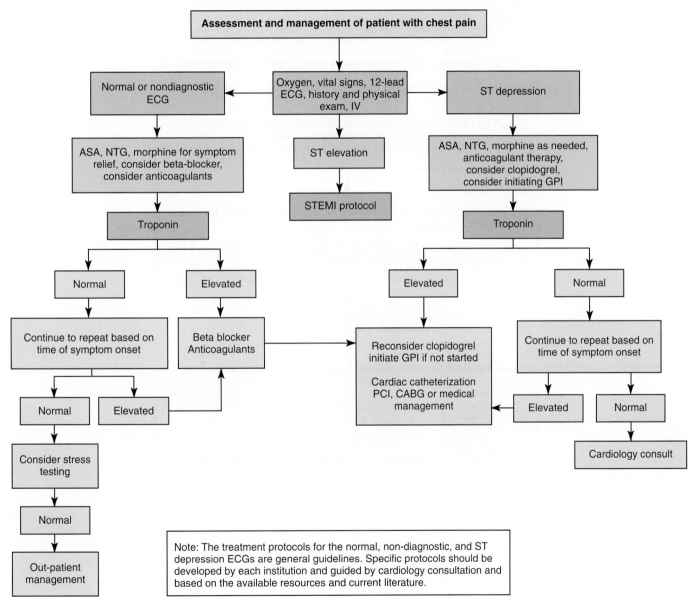

FIGURE 19-5 Initial assessment and management of patient with chest pain.

Text to be continued on p. 336

Management of suspected acute coronary syndrome

Chewable aspirin 162 to 325 mg.

Nitroglycerin 0.4 mg by sublingual tablet or lingual aerosol, repeat approximately every 5 minutes as necessary, for a total dose of three tablets or three lingual aerosol applications.

AND

If nitroglycerin is not effective after the third dose or the pain is severe administer morphine sulfate 2 to 4 mg IV slowly over 3 to 5 minutes and repeat in 5 to 10 minutes as necessary, up to a total dose of 10 to 20 mg.

Nitroglycerin infusion at a rate of 5μg/min and increase the rate of infusion by 5μg/min every 5 to 10 minutes until one of the following occurs, at which time stop increasing the infusion rate and continue it at its current rate:
- The chest pain or the symptoms of congestive heart failure are relieved
- The mean arterial blood pressure drops by 10% in a normotensive patient
- The mean arterial blood pressure drops by 30% in a hypertensive patient

AND

If the mean arterial blood pressure drops below 80mm Hg or the systolic blood pressure drops below 90 mm Hg at any time:
- Slow or temporarily stop the IV infusion of nitroglycerin

Consider diazepam 2.5 to 5 mg IV slowly, or lorazepam 0.5 to 1 mg IV slowly if significant anxiety

Administer promethazine hydrochloride 12.5 to 25 mg IV or ondansetron 4 mg IV as needed for nausea and vomiting

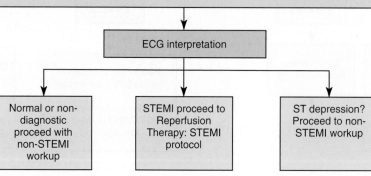

ECG interpretation

| Normal or non-diagnostic proceed with non-STEMI workup | STEMI proceed to Reperfusion Therapy: STEMI protocol | ST depression? Proceed to non-STEMI workup |

FIGURE 19-6 Management of suspected acute coronary syndrome.

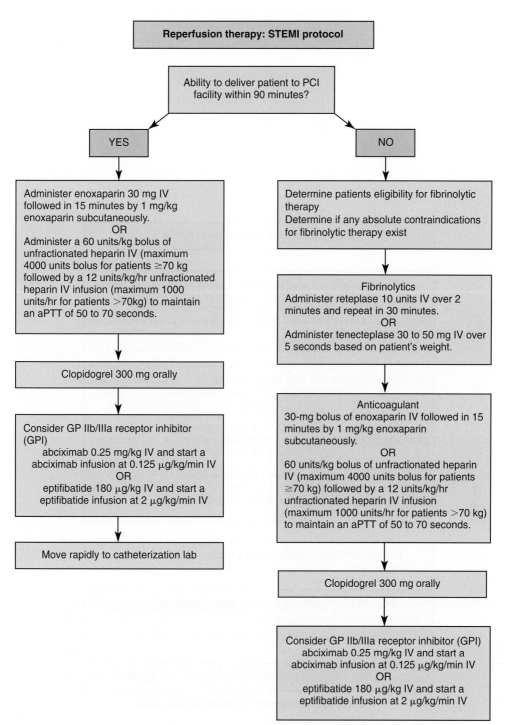

FIGURE 19-7 Reperfusion therapy: STEMI protocol.

Management of congestive heart failure

- Place the patient in a semi-reclining or full upright position, if possible, while reassuring the patient and loosening any tight clothing.
- Secure the airway and administer high-concentration oxygen.
- Reassess the patient's vital signs, including the respiratory and circulatory status.

Administer nitroglycerin 0.4 mg by sublingual tablet or lingual aerosol, and repeat every 5 to 10 minutes as needed
AND/OR
Start an IV infusion of nitroglycerin at a rate of 10 to 20 µg/min and increase the rate of infusion by 5 to 10 µg/min every 5 to 10 minutes until signs and symptoms of congestive heart failure improve or maximum dose of 400 µg/min is reached.

If the mean arterial blood pressure drops below 80 mm Hg or the systolic blood pressure drops below 90 mm Hg at any time: slow or temporarily stop the IV infusion of nitroglycerin

Institute continuous positive airway pressure (CPAP) ventilation

Consider a diuretic: administer furosemide 20 to 40 mg (0.25 to 0.50 mg/kg) IV slowly over 4 to 5 minutes

Consider an ACE inhibitor: administer captopril 6.25 to 12.5 mg sublingually

FIGURE 19-8 Management of congestive heart failure.

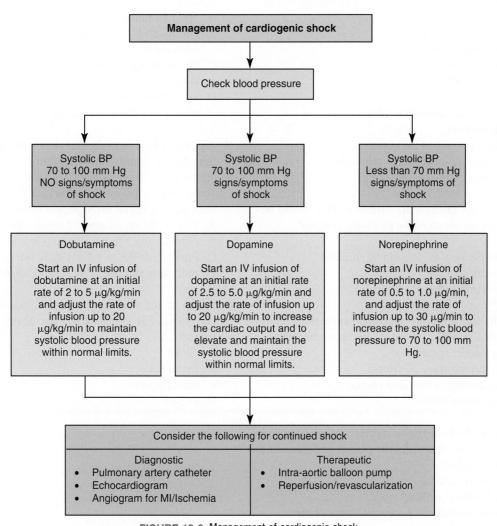

FIGURE 19-9 Management of cardiogenic shock.

CHAPTER REVIEW

1. The ultimate goal in the treatment of the patient suffering a myocardial infarction is to:
   A. administer aspirin to all patients with chest pain
   B. administer nitroglycerin as soon as possible
   C. identify the at risk patient as quickly as possible
   D. limit the amount of myocardial damage

2. The time-critical goal of patient arrival to administration of fibrinolytics is referred to as _____ time and should be within _____ minutes.
   A. ECG-to-needle, 30 minutes
   B. door-to-balloon, 30 minutes
   C. door-to-needle, 30 minutes
   D. door-to-needle, 90 minutes

3. Antiplatelet agents are administered to:
   A. lyse the thrombus
   B. maintain the patency of the vessel
   C. stop the formation of additional thrombus
   D. thin the blood to promote bleeding

4. The decision to use fibrinolytics instead of PCI should be based primarily on which of the following criteria?
   A. cost
   B. inability to perform PCI within 90 minutes
   C. insurance criteria
   D. insurance reimbursement

5. LMW heparin, warfarin, and abciximab exert their effect on the thrombus by which of the following mechanisms?
   A. inhibiting platelet aggregation
   B. inhibiting thromboxane A_1 release
   C. promoting healing of ruptured plaque
   D. promoting lysis of fibrin

6. The insertion of a balloon-tipped catheter into an occluded artery to fracture an atherosclerotic plaque and dilate the arterial lumen is called:
   A. coronary artery stenting
   B. directional coronary atherectomy
   C. percutaneous transluminal coronary angioplasty
   D. rotational atherectomy

7. The correct dosage of reteplase for thrombolytic therapy alone is:
   A. 5-U IV bolus in 1 minute, repeated in 30 minutes
   B. 10-U IV bolus in 2 minutes, repeated in 30 minutes
   C. 10-U IV bolus in 5 minutes, repeated in 60 minutes
   D. 20-U IV bolus in 3 minutes, repeated in 15 minutes

8. The correct dosage of tenecteplase for thrombolytic therapy alone is:
   A. 10-U IV bolus in 5 minutes, repeated in 60 minutes
   B. 30- to 40-U IV bolus in 2 minutes, repeated in 30 minutes
   C. 30- to 50-mg IV bolus in 5 seconds based on the patient's weight
   D. 30- to 50-mg IV bolus in 5 minutes based on the patient's weight in 1 minute, repeated in 30 minutes

9. A patient presents awake and alert with jugular vein distention during inspiration and pitting edema in the lower extremities. The patient's systolic blood pressure is 70 mm Hg by palpation. Which of the following steps is indicated for initial management of this patient?
   A. 250 to 500 mL of normal saline rapidly
   B. dobutamine 2 to 5 µg/kg/min iv
   C. furosemide 0.5 to 1.0 mg/kg iv slowly
   D. morphine sulphate 1 to 3 mg IV slowly

10. Which of the following treatments has become less used and somewhat controversial for acute congestive heart failure?
    A. CPAP
    B. furosemide
    C. nitroglycerin
    D. oxygen

A | Methods of Determining the QRS Axis

OBJECTIVES

Upon completion of all or part of this appendix, you should be able to complete the following objectives:

1. Describe in detail the steps in determining the QRS axis using one or more of the following methods:
   - The Two-Lead Method (Leads I and II)
   - The Three-Lead Method (Leads I, II, and aVF)
   - The Four-Lead Method (Leads I, II, III, and aVF)
   - The Six-Lead Method (Leads I, II, III, aVR, aVL, and aVF)
   - The "Perpendicular" Method

METHODS OF DETERMINING THE QRS AXIS

Various methods of determining the approximate position of the QRS axis in the frontal plane are available using the hexaxial reference figure. The methods presented in the following section are listed below.

Method A: The Two-Lead Method. This method uses leads I and II to make a rapid determination of whether the QRS axis is normal or abnormally deviated to the left or right. This is one of the fastest methods in determining the QRS axis. It is especially useful in the emergency situation to spot left axis deviation because the perpendicular of lead II lies on the −30° axis.

Method B: The Three-Lead Method. This method uses leads I, II, and aVF to make a rapid approximation of whether the QRS axis is normally or abnormally deviated to the left or right. The positivity or negativity of leads I and aVF are determined first to ascertain in which of the four quadrants the QRS axis lies. Then, determining the positivity or negativity of lead II helps to place the QRS axis in quadrant I or III within a 30° to 60° arc.

Method C: The Four-Lead Method. This method uses leads I, II, III, and aVF, and sometimes aVR in certain circumstances, to make a rapid determination of the QRS axis within a 30° arc.

Method D: The Six-Lead Method. This method uses leads I and aVF to determine in which quadrant the QRS axis lies. Then, depending on which quadrant the QRS axis lies in, leads II and aVR or leads III and aVL are used to determine the position of the QRS axis in the quadrant, within a 30° arc. This method is probably too slow for use in an emergency situation.

Method E: The "Perpendicular" Method. This method is a rapid determination of the QRS axis based on the perpendicular of a bipolar or unipolar limb lead with an equiphasic QRS complex, if one is present.

Method A: The Two-Lead Method

The two-lead method uses leads I and II to determine the general position of the QRS axis and to identify left axis deviation quickly.

Determine the net positivity or negativity of the QRS complexes in leads I and II (Table A-1).

If lead I is *positive* and:

A. Lead II is predominantly positive, the QRS axis is between −30° and +60°.

B. Lead II is equiphasic, the QRS axis is exactly −30°.
C. Lead II is predominantly negative, the QRS axis is between −30° and −90°.

If lead I is *negative* and:

D. Lead II is predominantly positive, the QRS axis is between +90° and +150°.
E. Lead II is equiphasic, the QRS axis is exactly +150°.
F. Lead II is predominantly negative, the QRS axis is greater than +150°.

TABLE A-1 Method A

Figure	Lead I	Lead II	Location of QRS Axis
A	+	+	−30° to +90°
B	+	±	−30°
C	+	−	−30° to −90°
D	−	+	+90° to +150°
E	−	±	+150°
F	−	−	>+150°

+, Predominantly positive; −, predominantly negative; ±, equiphasic

Method B: The Three-Lead Method

The three-lead method uses leads I, II, and aVF, and sometimes aVR in certain circumstances, to determine the general position of the QRS axis and to identify left and right axis deviation quickly.

Determine the net positivity or negativity of the QRS complexes in leads I, aVF, and II, in that order, and also aVR if lead I is negative (Table A-2).

If lead I is *positive* and:

A. Leads aVF and II are predominantly positive, the QRS axis is between 0° and +90°.
B. Lead aVF is predominantly negative and lead II is predominantly positive, the QRS axis is between 0° and −30°.
C. Lead aVF is predominantly negative and lead II is equiphasic, the QRS axis is exactly −30°.
D. Leads aVF and II are predominantly negative, the QRS axis is between −30° and −90°.

If Lead I is equiphasic and:

E. Leads aVF and II are predominantly negative, the QRS axis is exactly −90°.
F. Leads aVF and II are predominantly positive, the QRS axis is exactly +90°.

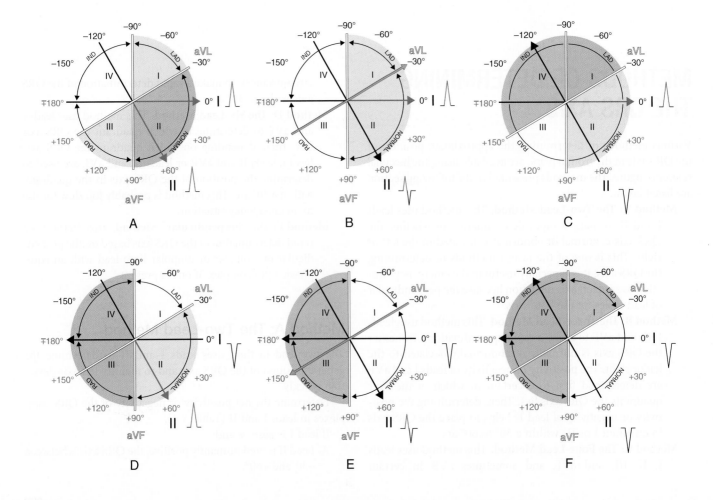

A   B   C

D   E   F

If Lead I is negative and:

G. 1. Leads aVF and II are predominantly positive, the QRS axis is between +90° and +150°.

2. If, in addition, aVR is also predominantly positive, the QRS axis is between +120° and +150°.

H. Lead aVF is predominantly positive and lead II is equiphasic, the QRS axis is exactly +150°.

I. Leads aVF and II are predominantly negative, the QRS axis is between −90°and −180°.

Method C: The Four-Lead Method

The four-lead method uses leads I, II, III, and aVF, and sometimes aVR in certain circumstances, to determine the QRS axis within 30°.

Determine the net positivity or negativity of the QRS complexes in leads I, III, aVF, and II, in that order, and also aVR if lead I is negative (Table A-3).

If Lead I is *positive* and:

A. Leads III, aVF, and II are predominantly positive, the QRS axis is between +30° and +90°.

B. Lead III is predominantly negative and leads aVF and II are predominantly positive, the QRS axis is between 0° and +30°.

C. Leads III and aVF are predominantly negative and lead II is predominantly positive, the QRS axis is between 0° and −30°.

D. Leads III and aVF are predominantly negative and lead II is equiphasic, the QRS axis is exactly −30°.

E. Leads III, aVF, and II are predominantly negative, the QRS axis is between −30°and −90°.

If Lead I is *equiphasic* and:

F. Leads III, aVF, and II are predominantly negative, the QRS axis is exactly −90°.

G. Leads III, aVF, and II are predominantly positive, the QRS axis is exactly +90°.

If lead I is *negative* and:

H. 1. Leads III, aVF, and II are predominantly positive, the QRS axis is between +90° and +150°.

2. If, in addition, aVR is also predominantly positive, the QRS axis is between +120° and +150°.

I. Leads III and aVF are predominantly positive and lead II is equiphasic, the QRS axis is exactly +150°.

J. Leads III, aVF, and II are predominantly negative, the QRS axis is between −90°and −150°.

TABLE A-2 Method B

Figure	Lead				Location of QRS axis
	I	**aVF**	**II**	**aVR**	
A	+	+	+		0° to +90°
B	+	−	+		0° to −30°
C	+	−	±		−30°
D	+	−	−		−30° to −90°
E	±	−	−		−90°
F	±	+	+		+90°
G (1)	−	+	+		+90° to +150°
G (2)	−	+	+	+	+120° to +150°
H	−	+	±		+150°
I	−	−	−		−90° to −180°

+, Predominantly positive; −, predominantly negative; ±, equiphasic

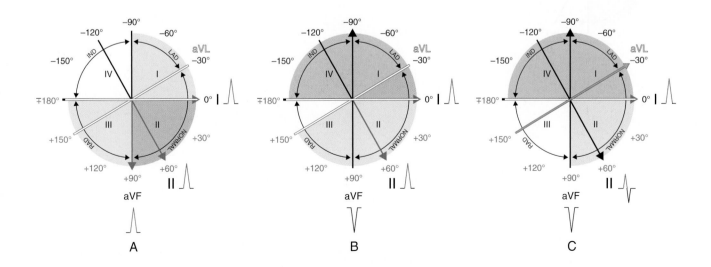

A   B   C

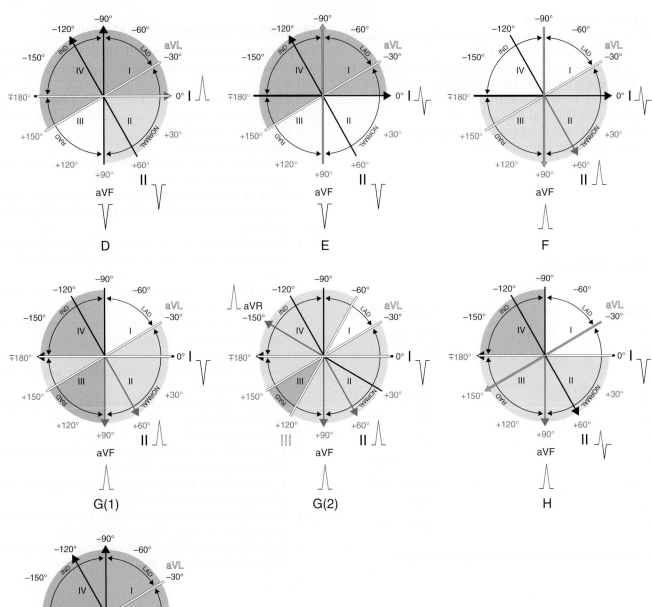

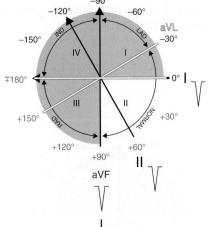

TABLE A-3 Method C

Figure	Leads					Location of QRS Axis
	I	III	aVF	II	aVR	
A	+	+	+	+		+30° to +90°
B	+	−	+	+		0° to +30°
C	+	−	−	+		0° to −30°
D	+	−	−	±		−30°
E	+	−	−	−		−30° to −90°
F	±	−	−	−		−90°
G	±	+	+	+		+90°
H (1)	−	+	+	+		+90° to +150°
H (2)	−	+	+	+	+	+120° to +150°
I	−	+	+	±		+150°
J	−	−	−	−		−90° to −150°

+, Predominantly positive; −, predominantly negative; ±, equiphasic.

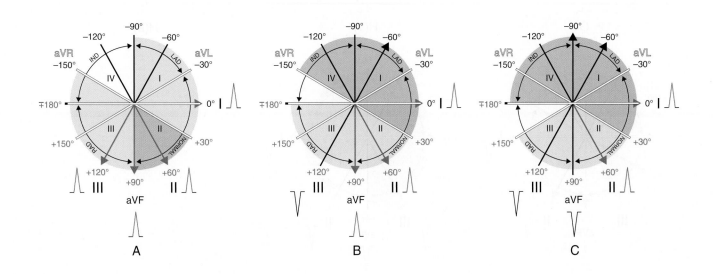

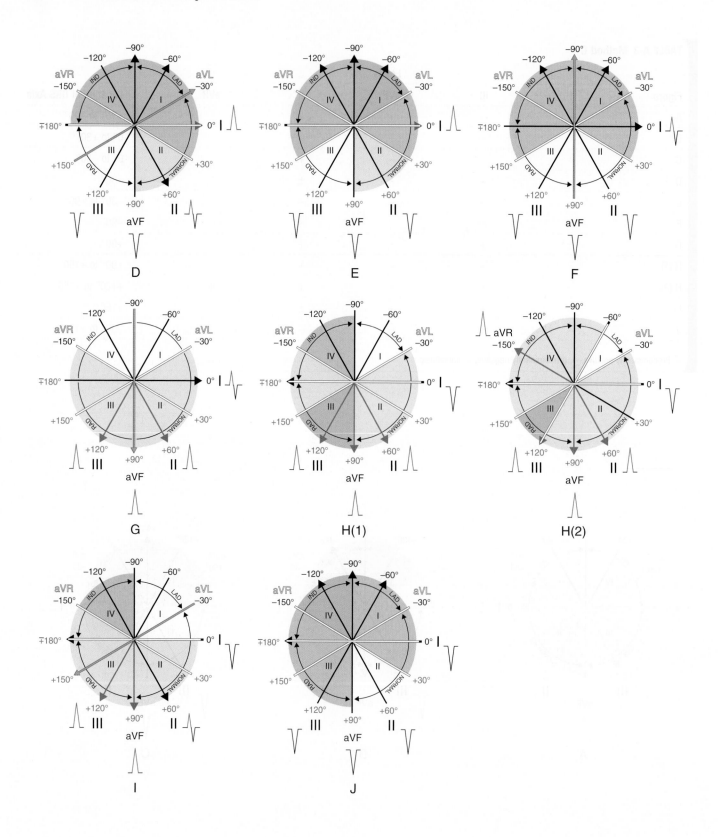

Method D: The Six-Lead Method

The two-step, six-lead method uses leads I and aVF in step 1 to determine in which quadrant the QRS axis lies. Then, in step 2, depending on the quadrant initially determined, leads II and aVR or leads III and aVL are used to determine the 30° arc in which the QRS axis lies.

Step 1. Determine the quadrant in which the QRS axis lies (Table A-4).

Determine the net positivity and negativity of the QRS complexes in leads I and aVF.

If lead I is *positive* and:

1A. Lead aVF is predominantly positive, the QRS axis is in quadrant II (0° to +90°).

1B. Lead aVF is equiphasic, the QRS axis is exactly 0°.

1C. Lead aVF is predominantly negative, the QRS axis is in quadrant I (0° to −90°).

If lead I is *equiphasic* and:

1D. Lead aVF is predominantly positive, the QRS axis is exactly +90°.

1E. Lead aVF is predominantly negative, the QRS axis is exactly −90°.

If lead I is *negative* and:

1F. Lead aVF is predominantly positive, the QRS axis is in quadrant III (+90° to +180°).

1G. Lead aVF is equiphasic, the QRS axis is exactly ±180°.

1H. Lead aVF is predominantly negative, the QRS axis is in quadrant IV (−90° to −180°).

TABLE A-4 Method D: Step 1, A-H

	Leads			
Figure	I	aVF	Location of QRS Axis	Quadrant
1A	+	+	0° to +90°	II
1B	+	±	0°	
1C	+	−	0° to +90°	I
1D	±	+	0° to +180°	
1E	±	−	190°	
1F	−	+	+90° to +180°	III
1G	−	±	±180°	
1H	−	−	−90° to −180°	IV

+, Predominantly positive; −, predominantly negative; ±, equiphasic.

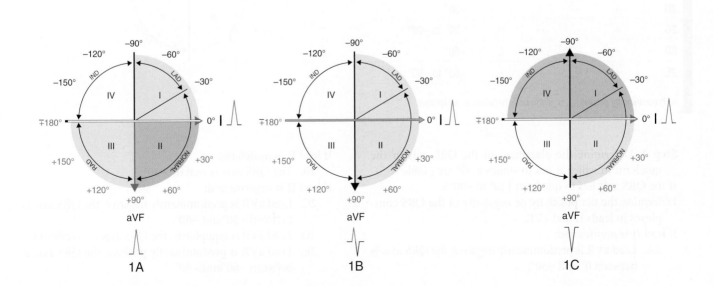

1A   1B   1C

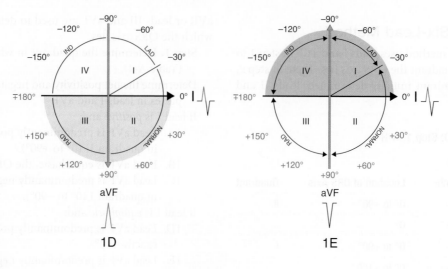

1D   1E

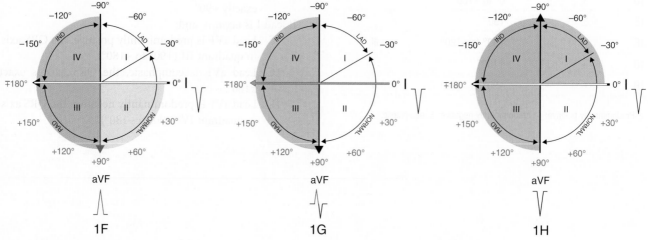

1F   1G   1H

TABLE A-5 Method D: Step 2, A-E

		Leads			
Figure	I	aVF	II	aVR	Location of QRS Axis
2A	+	−	+	−	0° to −30°
2B	+	−	±		−30°
2C	+	−	−	−	−30° to −60°
2D	+	−	−	±	−60°
2E	+	−	−	+	−60° to −90°

+, Predominantly positive; −, predominantly negative; ±, equiphasic.

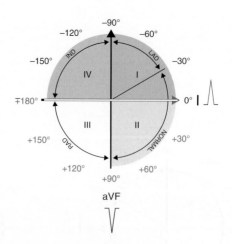

Step 2. Determine the placement of the QRS axis in the quadrant in which it lies to within a 30° arc (Table A-5).

If the QRS axis lies in quadrant I (0° to −90°):

Determine the net positivity or negativity of the QRS complexes in leads II and aVR.

If lead II is *positive* and:

    2A. Lead aVR is predominantly negative, the QRS axis is between 0° and −30°.

If lead II is *equiphasic:*

    2B. The QRS axis is exactly −30°.

If lead II is *negative* and:

    2C. Lead aVR is predominantly negative, the QRS axis is between −30°and −60°.

    2D. Lead aVR is equiphasic, the QRS axis is exactly −60°.

    2E. Lead aVR is predominantly positive, the QRS axis is between −60°and −90°.

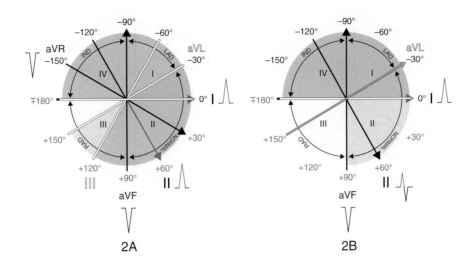

2A

2B

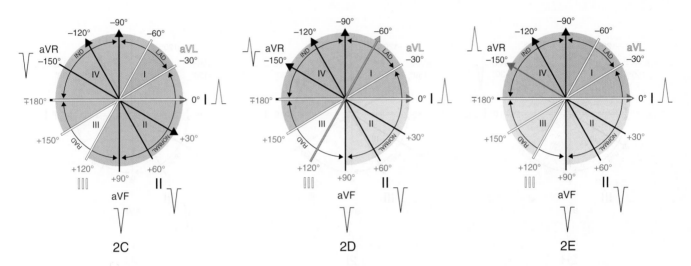

2C

2D

2E

If the QRS axis lies in quadrant II (0° to +90°):

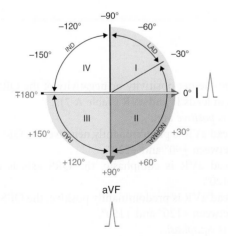

Determine the net positivity or negativity of the QRS complexes in leads III and aVL (Table A-6).

If lead III is *positive* and:

2F. Lead aVL is predominantly positive, the QRS axis is between +30° and +60°.

TABLE A-6 **Method D: Step 2, F-J**

	Leads				
Figure	I	aVF	III	aVL	Location of QRS Axis
2F	+	+	+	+	+30° to +60°
2G	+	+	+	±	+60°
2H	+	+	+	−	+60° to +90°
2I	+	+	±	+	+30°
2J	+	+	−	+	0° to +30°

+, Predominantly positive; −, predominantly negative; ±, equiphasic.

2G. Lead aVL is equiphasic, the QRS axis is exactly +60°.

2H. Lead aVL is predominantly negative, the QRS axis is between +60° and +90°.

If lead III is *equiphasic* and:

2I. Lead aVL is predominantly positive, the QRS axis is exactly +30°.

If Lead III is *negative* and:

2J. Lead aVL is predominantly positive, the QRS axis is between 0° and +30°.

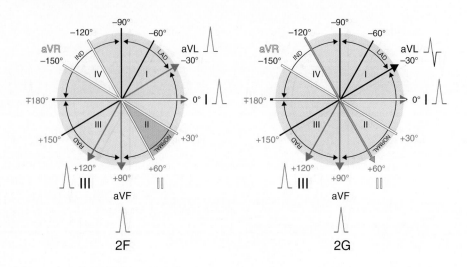

2F

2G

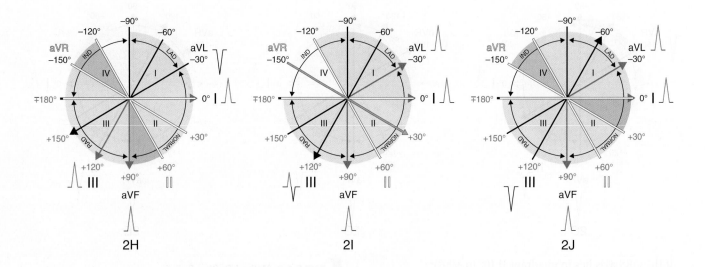

2H

2I

2J

If the QRS axis lies in quadrant III (+90° to +180°):

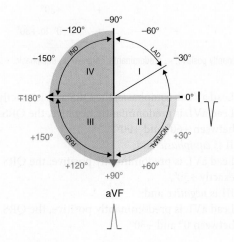

Determine the net positivity or negativity of the QRS complexes in leads II and aVR (Table A-7).

If lead II is *positive* and:

2K. Lead aVR is predominantly negative, the QRS axis is between +90° and +120°.

2L. Lead aVR is equiphasic, the QRS axis is exactly +120°.

2M. Lead aVR is predominantly positive, the QRS axis is between +120° and +150°.

If lead II is *equiphasic*:

2N. The QRS axis is exactly +150°.

If lead II is *negative* and:

2O. Lead aVR is predominantly positive, the QRS axis is between +150° and +180°.

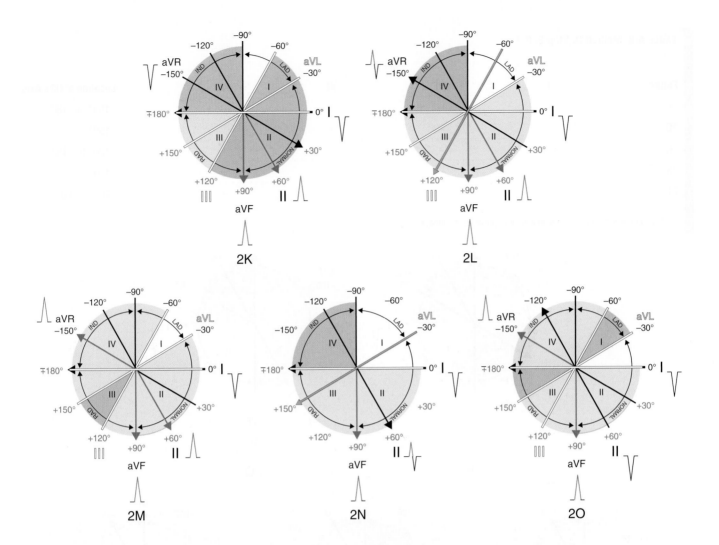

2K 2L 2M 2N 2O

If the QRS axis lies in quadrant IV (−90° to −180°):

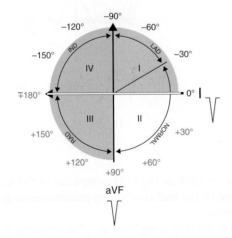

Determine the net positivity or negativity of the QRS complexes in leads III and aVL (Table A-8).

If lead III is *positive* and:
  2P. Lead aVL is predominantly negative, the QRS axis is between −150°and −180°.

TABLE A-7 Method D: Step 2, K-O

| | Leads | | | | |
Figure	I	aVF	II	aVR	Location of QRS Axis
2K	−	+	+	−	+90° to +120°
2L	−	+	+	±	+120°
2M	−	+	+	+	+120° to +150°
2N	−	+	±		+150°
2O	−	+	−	+	+150° to +180°

+, Predominantly positive; −, predominantly negative; ±, equiphasic.

If lead III is *equiphasic*:
  2Q. The QRS axis is exactly −150°.
If lead III is *negative* and:
  2R. Lead aVL is predominantly negative, the QRS axis is between −120°and −150°.
  2S. Lead aVL is equiphasic, the QRS axis is exactly −120°.
  2T. Lead aVL is predominantly positive, the QRS axis is between −90°and −120°.

TABLE A-8 Method D: Step 2, P-T

| Figure | Leads | | | | Location of QRS Axis |
	I	aVF	III	aVL	
2P	−	−	+	−	−150° to −180°
2Q	−	−	±		−150°
2R	−	−	−	−	−120° to −150°
2S	−	−	−	±	−120°
2T	−	−	−	+	−90° to −120°

+, Predominantly positive; −, predominantly negative; ±, equiphasic.

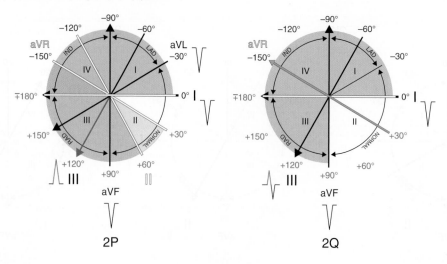

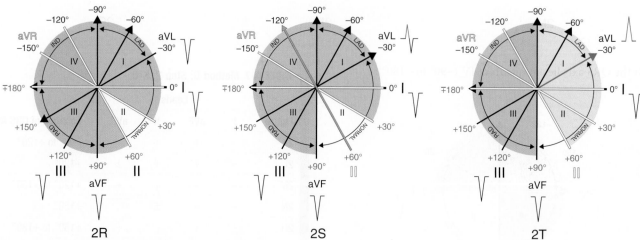

Method E: The "Perpendicular" Method

The "perpendicular" method uses the perpendicular of a lead with equiphasic or almost equiphasic QRS complexes to determine the position of the QRS axis (Table A-9).

Step 1. Identify the lead with equiphasic (or almost equiphasic) QRS complexes, and label it "A" on the hexaxial reference figure.

and

Determine the perpendicular to this lead, and label it "B."

Step 2. Identify the lead axis that lies parallel to the perpendicular "B," and label it "C."

and

Determine whether the QRS complexes in the lead represented by the lead axis "C" are predominantly positive or negative.

Step 3. If the QRS complexes are predominantly positive in the lead represented by lead axis "C," the QRS axis lies in the direction of the positive pole of lead axis "C."

Step 4. If the QRS complexes are predominantly negative in the lead represented by lead axis "C," the QRS axis lies in the direction of the negative pole of lead axis "C."

TABLE A-9 Method E

	Poles of Lead Axis	"C" Lead Positive	"C" Lead Negative
Lead "A"	Lead Axis "C"	1	2
I	aVF	+90°	−90°
II	aVL	−30°	+150°
III	aVR	−150°	+30°
aVR	III	+120°	−60°
aVL	II	+60°	−120°
aVF	I	0°	±180°

+, Predominantly positive; −, predominantly negative; ±, equiphasic.

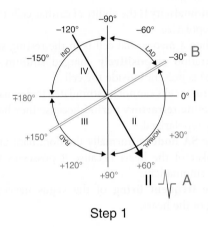

Step 1

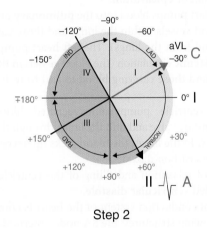

Step 2

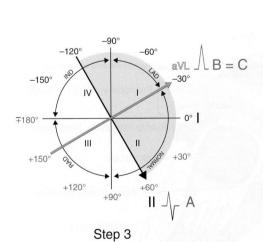

Step 3

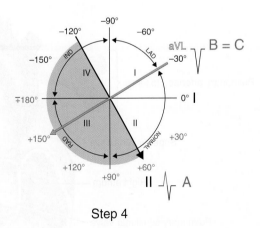

Step 4

CHAPTER 1

1. (B) The inner layer of the serous pericardium is called the *visceral pericardium* or **epicardium.**
2. (C) The **right** heart pumps blood into the **pulmonary** circulation (the blood vessels within the lungs and those carrying blood to and from the lungs). The **left** heart pumps blood into the **systemic** circulation (the blood vessels in the rest of the body and those carrying blood to and from the body).
3. (C) The right ventricle pumps unoxygenated blood through the **pulmonic** valve and into the lungs through the **pulmonary** artery. In the lungs, the blood picks up oxygen and releases excess carbon dioxide.
4. (C) The period of relaxation and filling of the ventricles with blood is called **ventricular diastole.**
5. (C) The electrical conduction system of the heart is composed of the following structures: the SA node, internodal atrial conduction tracts, AV junction, **bundle branches**, and the Purkinje network. The coronary sinus, atrial septa, and vagus nerve are not components of the electrical conduction system.
6. (A) **Automaticity** is the ability of cardiac cells to spontaneously depolarize.
7. (D) When a myocardial cell is in the resting state, a high concentration of **positively** charged **sodium** ions (Na^+) (cations) is present outside the cell.
8. (A) Cardiac cells cannot be stimulated to depolarize during the **absolute refractory period** because they have not sufficiently repolarized.
9. (D) The **SA node** is normally the dominant and primary pacemaker of the heart because it possesses the highest level of automaticity.
10. (A) The **frequent firing** of the vagus nerve will cause slowing of the heart.
11.

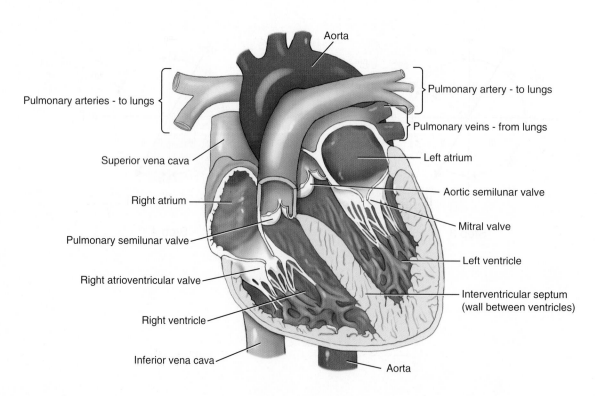

Aorta

Pulmonary arteries - to lungs

Pulmonary artery - to lungs

Pulmonary veins - from lungs

Superior vena cava

Left atrium

Right atrium

Aortic semilunar valve

Pulmonary semilunar valve

Mitral valve

Left ventricle

Right atrioventricular valve

Interventricular septum
(wall between ventricles)

Right ventricle

Inferior vena cava

Aorta

CHAPTER 2

1. (A) The ECG is a record of the electrical activity (electric current) generated by the **depolarization and repolarization of the atria and ventricles.** The electrical impulses responsible for initiating depolarization of the atria and ventricles are too small to be detected by the ECG electrodes; and the mechanical contraction and relaxation of the atria and ventricles do not generate electrical activity.

2. (D) Dark vertical lines are **0.20 second** (5 mm) apart, whereas light vertical lines are **0.04 second** (1 mm) apart.

3. (B) The sensitivity of the ECG machine is calibrated so that a **1-millivolt** electrical signal produces a **10-mm** deflection on the ECG, equivalent to two large squares on the ECG paper.

4. (B) Atrial depolarization is recorded as the P wave, **ventricular depolarization as the QRS complex,** atrial repolarization as the atrial T wave, **and ventricular repolarization as the T wave.**

5. (D) Atrial depolarization is recorded as the P wave, ventricular depolarization as the QRS complex, atrial repolarization as the atrial T wave, **and ventricular repolarization as the T wave.**

6. (C) Muscle tremors, poor electrode contact, external chest compressions and turning the gain up can all cause artifacts on an ECG tracing. However, **the most common cause of artefact is poor electrode contact with the skin** usually due to diaphoresis or hair.

7. (D) An EGG lead composed of a single positive electrode and a zero reference point (the central terminal) is called a **unipolar lead.**

8. (C) Monitoring lead II is obtained by attaching the negative electrode to **the right arm** and the positive electrode to the **left leg.**

9. (D) If the positive ECG electrode is attached to the left leg or lower left anterior chest, all of the electric currents generated in the heart that flow toward the positive electrode will be recorded as **positive (upright)** deflections. The electric currents flowing away from the positive electrode will be recorded as negative (inverted) deflections.

10. (D) Monitoring lead MCL$_1$ is obtained by attaching the positive **electrode to the right side of the anterior chest in the fourth intercostal space just right of the sternum.**

CHAPTER 3

1. (B) Increased left atrial pressure resulting in left atrial dilatation and hypertrophy as found in **hypertension, mitral and aortic valvular disease, acute MI.** Pulmonary edema secondary to left heart failure may also cause wide, notched P waves.

2. (D) The normal PR interval is between **0.12 and 0.20 second.**

3. (D) An ectopic P wave represents atrial depolarization occurring in an **abnormal direction** or **sequence** or both.

4. (B) A normal QRS complex represents normal **depolarization of the ventricles.**

5. (D) The time from the onset of the QRS complex to the peak of the R wave is the **ventricular activation time** (VAT). The VAT represents the time taken for depolarization of the interventricular septum plus depolarization of the ventricle from the endocardium to the epicardium under the facing lead.

6. (B) The **atrio-His fibers** is an accessory conduction pathway that connects the atria with the lowest part of the AV node near the bundle of His and not with the ventricles directly, as do the other accessory conduction pathways. For this reason it does not cause ventricular preexcitation but preexcitation of the bundle of His (i.e., atrio-His preexcitation). Delta waves are absent.

7. (C) Abnormal ventricular repolarization (the **T wave**) may result from myocardial ischemia, acute MI, myocarditis, pericarditis, ventricular enlargement (hypertrophy), electrolyte imbalance (e.g., excess serum potassium), or administration of certain cardiac drugs (e.g., quinidine, procainamide).

8. (C) An abnormally tall U wave may be present in **hypokalemia, cardiomyopathy**, and left ventricular hypertrophy and may follow administration of digitalis, quinidine, and procainamide.

9. (C) A **prolonged PR interval** (one that is greater in duration than 0.20 second) indicates that a delay of progression of the electrical impulse through the AV node, bundle of His, or, rarely, the bundle branches is present.

10. (C) An abnormal ST segment indicates **abnormal ventricular repolarization**, a common consequence of myocardial ischemia and acute MI. It is also present in ventricular fibrosis or aneurysm, pericarditis, left ventricular enlargement (hypertrophy), and administration of digitalis.

CHAPTER 4

1. (B) The **heart rate calculator ruler**, is most accurate if the rhythm is regular method, or the triplicate method.

2. (A) The 6-second count method can be used when the rhythm is either regular or **irregular**.

3. (B) The heart rate is 75 beats/min. Provided the ECG has a regular rate, one method to determine the rate is to count the large squares (0.20-second squares) between the peaks of two consecutive **R** waves and divide this number into 300.

4. (D) The rate of the P waves is usually **the same as that of the QRS complexes**, but sometimes it may be **less**: if an AV block is present, it may be **greater**.

5. (A) If QRS complexes are present but do not regularly precede or follow the P waves, **a complete AV block**

(third-degree AV block) is present. Another term used to describe the condition when QRS complexes occur totally unrelated to the P, P′, or F waves is *atrioventricular (AV) dissociation.*

6. (B) If atrial flutter or fibrillation waves are present, the electrical impulses responsible for them have originated in the **atria**.

7. (B) If the P waves are inverted in lead II, the electrical impulses responsible for the P waves most likely have originated in the **lower atria**.

8. (D) A PR interval of less than 0.12 second is usually present in an atrial arrhythmia arising in the atria near the AV junction and in a junctional arrhythmia. It is also present in ventricular preexcitation and atrio-His preexcitation.

9. (A) If the QRS complexes are 0.12 second or less in duration, the electrical impulses responsible for the QRS complexes most likely have originated in the **SA node**, atria, or AV junction.

10. (D) A QRS originating in the Purkinje network will travel through slower and abnormal pathways; it will have a **bizarre shape** and duration **greater than 0.12 second**.

CHAPTER 5

1. (C) Typically, the heart rate **increases** during inspiration and **decreases** during expiration.

2. (B) The most common type of sinus arrhythmia, the one related to respiration, is a normal phenomenon commonly seen in children, young adults, and elderly individuals. It is caused by the **inhibitory vagal effect** of respiration on the SA node.

3. (C) Another less common type of sinus arrhythmia is not related to respiration. It may occur in healthy individuals but is more commonly found in adult patients **with heart disease or acute MI** and in those **on digitalis** or morphine.

4. (C) A dysrhythmia originating in the SA node with a regular rate of less than 60 beats per minute is called **sinus bradycardia.**

5. (A) Sinus bradycardia may be caused by **excessive inhibitory vagal tone on the SA node, decrease in sympathetic tone on the SA node**, and **hypothermia**, among other things.

6. (C) A mild sinus bradycardia has a heart beat of 50 to 59 beats per minute.

7. (B) A patient with marked sinus bradycardia who is symptomatic will likely have **hypotension and decreased cerebral perfusion.**

8. (A) Symptomatic sinus tachycardia is best treated with **addressing the underlying cause.**

9. (C) **Sinus arrest** is an arrhythmia caused by episodes of failure in the automaticity of the SA node resulting in bradycardia or asystole.

10. (B) **Digitalis** is the most common cause of sinoatrial exit block. Beta-blockers and quinidine may also cause this condition.

CHAPTER 6

1. (D) An arrhythmia originating in pacemakers that shifts back and forth between the SA node and an ectopic pacemaker in the atria or AV junction is called a **wandering atrial pacemaker.** It is characterized by P waves of varying size, shape, and direction in any given lead.

2. (D) The arrhythmia described in question No. 1 may normally be seen in **the very young,** the elderly, and athletes.

3. (A) An extra atrial complex consisting of a positive P wave in lead II followed by a normal or abnormal QRS complex, occurring earlier than the next beat of the underlying rhythm, is called **a premature atrial complex.** It is usually followed by a noncompensatory pause.

4. (B) A nonconducted or blocked PAC is **a P′ wave that is not followed by a QRS complex.**

5. (D) The QRS complex of a PAC usually resembles that of **the underlying rhythm.**

6. (B) Two PACs in a row are called **a couplet.**

7. (B) An arrhythmia originating in an ectopic pacemaker in the atria node with an atrial rate between 160 and 240 beats per minute is called **atrial tachycardia.**

8. (D) The **reduction in cardiac output** accompanying atrial tachycardia can cause syncope, light-headedness, and dizziness. In patients with coronary artery disease, it can also cause angina, congestive heart failure, or an acute MI.

9. (D) Atrial flutter is characterized by **flutter waves with a sawtooth appearance** occurring at a rate of 240 to 360 per minute.

10. (A) **Atrial fibrillation** is characterized by multiple dissimilar, small atrial f waves occurring at a rate of 350 to 600 per minute.

CHAPTER 7

1. (A) Absent P′ waves in a junctional dysrhythmia indicate that **atrial depolarizations** have not occurred because of a retrograde AV block between the ectopic pacemaker site in the AV junction and the atria and/or occur during the QRS complex.

2. (C) If the ectopic pacemaker in the AV junction discharges too soon after the preceding QRS complex, **the premature P′ wave may not be followed by a QRS complex.**

3. (B) An extra QRS that originates from an ectopic pacemaker in the AV junction, occurring before the next expected beat of the underlying rhythm, is called a **premature junctional complex**, or **PJC.**

4. (C) The QRS complex of a PJC usually resembles that of the underlying rhythm, being 0.10 second or less in duration. The QRS complex, however, may be 0.12 second or

greater in duration and resemble that of a premature ventricular contraction if aberrant ventricular conduction is present. The QRS complex may precede or follow the P′ wave with which it is associated.

5. (C) The pause following the PJC is **compensatory,** unlike that following the PAC, because the retrograde P′ of the PJC does not depolarize the SA node. The next QRS complex occurs sooner than expected because the SA node has **not been reset**.

6. (C) More than four to six PJCs per minute may indicate an **enhanced automaticity** or a **reentry mechanism** in the **AV junction** and that more serious **junctional arrhythmias may occur** but this is **not a normal variant.**

7. (B) A dysrhythmia originating in an escape pacemaker in the AV junction with a regular rate greater than 100 beats per minute is called a **junctional tachycardia.**

8. (A) By definition any dysrhythmia that originates above the ventricles and has a rate greater than 150 beats per minute is termed **supraventricular tachycardia** (PSVT). Paroxysmal supraventricular tachycardias are more clinical significant because of their abrupt onset and significant symptomatology.

9. (C) Paroxysmal supraventricular tachycardia is characterized by a heart rate between 160 and 240 beats per minute and **an abrupt onset and termination.** The electrophysiological mechanism responsible for PSVT is a reentry mechanism involving the AV node.

10. (D) When the rate of supraventricular tachycardia is high and when there are ventricular conduction delays, SVT is difficult to distinguish from **ventricular tachycardia.**

CHAPTER 8

1. (D) An unexpected abnormally wide and bizarre QRS complex originating in an ectopic site in the ventricles is called a **PVC.**

2. (D) Premature ventricular contractions that originate from a single ectopic pacemaker site are called **unifocal.**

3. (D) A PVC may **trigger ventricular fibrillation if it occurs on the T wave** or **depolarize the SA node,** momentarily suppressing it, so that the next P wave of the underlying rhythm appears later than expected. A PVC occurring simultaneously with a normal QRS forms a fusion beat.

4. (B) A noncompensatory pause is usually **2** times the preceding R-R interval.

5. (D) A QRS that has characteristics of both the PVC and a QRS complex of the underlying rhythm is called a **ventricular fusion beat.**

6. (C) Groups of two PVCs are called **couplets.** Three PVCs in a row is a **run of V-Tach.**

7. (C) A form of ventricular tachycardia characterized by QRS complexes that gradually change back and forth from one shape, size, and direction to another over a series of beats is called **torsades de pointes.**

8. (C) **Ventricular fibrillation** is a life-threatening arrhythmia requiring immediate defibrillation which is most successful when the **fibrillatory waves are coarse.**

9. (A) Asymptomatic accelerated idioventricular rhythm is characterized by a ventricular rate between 40 and 100 beats/min. It is often **acute myocardial infarction.**

10. (D) A ventricular rhythm with a rate less than 40 beats/min is a **ventricular escape rhythm.**

CHAPTER 9

1. (A) A dysrhythmia that occurs commonly in acute inferior myocardial infarction because of the effect of an increase in vagal tone and ischemia on the AV node is called a **first-degree AV block.**

2. (B) A dysrhythmia in which there is a progressive delay following each P wave in the conduction of electrical impulses through the AV node until the conduction of the electrical impulses is completely blocked is called a **second-degree, type I AV block** or Wenckebach block.

3. (A) Second-degree, type I AV block is usually transient and reversible and asymptomatic, yet the patient should be monitored and observed because **it can progress to a higher degree AV block**. It is more commonly associated with an acute inferior wall MI.

4. (C) A dysrhythmia in which a complete block of conduction of electrical impulses occurs in one bundle branch and an intermittent block in the other is called a **second-degree, type II AV block.**

5. (D) **Temporary cardiac pacing** is indicated immediately in a symptomatic second-degree, type II AV block that occurs following an acute anteroseptal MI.

6. (C) A second-degree, advanced AV block has an AV conduction ratio of 3 : 1 **or greater** (i.e., 3 : 1, 4 : 1, 6 : 1, 8 : 1, or greater).

7. (C) The absence of conduction of electrical impulses through the AV node, bundle of His, or bundle branches, characterized by independent beating of the atria and ventricles, is called a **third-degree AV block.**

8. (D) An escape pacemaker in the AV junction has an inherent firing rate of **40 to 60 beats/min.**

9. (A) If an AV junctional or ventricular escape pacemaker does not take over following a sudden onset of third-degree AV block, asystole will occur. No pulse is generated and **cardiac arrest** occurs.

10. (B) The clinical significance of atrioventricular blocks is due primarily to their resultant effect on heart rate, which is that of the **ventricular response** from the escape pacemaker.

CHAPTER 10

1. (D) In a patient with symptomatic bradycardia and an ECG showing a second-degree, type II AV block, you

should administer oxygen, start an IV line, and begin **transcutaneous pacing.** Administration of atropine would be reasonable if TPC was not immediately available. There is no role for a vasopressor at this point and an antiarrhythmic would not be indicated.

2. (A) Patients with symptomatic sinus tachycardia should be treated with the **appropriate treatment for the underlying cause of the tachycardia** (i.e., anxiety, exercise, pain, fever, congestive heart failure, hypoxemia, hypovolemia, hypotension, or shock).

3. (D) If a patient is stable with an ECG showing PSVT after administering oxygen and starting an IV line, you should **attempt vagal maneuvers.** Make sure to verify the absence of known carotid artery disease or carotid bruits before attempting carotid sinus massage.

4. (B) Your patient presents with chest pain and signs and symptoms of an acute MI. His ECG shows atrial tachycardia without a block. After administering oxygen and starting an IV line, you should immediately **consider a loading dose of amiodarone.**

5. (A) Adenosine may slow the rate of an unknown narrow complex QRS tachycardia thought initially to be SVT only to reveal an underlying rhythm of atrial tachycardia, atrial fibrillation, or atrial flutter. It should be administered as fast as possible followed by bolus of saline to ensure it reaches the heart. It may now always convert the rhythm thus requiring other agents or electrical therapy be considered.

6. (C) A patient with atrial fibrillation of less than 48 hours in duration, who is hemodynamically unstable and hypotensive, should be **immediately cardioverted and receive a loading dose of amiodarone.**

7. (B) Your patient is conscious and hemodynamically stable, with a pulse and an ECG showing monomorphic ventricular tachycardia. After administering oxygen and starting an IV, you should perform the following: **administer a 150-mg loading dose of amiodarone IV.**

8. (D) If your patient in question number 7 begins to complain of chest pain and then becomes pulseless, you should immediately deliver **defibrillation** of 360 joules.

9. (B) Pulseless electrical activity is the absence of a detectable pulse and blood pressure in the presence of electrical activity of the heart on the ECG. It may result from a complete absence of ventricular contractions or marked decrease in cardiac output because of a variety of causes, such as hypovolemia, cardiac rupture, pericardial tamponade, hypothermia, and so forth. It is not a specific rhythm; however, it is associated with rhythms that would otherwise be expected to produce a pulse. Therefore **normal sinus rhythm** would be associated with PEA.

10. (D) Once return of spontaneous circulation occurs, the primary goal is to **treat the underlying cause to avoid a recurrence of the arrest.** While ensuring the ABCs are intact and that vascular access is good, they are only components of the overall goal. Rewarming is not indicated immediately following cardiac arrest unless severe hypothermia is thought to be the cause.

CHAPTER 11

1. (A) The electrode attached to the right leg is a **ground** electrode to provide a path of least resistance for electrical interference in the body.

2. (A) A **bipolar** lead represents the difference in electrical potential between two electrodes.

3. (D) The 'a' in aVR, aVL, and aVF stands for **augmented.**

4. (B) The electrical currents of **Lead I + Lead III = Lead II** is called *Einthoven's law.*

5. (B) Lead aVL is obtained by measuring the electric current between the positive electrode attached to the **left arm** and the central terminal formed by the electrodes attached to the **right arm and left leg.**

6. (B) A **precordial** lead measures the difference in electrical potential between a chest electrode and the central terminal.

7. (D) The placement of the positive chest electrode is as follows:
   V_1-right side of the sternum in the fourth intercostal space
   V_2-left side of the sternum in the fourth intercostal space
   V_3-midway between V_2 and V_4
   V_4-left **midclavicular line in the fifth intercostal space**
   V_5-left anterior axillary line at the same level as V_4
   V_6-left midaxillary line at the same level as V_4

8. (B) The placement of the positive chest electrode is as follows:
   V_1-right side of the sternum in the fourth intercostal space
   V_2-**left side of the sternum in the fourth intercostal space**
   V_3-midway between V_2 and V_4
   V_4-left midclavicular line in the fifth intercostal space
   V_5-left anterior axillary line at the same level as V_4
   V_6-left midaxillary line at the same level as V_4

9. (C) For V_{6R}, the positive chest electrode is **placed at the right midaxillary line at the same level as V_{4R}.** The location of V_{4R} is in the midclavicular line in the right fifth intercostal space.

10. (B) Leads II, III, and aVF face the **inferior** or diaphragmatic surface of the heart.

CHAPTER 12

1. (B) The mean of all vectors generated during the depolarization of the ventricles is the **QRS** axis. That of the atria is the P axis and that of repolarization is the T axis.

2. (D) An electric current flowing toward the positive pole produces **a positive deflection** on the ECG.

3. (A) The more parallel the electric current is to the axis of the lead, the **larger** the deflection. The more perpendicular, the smaller the deflection.

4. (B) A predominantly negative QRS complex indicates that the **positive** pole of the vector of the QRS axis lies somewhere on the **negative** side of the perpendicular axis.

5. (B) A QRS complex with right axis deviation is **greater than +90°.**

6. (B) Left axis deviation with a QRS axis greater than −30° occurs in adults in the following cardiac disorders:
   —left ventricular enlargement and hypertrophy caused by:
   —**hypertension**
   —**aortic stenosis**
   —**ischemic heart disease**
   —left bundle branch block and left anterior fascicular block

7. (D) Right axis deviation occurs in adults with **right ventricular hypertrophy.**

8. (A) A QRS axis **greater than +90°** (right axis deviation) occurs in adults with the following cardiac and pulmonary disorders: COPD, pulmonary embolism, congenital heart disease, cor pulmonale, and severe pulmonary hypertension.

9. (D) QRS axis is significantly beneficial in differentiating ventricular versus supraventricular **tachycardia with wide QRS complexes.**

10. (B) If the QRS complexes are predominantly positive in lead aVF, the QRS axis is between **0 and +90°.**

CHAPTER 13

1. (D) The time from the onset of the QRS complex to the peak of the R wave in the QRS complex is called **the ventricular activation time** (VAT)

2. (B) The anterior portion of the septum is supplied with blood from the **left anterior descending coronary artery.**

3. (D) The main blood supply of the AV node and proximal part of the bundle of His is the AV node artery, which arises from the **right coronary artery** in 85% to 90% of the hearts. In the rest of the hearts, the AV node artery arises from the left circumflex coronary artery.

4. (B) Common causes of bundle branch and fascicular blocks are cardiomyopathy, **ischemic heart disease,** idiopathic degenerative disease of the electrical conduction system, severe left ventricular hypertrophy, and, of course, acute MI.

5. (A) In the setting of an acute MI, a right bundle branch block occurs primarily in an **anteroseptal MI,** and rarely in an inferior MI.

6. (B) In patients with an acute MI complicated by a bundle branch block, **the incidence of pump failure and ventricular arrhythmias is much higher** than in those not so complicated.

7. (C) Common causes of chronic right bundle branch blocks include **myocarditis, cardiomyopathy, and cardiac surgery.**

8. (B) In a right bundle branch block, the QRS complex in lead V₁ is **wide with a classic triphasic rSR′ pattern.**

9. (B) When the electrical impulses are prevented from directly entering the anterior and lateral walls of the left ventricle, the condition is called a **left anterior fascicular block.**

10. (C) The most ominous bifascicular block is a RBBB with **left posterior fascicular block.**

CHAPTER 14

1. (C) **Symptomatic bradydysrhythmias** such as third-degree AVB and advanced AVB are indications for permanent pacemaker insertion. Digitalis toxicity and complications related to acute myocardial infarction are usually treated with temporary pacemakers. Pacemakers are not indicated in the treatment of PVCs.

2. (A) As scar tissue builds up around the pacemaker tip of the electrode, it affects the ability of the electrode to **sense** the electrical activity of the heart.

3. (A) **Demand pacemakers** fire when the intrinsic heart rate falls below the lower set limit. Fixed rate pacemakers fire at a preset rate regardless of the underlying heart rate.

4. (D) **RBBB appearance** because the electrode lies within the right ventricle. The QRS duration will exceed .12 seconds, and there is no normal P generated by a pacemaker QRS complex.

5. (B) **DDD.** Paces and sense, both atria and ventricles, and is inhibited by electrical activity in either. The first letter (D = Dual) indicates that it paces both atrial and ventricle. The second letter (D = Dual) indicates that is sense both the atrial and the ventricle. The third letter (D = Dual) indicates that it is inhibited by electrical discharge from either the atria and/or ventricle.

6. (D) **The ventricular refractory** period is that time following the discharge of a ventricular pacer spike during which the pacemaker will not fire again. This is seen in a pacemaker that has ventricular pacer spikes. The lower limit is the maximum time the pacemaker will allow between consecutive R waves before discharging the pacemaker. Absolute and relative refractory period are terms that relate to normal repolarization of the ventricles and is unrelated to pacemakers.

7. (B) The application of the insulated circular magnet **causes the pacemaker to go into default fixed-rate mode,** which should allow visualization of pacer spikes on the ECG if the pacemaker battery and lead are functioning.

8. (C) ICDs are indicated for nonreversible cause of VT. Digitalis toxicity can be treated by withholding the drug and administering Digibind if indicated.

9. (A) **ICDs and pacemakers can be interrogated by an external device,** which can download the generators internal parameters such as sensing and pacing rate, along with the energy that will be used for cardioversion/defibrillation. Only ICDs can cardiovert and overdrive pace. The electrode of the ICD is different than that of the pacemaker as it has a larger surface area to allow it to pass the higher current to the endocardium.

10. (C) Abrupt increase in ICD firing can occur for a host of reasons, which include lead fracture, oversensing of T waves, tachydysrhythmias, or actual ventricular tachycardia. A dead battery would result in a lack of firing. Bradycardia would result in a pacing activity, which would not be as noticeable as ICD firing. Regardless **the patient must be placed on cardiac monitoring** to determine the underlying cardiac activity. He would not necessarily have to suffer cardiac arrest for the ICD to fire.

CHAPTER 15

1. (C) A chronic condition of the heart characterized by an increase in the thickness of a chamber's myocardial wall secondary to the increase in the size of the muscle fibers is called **hypertrophy.** Dilation is enlargement of the chamber while atrophy is thinning of the muscle wall. Stenosis refers to stiffening or scarring, which usually occurs to valves.
2. (A) A patient with mitral valve insufficiency or left heart failure may develop **left atrial and ventricular enlargement.**
3. (C) Left ventricular hypertrophy, a condition usually caused by increased pressure or volume in the left ventricle, is often found in **systemic hypertension, acute MI,** mitral insufficiency, hypertrophic cardiomyopathy, and aortic stenosis or insufficiency. The other listed answers are associated with right ventricular hypertrophy.
4. (D) **Pericarditis** is an inflammatory disease directly involving the epicardium, with deposition of inflammatory cells and a variable amount of serous, fibrous, purulent, or hemorrhagic exudate within the sac surrounding the heart.
5. (A) In a diffuse pericarditis, the ST segment is elevated in **all leads except aVR and V$_1$.**
6. (C) **Hyperkalemia** is an excess of serum potassium above normal levels of 3.5 to 5.0 milliequivalents per liter (mEq/L).
7. (D) The ECG changes that occur at various levels of excess serum potassium are: **the QRS complexes widen and the T waves become tall**; the ST segments disappear and the T waves become peaked; and the PR intervals become prolonged and a "sine wave" QRS-ST-T pattern appears.
8. (C) A medication normally prescribed to heart patients, which when taken in excess causes depression of myocardial contractility, AV block, ventricular asystole, PVCs, and ventricular tachycardia and fibrillation, is **procainamide.**
9. (A) The ECG changes in acute pulmonary embolism include **a QRS axis of greater than +90°.**
10. (B) The Osborn wave is a sign of **hypothermia.**

CHAPTER 16

1. (B) The artery that arises from the left main coronary artery at an obtuse angle and runs posteriorly along the left atrioventricular groove to end in back of the left ventricle is called the **left circumflex** coronary artery. This is the case

in 85% to 90% of hearts. In the remaining percentage, the left circumflex coronary artery continues along the atrioventricular groove to become the posterior descending coronary artery while giving rise to the posterior left ventricular arteries and the AV node artery.
2. (C) The SA node is supplied with blood by the sinoatrial node artery, which arises from either **the left circumflex coronary artery** (in 40% to 50% of hearts) or **the right coronary artery** (in 50% to 60% of hearts).
3. (D) The most common cause of myocardial ischemia or infarction is caused by an **occlusion of an atherosclerotic coronary artery.** Other causes include coronary artery spasm, increased myocardial workload, toxic exposure to cocaine or ethanol, decreased level of oxygen in the blood delivered to the myocardium, and decreased coronary artery blood flow from whatever cause.
4. (D) The increase in existing angina from a CCSC class II to a class III indicates the **onset of unstable angina.**
5. (C) The most common cause of acute MI (occurring in about 90% of acute MIs) is a **coronary thrombosis.**
6. (A) Upon revascularization or reoxygenation, necrotic cells **do not return to normal function.**
7. (D) A myocardial infarction in which the zone of infarction involves the entire full thickness of the ventricular wall, from the endocardium to the epicardial surface, is called a **transmural infarction.**
8. (B) The "window" theory provides an explanation for the appearance of **pathologic Q waves** through which the facing lead views the Q wave of the normal myocardium on the opposite side of the infarction.
9. (C) Inverted or tall peaked T waves in the facing leads during the early phase of an acute MI are an indication of **ischemia.** Necrosis and infarction are signified by the presence of pathologic Q waves and injury by ST-segment elevation.
10. (D) The most likely cause of an inferior MI is an occlusion of the posterior left ventricular arteries, which in the majority of persons branch from the **right coronary artery.**

CHAPTER 17

1. (A) A **localized anterior myocardial infarction** presents early with ST-segment elevation with tall T waves and taller than normal R waves in the midprecordial leads V$_3$ and V$_4$, and late with QS complexes with T wave inversion in leads V$_3$ and V$_4$.
2. (C) A **lateral myocardial infarction** presents early with ST segment depression in leads II, III, and aVF and ST-segment elevation, tall T waves, and taller than normal R waves in leads I, aVL, and the left precordial lead V$_5$ or V$_6$ or both.
3. (D) A **septal myocardial infarction** involves both the anterior wall of the left ventricle overlying the interventricular septum and the anterior two thirds of the interventricular septum.

4. (D) A **septal myocardial infarction** presents late with QS complexes with T wave inversions in leads V_1-V_2 and absent normal "septal" q waves in leads II, III, and aVF.

5. (B) An **anterolateral myocardial infarction** presents early with ST-segment elevation, tall T waves, and taller than normal R waves in leads I and aVL and the precordial leads V_3-V_6 and ST-segment depression in leads II, III, and aVF.

6. (C) An **extensive anterior myocardial infarction** results from occlusion of the LAD proximal to the marginal and diagonal branches. Occlusion more distally in the LAD of the ventricular perforator arteries results in a septal infarct. Posterior MIs occur from either occlusion of the RCA or the distal circumflex while inferior wall MIs occur from occlusion of the posterior left ventricular branches of the RCA.

7. (B) An **inferior myocardial infarction** involves the posterior left ventricular arteries arising from the right coronary artery or the left circumflex coronary artery of the left coronary artery.

8. (B) An **inferior myocardial infarction** presents early with ST-segment elevation, tall T waves, and taller than normal R waves in leads II, III, and aVF and ST-segment depression in leads I and aVL.

9. (C) A **posterior myocardial infarction** presents late with large R waves and tall T waves in leads V_1-V_4, an R wave ≥ 0.04 seconds in width with slurring and notching in V_1, and an R/S ratio of ≥ 1 in V_1.

10. (A) An **inferior myocardial infarction** is noted by the presence of ST-segment elevation, tall T waves, and taller than normal R waves in leads II, III, and aVF; ST-segment elevation in V_{4R}; and ST-segment depression in leads I and aVL.

CHAPTER 18

1. (D) **Recognizing the signs and symptoms of ACS** is the single most important factor both for the patient and clinician in avoiding unrecognized myocardial infarctions.

2. (A) **Anginal equivalents** are symptoms other than typical chest pain that are consistent with ACS. They occur more commonly in the elderly, diabetic, and in women. A silent MI is one in which a myocardial infarction occurs but the patient had no symptoms.

3. (C) **Increased sympathetic discharge** is a response to ischemia, hypoxia, and pain and results in the changes in vital signs and other signs and symptoms exhibited by the ACS patient.

4. (A) The typical ACS chest pain is a crushing, **heavy pressure**, substernal pain that lasts more than 5 minutes and is not associated with breathing or movement.

5. (C) In the early phases of CHF, pulmonary edema causes **dyspnea with exertion.** As it progresses the dyspnea worsens and occurs while at rest and laying down. Chest pain and cough are not specific to the condition.

6. (C) The skin of the ACS patient is usually **pale, cool, and clammy** due to the increased sympathetic discharge causing vasoconstriction and sweating.

7. (C) An S_3 **represents turbulent blood impacting a dysfunctional ventricular** wall during an acute MI.

8. (A) Generalized edema throughout the body is referred to as **anasarca.** Pretibial edema is found over the anterior lower leg. Presacral edema is found over the lower lumbar region.

9. (C) This patient is most likely suffering from **right heart failure.** In right heart failure the lungs are usually clear and the blood pressure is low. In cardiogenic shock the blood pressure is low. None of these findings would be present in an uncomplicated MI.

10. (D) The patient with a nondiagnostic 12-lead ECG must have a risk stratification performed. This will include **a combination of history and cardiac markers** to make the diagnosis of non-ST elevated MI. Neither one alone is sufficient to make the diagnosis and serial ECGs will not result in changes.

CHAPTER 19

1. (D) When caring for a patient suffering a myocardial infarction all treatment is designed to **limit the amount of myocardial damage.** This is accomplished by rapid identification, early administration of nitroglycerin, antiplatelets, and reperfusion therapy.

2. (C) The goal for administering fibrinolytics is referred to as **door-to-needle** time and should occur within **30 minutes.**

3. (C) Antiplatelet agents **stop the formation of additional thrombus** by blocking substances such as thromboxane. Fibrinolytics lyse the thrombus and only PTCS mechanically opens the vessels. The goal is *not* to thin the blood but only to stop additional thrombus formation.

4. (B) PCI is the preferred technique for reperfusion and should generally only be deferred if it cannot be performed or there is an **inability to perform PCI within 90 minutes.** The other listed reasons should never play a role in deciding which modality to use.

5. (A) LMW heparin, warfarin, and abciximab exert their effect on the thrombus by **inhibiting platelet aggregation.** Aspirin exerts it effect by inhibiting thromboxane A_1 release and reteplase exerts it effect by promoting lysis of fibrin.

6. (C) **Percutaneous transluminal coronary angioplasty** (PTCA) is a procedure in which a balloon-tipped catheter is inserted into an occluded artery and then the balloon is inflated, thereby fracturing the atherosclerotic plaque and dilating the arterial lumen. This procedure is also referred to as *balloon angioplasty.*

7. (B) The correct dosage of reteplase for thrombolytic therapy is **10-U IV bolus in 2 minutes, repeated in 30 minutes.** When reteplase is given in conjunction with antithrombin therapy, such as the administration

of a GP IIb/IIIa receptor inhibitor, the correct dosage is 5-U IV bolus of reteplase in 2 minutes, repeated in 30 minutes.

8. (C) The correct dosage of tenecteplase for thrombolytic therapy is **a 30- to 50-mg IV bolus in 5 seconds based on the patient's weight**. When tenecteplase is given in conjunction with GP IIb/IIIa receptor inhibitor, the correct dosage is half of the above calculated dosage.

9. (A) Morphine sulfate, nitroglycerin, and diuretics should be avoided in patients with possible acute right ventricular myocardial infarction. Normal saline should help restore cardiac output and elevate the systolic blood pressure to 90 to 100 mm Hg. If normal saline is ineffective, dobutamine is indicated **at a dosage of 2 to 20 µg/kg/min.**

10. (B) The routine use of **furosemide** has become controversial in the treatment of congestive heart failure. Research has shown that early and aggressive use of nitrates and CPAP are superior and therefore furosemide is being used less often.

Rhythm Interpretation: Self-Assessment

DYSRHYTHMIAS

1.

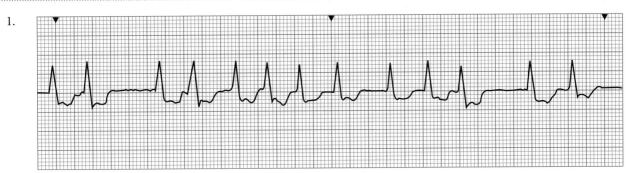

Rate: _____ PRI: _____

Rhythm: _____ QRS: _____

P Waves: _____ Interp: _____

2.

Rate: _____ PRI: _____

Rhythm: _____ QRS: _____

P Waves: _____ Interp: _____

3.

Rate: _____ PRI: _____

Rhythm: _____ QRS: _____

P Waves: _____ Interp: _____

4.

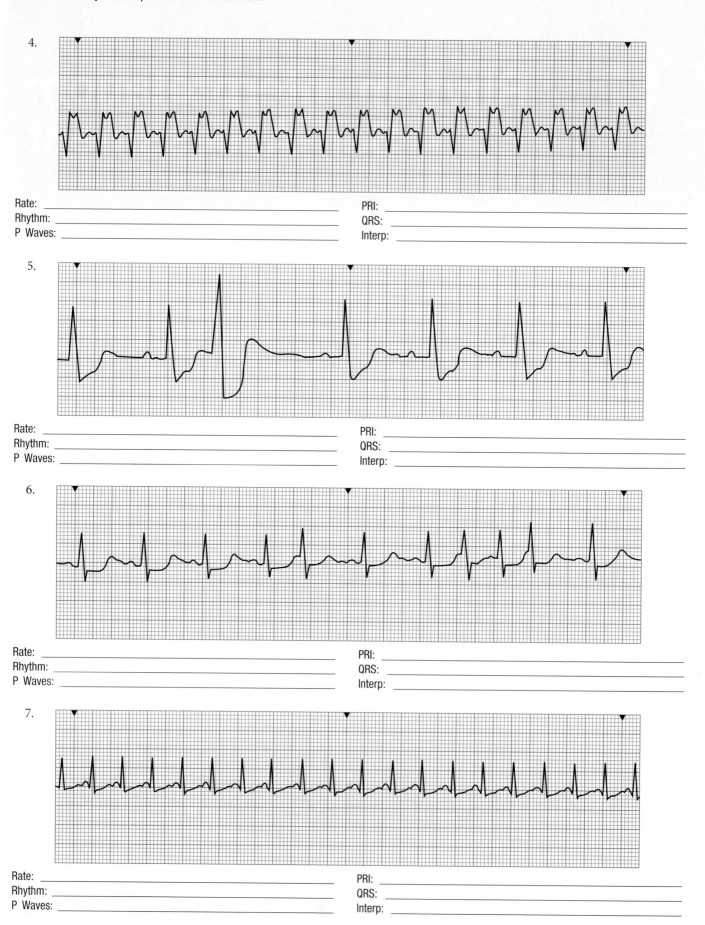

Rate: _____ PRI: _____

Rhythm: _____ QRS: _____

P Waves: _____ Interp: _____

5.

Rate: _____ PRI: _____

Rhythm: _____ QRS: _____

P Waves: _____ Interp: _____

6.

Rate: _____ PRI: _____

Rhythm: _____ QRS: _____

P Waves: _____ Interp: _____

7.

Rate: _____ PRI: _____

Rhythm: _____ QRS: _____

P Waves: _____ Interp: _____

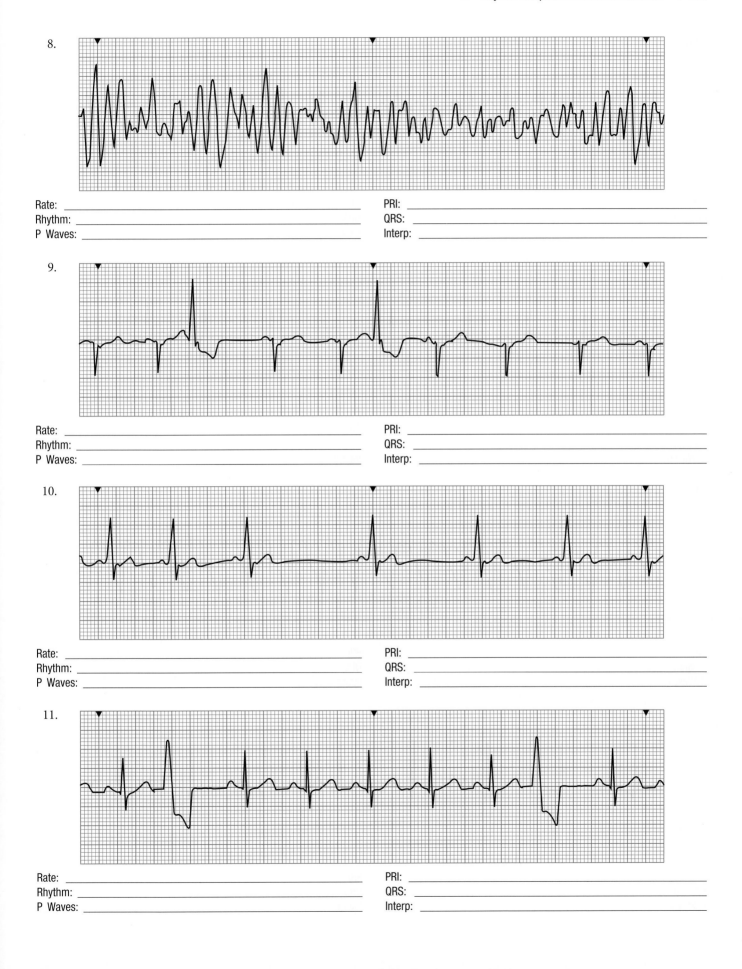

8.

Rate: _____   PRI: _____
Rhythm: _____   QRS: _____
P Waves: _____   Interp: _____

9.

Rate: _____   PRI: _____
Rhythm: _____   QRS: _____
P Waves: _____   Interp: _____

10.

Rate: _____   PRI: _____
Rhythm: _____   QRS: _____
P Waves: _____   Interp: _____

11.

Rate: _____   PRI: _____
Rhythm: _____   QRS: _____
P Waves: _____   Interp: _____

12.

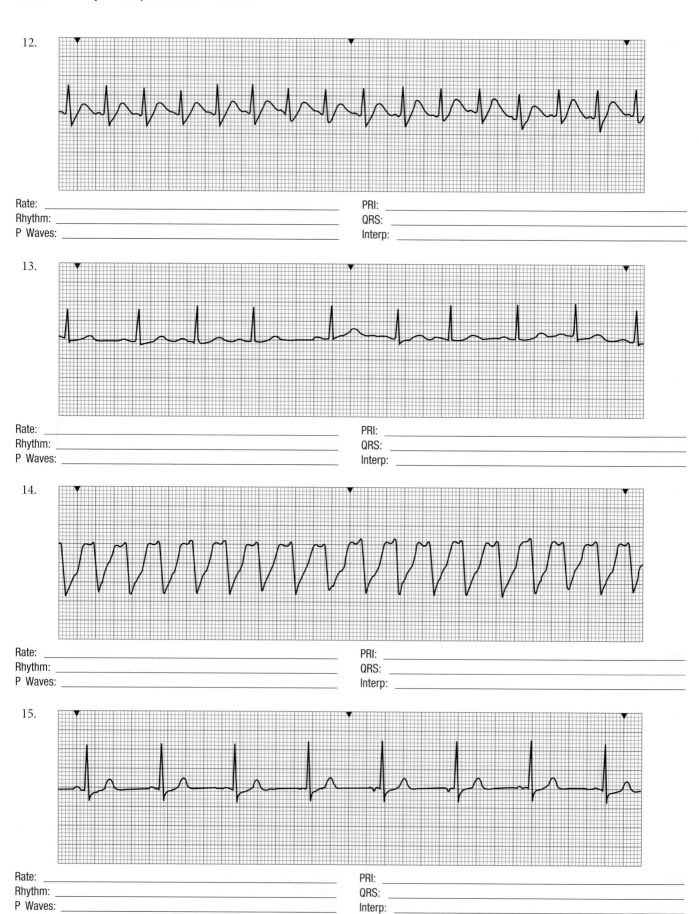

Rate: _____   PRI: _____
Rhythm: _____   QRS: _____
P Waves: _____   Interp: _____

13.

Rate: _____   PRI: _____
Rhythm: _____   QRS: _____
P Waves: _____   Interp: _____

14.

Rate: _____   PRI: _____
Rhythm: _____   QRS: _____
P Waves: _____   Interp: _____

15.

Rate: _____   PRI: _____
Rhythm: _____   QRS: _____
P Waves: _____   Interp: _____

16.

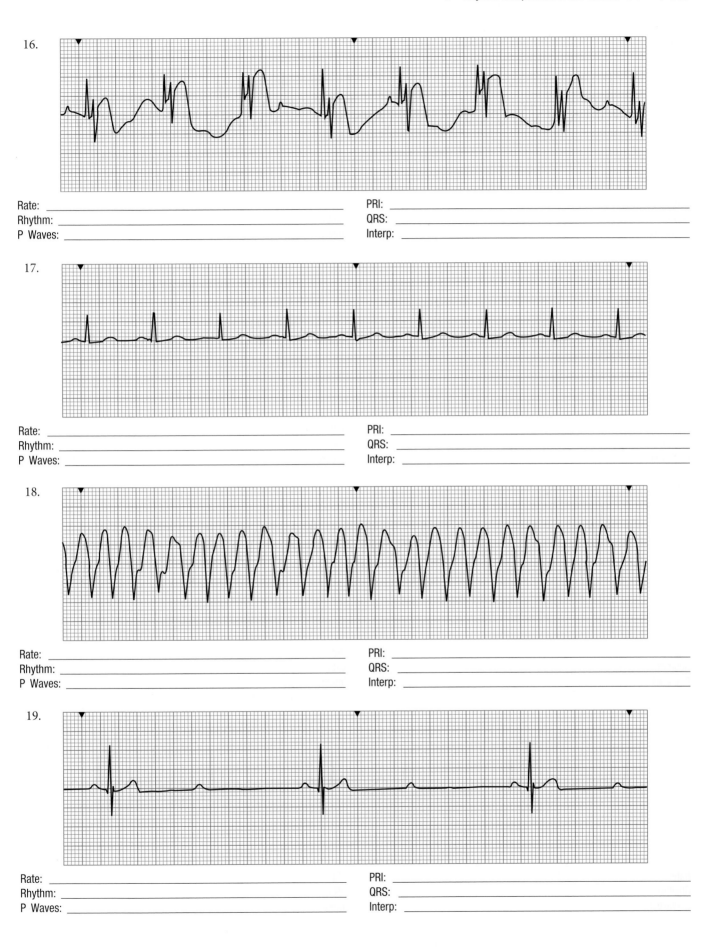

Rate: _____   PRI: _____
Rhythm: _____   QRS: _____
P Waves: _____   Interp: _____

17.

Rate: _____   PRI: _____
Rhythm: _____   QRS: _____
P Waves: _____   Interp: _____

18.

Rate: _____   PRI: _____
Rhythm: _____   QRS: _____
P Waves: _____   Interp: _____

19.

Rate: _____   PRI: _____
Rhythm: _____   QRS: _____
P Waves: _____   Interp: _____

20.

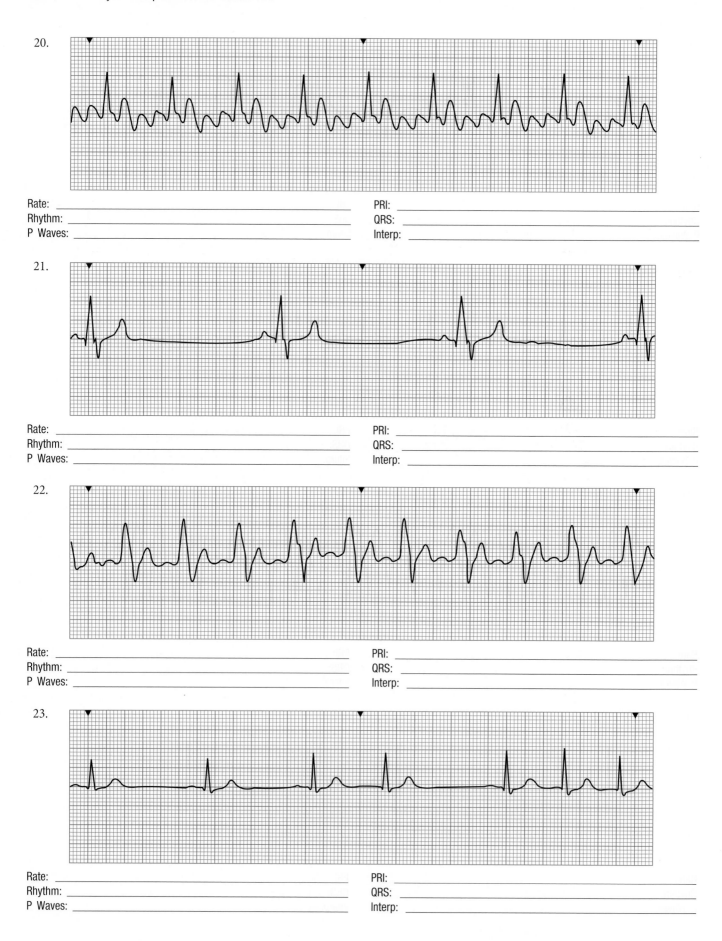

Rate: _____ PRI: _____
Rhythm: _____ QRS: _____
P Waves: _____ Interp: _____

21.

Rate: _____ PRI: _____
Rhythm: _____ QRS: _____
P Waves: _____ Interp: _____

22.

Rate: _____ PRI: _____
Rhythm: _____ QRS: _____
P Waves: _____ Interp: _____

23.

Rate: _____ PRI: _____
Rhythm: _____ QRS: _____
P Waves: _____ Interp: _____

24.

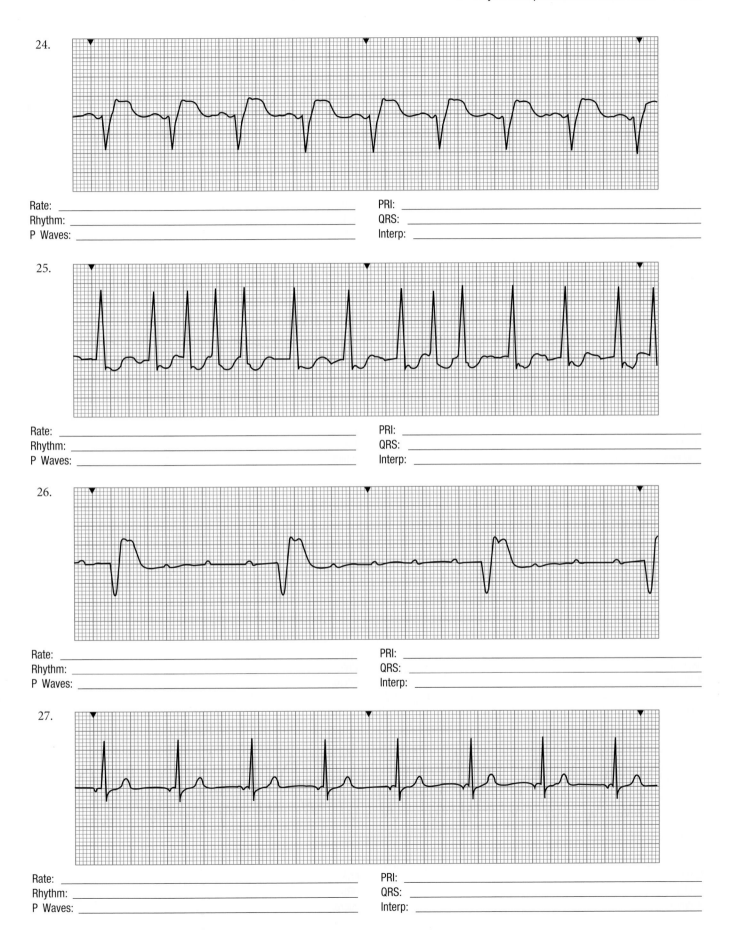

Rate: _____

Rhythm: _____

P Waves: _____

PRI: _____

QRS: _____

Interp: _____

25.

Rate: _____

Rhythm: _____

P Waves: _____

PRI: _____

QRS: _____

Interp: _____

26.

Rate: _____

Rhythm: _____

P Waves: _____

PRI: _____

QRS: _____

Interp: _____

27.

Rate: _____

Rhythm: _____

P Waves: _____

PRI: _____

QRS: _____

Interp: _____

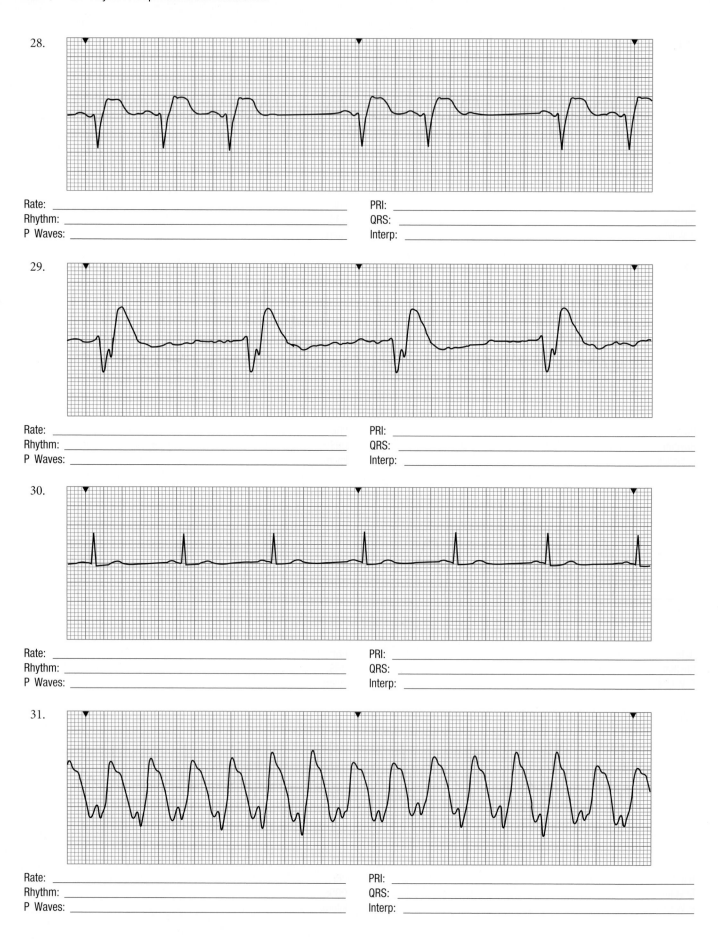

28.

Rate: _____ PRI: _____
Rhythm: _____ QRS: _____
P Waves: _____ Interp: _____

29.

Rate: _____ PRI: _____
Rhythm: _____ QRS: _____
P Waves: _____ Interp: _____

30.

Rate: _____ PRI: _____
Rhythm: _____ QRS: _____
P Waves: _____ Interp: _____

31.

Rate: _____ PRI: _____
Rhythm: _____ QRS: _____
P Waves: _____ Interp: _____

32.

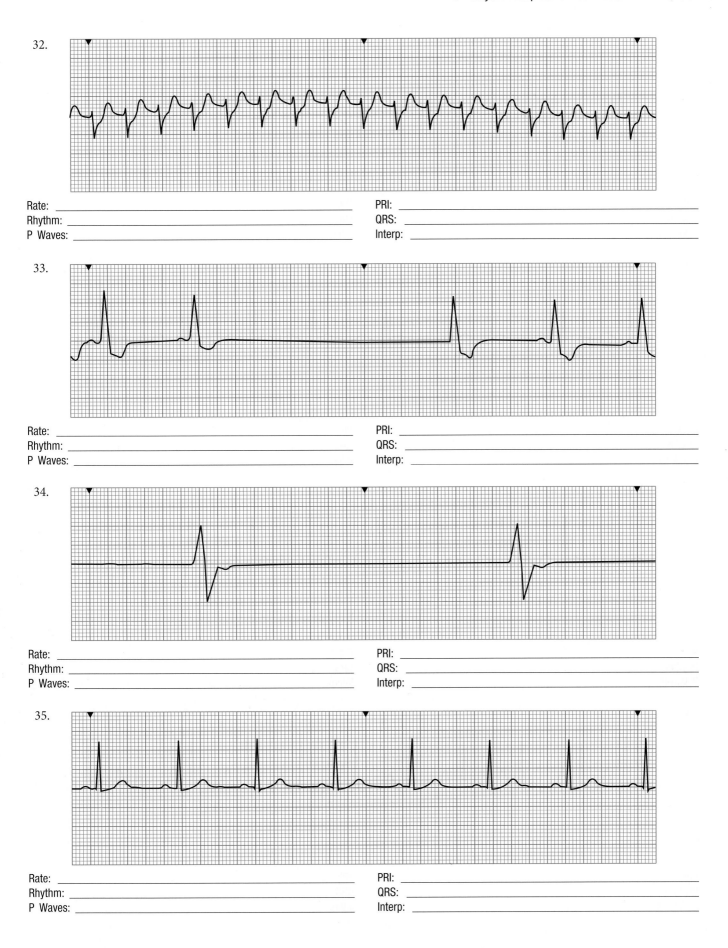

Rate: _____   PRI: _____
Rhythm: _____   QRS: _____
P Waves: _____   Interp: _____

33.

Rate: _____   PRI: _____
Rhythm: _____   QRS: _____
P Waves: _____   Interp: _____

34.

Rate: _____   PRI: _____
Rhythm: _____   QRS: _____
P Waves: _____   Interp: _____

35.

Rate: _____   PRI: _____
Rhythm: _____   QRS: _____
P Waves: _____   Interp: _____

36.

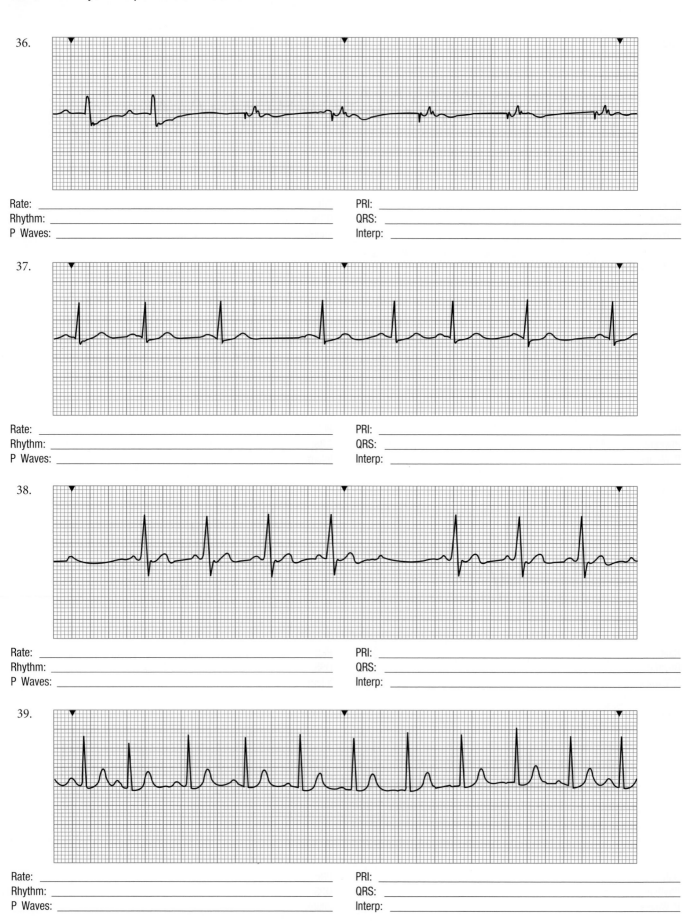

Rate: _____

Rhythm: _____

P Waves: _____

PRI: _____

QRS: _____

Interp: _____

37.

Rate: _____

Rhythm: _____

P Waves: _____

PRI: _____

QRS: _____

Interp: _____

38.

Rate: _____

Rhythm: _____

P Waves: _____

PRI: _____

QRS: _____

Interp: _____

39.

Rate: _____

Rhythm: _____

P Waves: _____

PRI: _____

QRS: _____

Interp: _____

40.

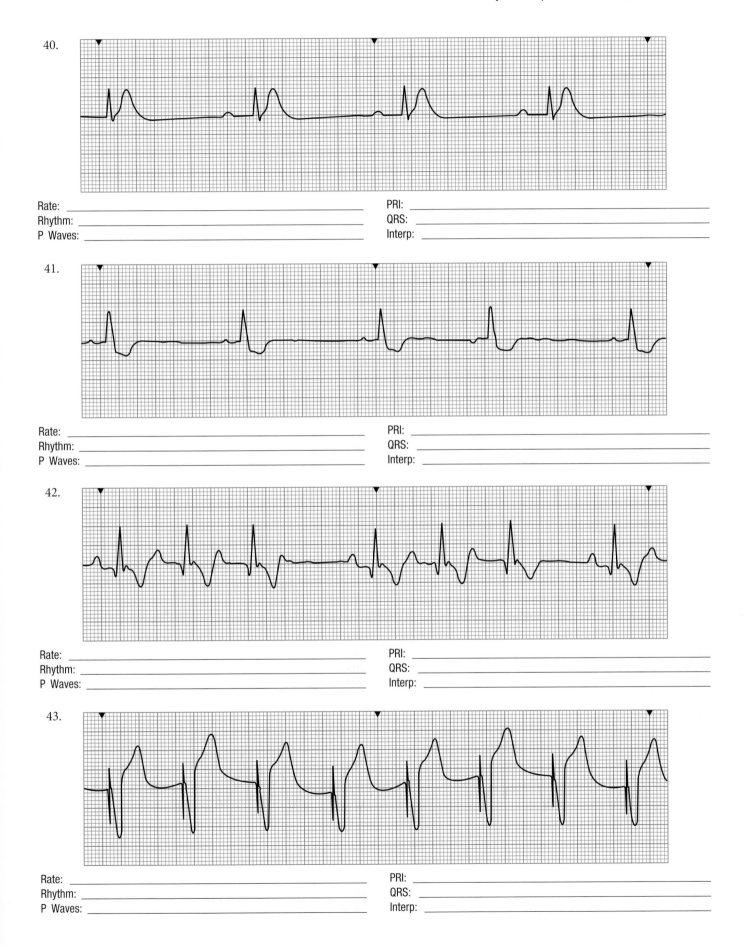

Rate: _____   PRI: _____
Rhythm: _____   QRS: _____
P Waves: _____ Interp: _____

41.

Rate: _____   PRI: _____
Rhythm: _____   QRS: _____
P Waves: _____ Interp: _____

42.

Rate: _____   PRI: _____
Rhythm: _____   QRS: _____
P Waves: _____ Interp: _____

43.

Rate: _____   PRI: _____
Rhythm: _____   QRS: _____
P Waves: _____ Interp: _____

44.

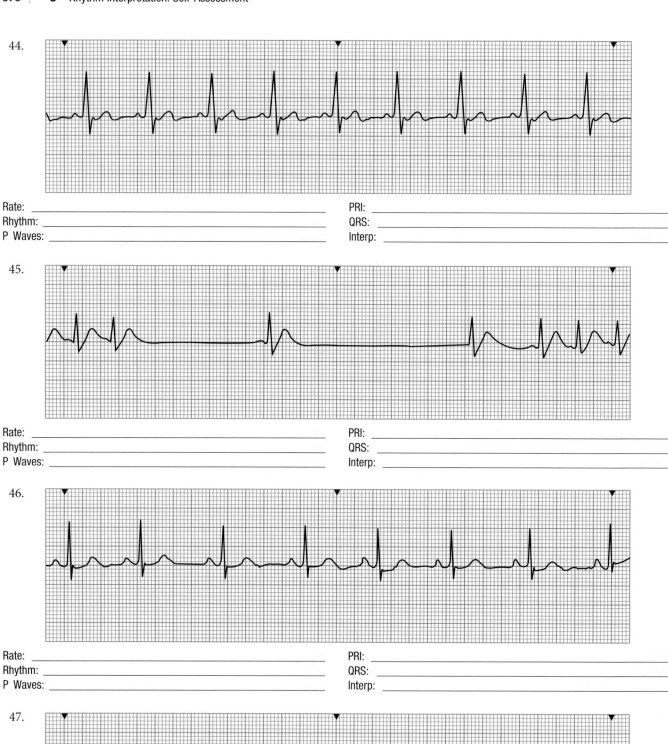

Rate: _____ PRI: _____
Rhythm: _____ QRS: _____
P Waves: _____ Interp: _____

45.

Rate: _____ PRI: _____
Rhythm: _____ QRS: _____
P Waves: _____ Interp: _____

46.

Rate: _____ PRI: _____
Rhythm: _____ QRS: _____
P Waves: _____ Interp: _____

47.

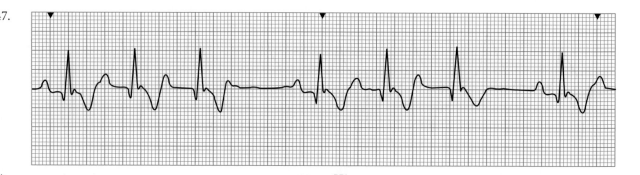

Rate: _____ PRI: _____
Rhythm: _____ QRS: _____
P Waves: _____ Interp:

48.

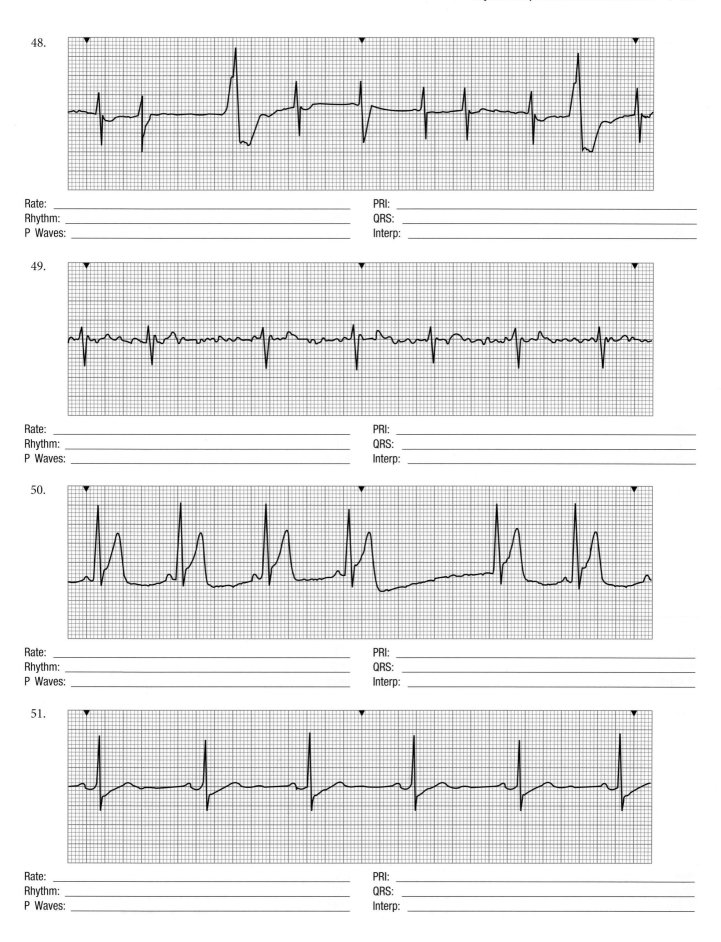

Rate: _____ PRI: _____
Rhythm: _____ QRS: _____
P Waves: _____ Interp: _____

49.

Rate: _____ PRI: _____
Rhythm: _____ QRS: _____
P Waves: _____ Interp: _____

50.

Rate: _____ PRI: _____
Rhythm: _____ QRS: _____
P Waves: _____ Interp: _____

51.

Rate: _____ PRI: _____
Rhythm: _____ QRS: _____
P Waves: _____ Interp: _____

52.

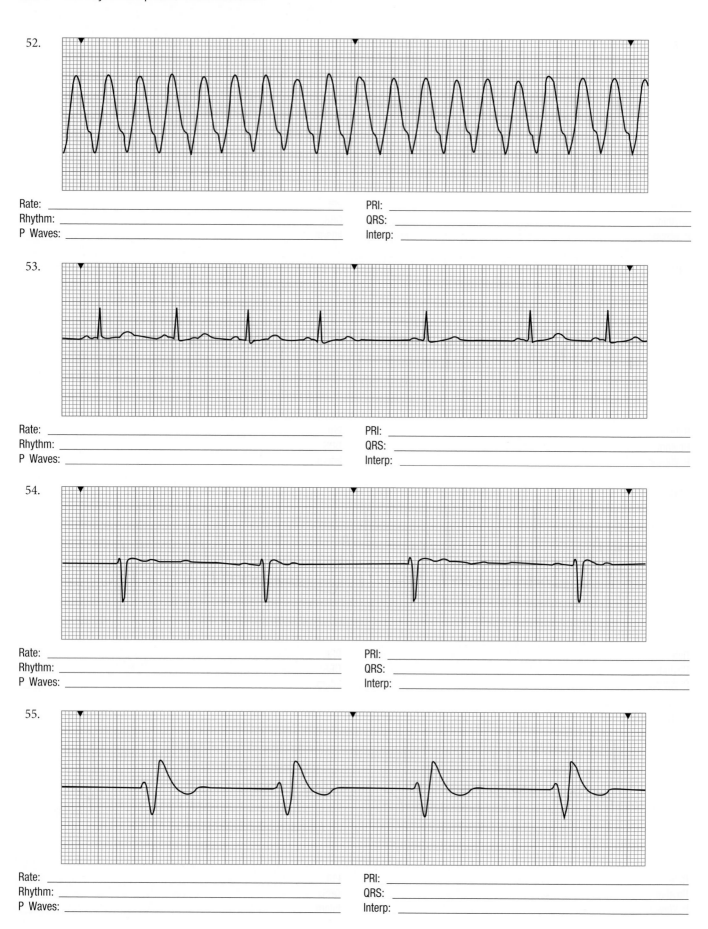

Rate: _____   PRI: _____
Rhythm: _____   QRS: _____
P Waves: _____   Interp: _____

53.

Rate: _____   PRI: _____
Rhythm: _____   QRS: _____
P Waves: _____   Interp: _____

54.

Rate: _____   PRI: _____
Rhythm: _____   QRS: _____
P Waves: _____   Interp: _____

55.

Rate: _____   PRI: _____
Rhythm: _____   QRS: _____
P Waves: _____   Interp: _____

56.

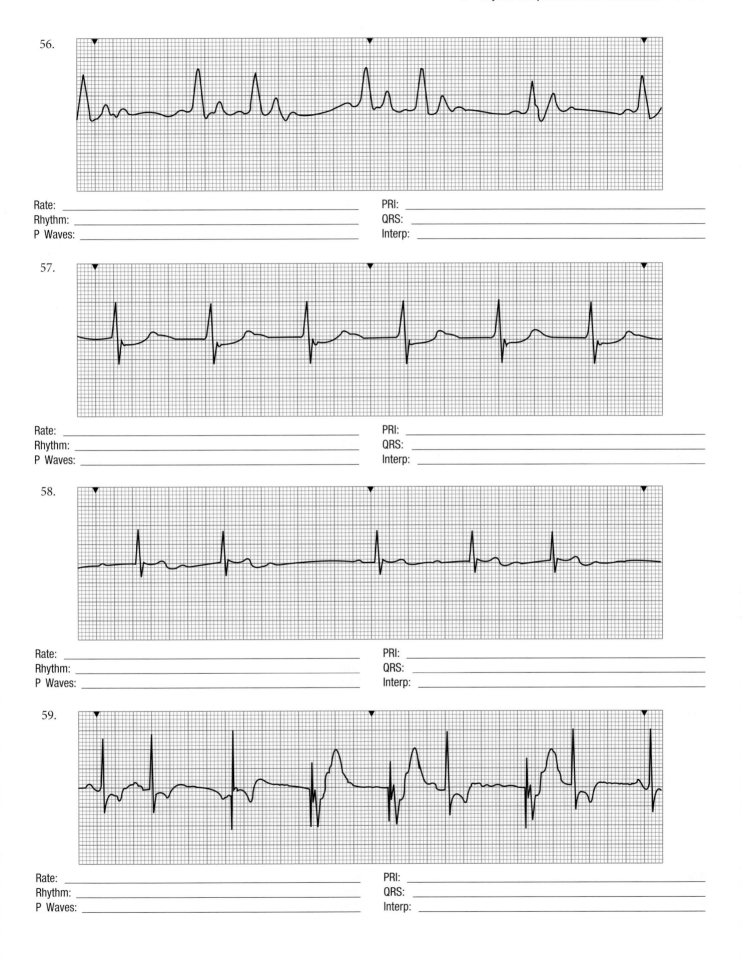

Rate: _____   PRI: _____
Rhythm: _____   QRS: _____
P Waves: _____   Interp: _____

57.

Rate: _____   PRI: _____
Rhythm: _____   QRS: _____
P Waves: _____   Interp: _____

58.

Rate: _____   PRI: _____
Rhythm: _____   QRS: _____
P Waves: _____   Interp: _____

59.

Rate: _____   PRI: _____
Rhythm: _____   QRS: _____
P Waves: _____   Interp: _____

60.

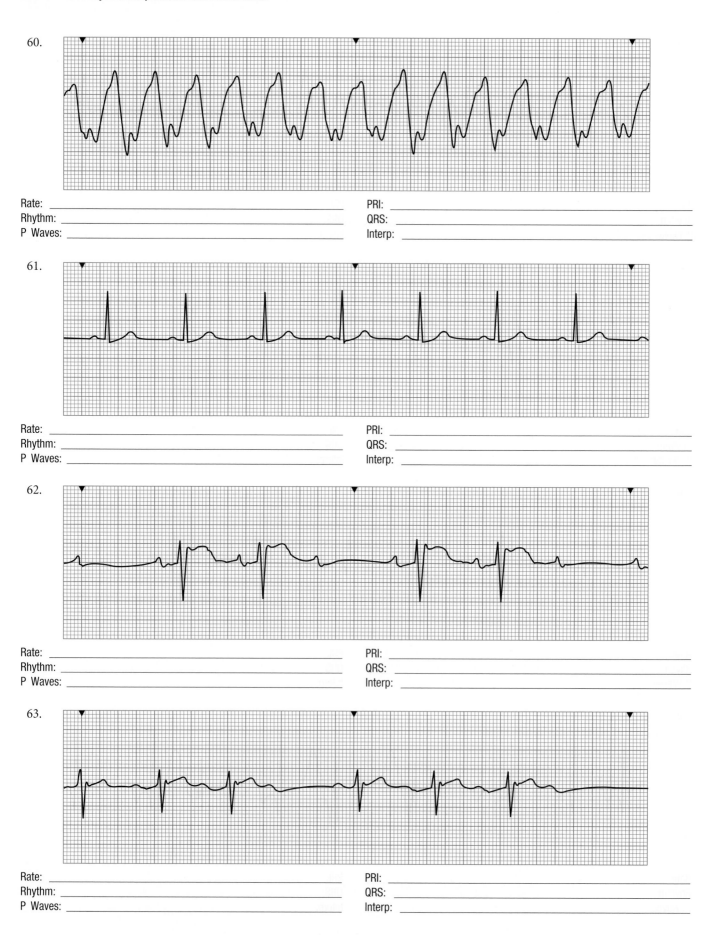

Rate: _____ PRI: _____
Rhythm: _____ QRS: _____
P Waves: _____ Interp: _____

61.

Rate: _____ PRI: _____
Rhythm: _____ QRS: _____
P Waves: _____ Interp: _____

62.

Rate: _____ PRI: _____
Rhythm: _____ QRS: _____
P Waves: _____ Interp: _____

63.

Rate: _____ PRI: _____
Rhythm: _____ QRS: _____
P Waves: _____ Interp: _____

64.

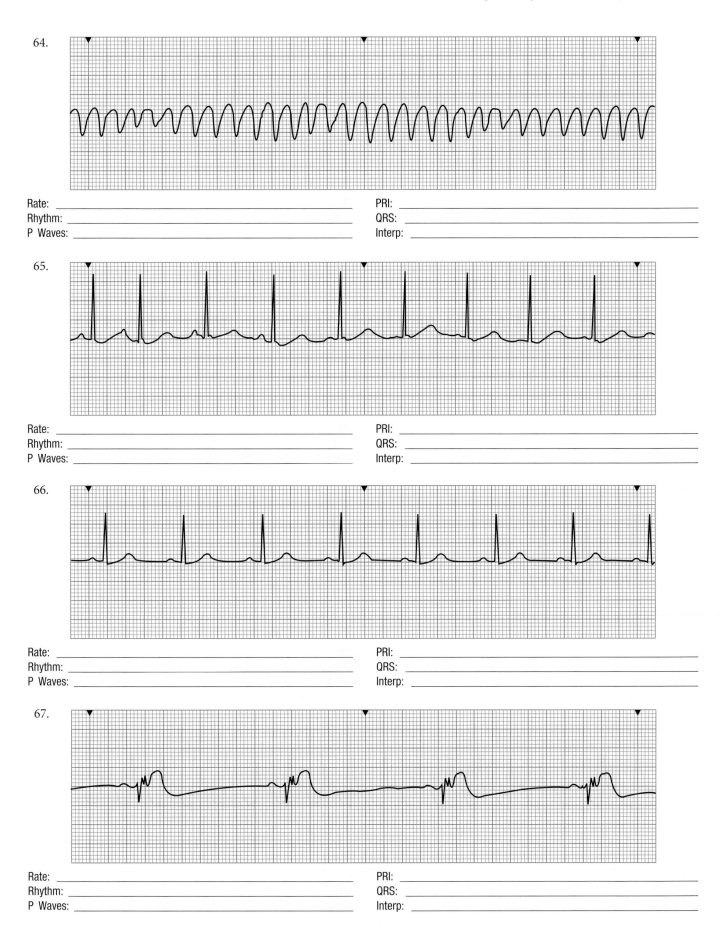

Rate: _____   PRI: _____
Rhythm: _____   QRS: _____
P Waves: _____   Interp: _____

65.

Rate: _____   PRI: _____
Rhythm: _____   QRS: _____
P Waves: _____   Interp: _____

66.

Rate: _____   PRI: _____
Rhythm: _____   QRS: _____
P Waves: _____   Interp: _____

67.

Rate: _____   PRI: _____
Rhythm: _____   QRS: _____
P Waves: _____   Interp: _____

68.

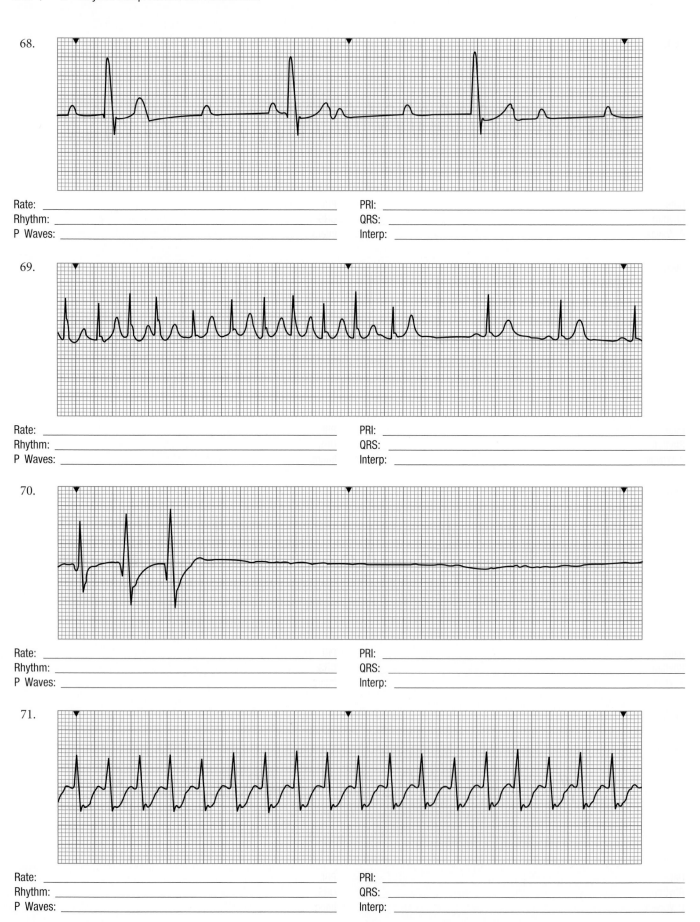

Rate: _____   PRI: _____
Rhythm: _____   QRS: _____
P Waves: _____   Interp: _____

69.

Rate: _____   PRI: _____
Rhythm: _____   QRS: _____
P Waves: _____   Interp: _____

70.

Rate: _____   PRI: _____
Rhythm: _____   QRS: _____
P Waves: _____   Interp: _____

71.

Rate: _____   PRI: _____
Rhythm: _____   QRS: _____
P Waves: _____   Interp: _____

72.

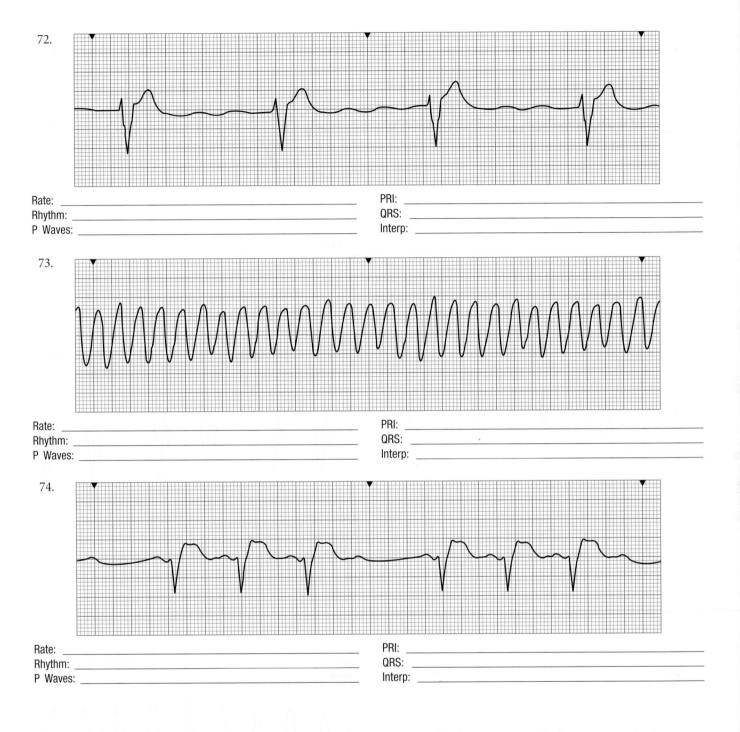

Rate: _____   PRI: _____

Rhythm: _____   QRS: _____

P Waves: _____   Interp: _____

73.

Rate: _____   PRI: _____

Rhythm: _____   QRS: _____

P Waves: _____   Interp: _____

74.

Rate: _____   PRI: _____

Rhythm: _____   QRS: _____

P Waves: _____   Interp: _____

75.

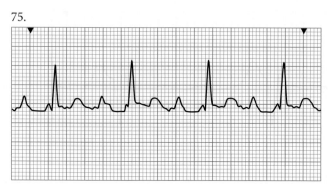

Rate: _____

Rhythm: _____

P Waves: _____

PRI: _____

QRS: _____

Interp: _____

76.

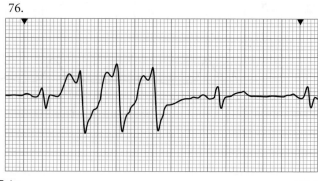

Rate: _____

Rhythm: _____

P Waves: _____

PRI: _____

QRS: _____

Interp: _____

77.

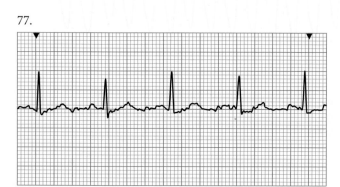

Rate: _____

Rhythm: _____

P Waves: _____

PRI: _____

QRS: _____

Interp: _____

78.

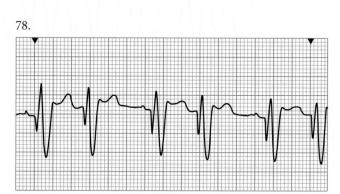

Rate: _____

Rhythm: _____

P Waves: _____

PRI: _____

QRS: _____

Interp: _____

79.

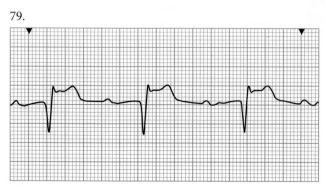

Rate: _____

Rhythm: _____

P Waves: _____

PRI: _____

QRS: _____

Interp: _____

80.

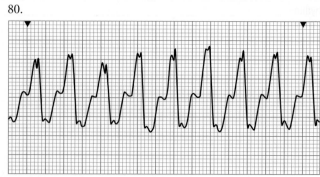

Rate: _____

Rhythm: _____

P Waves: _____

PRI: _____

QRS: _____

Interp: _____

81.

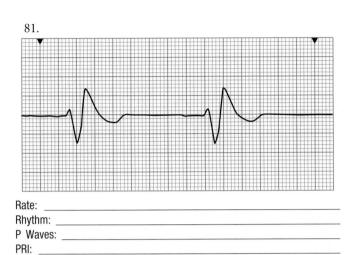

Rate: _____
Rhythm: _____
P Waves: _____
PRI: _____
QRS: _____
Interp: _____

82.

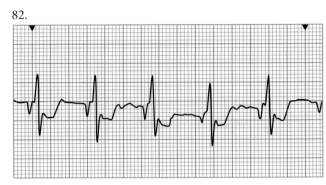

Rate: _____
Rhythm: _____
P Waves: _____
PRI: _____
QRS: _____
Interp: _____

83.

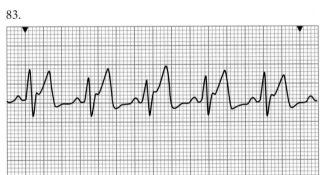

Rate: _____
Rhythm: _____
P Waves: _____
PRI: _____
QRS: _____
Interp: _____

84.

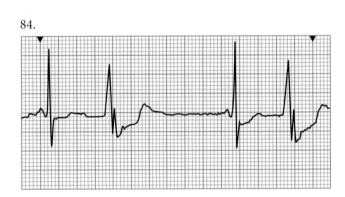

Rate: _____
Rhythm: _____
P Waves: _____
PRI: _____
QRS: _____
Interp: _____

85.

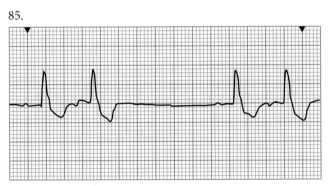

Rate: _____
Rhythm: _____
P Waves: _____
PRI: _____
QRS: _____
Interp: _____

86.

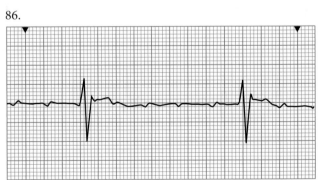

Rate: _____
Rhythm: _____
P Waves: _____
PRI: _____
QRS: _____
Interp: _____

87.

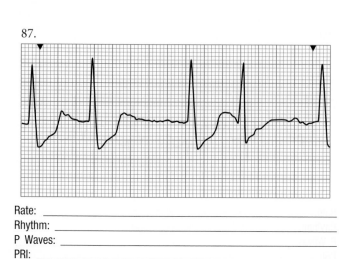

Rate: _____
Rhythm: _____
P Waves: _____
PRI: _____
QRS: _____
Interp: _____

88.

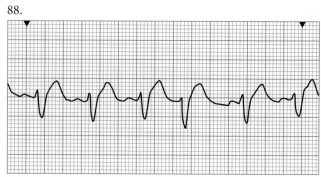

Rate: _____
Rhythm: _____
P Waves: _____
PRI: _____
QRS: _____
Interp: _____

89.

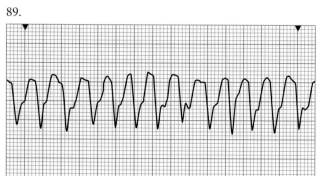

Rate: _____
Rhythm: _____
P Waves: _____
PRI: _____
QRS: _____
Interp: _____

90.

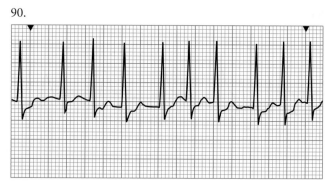

Rate: _____
Rhythm: _____
P Waves: _____
PRI: _____
QRS: _____
Interp: _____

91.

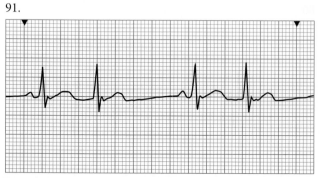

Rate: _____
Rhythm: _____
P Waves: _____
PRI: _____
QRS: _____
Interp: _____

92.

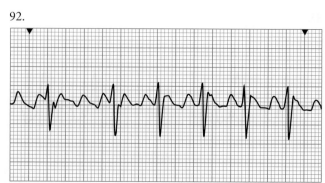

Rate: _____
Rhythm: _____
P Waves: _____
PRI: _____
QRS: _____
Interp: _____

93.

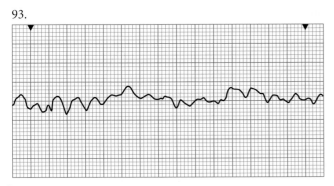

Rate: _____
Rhythm: _____
P Waves: _____
PRI: _____
QRS: _____
Interp: _____

94.

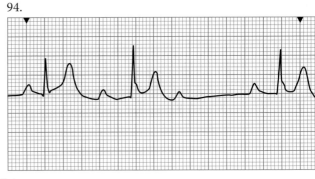

Rate: _____
Rhythm: _____
P Waves: _____
PRI: _____
QRS: _____
Interp: _____

95.

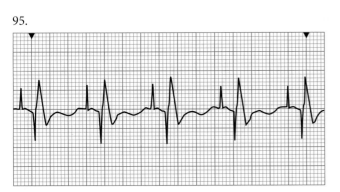

Rate: _____
Rhythm: _____
P Waves: _____
PRI: _____
QRS: _____
Interp: _____

96.

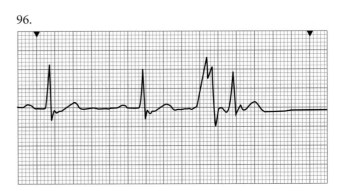

Rate: _____
Rhythm: _____
P Waves: _____
PRI: _____
QRS: _____
Interp: _____

97.

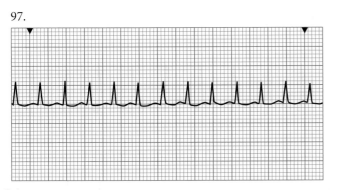

Rate: _____
Rhythm: _____
P Waves: _____
PRI: _____
QRS: _____
Interp: _____

98.

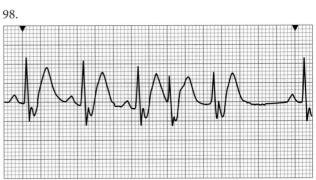

Rate: _____
Rhythm: _____
P Waves: _____
PRI: _____
QRS: _____
Interp: _____

99.

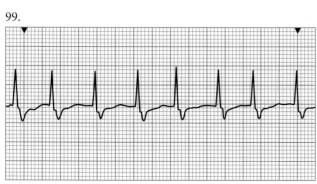

Rate: _____
Rhythm: _____
P Waves: _____
PRI: _____
QRS: _____
Interp: _____

100.

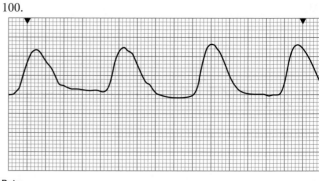

Rate: _____
Rhythm: _____
P Waves: _____
PRI: _____
QRS: _____
Interp: _____

101.

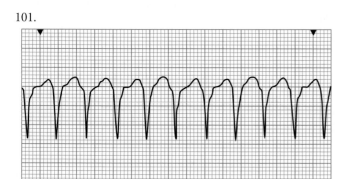

Rate: _____
Rhythm: _____
P Waves: _____
PRI: _____
QRS: _____
Interp: _____

102.

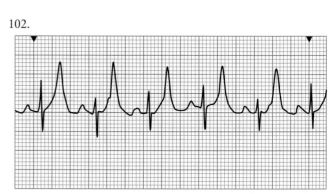

Rate: _____
Rhythm: _____
P Waves: _____
PRI: _____
QRS: _____
Interp: _____

103.

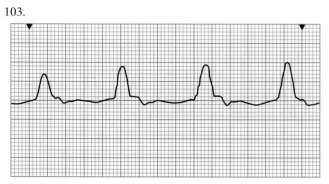

Rate: _____
Rhythm: _____
P Waves: _____
PRI: _____
QRS: _____
Interp: _____

104.

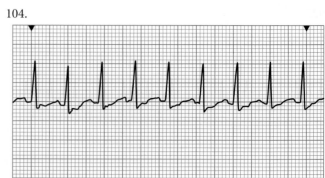

Rate: _____
Rhythm: _____
P Waves: _____
PRI: _____
QRS: _____
Interp: _____

105.

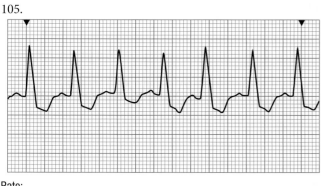

Rate: _____
Rhythm: _____
P Waves: _____
PRI: _____
QRS: _____
Interp: _____

106.

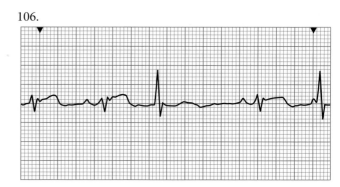

Rate: _____
Rhythm: _____
P Waves: _____
PRI: _____
QRS: _____
Interp: _____

107.

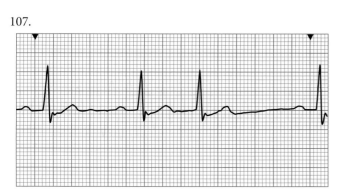

Rate: _____
Rhythm: _____
P Waves: _____
PRI: _____
QRS: _____
Interp: _____

108.

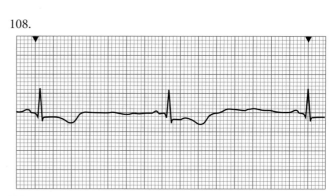

Rate: _____
Rhythm: _____
P Waves: _____
PRI: _____
QRS: _____
Interp: _____

109.

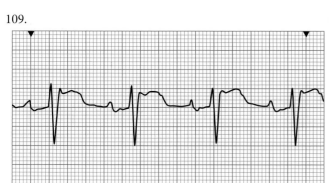

Rate: _____
Rhythm: _____
P Waves: _____
PRI: _____
QRS: _____
Interp: _____

110.

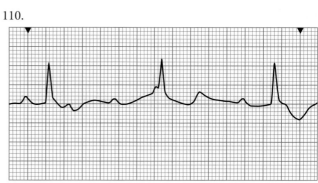

Rate: _____
Rhythm: _____
P Waves: _____
PRI: _____
QRS: _____
Interp: _____

111.

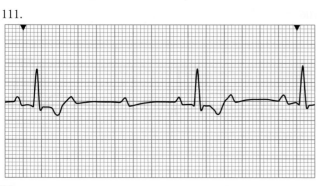

Rate: _____

Rhythm: _____

P Waves: _____

PRI: _____

QRS: _____

Interp: _____

112.

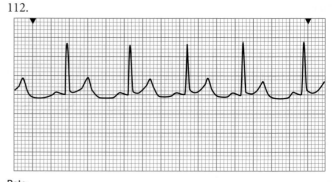

Rate: _____

Rhythm: _____

P Waves: _____

PRI: _____

QRS: _____

Interp: _____

113.

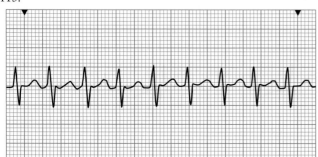

Rate: _____

Rhythm: _____

P Waves: _____

PRI: _____

QRS: _____

Interp: _____

114.

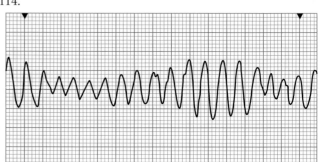

Rate: _____

Rhythm: _____

P Waves: _____

PRI: _____

QRS: _____

Interp: _____

115.

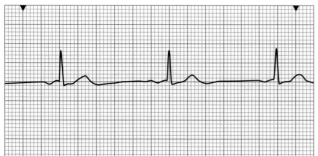

Rate: _____

Rhythm: _____

P Waves: _____

PRI: _____

QRS: _____

Interp: _____

116.

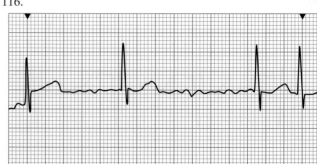

Rate: _____

Rhythm: _____

P Waves: _____

PRI: _____

QRS: _____

Interp: _____

117.

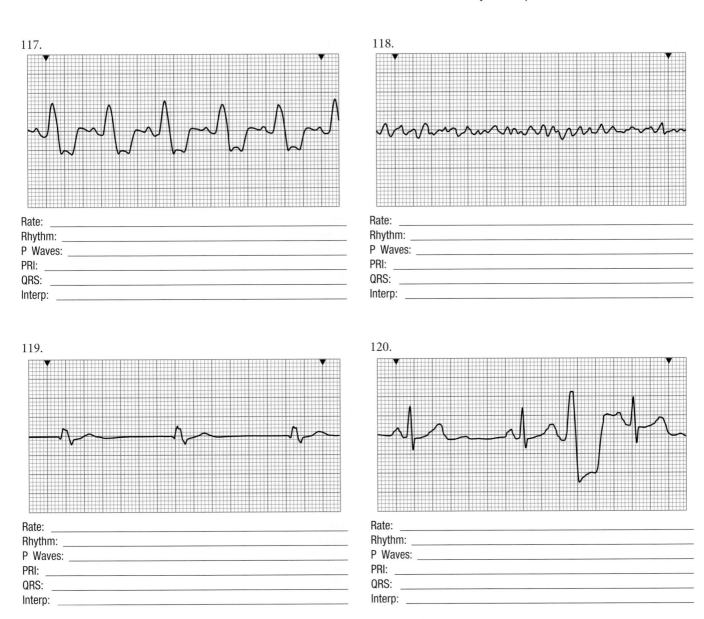

Rate: _____
Rhythm: _____
P Waves: _____
PRI: _____
QRS: _____
Interp: _____

118.

Rate: _____
Rhythm: _____
P Waves: _____
PRI: _____
QRS: _____
Interp: _____

119.

Rate: _____
Rhythm: _____
P Waves: _____
PRI: _____
QRS: _____
Interp: _____

120.

Rate: _____
Rhythm: _____
P Waves: _____
PRI: _____
QRS: _____
Interp: _____

121.

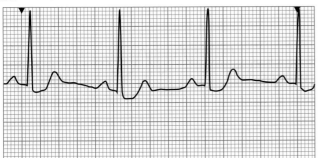

Rate: _____
Rhythm: _____
P Waves: _____
PRI: _____
QRS: _____
Interp: _____

122.

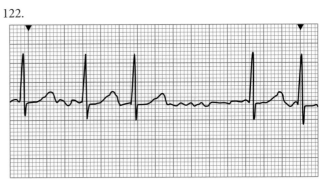

Rate: _____
Rhythm: _____
P Waves: _____
PRI: _____
QRS: _____
Interp: _____

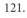

123.

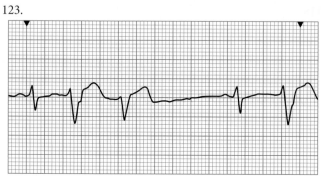

Rate: _____

Rhythm: _____

P Waves: _____

PRI: _____

QRS: _____

Interp: _____

124.

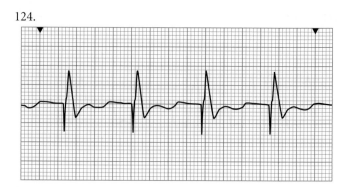

Rate: _____

Rhythm: _____

P Waves: _____

PRI: _____

QRS: _____

Interp: _____

125.

Rate: _____

Rhythm: _____

P Waves: _____

PRI: _____

QRS: _____

Interp: _____

126.

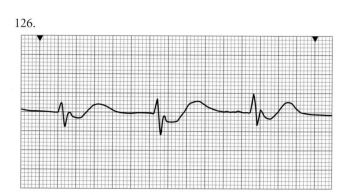

Rate: _____

Rhythm: _____

P Waves: _____

PRI: _____

QRS: _____

Interp: _____

127.

Rate: _____

Rhythm: _____

P Waves: _____

PRI: _____

QRS: _____

Interp: _____

128.

Rate: _____

Rhythm: _____

P Waves: _____

PRI: _____

QRS: _____

Interp: _____

129.

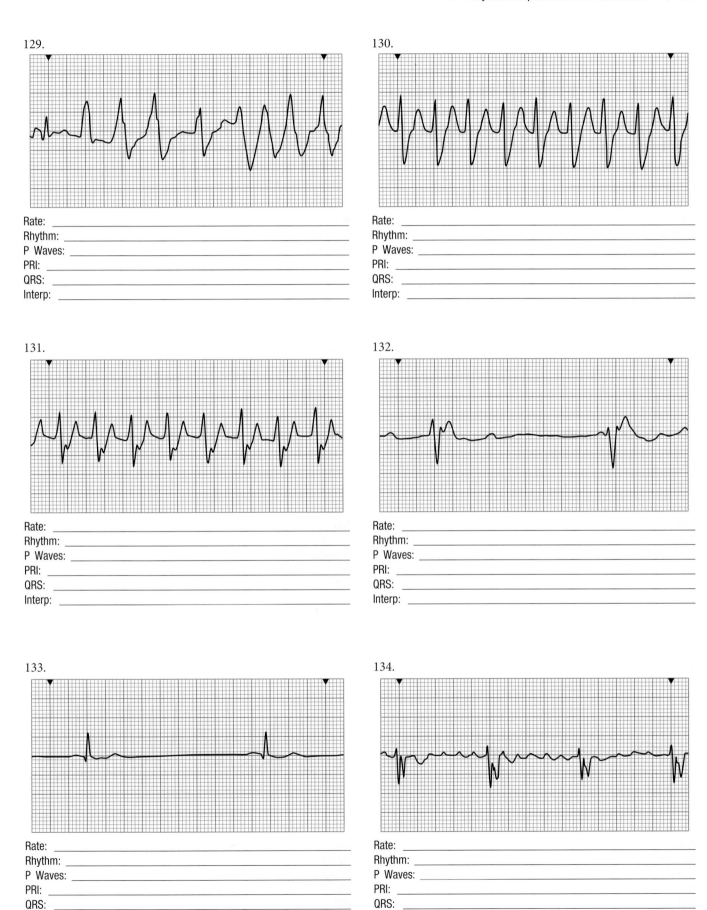

Rate: _____
Rhythm: _____
P Waves: _____
PRI: _____
QRS: _____
Interp: _____

130.

Rate: _____
Rhythm: _____
P Waves: _____
PRI: _____
QRS: _____
Interp: _____

131.

Rate: _____
Rhythm: _____
P Waves: _____
PRI: _____
QRS: _____
Interp: _____

132.

Rate: _____
Rhythm: _____
P Waves: _____
PRI: _____
QRS: _____
Interp: _____

133.

Rate: _____
Rhythm: _____
P Waves: _____
PRI: _____
QRS: _____
Interp: _____

134.

Rate: _____
Rhythm: _____
P Waves: _____
PRI: _____
QRS: _____
Interp: _____

135.

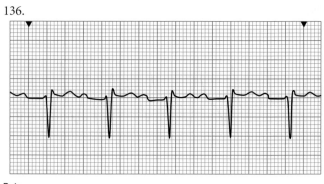

Rate: _____
Rhythm: _____
P Waves: _____
PRI: _____
QRS: _____
Interp: _____

136.

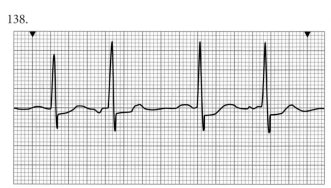

Rate: _____
Rhythm: _____
P Waves: _____
PRI: _____
QRS: _____
Interp: _____

137.

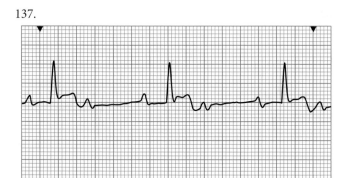

Rate: _____
Rhythm: _____
P Waves: _____
PRI: _____
QRS: _____
Interp: _____

138.

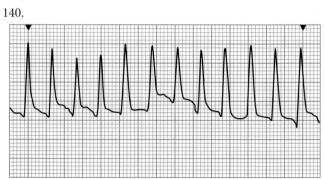

Rate: _____
Rhythm: _____
P Waves: _____
PRI: _____
QRS: _____
Interp: _____

139.

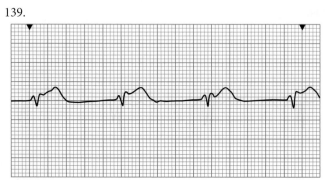

Rate: _____
Rhythm: _____
P Waves: _____
PRI: _____
QRS: _____
Interp: _____

140.

Rate: _____
Rhythm: _____
P Waves: _____
PRI: _____
QRS: _____
Interp: _____

141.

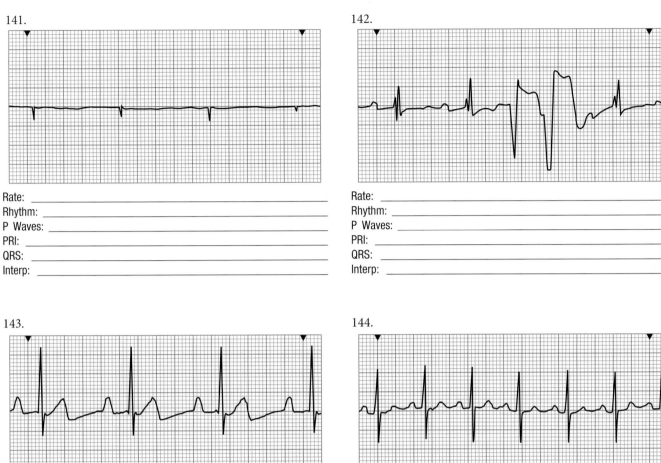

Rate: _____
Rhythm: _____
P Waves: _____
PRI: _____
QRS: _____
Interp: _____

142.

Rate: _____
Rhythm: _____
P Waves: _____
PRI: _____
QRS: _____
Interp: _____

143.

Rate: _____
Rhythm: _____
P Waves: _____
PRI: _____
QRS: _____
Interp: _____

144.

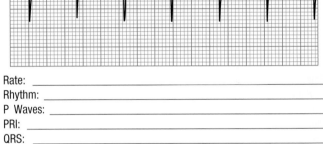

Rate: _____
Rhythm: _____
P Waves: _____
PRI: _____
QRS: _____
Interp: _____

145.

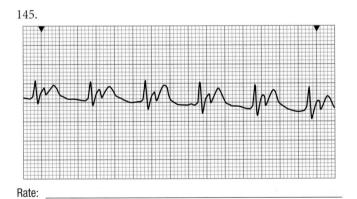

Rate: _____
Rhythm: _____
P Waves: _____
PRI: _____
QRS: _____
Interp: _____

146.

Rate: _____
Rhythm: _____
P Waves: _____
PRI: _____
QRS: _____
Interp: _____

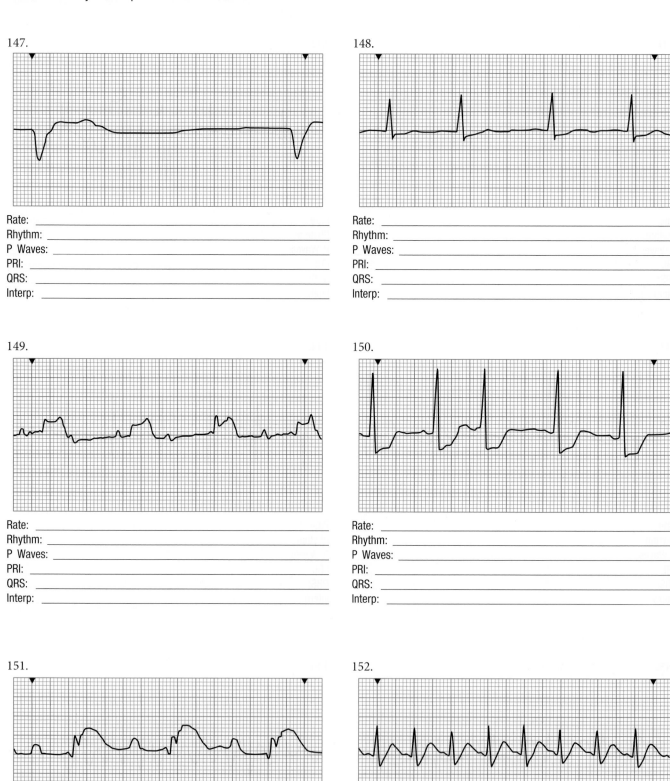

147.

Rate: _____
Rhythm: _____
P Waves: _____
PRI: _____
QRS: _____
Interp: _____

148.

Rate: _____
Rhythm: _____
P Waves: _____
PRI: _____
QRS: _____
Interp: _____

149.

Rate: _____
Rhythm: _____
P Waves: _____
PRI: _____
QRS: _____
Interp: _____

150.

Rate: _____
Rhythm: _____
P Waves: _____
PRI: _____
QRS: _____
Interp: _____

151.

Rate: _____
Rhythm: _____
P Waves: _____
PRI: _____
QRS: _____
Interp: _____

152.

Rate: _____
Rhythm: _____
P Waves: _____
PRI: _____
QRS: _____
Interp: _____

153.

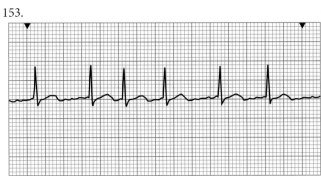

Rate: _____
Rhythm: _____
P Waves: _____
PRI: _____
QRS: _____
Interp: _____

154.

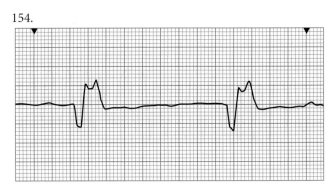

Rate: _____
Rhythm: _____
P Waves: _____
PRI: _____
QRS: _____
Interp: _____

155.

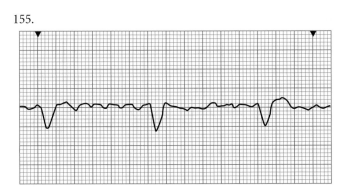

Rate: _____
Rhythm: _____
P Waves: _____
PRI: _____
QRS: _____
Interp: _____

156.

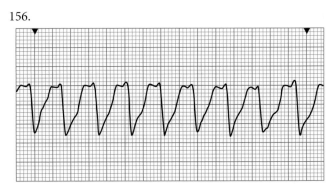

Rate: _____
Rhythm: _____
P Waves: _____
PRI: _____
QRS: _____
Interp: _____

157.

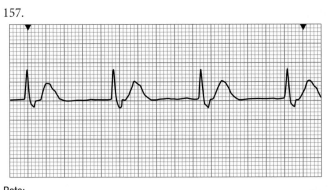

Rate: _____
Rhythm: _____
P Waves: _____
PRI: _____
QRS: _____
Interp: _____

158.

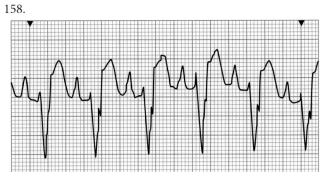

Rate: _____
Rhythm: _____
P Waves: _____
PRI: _____
QRS: _____
Interp: _____

159.

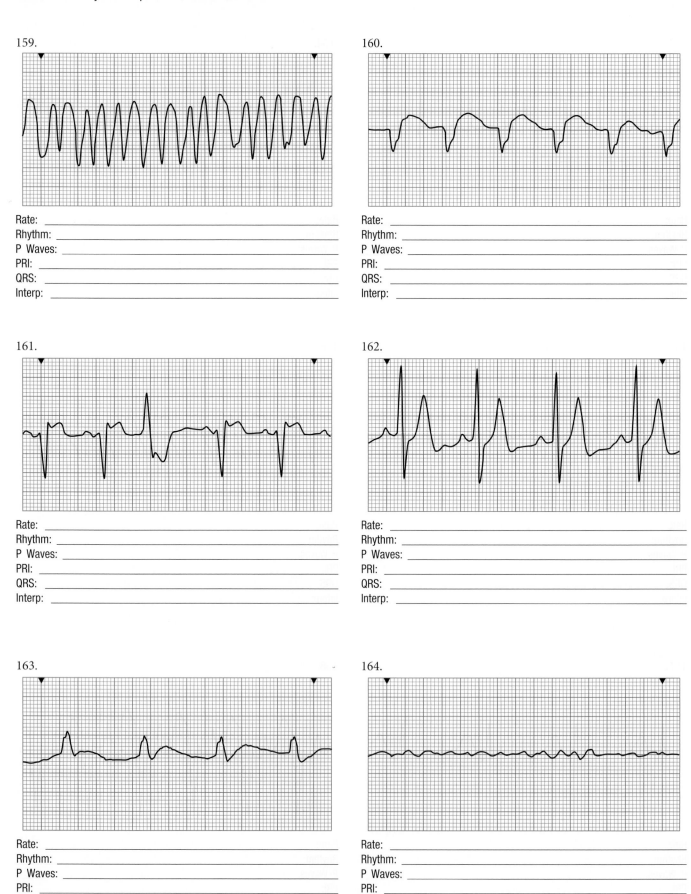

Rate: _____

Rhythm: _____

P Waves: _____

PRI: _____

QRS: _____

Interp: _____

160.

Rate: _____

Rhythm: _____

P Waves: _____

PRI: _____

QRS: _____

Interp: _____

161.

Rate: _____

Rhythm: _____

P Waves: _____

PRI: _____

QRS: _____

Interp: _____

162.

Rate: _____

Rhythm: _____

P Waves: _____

PRI: _____

QRS: _____

Interp: _____

163.

Rate: _____

Rhythm: _____

P Waves: _____

PRI: _____

QRS: _____

Interp: _____

164.

Rate: _____

Rhythm: _____

P Waves: _____

PRI: _____

QRS: _____

Interp: _____

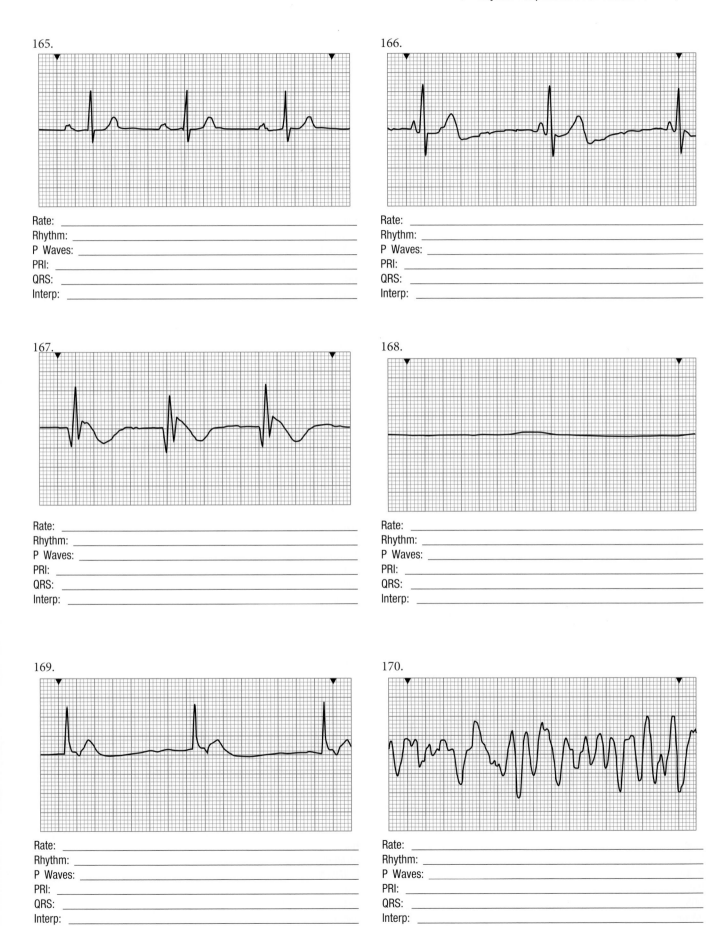

165.

Rate: _____
Rhythm: _____
P Waves: _____
PRI: _____
QRS: _____
Interp: _____

166.

Rate: _____
Rhythm: _____
P Waves: _____
PRI: _____
QRS: _____
Interp: _____

167.

Rate: _____
Rhythm: _____
P Waves: _____
PRI: _____
QRS: _____
Interp: _____

168.

Rate: _____
Rhythm: _____
P Waves: _____
PRI: _____
QRS: _____
Interp: _____

169.

Rate: _____
Rhythm: _____
P Waves: _____
PRI: _____
QRS: _____
Interp: _____

170.

Rate: _____
Rhythm: _____
P Waves: _____
PRI: _____
QRS: _____
Interp: _____

171.

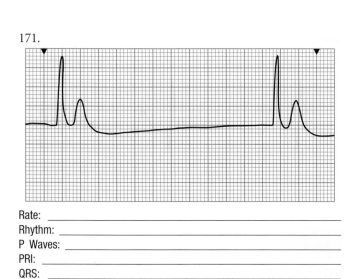

Rate: _____
Rhythm: _____
P Waves: _____
PRI: _____
QRS: _____
Interp: _____

172.

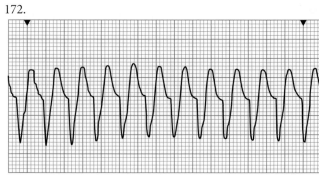

Rate: _____
Rhythm: _____
P Waves: _____
PRI: _____
QRS: _____
Interp: _____

173.

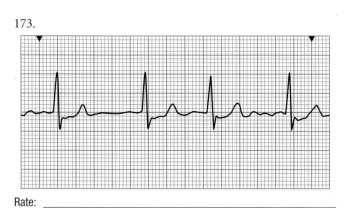

Rate: _____
Rhythm: _____
P Waves: _____
PRI: _____
QRS: _____
Interp: _____

174.

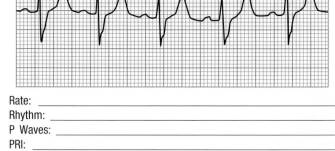

Rate: _____
Rhythm: _____
P Waves: _____
PRI: _____
QRS: _____
Interp: _____

175.

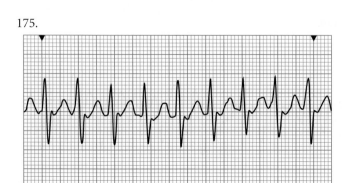

Rate: _____
Rhythm: _____
P Waves: _____
PRI: _____
QRS: _____
Interp: _____

176.

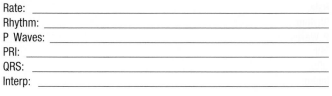

Rate: _____
Rhythm: _____
P Waves: _____
PRI: _____
QRS: _____
Interp: _____

177.

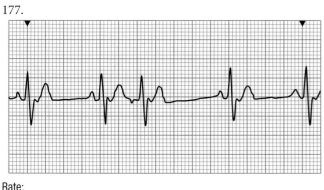

Rate: _____
Rhythm: _____
P Waves: _____
PRI: _____
QRS: _____
Interp: _____

178.

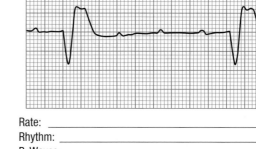

Rate: _____
Rhythm: _____
P Waves: _____
PRI: _____
QRS: _____
Interp: _____

179.

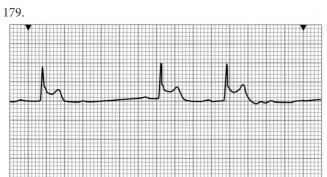

Rate: _____
Rhythm: _____
P Waves: _____
PRI: _____
QRS: _____
Interp: _____

180.

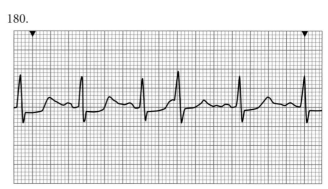

Rate: _____
Rhythm: _____
P Waves: _____
PRI: _____
QRS: _____
Interp: _____

181.

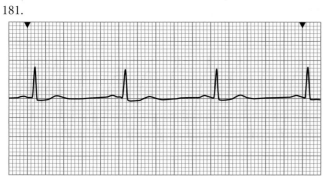

Rate: _____
Rhythm: _____
P Waves: _____
PRI: _____
QRS: _____
Interp: _____

182.

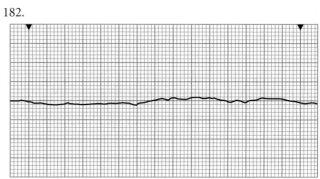

Rate: _____
Rhythm: _____
P Waves: _____
PRI: _____
QRS: _____
Interp: _____

183.

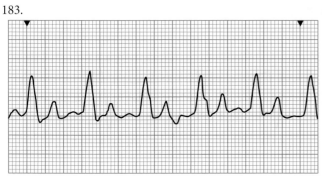

Rate: _____

Rhythm: _____

P Waves: _____

PRI: _____

QRS: _____

Interp: _____

184.

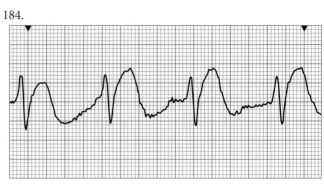

Rate: _____

Rhythm: _____

P Waves: _____

PRI: _____

QRS: _____

Interp: _____

185.

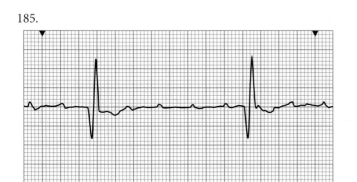

Rate: _____

Rhythm: _____

P Waves: _____

PRI: _____

QRS: _____

Interp: _____

186.

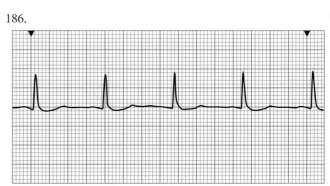

Rate: _____

Rhythm: _____

P Waves: _____

PRI: _____

QRS: _____

Interp: _____

187.

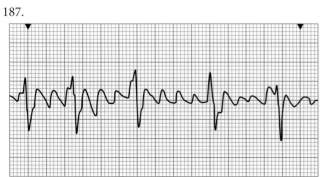

Rate: _____

Rhythm: _____

P Waves: _____

PRI: _____

QRS: _____

Interp: _____

188.

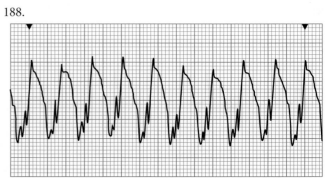

Rate: _____

Rhythm: _____

P Waves: _____

PRI: _____

QRS: _____

Interp: _____

189.

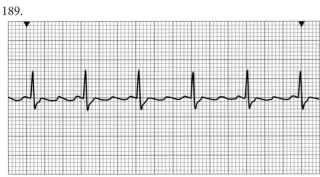

Rate: _____
Rhythm: _____
P Waves: _____
PRI: _____
QRS: _____
Interp: _____

190.

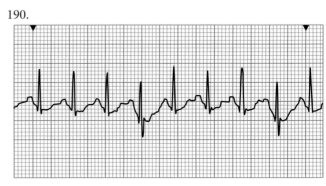

Rate: _____
Rhythm: _____
P Waves: _____
PRI: _____
QRS: _____
Interp: _____

191.

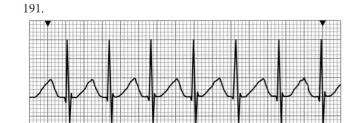

Rate: _____
Rhythm: _____
P Waves: _____
PRI: _____
QRS: _____
Interp: _____

192.

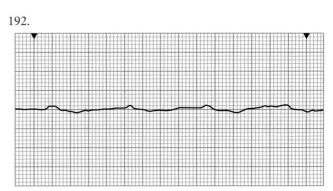

Rate: _____
Rhythm: _____
P Waves: _____
PRI: _____
QRS: _____
Interp: _____

193.

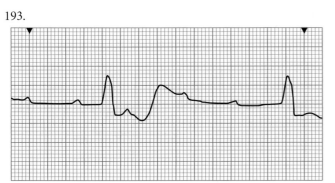

Rate: _____
Rhythm: _____
P Waves: _____
PRI: _____
QRS: _____
Interp: _____

194.

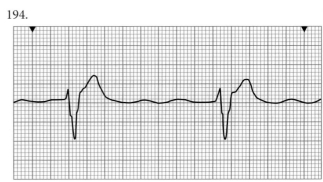

Rate: _____
Rhythm: _____
P Waves: _____
PRI: _____
QRS: _____
Interp: _____

195.

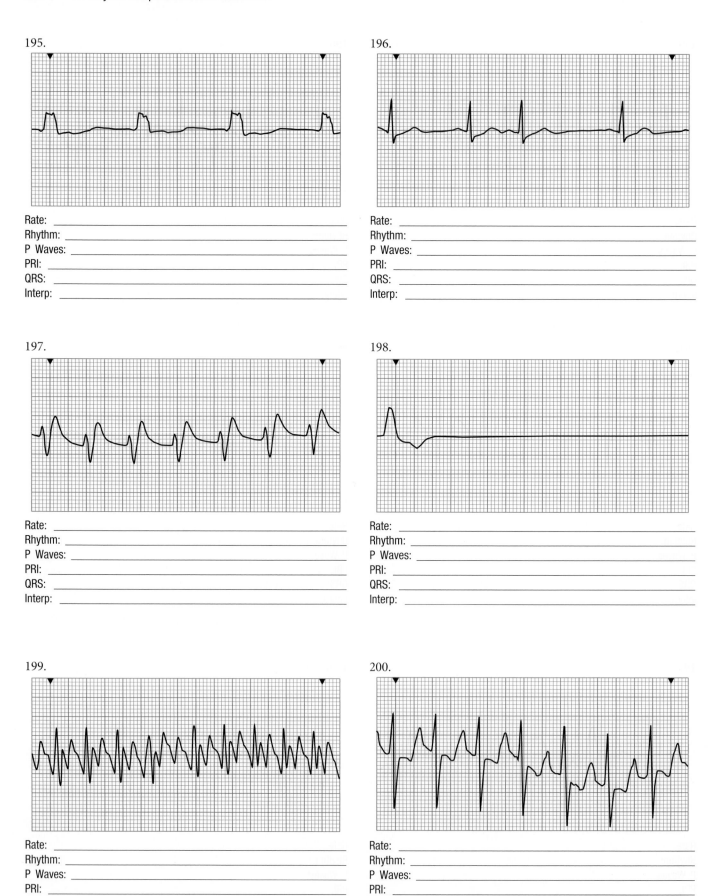

Rate: _____
Rhythm: _____
P Waves: _____
PRI: _____
QRS: _____
Interp: _____

196.

Rate: _____
Rhythm: _____
P Waves: _____
PRI: _____
QRS: _____
Interp: _____

197.

Rate: _____
Rhythm: _____
P Waves: _____
PRI: _____
QRS: _____
Interp: _____

198.

Rate: _____
Rhythm: _____
P Waves: _____
PRI: _____
QRS: _____
Interp: _____

199.

Rate: _____
Rhythm: _____
P Waves: _____
PRI: _____
QRS: _____
Interp: _____

200.

Rate: _____
Rhythm: _____
P Waves: _____
PRI: _____
QRS: _____
Interp: _____

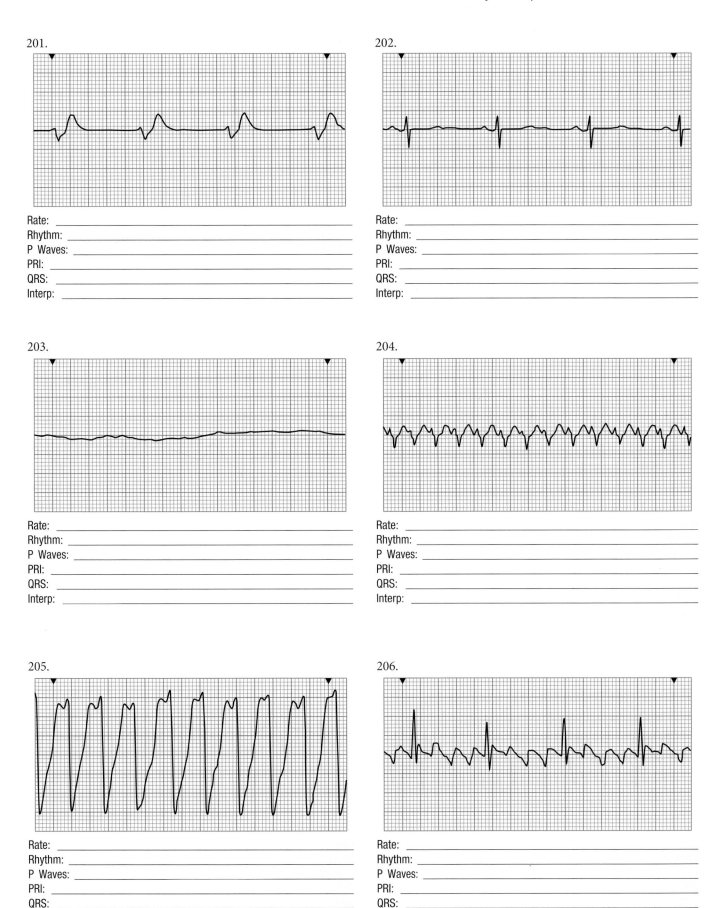

201.

Rate: _____
Rhythm: _____
P Waves: _____
PRI: _____
QRS: _____
Interp: _____

202.

Rate: _____
Rhythm: _____
P Waves: _____
PRI: _____
QRS: _____
Interp: _____

203.

Rate: _____
Rhythm: _____
P Waves: _____
PRI: _____
QRS: _____
Interp: _____

204.

Rate: _____
Rhythm: _____
P Waves: _____
PRI: _____
QRS: _____
Interp: _____

205.

Rate: _____
Rhythm: _____
P Waves: _____
PRI: _____
QRS: _____
Interp: _____

206.

Rate: _____
Rhythm: _____
P Waves: _____
PRI: _____
QRS: _____
Interp: _____

207.

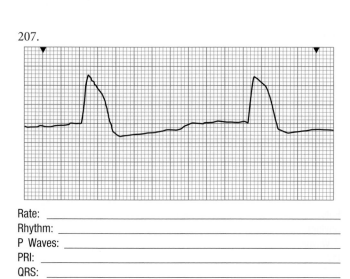

Rate: _____
Rhythm: _____
P Waves: _____
PRI: _____
QRS: _____
Interp: _____

208.

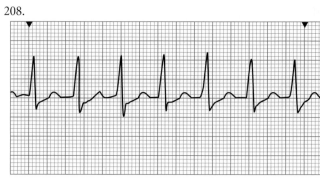

Rate: _____
Rhythm: _____
P Waves: _____
PRI: _____
QRS: _____
Interp: _____

209.

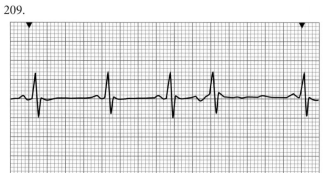

Rate: _____
Rhythm: _____
P Waves: _____
PRI: _____
QRS: _____
Interp: _____

210.

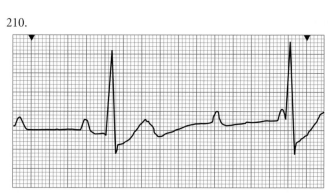

Rate: _____
Rhythm: _____
P Waves: _____
PRI: _____
QRS: _____
Interp: _____

211.

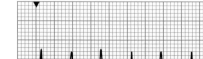
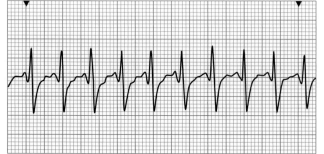

Rate: _____
Rhythm: _____
P Waves: _____
PRI: _____
QRS: _____
Interp: _____

212.

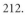
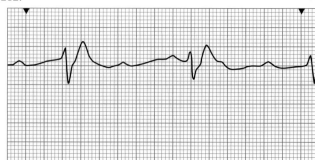

Rate: _____
Rhythm: _____
P Waves: _____
PRI: _____
QRS: _____
Interp: _____

213.

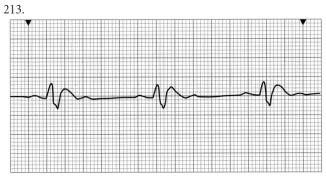

Rate: _____
Rhythm: _____
P Waves: _____
PRI: _____
QRS: _____
Interp: _____

214.

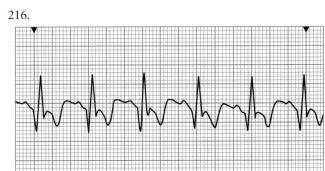

Rate: _____
Rhythm: _____
P Waves: _____
PRI: _____
QRS: _____
Interp: _____

215.

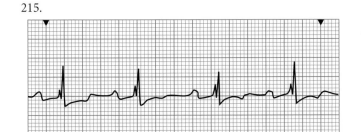

Rate: _____
Rhythm: _____
P Waves: _____
PRI: _____
QRS: _____
Interp: _____

216.

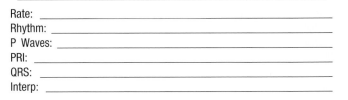

Rate: _____
Rhythm: _____
P Waves: _____
PRI: _____
QRS: _____
Interp: _____

217.

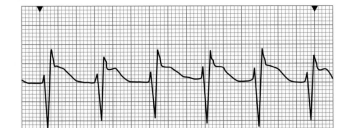

Rate: _____
Rhythm: _____
P Waves: _____
PRI: _____
QRS: _____
Interp: _____

218.

Rate: _____
Rhythm: _____
P Waves: _____
PRI: _____
QRS: _____
Interp: _____

219.

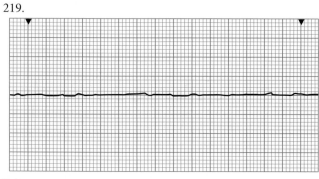

Rate: _____

Rhythm: _____

P Waves: _____

PRI: _____

QRS: _____

Interp: _____

220.

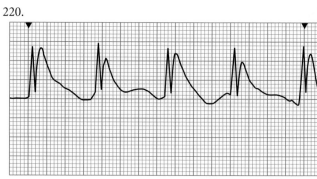

Rate: _____

Rhythm: _____

P Waves: _____

PRI: _____

QRS: _____

Interp: _____

221.

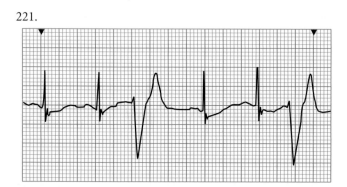

Rate: _____

Rhythm: _____

P Waves: _____

PRI: _____

QRS: _____

Interp: _____

222.

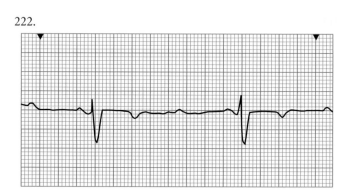

Rate: _____

Rhythm: _____

P Waves: _____

PRI: _____

QRS: _____

Interp: _____

223.

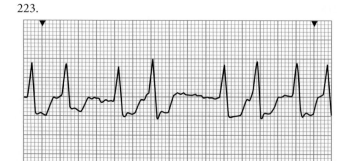

Rate: _____

Rhythm: _____

P Waves: _____

PRI: _____

QRS: _____

Interp: _____

224.

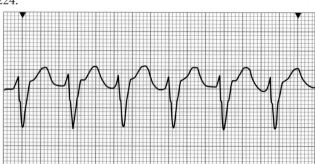

Rate: _____

Rhythm: _____

P Waves: _____

PRI: _____

QRS: _____

Interp: _____

II. BUNDLE BRANCH AND FASCICULAR BLOCKS

225.

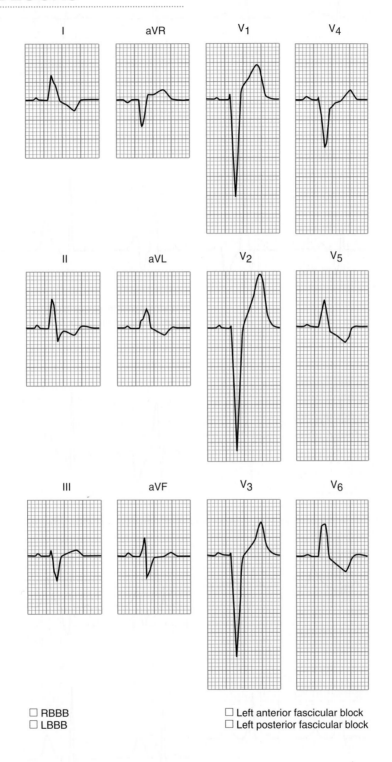

☐ RBBB
☐ LBBB

☐ Left anterior fascicular block
☐ Left posterior fascicular block

226.

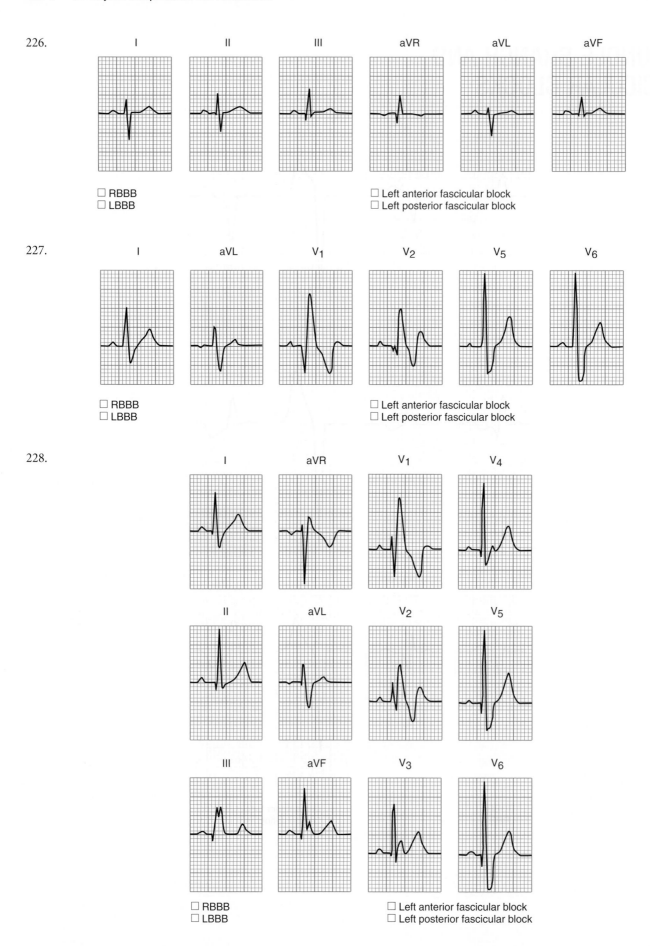

| I | II | III | aVR | aVL | aVF |

☐ RBBB
☐ LBBB

☐ Left anterior fascicular block
☐ Left posterior fascicular block

227.

| I | aVL | V₁ | V₂ | V₅ | V₆ |

☐ RBBB
☐ LBBB

☐ Left anterior fascicular block
☐ Left posterior fascicular block

228.

I	aVR	V₁	V₄
II	aVL	V₂	V₅
III	aVF	V₃	V₆

☐ RBBB
☐ LBBB

☐ Left anterior fascicular block
☐ Left posterior fascicular block

229.

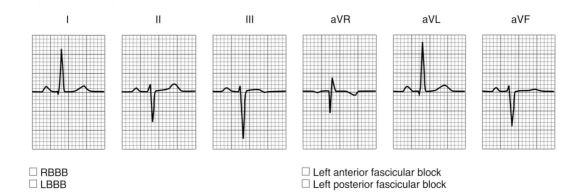

☐ RBBB   ☐ Left anterior fascicular block
☐ LBBB   ☐ Left posterior fascicular block

III. MYOCARDIAL INFARCTIONS

230.

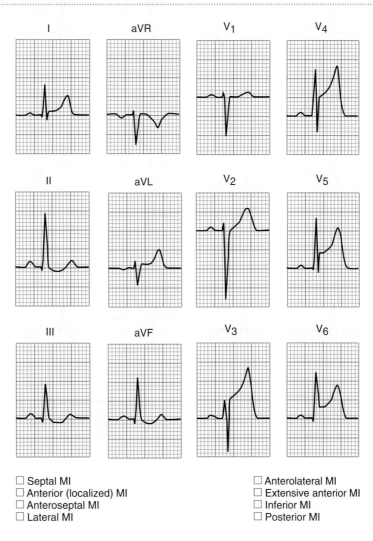

☐ Septal MI   ☐ Anterolateral MI
☐ Anterior (localized) MI   ☐ Extensive anterior MI
☐ Anteroseptal MI   ☐ Inferior MI
☐ Lateral MI   ☐ Posterior MI

231.

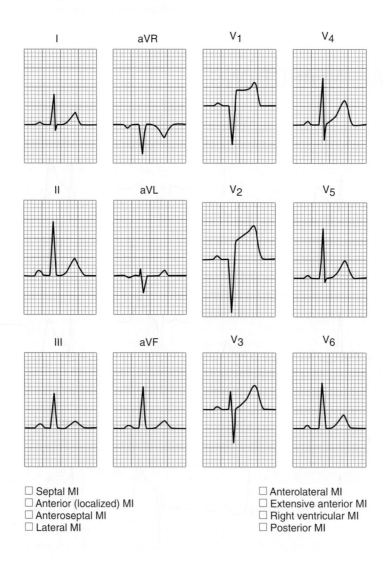

☐ Septal MI
☐ Anterior (localized) MI
☐ Anteroseptal MI
☐ Lateral MI

☐ Anterolateral MI
☐ Extensive anterior MI
☐ Right ventricular MI
☐ Posterior MI

232.

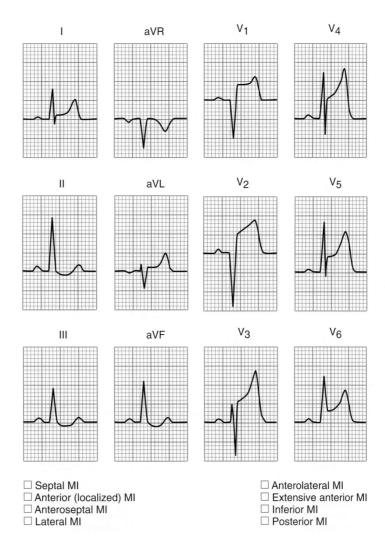

☐ Septal MI
☐ Anterior (localized) MI
☐ Anteroseptal MI
☐ Lateral MI

☐ Anterolateral MI
☐ Extensive anterior MI
☐ Inferior MI
☐ Posterior MI

233.

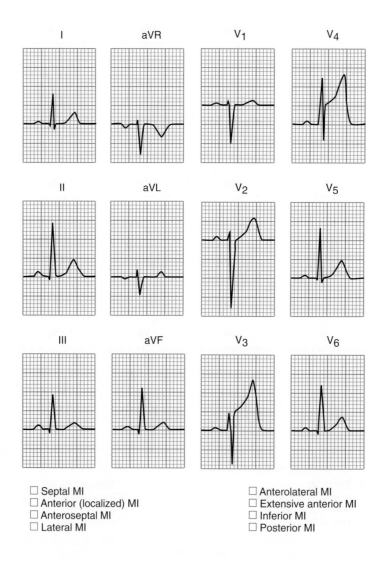

☐ Septal MI
☐ Anterior (localized) MI
☐ Anteroseptal MI
☐ Lateral MI

☐ Anterolateral MI
☐ Extensive anterior MI
☐ Inferior MI
☐ Posterior MI

234.

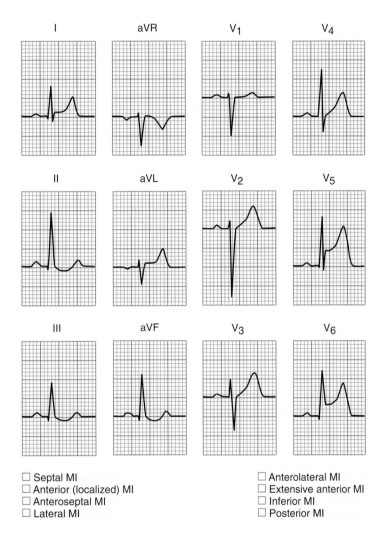

I	aVR	V₁	V₄
II	aVL	V₂	V₅
III	aVF	V₃	V₆

☐ Septal MI
☐ Anterior (localized) MI
☐ Anteroseptal MI
☐ Lateral MI

☐ Anterolateral MI
☐ Extensive anterior MI
☐ Inferior MI
☐ Posterior MI

235.

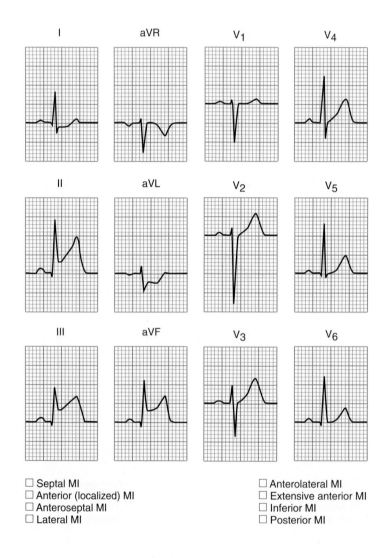

☐ Septal MI
☐ Anterior (localized) MI
☐ Anteroseptal MI
☐ Lateral MI

☐ Anterolateral MI
☐ Extensive anterior MI
☐ Inferior MI
☐ Posterior MI

236.

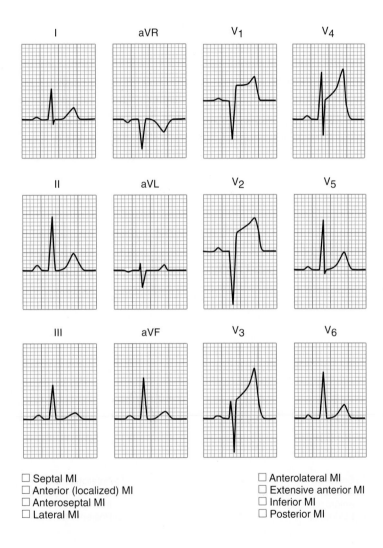

I	aVR	V₁	V₄
II	aVL	V₂	V₅
III	aVF	V₃	V₆

☐ Septal MI
☐ Anterior (localized) MI
☐ Anteroseptal MI
☐ Lateral MI

☐ Anterolateral MI
☐ Extensive anterior MI
☐ Inferior MI
☐ Posterior MI

237.

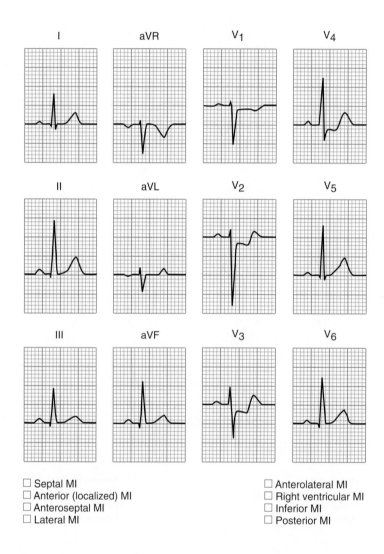

I   aVR   V₁   V₄
II   aVL   V₂   V₅
III   aVF   V₃   V₆

☐ Septal MI
☐ Anterior (localized) MI
☐ Anteroseptal MI
☐ Lateral MI

☐ Anterolateral MI
☐ Right ventricular MI
☐ Inferior MI
☐ Posterior MI

238.

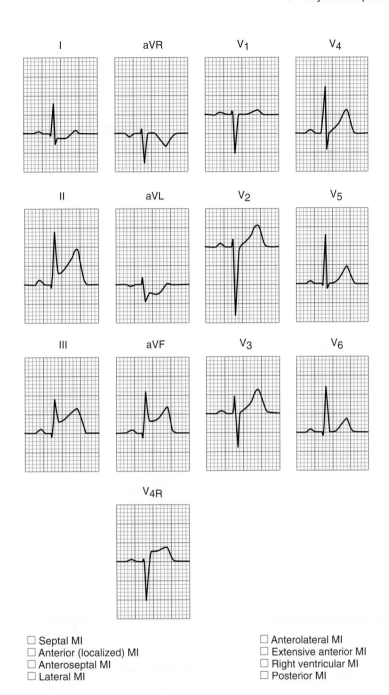

☐ Septal MI
☐ Anterior (localized) MI
☐ Anteroseptal MI
☐ Lateral MI

☐ Anterolateral MI
☐ Extensive anterior MI
☐ Right ventricular MI
☐ Posterior MI

IV. QRS AXES

239.

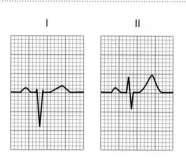

  ☐ QRS axis: −30° to −90°   ☐ QRS axis: 0° to +30°
  ☐ QRS axis: +90° to +150°   ☐ QRS axis: +150°
  ☐ QRS axis: +90°   ☐ QRS axis: 0° to −30°

240.

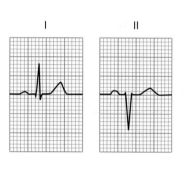

  ☐ QRS axis: −30° to −90°   ☐ QRS axis: 0° to +30°
  ☐ QRS axis: +90° to +150°   ☐ QRS axis: +150°
  ☐ QRS axis: +90°   ☐ QRS axis: 0° to −30°

241.

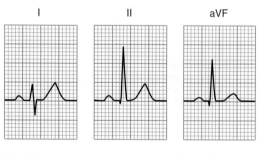

  ☐ QRS axis: −30° to −90°   ☐ QRS axis: 0° to +30°
  ☐ QRS axis: +90° to +150°   ☐ QRS axis: +150°
  ☐ QRS axis: +90°   ☐ QRS axis: 0° to −30°

242.

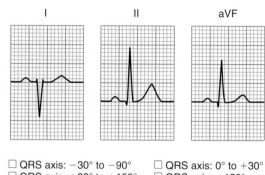

  ☐ QRS axis: −30° to −90°   ☐ QRS axis: 0° to +30°
  ☐ QRS axis: +90° to +150°   ☐ QRS axis: +150°
  ☐ QRS axis: +90°   ☐ QRS axis: 0° to −30°

243.

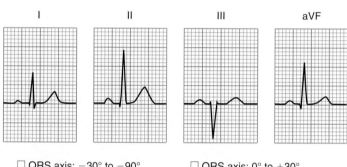

  ☐ QRS axis: −30° to −90°   ☐ QRS axis: 0° to +30°
  ☐ QRS axis: +90° to +150°   ☐ QRS axis: +150°
  ☐ QRS axis: +90°   ☐ QRS axis: 0° to −30°

244.

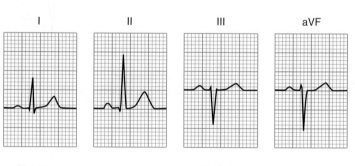

  ☐ QRS axis: −30° to −90°   ☐ QRS axis: 0° to +30°
  ☐ QRS axis: +90° to +150°   ☐ QRS axis: +150°
  ☐ QRS axis: +90°   ☐ QRS axis: 0° to −30°

V. ECG CHANGES: DRUG AND ELECTROLYTE

245.

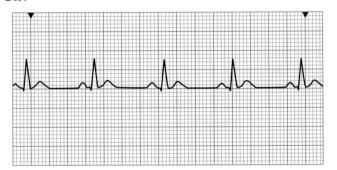

- ☐ Hyperkalemia
- ☐ Hypokalemia
- ☐ Hypercalcemia
- ☐ Hypocalcemia
- ☐ Digitalis effect
- ☐ Procainamide/quinidine toxicity

246.

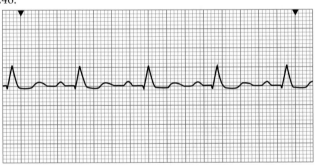

- ☐ Hyperkalemia
- ☐ Hypokalemia
- ☐ Hypercalcemia
- ☐ Hypocalcemia
- ☐ Digitalis effect
- ☐ Procainamide/quinidine toxicity

247.

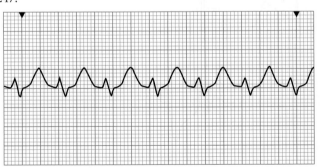

- ☐ Hyperkalemia
- ☐ Hypokalemia
- ☐ Hypercalcemia
- ☐ Hypocalcemia
- ☐ Digitalis effect
- ☐ Procainamide/quinidine toxicity

248.

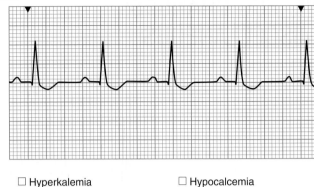

- ☐ Hyperkalemia
- ☐ Hypokalemia
- ☐ Hypercalcemia
- ☐ Hypocalcemia
- ☐ Digitalis effect
- ☐ Procainamide/quinidine toxicity

249.

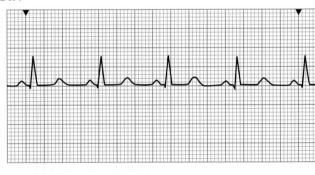

- ☐ Hyperkalemia
- ☐ Hypokalemia
- ☐ Hypercalcemia
- ☐ Hypocalcemia
- ☐ Digitalis effect
- ☐ Procainamide/quinidine toxicity

250.

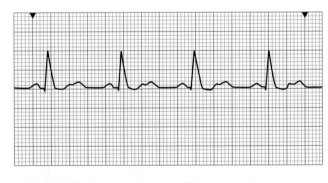

- ☐ Hyperkalemia
- ☐ Hypokalemia
- ☐ Hypercalcemia
- ☐ Hypocalcemia
- ☐ Digitalis effect
- ☐ Procainamide/quinidine toxicity

VI. ECG CHANGES: MISCELLANEOUS

251.

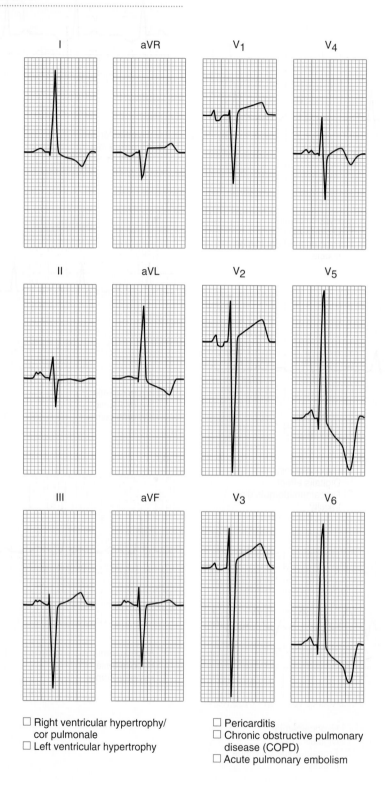

☐ Right ventricular hypertrophy/
   cor pulmonale
☐ Left ventricular hypertrophy

☐ Pericarditis
☐ Chronic obstructive pulmonary
   disease (COPD)
☐ Acute pulmonary embolism

252.

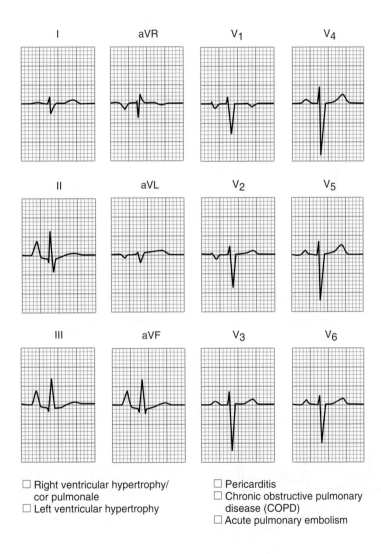

I aVR V₁ V₄

II aVL V₂ V₅

III aVF V₃ V₆

☐ Right ventricular hypertrophy/
   cor pulmonale
☐ Left ventricular hypertrophy

☐ Pericarditis
☐ Chronic obstructive pulmonary
   disease (COPD)
☐ Acute pulmonary embolism

253.

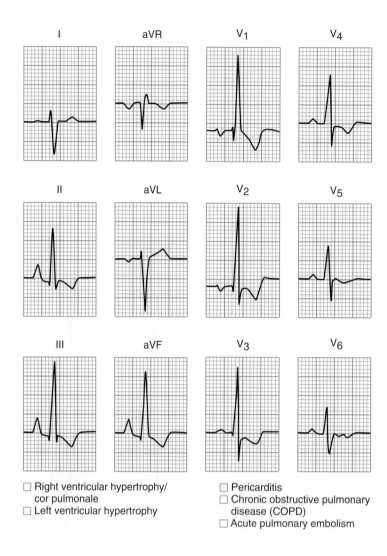

☐ Right ventricular hypertrophy/
cor pulmonale
☐ Left ventricular hypertrophy

☐ Pericarditis
☐ Chronic obstructive pulmonary
disease (COPD)
☐ Acute pulmonary embolism

254.

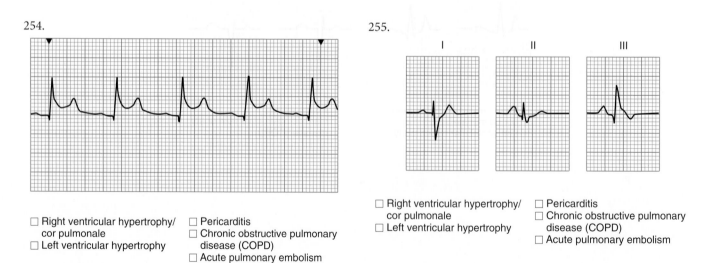

☐ Right ventricular hypertrophy/
cor pulmonale
☐ Left ventricular hypertrophy

☐ Pericarditis
☐ Chronic obstructive pulmonary
disease (COPD)
☐ Acute pulmonary embolism

255.

☐ Right ventricular hypertrophy/
cor pulmonale
☐ Left ventricular hypertrophy

☐ Pericarditis
☐ Chronic obstructive pulmonary
disease (COPD)
☐ Acute pulmonary embolism

256.

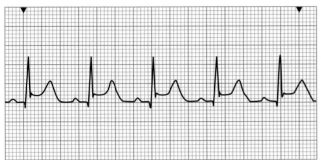

☐ Hypothermia
☐ Nodoventricular/fasciculo-
   ventricular preexcitation

☐ Ventricular preexcitation
☐ Early repolarization
☐ Atrio-His preexcitation

257.

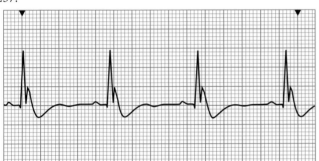

☐ Hypothermia
☐ Nodoventricular/fasciculo-
   ventricular preexcitation

☐ Ventricular preexcitation
☐ Early repolarization
☐ Atrio-His preexcitation

258.

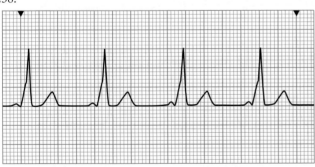

☐ Hypothermia
☐ Nodoventricular/fasciculo-
   ventricular preexcitation

☐ Ventricular preexcitation
☐ Early repolarization
☐ Atrio-His preexcitation

259.

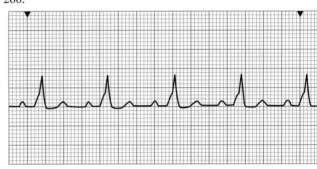

☐ Hypothermia
☐ Nodoventricular/fasciculo-
   ventricular preexcitation

☐ Ventricular preexcitation
☐ Early repolarization
☐ Atrio-His preexcitation

260.

☐ Hypothermia
☐ Nodoventricular/fasciculo-
   ventricular preexcitation

☐ Ventricular preexcitation
☐ Early repolarization
☐ Atrio-His preexcitation

VII. SCENARIOS

Scenario 1

The ambulance is dispatched to a local shopping center for a female who has "fainted." On arrival you find a 62-year-old female, who is alert and oriented. She is sitting on a chair accompanied by her daughter. She states she just completed her home peritoneal dialysis when she decided to go shopping. The patient states she has a history of renal failure, CHF, and takes "a water pill, potassium, and a baby aspirin." She denies any allergies. On examination you find the patient's skin warm, pink, and moist. Lungs are clear bilaterally. BP 104/60, P 62 and regular, R 24, and O_2 saturations 95%. You apply the cardiac monitor and see the following rhythm:

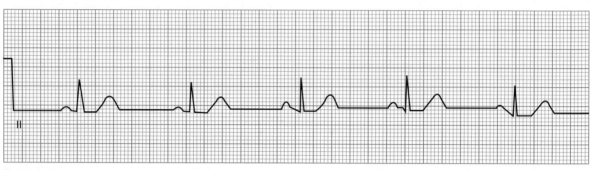

Scenario 1

261. The monitor reveals:
    A. normal sinus rhythm
    B. sinus arrhythmia
    C. sinus bradycardia
    D. wandering atrial pacemaker

Because of the syncopal episode you elect to obtain a 12-lead.

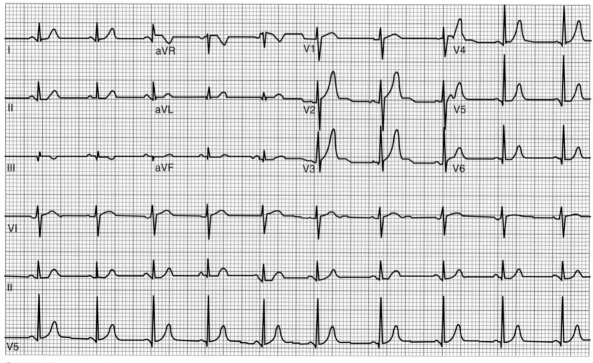

Scenario 1

262. The most striking finding on this patient's 12-Lead ECG is:
   A. anterior wall ST elevation
   B. peaked T waves in the precordial leads
   C. poor R wave progression across the precordial leads
   D. prolonged QT interval
263. The changes noted in question 2 are caused by:
   A. coronary artery occlusion
   B. hyperkalemia
   C. hypocalcemia
   D. hypothermia

Scenario 2

A 33-year-old female comes to the emergency room with complaints of her "sudden onset of heart pounding and missing beats." She states she has had this before once or twice but this is the worst one. She denies chest pain, but does say she feels weak. She has a history of insulin-dependent diabetes, but is very compliant with her testing and medications. She states she does not take any other medicines and is allergic to PCN. She is A & O x4, skin warm, pink, and dry. BP 110/70, P weak and rapid, and RR 24. After applying the monitor you see the following:

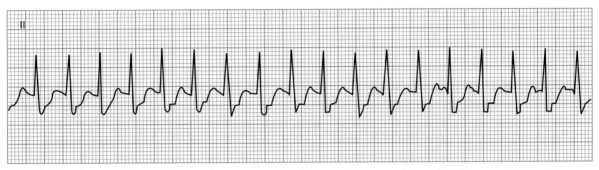

Scenario 2

264. The dysrhythmia is most likely:
   A. atrial flutter with 1:1 conduction
   B. atrial tachycardia
   C. paroxysmal supraventricular tachycardia
   D. sinus tachycardia
265. If the patient was stable but the QRS were wide, what step would assist in differentiating this rhythm from ventricular tachycardia?
   A. 12-Lead ECG
   B. administration of 6 mg adenosine IV
   C. administration of 150 mg amiodarone IV
   D. vagal maneuvers

266. This dysrhythmia is caused by:
   A. early repolarization of the AV node
   B. ectopic focus in the atria firing rapidly
   C. partial block of conduction through the AV node
   D. reentry mechanism from the AV node into the accessory pathways between the SA and AV node

Scenario 3

An 82-year-old man comes to ED complaining of flulike symptoms. He is concerned because he has not been able to get the immunization and was instructed to do so by his physician. He complains of nausea, some slight difficulty breathing, chills, and chest tightness. His skin is pale, cool, and clammy. BP 94/64, P 50 weak and regular, RR 20. He does not remember his medication but his son is bringing them in. He needs assistance getting onto the ED cart. Once on the monitor you find the following:

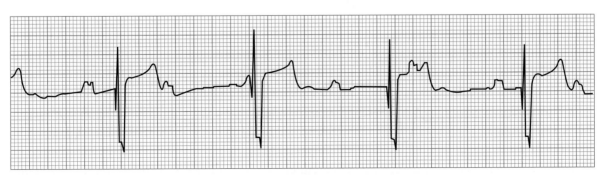

Scenario 3

267. The rhythm on the monitor is:
    A. first AVB
    B. second AVB Type I
    C. second AVB Type II
    D. third AVB
268. The QRS most likely originates from:
    A. AV node
    B. bundle of His
    C. Purkinje network
    D. SA node
269. The most appropriate initial therapy for this condition is:
    A. administration of 1 mg atropine
    B. administration of 1 mg epinephrine
    C. initiate transcutaneous pacing
    D. lay the patient supine and administer oxygen and establish vascular access

Scenario 4

You are called to an office building for a 57-year-old man with dizziness. His secretary states that the patient came in all week with a cold. Today when he got up to go to a meeting he fell to the floor, but did not lose consciousness. You find him sitting in a chair. He seems a little confused, but states he is "perfectly healthy" other than this sinus "thing." He has been taking over-the-counter decongestants and Tylenol, but takes no other medication. His skin is pale, cool, and clammy. BP 80/56, P absent at wrist, RR 18, and O_2 saturations 96%. You see the following rhythm on the monitor:

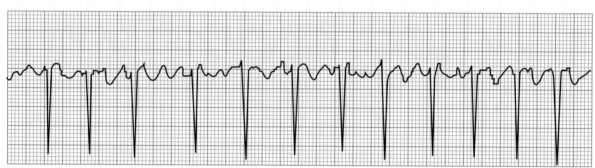

Scenario 4

270. The rhythm on the monitor is:
    A. atrial fib/flutter with rapid ventricular response
    B. multiatrial tachycardia
    C. paroxysmal supraventricular tachycardia
    D. sinus tachycardia with PACs
271. The regularity of this rhythm is referred to as:
    A. regular
    B. patterned irregularity
    C. unpatterned irregularity
    D. grossly or irregularly irregular

272. The most likely cause for the dysrhythmia in this patient is:
    A. acute myocardial infarction
    B. adrenergic stimulation from decongestants
    C. dehydration
    D. reentrant mechanism in the AV node

Scenario 5

You have responded to a cardiac arrest. After 2 minutes of CPR, the monitor shows ventricular fibrillation and you defibrillate at 360 J and resume CPR for another 2 minutes. At this point vascular access has been obtained and you stop CPR to analyze the rhythm and check for a pulse. You note no pulse and see the following on the monitor:

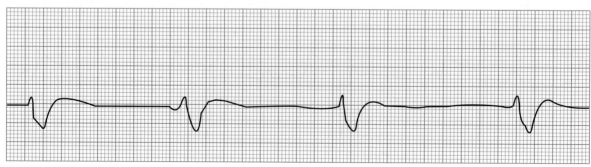

Scenario 5

273. The rhythm is:
    A. asystole
    B. PEA
    C. ventricular escape rhythm
    D. ventricular fibrillation
274. The next steps in resuscitation include:
    A. check for signs of life and if prolonged "down time" consider discontinuing efforts
    B. continue CPR, administer 1 mg atropine, 1 mg epinephrine, and 150 mg amiodarone, and recheck rhythm in 2 minutes
    C. continue CPR, administer 40 units vasopressin, and recheck rhythm in 2 minutes
    D. immediate defibrillation with 360 J

275. The goal of defibrillation in cardiac arrest resuscitation is to:
    A. electrically obliterate the source of myocardial ischemia
    B. repolarize the entire myocardium simultaneously
    C. stimulate the pacemaker cells to fire
    D. terminate VF/VT

Scenario 6

The ambulance is dispatched for a 36-year-old business executive who became ill during a board meeting. He complains of a dull aching pain to his left shoulder and chest, with radiation to his upper back. He states he has had some nausea and heartburn all week, so he has been taking antacids. He noticed some discomfort in his shoulder yesterday, but attributed it to a pulled muscle. He takes NSAIDs for routine pain, but nothing prescribed. He smokes one pack a day. BP 158/90, P 88, RR 18. His cardiac rhythm shows the following, and a 12-lead ECG is taken.

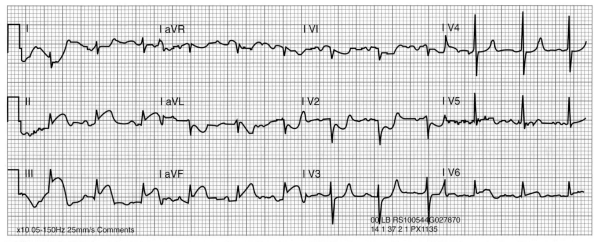

Scenario 6

276. The 12-Lead ECG is diagnostic of:
    A. acute anterior wall myocardial infarction
    B. acute inferior wall myocardial infarction
    C. acute inferior-lateral wall myocardial infarction with posterior extension
    D. unstable angina
277. The most likely coronary artery involved is the:
    A. distal left circumflex
    B. left anterior descending
    C. left main coronary artery
    D. right coronary artery
278. Initial care for this patient should include:
    A. a rapid assessment for PCI candidacy
    B. administration of β-blockers
    C. administration of heparin
    D. administration of morphine sulphate for pain

Scenario 7

EMS is called to the nursing home for a 92-year-old female who has had a fever for 4 days and appears to have become less responsive. Staff states that the patient had a couple episodes of vomiting with the fever. The patient is not normally oriented, but is pleasant and converses. Today she appears agitated, does not socialize, and pushed her granddaughter when she came to visit. She has a history of CHF, emphysema, and dementia. Her skin is pale, warm, and dry. BP 178/80, P 45, R 26, O_2 Saturation 97 on 2 L O_2 via nasal cannula. Your monitor shows the following:

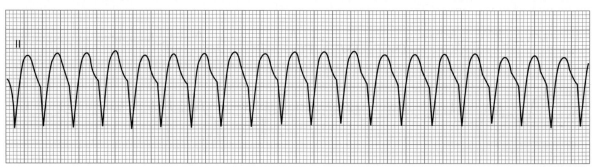

Scenario 7

279. The rhythm on the monitor is:
    A. sinus rhythm with sinus arrest
    B. second AVB Type I (Wenckebach)
    C. second AVB Type II
    D. advanced second AVB
280. The conduction ratio of this dysrhythmia is:
    A. 1:2
    B. 2:1
    C. 2:3
    D. 3:2

281. The most likely cause of the dysrhythmia in this patient is:
    A. conduction defect not associated with any acute cause
    B. dehydration
    C. digitalis toxicity
    D. hypoxia

Scenario 8

A 50-year-old male presents to triage in the ED with vague complaints of not feeling well. He becomes unresponsive with a pulse. The code team arrives and places the defibrillator patches on the patient and the following rhythm is present:

II

Scenario 8

282. The rhythm is most likely:
    A. supraventricular tachycardia
    B. torsades de pointes
    C. ventricular fibrillation
    D. ventricular tachycardia

283. The most appropriate initial step in this patient's resuscitation is:
    A. apply high flow oxygen and assist ventilation if necessary
    B. establish vascular access and administer 150 mg amiodarone
    C. immediate defibrillate the patient with 360 J
    D. perform synchronized cardioversion at 100 J

Following the procedure performed in question 283, a 12-Lead ECG is obtained and reveals the following:

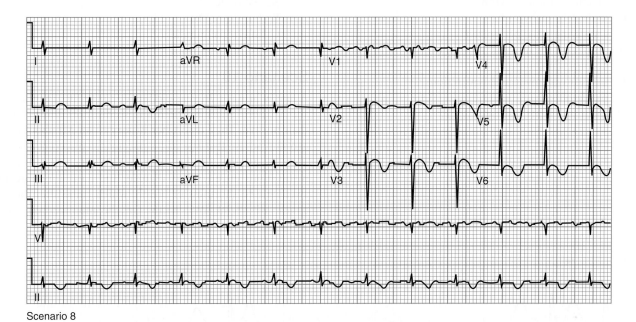

Scenario 8

284. Which of the following best describes the 12-Lead ECG findings:
    A. acute anterior wall myocardial infarction
    B. acute anteroseptal wall myocardial infarction
    C. acute inferior wall myocardial infarction
    D. anterolateral wall ischemia

Scenario 9

A 63-year-old male complains of chest pain for last 2 days. He states he has no medical problems. He also states he has had some nausea and vomiting. When it didn't resolve, he became concerned and came to the doctor's office. He appears to be in good health. States he still works full time as an accountant and denies undue stress or lifestyle changes. BP 158/78, P75, RR18, O_2 saturations 98%.

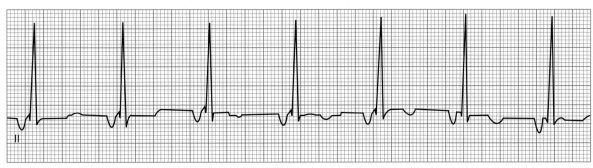

Scenario 9

285. The monitor reveals:
    A. junctional tachycardia
    B. junctional escape rhythm
    C. multiatrial tachycardia
    D. wandering atrial pacemaker
286. In this patient the most likely cause of the dysrhythmia is:
    A. decongestant abuse
    B. inferior wall myocardial infarction
    C. pericarditis
    D. rheumatic heart disease

287. This dysrhythmia is due to disruption of normal conduction in the:
    A. AV node
    B. bundle of His
    C. interatrial bundles
    D. Purkinje network

Scenario 10

A family brings a 76-year-old female to the ER. They state that she has been unusually tired and seems more short of breath than normal. They report her history of an MI about 6 years ago and advise that she had a pacemaker placed at that time. They report that she has been healthy since that time. Her medications include nitro, digoxin, and Lasix for some ankle swelling and shortness of breath, which came after the heart attack. BP 96/40, P45, RR18. On the monitor you see the following:

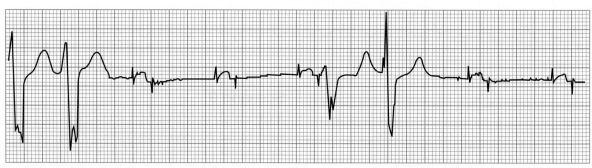

Scenario 10

288. What type of pacemaker does the patient have?
    A. AAI
    B. DDI
    C. VDD
    D. VVI
289. The condition exhibited by the pacemaker malfunction is called:
    A. automatic demand mode
    B. failure to sense
    C. failure to capture
    D. failure to sense and capture

290. Which of the following would not be indicated in initial care of this patient?
    A. administration of supplemental oxygen
    B. initiation of transcutaneous pacing
    C. large volume fluid resuscitation for shock
    D. obtaining STAT cardiology consult for evaluation of her pacemaker

I. DYSRHYTHMIAS

1. **Rate:** 126 beats/min.[†]
   Rhythm: Irregular.
   P Waves: None; fine atrial fibrillation waves are present.
   PR Int: None.
   QRS: 0.10 sec.
   Intrp: Atrial fibrillation (fine).

2. **Rate:** 33 beats/min.
   Rhythm: Irregular.
   P Waves: Present; the first, second, third, and fifth P waves are followed by QRS complexes.
   PR Int: 0.22 to 0.36 sec. The PR intervals progressively increase until a QRS complex fails to follow the P wave.
   QRS: 0.10 sec.
   Intrp: Sinus rhythm with second-degree, Type I AV block (Wenckebach).

3. **Rate:** 41 beats/min.
   Rhythm: Irregular.
   P Waves: Present; precede each QRS complex.
   PR Int: 0.16 sec.
   QRS: 0.08 sec.
   Intrp: Sinus bradycardia with sinus arrhythmia.

4. **Rate:** 170 beats/min.
   Rhythm: Regular.
   P Waves: Present; precede each QRS complex.
   PR Int: 0.12 sec.
   QRS: About 0.12 sec.
   Intrp: Atrial tachycardia with wide QRS complexes.

5. **Rate:** 62 beats/min.
   Rhythm: Irregular.
   P Waves: Present; precede the second, fourth, fifth, sixth, and seventh QRS complexes. The P waves are abnormal (0.16 sec in duration and notched).
   PR Int: 0.26 sec.

   QRS: 0.12 sec (all QRS complexes except the third QRS complex); 0.14 sec (third QRS complex).
   Intrp: Sinus rhythm with first-degree AV block, bundle branch block, and an isolated premature ventricular complex.

6. **Rate:** 107 beats/min.
   Rhythm: Irregular.
   P Waves: Present; precede all QRS complexes except the fifth, eighth, ninth, and tenth QRS complexes.
   PR Int: 0.16 sec.
   QRS: 0.09 to 0.10 sec.
   Intrp: Normal sinus rhythm with premature junctional complexes (fifth, eighth, ninth, and tenth QRS complexes) occurring singly and in group beats; the latter may be considered a short episode of junctional tachycardia.

7. **Rate:** 182 beats/min.
   Rhythm: Regular.
   P Waves: Present; precede each QRS complex.
   PR Int: 0.08 sec.
   QRS: 0.09 sec.
   Intrp: Atrial tachycardia.

8. **Rate:** Unmeasurable.
   Rhythm: Irregular.
   P Waves: None; coarse ventricular fibrillation waves are present.
   PR Int: None.
   QRS: None.
   Intrp: Ventricular fibrillation (coarse).

9. **Rate:** 89 beats/min.
   Rhythm: Irregular.
   P Waves: Present; precede all except the third and sixth QRS complexes. The shape and direction of the P waves vary from positive to negative.
   PR Int: 0.6 to 0.12 sec.
   QRS: 0.10 sec (all QRS complexes except the third and sixth QRS complexes); 0.12 sec (third and sixth QRS complexes).
   Intrp: Wandering atrial pacemaker with unifocal (uniform) premature ventricular complexes.

---

*Because of the possible distortion of the ECGs during printing, the measurement of the ECG components may vary slightly.
[†]The heart rates were calculated using R-R interval method 3.

10. **Rate:** 61 beats/min.
    Rhythm: Irregular.
    P Waves: Present; precede each QRS complex.
    PR Int: 0.12 sec.
    QRS: 0.14 sec.
    Intrp: Sinus arrhythmia.
11. **Rate:** 89 beats/min.
    Rhythm: Irregular.
    P Waves: Present; precede all QRS complexes except the second and eighth QRS complexes.
    PR Int: About 0.16 sec.
    QRS: 0.08 sec (all QRS complexes except the second and eighth QRS complexes); 0.12 sec (second and eighth QRS complexes).
    Intrp: Normal sinus rhythm with isolated unifocal (uniform) premature ventricular complexes.
12. **Rate:** 145 beats/min.
    Rhythm: Regular.
    P Waves: Present; precede each QRS complex.
    PR Int: About 0.10 sec.
    QRS: 0.08 sec.
    Intrp: Sinus tachycardia.
13. **Rate:** 87 beats/min.
    Rhythm: Irregular.
    P Waves: Present; precede each QRS complex.
    PR Int: 0.18 sec.
    QRS: 0.06 sec.
    Intrp: Sinus arrhythmia.
14. **Rate:** 164 beats/min.
    Rhythm: Regular.
    P Waves: None.
    PR Int: None.
    QRS: 0.12 sec.
    Intrp: Ventricular tachycardia.
15. **Rate:** 74 beats/min.
    Rhythm: Regular.
    P Waves: Present; precede each QRS complex; shape and direction vary from positive to negative.
    PR Int: 0.08 to 0.12 sec.
    QRS: 0.08 sec.
    Intrp: Wandering atrial pacemaker.
16. **Rate:** 70 beats/min (atrial rate: 52 beats/min).
    Rhythm: Regular.
    P Waves: Present, but have no set relation to the QRS complexes.
    PR Int: None.
    QRS: 0.14 sec.
    Intrp: Accelerated idioventricular rhythm with AV dissociation.
17. **Rate:** 83 beats/min.
    Rhythm: Regular.
    P Waves: Present; precede each QRS complex.
    PR Int: 0.16 sec.
    QRS: 0.06 sec.
    Intrp: Normal sinus rhythm.

18. **Rate:** 229 beats/min.
    Rhythm: Regular.
    P Waves: None.
    PR Int: None.
    QRS: 0.12 sec.
    Intrp: Ventricular tachycardia.
19. **Rate:** 26 beats/min.
    Rhythm: Regular.
    P Waves: Present; the first, third, and fifth P waves are followed by QRS complexes. AV conduction ratio is 2 : 1.
    PR Int: 0.19 sec.
    QRS: 0.10 sec.
    Intrp: Sinus rhythm with second-shape, 2 : 1 AV block.
20. **Rate:** 84 beats/min.
    Rhythm: Regular.
    P Waves: None; atrial flutter waves are present.
    PR Int: None.
    QRS: 0.10 sec.
    Intrp: Atrial flutter.
21. **Rate:** 30 beats/min.
    Rhythm: Regular.
    P Waves: Present; precede each QRS complex.
    PR Int: 0.17 to 0.18 sec.
    QRS: 0.14 sec.
    Intrp: Sinus bradycardia with bundle branch block.
22. **Rate:** 98 beats/min.
    Rhythm: Regular.
    P Waves: Present; precede each QRS complex.
    PR Int: About 0.16 sec.
    QRS: About 0.19 sec.
    Intrp: Normal sinus rhythm with bundle branch block.
23. **Rate:** 62 beats/min.
    Rhythm: Irregular.
    P Waves: Present; precede the first, second, third, and fifth QRS complexes.
    PR Int: 0.18 sec.
    QRS: 0.12 sec.
    Intrp: Normal sinus rhythm with premature junctional complexes.
24. **Rate:** 82 beats/min.
    Rhythm: Regular.
    P Waves: Present; precede each QRS complex. The P waves are abnormally wide.
    PR Int: 0.16 sec.
    QRS: 0.16 sec.
    Intrp: Normal sinus rhythm with bundle branch block.
25. **Rate:** 129 beats/min.
    Rhythm: Irregular.
    P Waves: None; fine atrial fibrillation waves are present.
    PR Int: None.
    QRS: About 0.10 sec.
    Intrp: Atrial fibrillation (fine).

26. **Rate:** 31 beats/min.
    Rhythm: Irregular.
    P Waves: Present; a QRS complex follows the first, fifth, and tenth P waves. AV conduction ratios are 4:1 and 5:1.
    PR Int: 0.34 sec.
    QRS: 0.16 sec.
    Intrp: Sinus rhythm with second-degree, advanced AV block and bundle branch block.

27. **Rate:** 75 beats/min.
    Rhythm: Regular.
    P Waves: Present; negative P waves precede each QRS complex.
    PR Int: 0.08 sec.
    QRS: 0.08 sec.
    Intrp: Accelerated junctional rhythm.

28. **Rate:** 62 beats/min.
    Rhythm: Irregular. The R-R intervals between the third and fourth QRS complexes and the fifth and sixth QRS complexes are twice the R-R interval of the underlying sinus rhythm.
    P Waves: Present; precede each QRS complex.
    PR Int: 0.18 sec.
    QRS: 0.18 sec.
    Intrp: Sinus rhythm with sinoatrial (SA) exit block and bundle branch block.

29. **Rate:** 37 beats/min.
    Rhythm: Regular.
    P Waves: None; atrial fibrillation waves are present.
    PR Int: None,
    QRS: About 0.24 sec.
    Intrp: Atrial fibrillation (fine) with ventricular escape rhythm.

30. **Rate:** 60 beats/min.
    Rhythm: Regular.
    P Waves: Present; precede each QRS complex.
    PR Int: 0.16 sec.
    QRS: 0.06 sec.
    Intrp: Normal sinus rhythm.

31. **Rate:** 135 beats/min.
    Rhythm: Regular.
    P Waves: None.
    PR Int: None.
    QRS: 0.26 sec.
    Intrp: Ventricular tachycardia.

32. **Rate:** 163 beats/min.
    Rhythm: Regular.
    P Waves: None.
    PR Int: None.
    QRS: 0.10 sec.
    Intrp: Junctional tachycardia.

33. **Rate:** 41 beats/min.
    Rhythm: Irregular.
    P Waves: Present; precede the first, second, fourth, and fifth QRS complexes. The R-R interval between the second and fourth QRS complexes is four times the R-R interval of the underlying sinus rhythm.
    PR Int: 0.14 sec.
    QRS: 0.12 sec.
    Intrp: Sinus rhythm with sinoatrial (SA) exit block and an isolated junctional escape beat (third QRS complex).

34. **Rate:** 17 beats/min.
    Rhythm: Undeterminable.
    P Waves: None.
    PR Int: None.
    QRS: 0.16 sec.
    Intrp: Ventricular escape rhythm.

35. **Rate:** 70 beats/min.
    Rhythm: Regular.
    P Waves: Present; precede each QRS complex.
    PR Int: 0.16 sec.
    QRS: 0.06 sec.
    Intrp: Normal sinus rhythm.

36. **Rate:** 64 beats/min.
    Rhythm: Irregular.
    P Waves: Present; precede the first and second QRS complexes. Pacemaker spikes precede the rest of the QRS complexes.
    PR Int: 0.26 sec.
    QRS: 0.08 sec (first and second QRS complexes); 0.12 sec (third, fourth, fifth, sixth, and seventh QRS complexes).
    Intrp: Sinus rhythm with first-degree AV block followed by ventricular asystole and a ventricular demand pacemaker rhythm.

37. **Rate:** 72 beats/min.
    Rhythm: Irregular.
    P Waves: Present; precede each QRS complex.
    PR Int: 0.16 sec.
    QRS: 0.08 sec.
    Intrp: Sinus arrhythmia.

38. **Rate:** 75 beats/min.
    Rhythm: Irregular.
    P Waves: Present; all but the first and sixth P waves are followed by QRS complexes. AV conduction ratio is 5:4.
    PR Int: 0.12 to 0.14 sec.
    QRS: 0.12 sec.
    Intrp: Sinus rhythm with second-degree, type II AV block.

39. **Rate:** 101 beats/min.
    Rhythm: Irregular.
    P Waves: Present; precede each QRS complex. The shape and direction of the P waves vary from positive to negative.
    PR Int: 0.12 to 0.18 sec.
    QRS: 0.06 sec.
    Intrp: Wandering atrial pacemaker.

40. **Rate:** 37 beats/min.
    Rhythm: Regular.
    P Waves: Present; precede each QRS complex.
    PR Int: 0.34 sec.
    QRS: 0.08 sec.
    Intrp: Sinus bradycardia with first-degree AV block.
41. **Rate:** 42 beats/min.
    Rhythm: Irregular.
    P Waves: Present; precede each QRS complex. The fourth P wave is negative; the rest are positive.
    PR Int: 0.18 to 0.20 sec.
    QRS: 0.16 sec.
    Intrp: Sinus bradycardia with bundle branch block and an isolated premature atrial complex.
42. **Rate:** 66 beats/min.
    Rhythm: Irregular.
    P Waves: Present; all the P waves except the fourth and eighth P waves are followed by QRS complexes.
    PR Int: 0.22 to 0.40 sec. The PR intervals progressively increase until a QRS complex fails to follow the P wave.
    QRS: 0.16 sec.
    Intrp: Sinus rhythm with second-degree, type I AV block (Wenckebach) and bundle branch block.
43. **Rate:** 74 beats/min.
    Rhythm: Regular.
    P Waves: None.
    PR Int: None.
    QRS: 0.12 sec.
    Intrp: Pacemaker rhythm (ventricular pacemaker).
44. **Rate:** 88 beats/min.
    Rhythm: Regular.
    P Waves: Present; precede each QRS complex.
    PR Int: 0.12 sec.
    QRS: 0.14 sec.
    Intrp: Normal sinus rhythm with bundle branch block.
45. **Rate:** 61 beats/min.
    Rhythm: Irregular.
    P Waves: Present; precede all but the fourth QRS complex.
    PR Int: 0.12 sec.
    QRS: 0.08 sec.
    Intrp: Sinus rhythm with sinus arrest and a premature junctional complex.
46. **Rate:** 71 beats/min.
    Rhythm: Slightly irregular.
    P Waves: Present; precede each QRS complex.
    PR Int: 0.18 sec.
    QRS: About 0.10 sec.
    Intrp: Sinus arrhythmia.
47. **Rate:** 66 beats/min.
    Rhythm: Irregular.
    P Waves: Present; all but the fourth and eighth P waves are followed by QRS complexes.

PR Int: 0.22 to 0.40 sec. The PR intervals progressively increase until a QRS complex fails to follow the P wave.
QRS: About 0.15 sec.
Intrp: Sinus rhythm with second-degree, type I AV block (Wenckebach) and bundle branch block.
48. **Rate:** 102 beats/min.
    Rhythm: Irregular.
    P Waves: None; fine atrial fibrillation waves are present.
    PR Int: None.
    QRS: About to 0.10 sec (first, fifth, seventh, eighth, ninth, and tenth QRS complexes); 0.12 to 0.16 sec (second, third, fourth, sixth, and tenth QRS complexes). The shape and direction of the second, third, and fourth QRS complexes differ from each other. The second QRS complex is similar to the sixth QRS complex; the fourth QRS complex is similar to the tenth QRS complex.
    Intrp: Atrial fibrillation (fine) with third-degree AV block, accelerated junctional rhythm, multifocal (multiform) PVCs (group beats), and a short burst of ventricular tachycardia. AV dissociation is present.
49. **Rate:** 63 beats/min.
    Rhythm: Irregular.
    P Waves: None; coarse atrial fibrillation waves are present.
    PR Int: None.
    QRS: 0.13 sec.
    Intrp: Atrial fibrillation (coarse) with bundle branch block.
50. **Rate:** 57 beats/min.
    Rhythm: Irregular. The R-R interval between the fourth and fifth QRS complexes is less than twice the R-R interval of the underlying sinus rhythm.
    P Waves: Present; precede all but the fifth QRS complex.
    PR Int: 0.12 sec.
    QRS: About 0.12 sec.
    Intrp: Sinus rhythm with sinus arrest and an isolated junctional escape beat.
51. **Rate:** 52 beats/min.
    Rhythm: Regular.
    P Waves: Present; precede each QRS complex.
    PR Int: 0.20 sec.
    QRS: 0.08 sec.
    Intrp: Normal sinus rhythm.
52. **Rate:** 183 beats/min.
    Rhythm: Regular.
    P Waves: None.
    PR Int: None.
    QRS: 0.16 sec.
    Intrp: Ventricular tachycardia.
53. **Rate:** 65 beats/min.
    Rhythm: Irregular.

P Waves: Present; precede each QRS complex.
PR Int: 0.16 sec.
QRS: 0.08 sec.
Intrp: Sinus arrhythmia.

54. **Rate:** 36 beats/min.
Rhythm: Regular.
P Waves: None.
PR Int: None.
QRS: 0.12 sec.
Intrp: Junctional escape rhythm.

55. **Rate:** 40 beats/min.
Rhythm: Regular.
P Waves: None.
PR Int: None.
QRS: 0.16 sec.
Intrp: Ventricular escape rhythm.

56. **Rate:** 59 beats/min.
Rhythm: Irregular.
P Waves: Present; the second, third, fifth, sixth, eighth, and tenth P waves are followed by QRS complexes. AV conduction ratios are 3:2 and 2:1.
PR Int: About 0.16 sec.
QRS: About 0.16 sec.
Intrp: Sinus rhythm with second-degree, type II 3:2 AV block and 2:1 AV block and bundle branch block.

57. **Rate:** 58 beats/min.
Rhythm: Regular.
P Waves: Present; negative P waves follow each QRS complex.
PR Int: None.
QRS: 0.16 sec.
Intrp: Junctional escape rhythm with bundle branch block.

58. **Rate:** 53 beats/min.
Rhythm: Irregular.
P Waves: Present; the first, second, fourth, fifth, and sixth P waves are followed by QRS complexes.
PR Int: 0.22 to 0.46 sec. The PR intervals progressively increase until a QRS complex fails to follow the P wave.
QRS: 0.08 sec.
Intrp: Sinus rhythm with second-degree, type I AV block (Wenckebach).

59. **Rate:** 80 beats/min.
Rhythm: Irregular.
P Waves: Present; precede the first, second, third, sixth, eighth, and ninth QRS complexes. The third P wave is negative; the fifth wave is buried in the preceding T wave. Pacemaker spikes precede the third, fourth, fifth, and seventh QRS complexes.
PR Int: 0.12 to 0.18 sec.
QRS: 0.07 sec (first, second, sixth, eighth, and ninth QRS complexes); 0.16 sec (fourth, fifth, and seventh QRS complexes). The third QRS complex is a fusion beat—a combination of the normally conducted QRS complex and the pacemaker induced ventricular QRS complex.
Intrp: Sinus rhythm with episodes of ventricular demand pacemaker rhythm.

60. **Rate:** 135 beats/min.
Rhythm: Regular.
P Waves: None.
PR Int: None.
QRS: About 0.32 to 0.36 sec.
Intrp: Ventricular tachycardia.

61. **Rate:** 70 beats/min.
Rhythm: Regular.
P Waves: Present; precede each QRS complex.
PR Int: 0.16 sec.
QRS: 0.06 sec.
Intrp: Normal sinus rhythm.

62. **Rate:** 52 beats/min.
Rhythm: Irregular.
P Waves: Present; the second, third, fifth, and sixth P waves are followed by QRS complexes. The AV conduction ratio is 3:2.
PR Int: 0.24 to 0.26 sec.
QRS: 0.16 sec.
Intrp: Sinus rhythm with second-degree, type II AV block and bundle branch block.

63. **Rate:** 64 beats/min.
Rhythm: Irregular.
P Waves: Present; the first, second, fourth, fifth, and sixth P waves are followed by QRS complexes.
PR Int: 0.24 to 0.36 sec. The PR intervals progressively increase until a QRS complex fails to follow the P wave.
QRS: 0.12 sec.
Intrp: Sinus rhythm with second-degree, type I AV block (Wenckebach).

64. **Rate:** 284 beats/min.
Rhythm: Regular.
P Waves: None.
PR Int: None.
QRS: About 0.20 sec.
Intrp: Ventricular tachycardia.

65. **Rate:** 87 beats/min.
Rhythm: Irregular.
P Waves: Present; precede each QRS complex.
PR Int: 0.12 to 0.16 sec.
QRS: 0.04 sec.
Intrp: Wandering atrial pacemaker.

66. **Rate:** 70 beats/min.
Rhythm: Regular.
P Waves: Present; precede each QRS complex.
PR Int: 0.16 sec.
QRS: 0.07 sec.
Intrp: Normal sinus rhythm.

67. **Rate:** 37 beats/min.
Rhythm: Regular.

P Waves: Present; precede each QRS complex.
PR Int: 0.20 sec.
QRS: 0.12 sec.
Intrp: Sinus bradycardia.

68. **Rate:** 30 beats/min (atrial rate: 82 beats/min).
Rhythm: Regular.
P Waves: Present, but have no set relation to the QRS complexes.
PR Int: None.
QRS: 0.14 sec.
Intrp: Third-degree AV block with wide QRS complexes.

69. **Rate:** 125 beats/min (average); 165 beats/min (first part); 79 beats/min (second part).
Rhythm: Irregular.
P Waves: Present; precede each QRS complex. In the first part, the P waves are superimposed on the preceding T waves.
PR Int: 0.16 sec.
QRS: About 0.08 sec.
Intrp: Paroxysmal supraventricular tachycardia with reversion to normal sinus rhythm.

70. **Rate:** 120 beats minute (three beats).
Rhythm: Regular (three beats).
P Waves: None.
PR Int: None.
QRS: 0.14 sec.
Intrp: Supraventricular tachycardia with wide QRS complexes or ventricular tachycardia followed by asystole.

71. **Rate:** 174 beats/min.
Rhythm: Regular.
P Waves: None.
PR Int: None.
QRS: 0.12 sec.
Intrp: Supraventricular tachycardia.

72. **Rate:** 36 beats/min.
Rhythm: Regular.
P Waves: None.
PR Int: None.
QRS: 0.18 sec.
Intrp: Junctional escape rhythm with bundle branch block or ventricular escape rhythm.

73. **Rate:** 263 beats/min.
Rhythm: Regular.
P Waves: None.
PR Int: None.
QRS: About 0.20 sec.
Intrp: Ventricular tachycardia.

74. **Rate:** 69 beats/min.
Rhythm: Irregular.
P Waves: Present; the second, third, fourth, sixth, seventh, and eighth P waves are followed by QRS complexes. AV conduction ratio is 4:3.
PR Int: 0.16 sec.
QRS: 0.20 sec.

Intrp: Sinus rhythm with second-degree, type II AV block and bundle branch block.

75. **Rate:** 72 beats/min.
Rhythm: Regular.
P Waves: P waves are present. A QRS complex follows every third P wave.
PR Int: 0.32 sec.
QRS: 0.08 sec.
Intrp: Sinus rhythm with first-degree AV block.

76. **Rate:** 104 beats/min.
Rhythm: Irregular.
P Waves: Present; precede the first, fifth, and sixth QRS complex.
PR Int: 0.18 sec.
QRS: 0.12 sec (first, fifth, and sixth complexes); about 0.16 sec (second, third, and fourth QRS complex).
Intrp: Sinus rhythm with and unifocal (uniform) premature ventricular complexes occurring in a burst of three (ventricular tachycardia); R-on-T phenomenon.

77. **Rate:** 82 beats/min.
Rhythm: Regular.
P Waves: Present; precede each QRS complex.
PR Int: About 0.16 sec.
QRS: 0.08 sec.
Intrp: Normal sinus rhythm.

78. **Rate:** 100 beats/min.
Rhythm: Irregular.
P Waves: Present; precede QRS complexes 1, 3, and 5.
PR Int: 0.12 sec.
QRS: About 0.20 sec.
Intrp: Sinus rhythm with bundle branch block and premature junctional complexes.

79. **Rate:** 56 beats/min.
Rhythm: Regular.
P Waves: Present; precede each QRS complex.
PR Int: 0.36 to 0.42 sec. The PR intervals progressively increase.
QRS: About 0.12 sec.
Intrp: Sinus rhythm with second-degree AV block (type undeterminable, probably type I AV block [Wenckebach]).

80. **Rate:** 181 beats/min.
Rhythm: Regular.
P Waves: None.
PR Int: None.
QRS: About 0.18 sec.
Intrp: Supraventricular tachycardia with wide QRS complexes or ventricular tachycardia.

81. **Rate:** 40 beats/min.
Rhythm: Undeterminable.
P Waves: None.
PR Int: None.
QRS: About 0.20 sec.
Intrp: Ventricular escape rhythm.

82. **Rate:** 94 beats/min.
   Rhythm: Regular.
   P Waves: Present; negative P waves precede each QRS complex.
   PR Int: 0.08 sec.
   QRS: 0.10 sec.
   Intrp: Accelerated junctional rhythm.
83. **Rate:** 94 beats/min.
   Rhythm: Regular.
   P Waves: Present; precede each QRS complex.
   PR Int: 0.12 sec.
   QRS: 0.12 sec.
   Intrp: Normal sinus rhythm.
84. **Rate:** 68 beats/min.
   Rhythm: Irregular.
   P Waves: Present; precede the first and third QRS complexes.
   PR Int: About 0.08 sec.
   QRS: 0.08 sec (first and third QS complex); 0.18 sec (second and fourth QRS complex).
   Intrp: Atrial rhythm with premature ventricular complexes (ventricular bigeminy).
85. **Rate:** 68 beats/min.
   Rhythm: Irregular.
   P Waves: Present; precede each QRS complex. The first and third P waves are positive; the second and fourth P waves are negative.
   PR Int: 0.20 sec.
   QRS: 0.12 sec.
   Intrp: Sinus rhythm with first-degree AV block, and premature atrial complexes (atrial bigeminy).
86. **Rate:** 34 beats/min (atrial rate: 163 beats/min).
   Rhythm: Undeterminable.
   P Waves: Present, but the negative P waves have no set relation to the QRS complexes.
   PR Int: None.
   QRS: 0.16 sec.
   Intrp: Third-degree AV block with wide QRS complexes.
87. **Rate:** 75 beats/min.
   Rhythm: Irregular.
   P Waves: None; fine atrial fibrillation waves are present.
   PR Int: None.
   QRS: 0.16 sec.
   Intrp: Atrial fibrillation (fine).
88. **Rate:** 107 beats/min.
   Rhythm: Irregular.
   P Waves: Present; precede each QRS complex.
   PR Int: 0.14 sec.
   QRS: 0.16 sec.
   Intrp: Sinus tachycardia with first-degree AV block, bundle branch block, and an isolated premature junctional complex (fourth QRS complex).
89. **Rate:** 230 beats/min.
   Rhythm: Slightly irregular.
   P Waves: None.

   PR Int: None.
   QRS: 0.20 sec.
   Intrp: Ventricular tachycardia.
90. **Rate:** 170 beats/min.
   Rhythm: Irregular.
   P Waves: None; fine atrial fibrillation waves are present.
   PR Int: None.
   QRS: 0.08 sec.
   Intrp: Atrial fibrillation (fine).
91. **Rate:** 80 beats/min.
   Rhythm: Irregular.
   P Waves: Present; precede the first and third QRS complexes.
   PR Int: 0.14 sec.
   QRS: 0.12 sec.
   Intrp: Sinus rhythm with bundle branch block and premature junctional complexes (bigeminy).
92. **Rate:** 115 beats/min.
   Rhythm: Irregular.
   P Waves: None; atrial flutter waves are present.
   PR Int: None.
   QRS: 0.12 sec.
   Intrp: Atrial flutter with variable conduction ratio.
93. **Rate:** Unmeasurable.
   Rhythm: Irregular.
   P Waves: None; coarse ventricular fibrillation waves are present.
   PR Int: None.
   QRS: None.
   Intrp: Ventricular fibrillation (coarse).
94. **Rate:** 46 beats/min.
   Rhythm: Irregular.
   P Waves: Present; the first, second, and fourth P waves are followed by QRS complexes.
   PR Int: 0.20 to 0.32 sec. The PR intervals progressively increase until a QRS complex fails to follow the P wave.
   QRS: 0.10 sec.
   Intrp: Sinus rhythm with second-degree, type I AV block (Wenckebach).
95. **Rate:** 82 beats/min.
   Rhythm: Regular.
   P Waves: None; atrial and ventricular pacemaker spikes are present.
   PR Int: None.
   QRS: 0.16 sec.
   Intrp: Pacemaker rhythm (AV sequential pacemaker).
96. **Rate:** 61 beats/min.
   Rhythm: Irregular.
   P Waves: Present; precede the first, second, and fourth QRS complexes.
   PR Int: 0.22 sec.
   QRS: 0.11 sec.
   Intrp: Normal sinus rhythm with first-degree AV block and isolated premature ventricular complex (third QRS complex).

97. **Rate:** 224 beats/min.
    Rhythm: Regular.
    P Waves: None.
    PR Int: None.
    QRS: 0.06 sec.
    Intrp: Supraventricular tachycardia.

98. **Rate:** 98 beats/min.
    Rhythm: Irregular.
    P Waves: Present; precede the first, second, third, and sixth QRS complexes.
    PR Int: 0.16 sec.
    QRS: 0.16 to 0.18 sec.
    Intrp: Normal sinus rhythm with bundle branch block and premature junctional complexes (group beats).

99. **Rate:** 136 beats/min.
    Rhythm: Regular.
    P Waves: Present; negative P waves follow each QRS complex.
    PR Int: None.
    QRS: 0.06 sec.
    Intrp: Junctional tachycardia.

100. **Rate:** 63 beats/min.
    Rhythm: None.
    P Waves: None; positive wide artifacts are present.
    PR Int: None.
    QRS: None.
    Intrp: Ventricular asystole with artifacts (chest compressions).

101. **Rate:** 184 beats/min.
    Rhythm: Regular.
    P Waves: None.
    PR Int: None.
    QRS: 0.10 sec.
    Intrp: Supraventricular tachycardia.

102. **Rate:** 102 beats/min.
    Rhythm: Regular.
    P Waves: Present; precede each QRS complex.
    PR Int: 0.16 sec.
    QRS: 0.06 sec.
    Intrp: Sinus tachycardia. Abnormally tall T waves characteristic of hyperkalemia are present.

103. **Rate:** 68 beats/min.
    Rhythm: Regular.
    P Waves: None.
    PR Int: None.
    QRS: About 0.22 sec.
    Intrp: Accelerated idioventricular rhythm.

104. **Rate:** 164 beats/min.
    Rhythm: Regular.
    P Waves: Present; precede each QRS complex.
    PR Int: 0.12 sec.
    QRS: 0.08 sec.
    Intrp: Atrial tachycardia.

105. **Rate:** 123 beats/min.
    Rhythm: Regular.

    P Waves: Present; precede each QRS complex.
    PR Int: 0.12 sec.
    QRS: 0.16 sec.
    Intrp: Sinus tachycardia with bundle branch block.

106. **Rate:** 76 beats/min.
    Rhythm: Irregular.
    P Waves: Present; precede the second and fourth QRS complex. The fifth QRS complex is superimposed on a P wave.
    PR Int: 0.16 sec.
    QRS: 0.08 sec (third and fifth QRS complexes); 0.12 sec (first, second, and fourth QRS complexes).
    Intrp: Normal sinus rhythm with bundle branch block and premature junctional complexes.

107. **Rate:** 61 beats/min.
    Rhythm: Irregular.
    P Waves: Present; precede the first, second, and fourth QRS complexes.
    PR Int: 0.24 sec.
    QRS: 0.10 sec.
    Intrp: Sinus rhythm with first-degree AV block and an isolated premature junctional complex.

108. **Rate:** 41 beats/min.
    Rhythm: Regular.
    P Waves: Present; precede each QRS complex.
    PR Int: About 0.14 sec.
    QRS: 0.08 sec.
    Intrp: Sinus bradycardia.

109. **Rate:** 69 beats/min.
    Rhythm: Regular.
    P Waves: Present; precede each QRS complex.
    PR Int: About 0.24 sec.
    QRS: 0.16 sec.
    Intrp: Sinus rhythm with first-degree AV block and bundle branch block.

110. **Rate:** 48 beats/min (atrial rate: 125 beats/min).
    Rhythm: Regular.
    P Waves: Present, but have no set relation to the QRS complexes.
    PR Int: None.
    QRS: 0.10 sec.
    Intrp: Third-degree AV block.

111. **Rate:** 41 beats/min.
    Rhythm: Irregular.
    P Waves: Present; the first, fourth, and sixth P waves are followed by QRS complexes. AV conduction ratios are 2:1 and 3:1.
    PR Int: 0.20 sec.
    QRS: 0.12 sec.
    Intrp: Sinus rhythm with second-degree, 2:1 and advanced AV block.

112. **Rate:** 92 beats/min.
    Rhythm: Regular.
    P Waves: Present; precede each QRS complex.
    PR Int: 0.14 sec.

QRS: About 0.08 sec.
Intrp: Normal sinus rhythm.

113. **Rate:** 161 beats/min.
Rhythm: Regular.
P Waves: None.
PR Int: None.
QRS: 0.08 sec.
Intrp: Supraventricular tachycardia.

114. **Rate:** 320 beats/min.
Rhythm: Slightly irregular.
P Waves: None.
PR Int: None.
QRS: 0.14 to 0.20 sec.
Intrp: Torsades de pointes.

115. **Rate:** 50 beats/min.
Rhythm: Regular.
P Waves: Present; precede each QRS complex.
PR Int: 0.16 sec.
QRS: 0.08 sec.
Intrp: Junctional escape rhythm.

116. **Rate:** 60 beats/min.
Rhythm: Irregular.
P Waves: None; fine atrial fibrillation waves are present.
PR Int: None.
QRS: 0.08 sec.
Intrp: Atrial fibrillation (fine).

117. **Rate:** 97 beats/min.
Rhythm: Regular.
P Waves: Present; precede each QRS complex.
PR Int: 0.16 sec.
QRS: 0.20 sec.
Intrp: Normal sinus rhythm with bundle branch block.

118. **Rate:** Unmeasurable.
Rhythm: Irregular.
P Waves: None; coarse ventricular fibrillation waves present.
PR Int: None.
QRS: None.
Intrp: Ventricular fibrillation (coarse).

119. **Rate:** 48 beats/min.
Rhythm: Regular.
P Waves: Present; follow each QRS complex.
PR Int: None.
QRS: About 0.16 sec.
Intrp: Junctional escape rhythm with bundle branch block or accelerated idioventricular rhythm.

120. **Rate:** 73 beats/min.
Rhythm: Irregular.
P Waves: Present; precede the first, second, and fourth QRS complexes.
PR Int: 0.18 sec.
QRS: 0.08 sec (first, second, and fourth QRS complexes); 0.16 sec (third QRS complex).
Intrp: Normal sinus rhythm with an isolated premature ventricular complex (interpolated).

121. **Rate:** 62 beats/min.
Rhythm: Regular.
P Waves: Present; precede each QRS complex.
PR Int: 0.20 sec.
QRS: About 0.08 sec.
Intrp: Normal sinus rhythm.

122. **Rate:** 78 beats/min.
Rhythm: Irregular.
P Waves: None; fine atrial fibrillation waves are present.
PR Int: None.
QRS: 0.08 sec.
Intrp: Atrial fibrillation (fine).

123. **Rate:** 87 beats/min.
Rhythm: Irregular.
P Waves: Present; precede the first and fourth QRS complexes.
PR Int: 0.16 sec.
QRS: 0.10 sec (first and fourth QRS complexes); about 0.16 to 0.18 sec (second, third, and fifth QRS complexes).
Intrp: Normal sinus rhythm with uniform premature ventricular complexes (group beats).

124. **Rate:** 80 beats/min.
Rhythm: Regular.
P Waves: None; ventricular pacemaker spikes are present.
PR Int: None.
QRS: 0.16 sec.
Intrp: Pacemaker rhythm (ventricular pacemaker).

125. **Rate:** 31 beats/min (atrial rate: 97 beats/min).
Rhythm: Undeterminable.
P Waves: Present, but have no set relation to the QRS complexes.
PR Int: None.
QRS: 0.12 to 0.14 sec.
Intrp: Third-degree AV block with wide QRS complexes.

126. **Rate:** 57 beats/min.
Rhythm: Regular.
P Waves: None.
PR Int: None.
QRS: About 0.16 sec.
Intrp: Junctional escape rhythm with bundle branch block.

127. **Rate:** 47 beats/min.
Rhythm: Regular.
P Waves: Present; precede each QRS complex.
PR Int: 0.48 sec.
QRS: 0.08 sec.
Intrp: Sinus bradycardia with first-degree AV block.

128. **Rate:** 149 beats/min.
Rhythm: Regular.
P Waves: Present; precede each QRS complex.
PR Int: Unmeasurable.
QRS: 0.08 sec.
Intrp: Atrial tachycardia.

129. **Rate:**   160 beats/min.
 Rhythm: Irregular.
 P Waves: Undeterminable.
 PR Int: Undeterminable.
 QRS: 0.12 sec (first QRS complex); ≥ 0.16 sec (rest of the QRS complexes).
 Intrp: A wide QRS complex followed by ventricular tachycardia.

130. **Rate:**   160 beats/min.
 Rhythm: Regular.
 P Waves: None.
 PR Int: None.
 QRS: 0.16 sec.
 Intrp: Supraventricular tachycardia.

131. **Rate:**   150 beats/min.
 Rhythm: Regular.
 P Waves: Present; follow each QRS complex.
 PR Int: None.
 QRS: 0.10 sec.
 Intrp: Junctional tachycardia.

132. **Rate:**   31 beats/min (atrial rate: unmeasurable).
 Rhythm: Undeterminable.
 P Waves: Present, but have no set relation to the QRS complexes.
 PR Int: None.
 QRS: About 0.15 sec.
 Intrp: Third-degree AV block with wide QRS complexes.

133. **Rate:**   31 beats/min.
 Rhythm: Undeterminable.
 P Waves: Present; precede each QRS complex.
 PR Int: 0.14 sec.
 QRS: 0.08 sec.
 Intrp: Sinus bradycardia.

134. **Rate:**   59 beats/min.
 Rhythm: Regular.
 P Waves: None; atrial flutter waves are present.
 PR Int: None.
 QRS: 0.16 sec.
 Intrp: Atrial flutter with bundle branch block.

135. **Rate:**   178 beats/min.
 Rhythm: Regular.
 P Waves: None.
 PR Int: None.
 QRS: 0.08 sec.
 Intrp: Supraventricular tachycardia.

136. **Rate:**   91 beats/min.
 Rhythm: Regular.
 P Waves: Present; precede each QRS complex.
 PR Int: 0.28 sec.
 QRS: 0.12 sec.
 Intrp: Sinus rhythm with first-degree AV block and bundle branch block.

137. **Rate:**   47 beats/min.
 Rhythm: Regular.

 P Waves: Present; the first, third, and fifth P waves are followed by QRS complexes.
 PR Int: 0.28 sec.
 QRS: 0.12 sec.
 Intrp: Sinus rhythm with second-degree, 2:1 AV block and bundle branch block.

138. **Rate:**   78 beats/min.
 Rhythm: Irregular.
 P Waves: Present; precede each QRS complex. The second and fourth P waves are abnormal, each in a different way.
 PR Int: About 0.22 sec (first and third PR intervals); about 0.16 second (second and fourth PR intervals).
 QRS: About 0.10 sec.
 Intrp: Sinus rhythm with multifocal premature atrial complexes.

139. **Rate:**   64 beats/min.
 Rhythm: Regular.
 P Waves: None.
 PR Int: None.
 QRS: About 0.10 sec.
 Intrp: Accelerated junctional rhythm.

140. **Rate:**   222 beats/min.
 Rhythm: Regular.
 P Waves: None.
 PR Int: None.
 QRS: 0.12 sec.
 Intrp: Supraventricular tachycardia with wide QRS complexes or ventricular tachycardia.

141. **Rate:**   None (pacemaker spikes: 63 beats/min).
 Rhythm: Regular.
 P Waves: None; pacemaker spikes are present.
 PR Int: None.
 QRS: None.
 Intrp: Asystole with pacemaker spikes without capture.

142. **Rate:**   99 beats/min.
 Rhythm: Irregular.
 P Waves: Present; precede the first, second, and fifth QRS complexes.
 PR Int: 0.28 sec.
 QRS: 0.10 sec (first, second, and fifth QRS complexes); 0.12 to 0.16 second (third and fourth QRS complexes).
 Intrp: Sinus rhythm with first-degree AV block and multifocal premature ventricular complexes (group beats).

143. **Rate:**   61 beats/min.
 Rhythm: Regular.
 P Waves: Present: precede each QRS complex. P waves are abnormally tall (P pulmonale).
 PR Int: 0.26 sec.
 QRS: 0.10 sec.
 Intrp: Sinus rhythm with first-degree AV block.

144. **Rate:** 114 beats/min.
Rhythm: Regular.
P Waves: Present; precede each QRS complex.
PR Int: 0.16 sec.
QRS: 0.08 sec.
Intrp: Sinus tachycardia.
145. **Rate:** 100 beats/min.
Rhythm: Regular.
P Waves: Present; retrograde P waves follow each QRS complex.
PR Int: None.
QRS: 0.10 sec.
Intrp: Junctional tachycardia.
146. **Rate:** Unmeasurable.
Rhythm: Irregular.
P Waves: None; coarse ventricular fibrillation waves are present.
PR Int: None.
QRS: None.
Intrp: Ventricular fibrillation (coarse).
147. **Rate:** 21 beats/min.
Rhythm: Undeterminable.
P Waves: None.
PR Int: None.
QRS: 0.20 sec.
Intrp: Ventricular escape rhythm.
148. **Rate:** 68 beats/min.
Rhythm: Irregular.
P Waves: None; fine atrial fibrillation waves are present.
PR Int: None.
QRS: 0.10 sec.
Intrp: Atrial fibrillation (fine).
149. **Rate:** 65 beats/min (atrial rate: 113 beats/min).
Rhythm: Regular.
P Waves: Present, but have no set relation to the QRS complexes.
PR Int: None.
QRS: Undeterminable.
Intrp: Third-degree AV block.
150. **Rate:** 88 beats/min.
Rhythm: Irregular.
P Waves: Present; precede each QRS complex. Third wave negative.
PR Int: About 0.14 sec.
QRS: About 0.08 sec.
Intrp: Normal sinus rhythm with an isolated premature junctional complex.
151. **Rate:** 55 beats/min.
Rhythm: Regular.
P Waves: Present; abnormally wide, positive P waves precede each QRS complex.
PR Int: About 0.40 sec.
QRS: About 0.10 sec.
Intrp: Sinus rhythm with first-degree AV block. Possible 2:1 AV block.

152. **Rate:** 148 beats/min.
Rhythm: Regular.
P Waves: Present; precede each QRS complex.
PR Int: Undeterminable; P waves are buried in the preceding QRS complexes.
QRS: 0.10 sec.
Intrp: Sinus tachycardia.
153. **Rate:** 118 beats/min.
Rhythm: Irregular.
P Waves: None; fine atrial fibrillation waves are present.
PR Int: None.
QRS: 0.08 sec.
Intrp: Atrial fibrillation (fine).
154. **Rate:** 36 beats/min.
Rhythm: Undeterminable.
P Waves: None.
PR Int: None.
QRS: About 0.16 sec.
Intrp: Ventricular escape rhythm.
155. **Rate:** 50 beats/min.
Rhythm: Regular.
P Waves: None; atrial flutter waves are present.
PR Int: None.
QRS: 0.16 sec.
Intrp: Atrial flutter with bundle branch block.
156. **Rate:** 163 beats/min.
Rhythm: Regular.
P Waves: None.
PR Int: None.
QRS: 0.16 sec.
Intrp: Ventricular tachycardia.
157. **Rate:** 63 beats/min.
Rhythm: Regular.
P Waves: Present; negative P waves follow each QRS complex.
PR Int: None.
QRS: About 0.08 sec.
Intrp: Accelerated junctional rhythm.
158. **Rate:** 103 beats/min.
Rhythm: Regular.
P Waves: Present: P waves precede each QRS complex. The P waves are abnormally tall (P pulmonale).
PR Int: 0.19 sec.
QRS: About 0.15 sec.
Intrp: Sinus tachycardia with bundle branch block.
159. **Rate:** 312 beats/min.
Rhythm: Slightly irregular.
P Waves: None.
PR Int: None.
QRS: 0.12 to 0.14 sec.
Intrp: Ventricular tachycardia (multiform).
160. **Rate:** 101 beats/min.
Rhythm: Regular.
P Waves: None.

PR Int: None.

QRS: 0.14 sec.

Intrp: Junctional tachycardia with wide QRS complexes or ventricular tachycardia.

161. **Rate:** 92 beats/min.

     Rhythm: Irregular.

     P Waves: Present; precede the first, second fourth, and fifth QRS complexes.

     PR Int: 0.14 sec.

     QRS: 0.16 sec.

     Intrp: Normal sinus rhythm with bundle branch block and an isolated premature ventricular complex (interpolated).

162. **Rate:** 70 beats/min.

     Rhythm: Regular.

     P Waves: Present; precede each QRS complex.

     PR Int: About 0.12 sec.

     QRS: 0.12 sec.

     Intrp: Normal sinus rhythm.

163. **Rate:** 72 beats/min.

     Rhythm: Regular.

     P Waves: None.

     PR Int: None.

     QRS: 0.12 to 0.16 sec.

     Intrp: Accelerated idioventricular rhythm.

164. **Rate:** Unmeasurable.

     Rhythm: Irregular.

     P Waves: None; fine ventricular waves are present.

     PR Int: None.

     QRS: None.

     Intrp: Ventricular fibrillation (fine).

165. **Rate:** 57 beats/min.

     Rhythm: Regular.

     P Waves: Present; precede each QRS complex.

     PR Int: 0.24 sec.

     QRS: About 0.10 sec.

     Intrp: Sinus bradycardia with first-degree AV block.

166. **Rate:** 43 beats/min.

     Rhythm: Regular.

     P Waves: Present; positive P waves precede each QRS complex.

     PR Int: 0.10 sec.

     QRS: About 0.10 sec.

     Intrp: Sinus bradycardia with atrio-His preexcitation.

167. **Rate:** 57 beats/min.

     Rhythm: Regular.

     P Waves: None.

     PR Int: None.

     QRS: About 0.16 sec.

     Intrp: Accelerated idioventricular rhythm.

168. **Rate:** None.

     Rhythm: None.

     P Waves: None.

     PR Int: None.

     QRS: None.

     Intrp: Asystole.

169. **Rate:** 43 beats/min.

     Rhythm: Regular.

     P Waves: Present; negative P waves follow each QRS complex.

     PR Int: None.

     QRS: About 0.10 sec.

     Intrp: Junctional escape rhythm.

170. **Rate:** Unmeasurable.

     Rhythm: Irregular.

     P Waves: None; coarse ventricular fibrillation waves are present.

     PR Int: None.

     QRS: None.

     Intrp: Ventricular fibrillation (coarse).

171. **Rate:** 25 beats/min.

     Rhythm: Undeterminable.

     P Waves: None.

     PR Int: None.

     QRS: 0.16 sec.

     Intrp: Junctional escape rhythm with wide QRS complexes.

172. **Rate:** 213 beats/min.

     Rhythm: Regular.

     P Waves: None.

     PR Int: None.

     QRS: 0.12 sec.

     Intrp: Supraventricular tachycardia with wide QRS complexes or ventricular tachycardia.

173. **Rate:** 70 beats/min.

     Rhythm: Irregular.

     P Waves: None; fine atrial fibrillation waves are present.

     PR Int: None.

     QRS: 0.10 sec.

     Intrp: Atrial fibrillation (fine).

174. **Rate:** 89 beats/min.

     Rhythm: Regular.

     P Waves: Present; precede each QRS complex.

     PR Int: About 0.18 sec.

     QRS: 0.12 sec.

     Intrp: Normal sinus rhythm with bundle branch block.

175. **Rate:** 165 beats/min.

     Rhythm: Regular.

     P Waves: None.

     PR Int: None.

     QRS: 0.10 sec.

     Intrp: Supraventricular tachycardia.

176. **Rate:** 48 beats/min.

     Rhythm: Regular.

     P Waves: Present; appear to precede each QRS complex.

     PR Int: 0.08 sec.

     QRS: 0.08 sec.

     Intrp: Sinus bradycardia with atrio-His preexcitation.

177. **Rate:** 79 beats/min.

     Rhythm: Irregular.

P Waves: Present; positive P waves precede the first, second, fourth, and fifth QRS complexes. A negative P wave precedes the third QRS complex.

PR Int: 0.12 sec (first, second, fourth, and fifth QRS complexes); 0.09 sec (third QRS complex).

QRS: 0.10 sec.

Intrp: Normal sinus rhythm with an isolated premature junctional complex.

178. **Rate:** 33 beats/min (atrial rate: 39 beats/min).
 Rhythm: Undeterminable.
 P Waves: Present; the first and fifth P waves are followed by QRS complexes. AV conduction ratio is 4:1.
 PR Int: Variable.
 QRS: 0.14 sec.
 Intrp: Third-degree heart block.

179. **Rate:** 59 beats/min.
 Rhythm: Irregular.
 P Waves: Present; the first, third, and fourth P waves are followed by QRS complexes.
 PR Int: 0.20 to 0.28 sec.
 QRS: About 0.05 sec.
 Intrp: Sinus rhythm with second-degree AV block (probably Type I [Wenckebach]).

180. **Rate:** 96 beats/min.
 Rhythm: Irregular. An incomplete compensatory pause follows the fourth QRS complex.
 P Waves: Present; precede the second, third, fifth, and sixth QRS complexes.
 PR Int: 0.18 sec.
 QRS: 0.10 sec.
 Intrp: Normal sinus rhythm with an isolated premature junctional complex.

181. **Rate:** 60 beats/min.
 Rhythm: Regular.
 P Waves: Present; precede each QRS complex.
 PR Int: 0.15 sec.
 QRS: 0.07 sec.
 Intrp: Normal sinus rhythm.

182. **Rate:** Unmeasurable.
 Rhythm: Irregular.
 P Waves: None.
 PR Int: None.
 QRS: None.
 Intrp: Asystole

183. **Rate:** 98 beats/min.
 Rhythm: Regular.
 P Waves: Present; precede each QRS complex.
 PR Int: About 0.20 sec.
 QRS: About 0.16 sec.
 Intrp: Normal sinus rhythm with bundle branch block.

184. **Rate:** 64 beats/min.
 Rhythm: Regular.
 P Waves: None.
 PR Int: None.

QRS: About 0.16 sec.
Intrp: Accelerated idioventricular rhythm.

185. **Rate:** 35 beats/min (atrial rate: 167 beats/min).
 Rhythm: Undeterminable.
 P Waves: Present, but have no set relation to the QRS complexes.
 PR Int: None.
 QRS: 0.12 sec.
 Intrp: Third-degree AV block with wide QRS complexes.

186. **Rate:** 79 beats/min.
 Rhythm: Regular.
 P Waves: Present; precede each QRS complex.
 PR Int: 0.15 sec.
 QRS: 0.08 sec.
 Intrp: Normal sinus rhythm.

187. **Rate:** 87 beats/min.
 Rhythm: Irregular.
 P Waves: None; atrial flutter waves are present. The AV conduction ratios vary.
 PR Int: None.
 QRS: 0.12 sec.
 Intrp: Atrial flutter.

188. **Rate:** 181 beats/min.
 Rhythm: Regular.
 P Waves: None.
 PR Int: None.
 QRS: About 0.22 sec.
 Intrp: Supraventricular tachycardia with wide QRS complexes or ventricular tachycardia.

189. **Rate:** 103 beats/min.
 Rhythm: Regular.
 P Waves: None; atrial flutter waves are present.
 PR Int: None.
 QRS: 0.06 sec.
 Intrp: Atrial flutter.

190. **Rate:** 161 beats/min.
 Rhythm: Regular.
 P Waves: Present; precede each QRS complex.
 PR Int: 0.12 sec.
 QRS: 0.08 sec.
 Intrp: Sinus tachycardia.

191. **Rate:** 130 beats/min.
 Rhythm: Regular.
 P Waves: None.
 PR Int: None.
 QRS: About 0.10 sec.
 Intrp: Supraventricular tachycardia.

192. **Rate:** Ventricular rate: none (atrial rate: 70 beats/min).
 Rhythm: Regular.
 P Waves: Present.
 PR Int: None.
 QRS: None.
 Intrp: Asystole (ventricular standstill).

193. **Rate:** 31 beats/min (atrial rate 106 beats/min).
 Rhythm: Undeterminable.

P Waves: Present, but have no set relation to the QRS complexes.

PR Int: None.

QRS: About 0.16 sec.

Intrp: Third-degree AV block with wide QRS complexes.

194. **Rate:** 36 beats/min.

Rhythm: Undeterminable.

P Waves: None.

PR Int: None.

QRS: 0.16 sec.

Intrp: Ventricular escape rhythm.

195. **Rate:** 59 beats/min.

Rhythm: Regular.

P Waves: Absent.

PR Int: 0.05 to 0.06 sec.

QRS: About 0.16 sec.

Intrp: Junctional escape rhythm with bundle branch block.

196. **Rate:** 71 beats/min.

Rhythm: Irregular. A complete compensatory pause follows the third QRS complex.

P Waves: Present; precede each QRS complex.

PR Int: 0.16 sec.

QRS: 0.08 sec.

Intrp: Normal sinus rhythm with an isolated premature atrial complex.

197. **Rate:** 122 beats/min.

Rhythm: Regular.

P Waves: None.

PR Int: None.

QRS: 0.12 sec.

Intrp: Junctional tachycardia

198. **Rate:** None.

Rhythm: None.

P Waves: None.

PR Int: None.

QRS: 0.16 sec.

Intrp: A single wide QRS complex, probably ventricular in origin, followed by asystole.

199. **Rate:** 169 beats/min.

Rhythm: Irregular.

P Waves: None; atrial flutter waves are present. The AV conduction ratios vary.

PR Int: None.

QRS: 0.08 sec.

Intrp: Atrial flutter with rapid ventricular response.

200. **Rate:** 128 beats/min.

Rhythm: Regular.

P Waves: Present; precede each QRS complex. The P waves are abnormally tall (P pulmonale).

PR Int: 0.24 sec.

QRS: About 0.12 sec.

Intrp: Sinus tachycardia with first-degree AV block and bundle branch block.

201. **Rate:** 63 beats/min.

Rhythm: Regular.

P Waves: None.

PR Int: None.

QRS: About 0.16 sec.

Intrp: Accelerated junctional rhythm with wide QRS complexes or accelerated idioventricular rhythm.

202. **Rate:** 60 beats/min.

Rhythm: Regular.

P Waves: Present; precede each QRS complex.

PR Int: 0.16 sec.

QRS: 0.07 sec.

Intrp: Normal sinus rhythm.

203. **Rate:** Unmeasurable.

Rhythm: None.

P Waves: None.

PR Int: None.

QRS: None.

Intrp: Asystole.

204. **Rate:** 238 beats/min.

Rhythm: Regular.

P Waves: None.

PR Int: None.

QRS: About 0.10 sec.

Intrp: Supraventricular tachycardia.

205. **Rate:** 165 beats/min.

Rhythm: Regular.

P Waves: None.

PR Int: None.

QRS: About 0.24 sec.

Intrp: Ventricular tachycardia.

206. **Rate:** 72 beats/min.

Rhythm: Regular.

P Waves: None; atrial flutter waves are present.

PR Int: None.

QRS: 0.08 sec.

Intrp: Atrial flutter.

207. **Rate:** 33 beats/min.

Rhythm: Undeterminable.

P Waves: None.

PR Int: None.

QRS: Unmeasurable; greater than 0.12 sec.

Intrp: Ventricular escape rhythm.

208. **Rate:** 126 beats/min.

Rhythm: Regular.

P Waves: None.

PR Int: None.

QRS: 0.11 sec.

Intrp: Sinus tachycardia with first-degree AV block.

209. **Rate:** 81 beats/min.

Rhythm: Irregular.

P Waves: Present; precede each QRS complex. The shape and direction of the fourth P wave differs from the others.

PR Int: 0.13 sec (first, second, third, and fifth PR intervals); 0.18 sec (fourth PR interval).

QRS: 0.10 sec (first, second, third, and fifth QRS complex).

Intrp: Normal sinus rhythm with an isolated premature atrial complex.

210. **Rate:** 31 beats/min (atrial rate: 83 beats/min).
 Rhythm: Undeterminable.
 P Waves: Present, but have no set relation to the QRS complexes.
 PR Int: None.
 QRS: About 0.14 sec.
 Intrp: Third-degree AV block with wide QRS complexes.

211. **Rate:** 180 beats/min.
 Rhythm: Regular.
 P Waves: Present; precede each QRS complex.
 PR Int: 0.08 sec.
 QRS: 0.12 sec.
 Intrp: Atrial tachycardia with atrio-His preexcitation and bundle branch block.

212. **Rate:** 45 beats/min (atrial rate 111 beats/min).
 Rhythm: Regular.
 P Waves: Present, but have no set relation to the QRS complexes.
 PR Int: None.
 QRS: 0.12 sec.
 Intrp: Third-degree AV block.

213. **Rate:** 52 beats/min.
 Rhythm: Regular.
 P Waves: Present; the first, third, and fifth P waves are followed by QRS complexes. The AV conduction ratio is 2:1.
 PR Int: 0.20 sec.
 QRS: 0.14 sec.
 Intrp: Sinus rhythm with second-degree, 2:1 AV block and bundle branch block.

214. **Rate:** 44 beats/min.
 Rhythm: Irregular.
 P Waves: None; atrial flutter waves are present. The AV conduction ratios vary.
 PR Int: None.
 QRS: About 0.14 sec.
 Intrp: Atrial flutter with wide QRS complexes.

215. **Rate:** 71 beats/min.
 Rhythm: Regular.
 P Waves: Present; precede each QRS complex.
 PR Int: 0.26 sec.
 QRS: 0.10 sec.
 Intrp: Sinus rhythm with first-degree AV block.

216. **Rate:** 103 beats/min.
 Rhythm: Regular.
 P Waves: Present; precede each QRS complex.
 PR Int: 0.12 sec.
 QRS: 0.14 sec.
 Intrp: Sinus tachycardia with bundle branch block.

217. **Rate:** 104 beats/min.
 Rhythm: Regular.
 P Waves: None.
 PR Int: None.

QRS: 0.14 sec.
 Intrp: Junctional tachycardia with wide QRS complexes.

218. **Rate:** 109 beats/min.
 Rhythm: Irregular.
 P Waves: Present; precede the first, second, third, fourth, and fifth QRS complexes.
 PR Int: 0.14 sec.
 QRS: 0.09 sec (first, second, third, fourth, and fifth QRS complexes); 0.11 sec (sixth QRS complex).
 Intrp: Normal sinus rhythm with premature ventricular complexes and a fusion beat (third QRS complex).

219. **Rate:** None.
 Rhythm: None.
 P Waves: None.
 PR Int: None.
 QRS: None.
 Intrp: Asystole.

220. **Rate:** 81 beats/min.
 Rhythm: Regular.
 P Waves: None.
 PR Int: None.
 QRS: 0.10 sec.
 Intrp: Accelerated junctional rhythm with possible Osborn waves.

221. **Rate:** 109 beats/min.
 Rhythm: Irregular.
 P Waves: Present; precede the first, second, fourth, and fifth QRS complexes.
 PR Int: About 0.14 sec.
 QRS: 0.09 sec (first, second, fourth, and fifth QRS complexes); 0.11 sec (third and sixth QRS complexes).
 Intrp: Normal sinus rhythm with unifocal (uniform) premature ventricular complexes (trigeminy).

222. **Rate:** 37 beats/min.
 Rhythm: Undeterminable.
 P Waves: Present; the second and fifth P waves are followed by QRS complexes. The third and sixth P waves are buried in the preceding T waves. The AV conduction ratio is 3:1.
 PR Int: 0.16 sec.
 QRS: 0.14 sec.
 Intrp: Sinus rhythm with second-degree, advanced AV block and bundle branch block.

223. **Rate:** 128 beats/min.
 Rhythm: Irregular.
 P Waves: None; final atrial fibrillation waves are present.
 PR Int: None.
 QRS: 0.12 to 0.16 sec.
 Intrp: Atrial fibrillation (fine) with bundle branch block.

224. **Rate:** 108 beats/min.
 Rhythm: Regular.
 P Waves: None.

PR Int: None.
QRS: 0.16 sec.
Intrp: Supraventricular tachycardia.

II. BUNDLE BRANCH AND FASCICULAR BLOCKS

225. Left bundle branch block.
226. Left posterior fascicular block.
227. Right bundle branch block.
228. Right bundle branch block with an intact interventricular septum.
229. Left anterior fascicular block.

III. MYOCARDIAL INFARCTIONS

230. Anterolateral myocardial infarction.
231. Septal myocardial infarction.
232. Extensive anterior myocardial infarction.
233. Anterior myocardial infarction.
234. Lateral myocardial infarction.
235. Inferior myocardial infarction.
236. Anteroseptal myocardial infarction.
237. Posterior myocardial infarction.
238. Right ventricular myocardial infarction.

IV. QRS AXES

239. QRS axis: +150°.
240. QRS axis: −30° to −90°.
241. QRS axis: +90°.
242. QRS axis: +90° to +150°.
243. QRS axis: 0° to +30°.
244. QRS axis: 0° to −30°.

V. ECG CHANGES: DRUG AND ELECTROLYTE

245. Hypercalcemia.
246. Procainamide/quinidine toxicity.
247. Hyperkalemia.
248. Digitalis effect.
249. Hypocalcemia.
250. Hypokalemia.

VI. ECG CHANGES: MISCELLANEOUS

251. Left ventricular hypertrophy.
252. Chronic obstructive pulmonary disease (COPD).
253. Right ventricular hypertrophy/cor pulmonale.
254. Pericarditis.
255. Acute pulmonary embolism.
256. Early repolarization.
257. Hypothermia.
258. Ventricular preexcitation.
259. Atrio-His preexcitation.
260. Nodoventricular/fasciculoventricular preexcitation.

VII. SCENARIOS

Scenario 1

261. (A) The rhythm is regular with P waves preceding each QRS complex. All P waves are identical. The rate is between 60 and 100 therefore **normal sinus rhythm.**

262. (B) The T waves in the precordial leads are **tall and peaked**. While the ST segment appears to be slightly elevated in V2 and V3, the ST segment is "upsloping," which is not characteristic of ischemia. The QT interval is normal at 352 ms.

263. (B) Peaked T waves are caused by **hyperkalemia.** Coronary artery occlusion results in ST elevation. Hypocalcemia causes QT interval prolongation. Hypothermia is manifested by prolonged PR and QT intervals, QRS complexes, and the presence of Osborn waves.

Scenario 2

264. (C) While it is true that atrial tachycardia and atrial flutter with 1:1 conduction are supraventricular tachycardias, this patient reports a sudden onset of the dysrhythmia, which places it in the special category of **paroxysmal supraventricular tachycardia.** There are no P waves, therefore sinus tachycardia is unlikely.

265. (A) A wide QRS complex tachycardia may be either supraventricular tachycardia with aberrant conduction or ventricular tachycardia. If the patient is stable, a **12-lead ECG** may used to determine the axis of the QRS and assist in the differentiation. Performing vagal maneuvers will not assist in the differentiation. Administration of adenosine to ventricular tachycardia is contraindicated and can result in asystole. Amiodarone will treat either dysrhythmia but will not aid in differentiating the two.

266. (D) The electrophysiologic mechanism responsible for PSVT is a **reentry mechanism involving the AV node alone, or the AV node in conjunction with an accessory conduction pathway.**

Scenario 3

267. (D) **Third atrioventricular heart block** is characterized by total dissociation between the P waves and the QRS complexes. Examination of the rhythm strip, marking the P waves and attempting to correlate them with any QRS complex makes it clear that no association exists. The wide QRS complex and rate are consistent with a ventricular escape rhythm or junctional escape rhythm with aberrant conduction.

268. (A) It is more probable that the **AV node** pacemaker has assumed the escape rhythm with aberrant conduction as ventricular escape rhythms are more often slower than 40.

269. (D) While the patient's blood pressure is slightly low, he is awake and conscious. Therefore, he is tolerating the relative bradycardia well. Initial care would include **laying him down, administering oxygen, and obtaining vascular access.** It would be prudent to apply a transcutaneous pacemaker on the patient so as to be prepared in the event his rate slowed. If he continues to tolerate this rate, he can await a cardiology consultation for pacemaker placement. In the event he were to deteriorate, sedation and transcutaneous pacing would be appropriate.

Scenario 4

270. (A) The rhythm is totally irregular, there are no discernable P waves, the baseline in the R-R interval appears to contain f waves and F waves. The QRS complex rate is 128, which is fast. This meets the criteria of **atrial fib/flutter with rapid ventricular response.**

271. (D) The R-R intervals vary across the strip without pattern. This is called **grossly or irregularly irregular.**

272. (B) The patient admits to taking cold medication containing decongestants. These agents contain antihistamine and other adrenergic stimulating chemicals. This combined with fatigue and mild dehydration results in **increased adrenergic stimulation of the atria,** which can precipitate atrial fibrillation.

Scenario 5

273. (C) There are no P waves. The QRS complex is wide and bizarre at a rate of 40. This is consistent with a **ventricular escape rhythm,** which is common following defibrillation. PEA is not a rhythm but is instead a condition.

274. (C) Since there is no pulse, CPR must be continued. The goal now is to encourage the rate to increase and produce a sustainable pulse. This is accomplished by **administering 40 units of vasopressin,** which is a potent vasoconstrictor. Vasopressin will additionally stimulate the heart's pacemakers to fire. It is too early to consider termination of resuscitation. Only VF/VT are susceptible to defibrillation. The administration of too many agents this early in the resuscitation is not warranted and until the heart's pacemaker is above the AV node, the administration of amiodarone or lidocaine could extinguish the ventricular escape rhythm resulting in asystole.

275. (D) When the heart is defibrillated, the entire myocardium is **depolarized** simultaneous. This results in asystole and the **termination of VF/VT.** At this point, if quality CPR has been performed and the heart is perfused, the goal is for one of the pacemaker sites to "awaken" and begin an organized rhythm, which produces a pulse.

Scenario 6

276. (C) The most notable finding on this 12-lead ECG is the marked ST elevation in leads II, III, and aVF, which is consistent with an acute inferior wall myocardial wall infarction. However, looking at the lateral precordial leads V_5 and V_6 reveals ST-segment elevation as well. Examination of V_1-V_3 reveals marked ST-segment depression. Together this indicates a myocardial infarction involving the inferior, lateral, and posterior wall of the left ventricle.

277. (A) The majority of inferior wall myocardial infarctions are caused by occlusion of the right coronary artery because 80% to 90% of hearts are "right artery" dominant. However, the lateral and posterior wall of the left ventricle are perfused by the left circumflex artery. Therefore, this heart is "left artery" dominant and the **occlusion is in the distal left circumflex.**

278. (A) The primary goal for patients suffering acute myocardial infarction is to limit ischemic time. Therefore the goal is to rapidly assess the patient for their **candidacy for either PCI or fibrinolytic therapy.** Oxygen, aspirin, and nitrates are the only medications included in the initial therapy of all acute coronary syndromes. The decision to administer the other agents listed is case dependent.

Scenario 7

279. (B) The rhythm is patterned irregularity. There are more P waves than QRS complexes, therefore there is an AVB present. The PR interval is 0.20 second in complex 2 and 0.24 second in complex 3. There is no QRS following the next P wave. This progressive lengthening of the PR interval and "dropped" QRS complex is characteristic of second **AVB Type I (Wenckebach).**

280. (D) The conduction ratio is always the number of P waves to QRS complexes. In this case there are three P wave to ever two QRS complexes. Therefore **3 : 2.**

281. (A) More than likely this is the **patient's underlying cardiac rhythm.** The rate is normal and would not be expected to result in hemodynamic compromise. This is common dysrhythmia in the elderly and does not require treatment.

Scenario 8

282. (D) While it is possible that a wide QRS complex tachycardia could be supraventricular tachycardia in the emergent situation, it **is prudent to assume the rhythm is ventricular tachycardia until proven otherwise.** The QRS complexes are uniform "monomorphic" and therefore do not meet the criteria for torsades de pointes.

Ventricular fibrillation would not produce a pulse and would appear totally chaotic on the monitor.

283. (D) Despite the presence of a pulse, the dysrhythmia has resulted in shock and must be terminated immediately. This is accomplished by administering a **synchronized cardioversion at 100 joules.** Defibrillation would be effective in terminating the dysrhythmia but the higher energy and lack of synchronized delivery are more likely to result in producing ventricular fibrillation.

284. (D) The presence of inverted T waves in leads V_1-V^6 are consistent with extensive myocardial ischemia. The ST segments in V_1-V_3 are up sloping, which is characteristic of ischemia. These are common findings after defibrillation or could represent an underlying acute coronary syndrome, which precipitated the dysrhythmia.

Scenario 9

285. (A) The rhythm is regular. P and P′ waves are present. The PR interval varies due to the varying location of the P waves. The QRS complex is less than 0.12 seconds. The conduction ratio is 1:1. The rate is 70. This is characteristic of **junctional tachycardia.** Junctional escape rhythm would have a rate between 40 and 60. Multiatrial tachycardia would have a rate greater than 100. A wandering atrial pacemaker requires the identification of three or more ectopic P waves.

286. (B) Damage to the AV, which occurs during an **inferior wall myocardial infarction,** is a common cause of this dysrhythmia. While it can occur in rheumatic heart disease, the patient's history is consistent with an acute coronary syndrome. Adrenergic agents and pericarditis are not associated with junctional tachycardia.

287. (A) Junctional tachycardia results from **disruption of normal conduction through the AV node.**

Scenario 10

288. (B) This is a dual-chamber pacemaker that senses and paces both the atria and ventricles and is inhibited by electrical activity from both sites. Therefore it is referred to as **D (dual-chamber sense), D (dual-chamber pace), I (inhibited).** The AAI pacemaker only senses and paces the atria. VDD senses the ventricles, paces both atria and ventricles, and is a demand pacemaker. VVI pacemakers only sense and pace the ventricle.

289. (C) There are pacer spikes without corresponding P′ and QRS complexes. This indicates the pacemaker is firing but the electrical discharge is not, resulting in depolarization of the myocardium. **This condition is referred to as failure to capture because the pacemaker is not "capturing" the myocardium.**

290. (C) The patient has a history of congestive heart failure, therefore **a large volume fluid resuscitation would be contraindicated.** While the patient's blood pressure is low, she is conscious and therefore cautious therapy would include supplemental oxygen, institution of transcutaneous pacing once the patient is sedated, and a cardiology consultation for evaluation of the malfunctioning pacemaker.

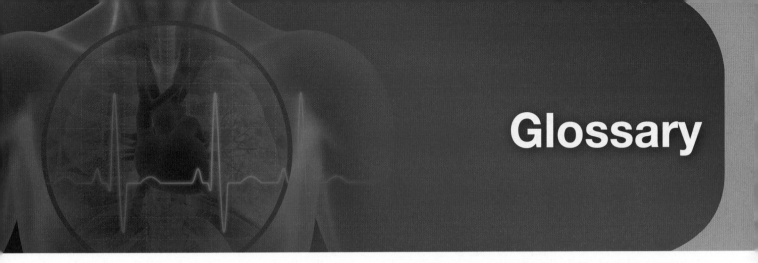

Glossary

A

ABCIXIMAB A platelet GP IIb/IIIa receptor inhibitor that blocks the GP IIb/IIIa receptors on activated platelets from binding to vWF and fibrinogen, thus inhibiting platelet adhesion and aggregation and further thrombus formation.

ABCs: AIRWAY, BREATHING, CIRCULATION The first steps in cardiopulmonary resuscitation whereby the patency of the airway, the adequacy of breathing, and the quality of the patient's circulation is assessed.

ABERRANCY See *Aberrant ventricular conduction (aberrancy).*

ABERRANT VENTRICULAR CONDUCTION (ABERRANCY) An electrical impulse originating in the SA node, atria, or AV junction that is temporarily conducted abnormally through the bundle branches, resulting in a bundle branch block. This is usually caused by the appearance of the electrical impulse at the bundle branches prematurely, before the bundle branches have been sufficiently repolarized. Aberrancy may occur with atrial fibrillation; atrial flutter; premature atrial and junctional complexes; and sinus, atrial, and junctional tachycardias. Also referred to simply as *ventricular aberrancy.*

ABSOLUTE REFRACTORY PERIOD (ARP) OF THE VENTRICLES The period of ventricular depolarization and most of ventricular repolarization during which the ventricles cannot be stimulated to depolarize. It begins with the onset of the QRS complex and ends at about the peak of the T wave.

ACCELERATED IDIOVENTRICULAR RHYTHM (AIVR) A dysrhythmia originating in an ectopic pacemaker in the ventricles with a rate between 40 and 100 beats per minute. Also referred to as *accelerated ventricular rhythm, idioventricular tachycardia,* and *slow ventricular tachycardia.*

ACCELERATED JUNCTIONAL RHYTHM A dysrhythmia originating in an ectopic pacemaker in the AV junction, with a rate between 60 and 100 beats per minute.

ACCELERATED RHYTHM Three or more consecutive beats originating in an ectopic pacemaker with a rate faster than the inherent rate of the escape pacemaker but less than 100 beats per minute. Examples are accelerated junctional rhythm and accelerated idioventricular rhythm (AIVR).

ACCELERATED VENTRICULAR RHYTHM See *Accelerated idioventricular rhythm (AIVR).*

ACCESSORY CONDUCTION PATHWAYS Several distinct abnormal electrical conduction pathways within the heart that bypass the AV node, the bundle of His, or both, thus allowing the electrical impulses to travel from the atria to the ventricles more rapidly than usual. They include the accessory atrioventricular (AV) pathways (the bundles of Kent), the atrio-His fibers, and the nodoventricular/fasciculoventricular fibers.

ACCESSORY ATRIOVENTRICULAR (AV) PATHWAYS (BUNDLES OF KENT) Abnormal accessory conduction pathways located between the atria and the ventricles that bypass the AV junction, resulting in the so-called Wolff-Parkinson-White (WPW) conduction. The result is an abnormally wide QRS complex with a delta wave and an abnormally short PR interval, the classic form of ventricular preexcitation. When this type of AV conduction is associated with a paroxysmal supraventricular tachycardia with normal QRS complexes, it is known as the Wolff-Parkinson-White syndrome. Three separate accessory AV pathways have been found: type A WPW conduction pathway, type B WPW conduction pathway, and posteroseptal WPW conduction pathway.

ACCESSORY AV PATHWAY CONDUCTION See *Accessory atrioventricular (AV) pathways (bundles of Kent).*

ACIDOSIS A disturbance in the acid-base balance of the body caused by excessive amounts of carbon dioxide (respiratory acidosis), lactic acid (metabolic acidosis), or both.

ACTIN One of the contractile protein filaments in myofibrils that give the myocardial cells the property of contractility. The other is myosin.

ACTION POTENTIAL See *Cardiac action potential.*

ACTIVASE Trade name for alteplase (t-PA), a thrombolytic agent.

ACUTE CORONARY SYNDROMES Include silent ischemia, stable and unstable angina, acute MI, and sudden cardiac death.

ACUTE MYOCARDIAL INFARCTION (ACUTE MI, AMI) A condition that is present when necrosis of the myocardium occurs because of prolonged and complete interruption of blood flow to the area. The area of the myocardium involved identifies the acute myocardial infarction: anterior MI, septal MI, lateral MI, anterior (localized) MI, anterolateral MI, anteroseptal MI, extensive anterior MI, inferior (diaphragmatic) MI, inferolateral MI, posterior MI, or right ventricular MI.

ADAMS-STOKES SYNDROME Sudden attacks of unconsciousness, with or without convulsions, caused by a sudden slowing or stopping of the heart beat.

ADENOSINE An antiarrhythmic used to convert paroxysmal supraventricular tachycardia (PSVT) with narrow QRS complexes and narrow-QRS-complex tachycardia of unknown origin (with pulse).

ADENOSINE DIPHOSPHATE (ADP) A substance released from platelets after the platelets are activated after damage to the blood vessel walls. Adenosine diphosphate promotes thrombus formation by stimulating platelet aggregation. Other substances released on platelet activation are serotonin and thromboxane A2.

ADP See *Adenosine diphosphate (ADP)*.

ADRENALIN Trade name for epinephrine. See *Epinephrine*.

ADRENERGIC Having the characteristics of the sympathetic nervous system; sympathomimetic.

ADVANCED AV BLOCK An AV block with a 3:1 or higher conduction ratio.

ADVANCED LIFE SUPPORT Emergency medical care beyond basic life support, including one or more of the following: starting an intravenous (IV) line, administering IV fluids, administering drugs, defibrillating, inserting an esophageal obturator airway or endotracheal tube, and monitoring and interpreting the ECG.

AFTERDEPOLARIZATION An abnormal condition of latent pacemaker and myocardial cells (nonpacemaker cells) in which spontaneous depolarization occurs because of a spontaneous and rhythmic increase in the level of phase 4 membrane action potential after a normal depolarization. If afterdepolarization occurs early in phase 4, it is called *early afterdepolarization*; if late in phase 4, it is called *delayed afterdepolarization*. This abnormal condition is also referred to as triggered activity.

AGONAL Occurring at the moment of or just before death.

AGONAL RHYTHM Cardiac dysrhythmia present in a dying heart. Ventricular escape rhythm.

ALTEPLASE (t-PA) A thrombolytic agent that converts plasminogen, a plasma protein, to plasmin, which in turn dissolves the fibrin binding the platelets together within a thrombus (fibrinolysis), causing the thrombus to break apart (thrombolysis). Trade name: Activase.

AMPLITUDE (VOLTAGE) With respect to ECGs, the height or depth of a wave or complex measured in millimeters (mm).

ANASCARA Generalized edema.

ANEURYSM Dilation of an artery (such as the aorta) or a chamber of the heart (such as the ventricle).

ANGINAL EQUIVALENTS Presence of associated symptoms in the absence of typical angina.

ANION An ion with a negative charge (e.g., Cl^-, PO_4^{---}, SO_4^{--}).

ANOXIA Absence or lack of oxygen.

ANTEGRADE (OR ANTEROGRADE) CONDUCTION Conduction of the electrical impulse in a forward direction, i.e., from the SA node or atria to the ventricles or from the AV junction to the ventricles.

ANTERIOR LEADS Leads I, aVL, and V_1-V_6.

ANTERIOR (LOCALIZED) MI A myocardial infarction commonly caused by occlusion of the diagonal arteries of the left anterior descending (LAD) coronary artery and characterized by early changes in the ST segments and T waves (i.e., ST elevation and tall, peaked T waves) and the appearance later of abnormal Q waves in leads V_3-V_4.

ANTERIOR MI A myocardial infarction caused by the occlusion of the left anterior descending (LAD) coronary artery or the left circumflex coronary artery or any of their branches, singly or in combination. Anterior MI includes septal, anterior (localized), anteroseptal, lateral, anterolateral, and extensive anterior myocardial infarctions and is characterized by early changes in the ST segments and T waves (i.e., ST elevation and tall, peaked T waves) and the appearance early or later of abnormal Q waves in two or all of leads I, aVL, and V_1-V_6, depending on the site of the infarction.

ANTEROLATERAL MI A myocardial infarction commonly caused by occlusion of the diagonal arteries of the left anterior descending (LAD) coronary artery alone or in conjunction with the anterolateral marginal artery of the left circumflex coronary artery and characterized by early changes in the ST segments and T waves (i.e., ST elevation and tall, peaked T waves) and the appearance later of abnormal Q waves in leads I, aVL, and V_3-V_6.

ANTEROSEPTAL MI A myocardial infarction commonly caused by occlusion of the left anterior descending (LAD) coronary artery involving both the septal perforator and diagonal arteries and characterized by early changes in the ST-segments and T waves (i.e., ST elevation and tall, peaked T waves) in leads V_1-V_4 and the appearance early of abnormal Q waves in leads V_1-V_2 and then later in leads V_3-V_4.

ANTICOAGULANT A substance that blocks the conversion of prothrombin to thrombin and inhibits the action of thrombin on fibrinogen, thus preventing the conversion of fibrinogen to fibrin threads.

ANTIPLATELET AGENT Any compound or drug that inhibits platelet adhesion and aggregation and further thrombus formation. Includes aspirin and platelet GP IIb/IIIa receptor inhibitors such as abciximab and eptifibatide.

AORTA The main trunk of the arterial system of the body consisting of the ascending aorta, the aortic arch, and the descending aorta. The descending aorta is further divided into the thoracic and abdominal aorta.

AORTIC DISSECTION Splitting of the media layer of the aorta, leading to the formation of a dissecting aneurysm.

AORTIC VALVE The one-way valve located between the left ventricle and the ascending aorta.

APEX OF THE HEART The pointed lower end of the heart formed by the pointed lower ends of the right and left ventricles.

ARTIFACTS Abnormal waves and spikes in an ECG that result from sources other than the electrical activity of the heart and interfere with or distort the components of the ECG. Common causes of artifacts are muscle tremor, alternating current (AC) interference, loose electrodes, interference related to biotelemetry, and external chest compression.

Artifacts are also referred to as electrical interference or noise.

ARTIFICIAL PACEMAKER An electronic device used to stimulate the heart to beat when the electrical conduction system of the heart malfunctions, causing bradycardia or ventricular asystole. An artificial pacemaker consists of an electronic pulse generator, a battery, and a wire lead that senses the electrical activity of the heart and delivers electrical impulses to the atria or ventricles or both when the pacemaker senses an absence of electrical activity.

ASPIRIN An antiplatelet agent.

ASYMPTOMATIC BRADYCARDIA A bradycardia with a systolic blood pressure greater than 90 to 100 mm Hg and stable and the absence of congestive heart failure, chest pain, dyspnea, signs and symptoms of decreased cardiac output, and premature ventricular complexes. Treatment may not be indicated even if the heart rate falls below 50 beats per minute.

ASYSTOLE Absence of electrical activity in the heart evidenced by lack of QRS complexes.

ATENOLOL A β-adrenergic blocking agent used primarily in the treatment of tachydysrhythmia, hypertension, angina pectoris, and acute MI.

ATHEROSCLEROTIC PLAQUE A lesion in the arterial wall that varies in size and composition from a well-demarcated, yellowish, raised area or swelling on the intimal surface of an artery, produced by subintimal fatty deposits (atheroma) to a large, protruding, dull, white, fibrous plaque filled with pools of gruel-like lipid and foam cells filled with lipid, surrounded by fibrous tissue, necrotic debris, various amounts of blood, and calcium, all covered by a fibrous cap.

ATRIAL AND VENTRICULAR DEMAND PACEMAKER An artificial pacemaker that paces either the atria or ventricles when there is no appropriate spontaneous underlying atrial or ventricular rhythm.

ATRIAL DEMAND PACEMAKER (AAI) An artificial pacemaker that senses spontaneously occurring P waves and paces the atria when they do not appear.

ATRIAL DEPOLARIZATION The electrical process of discharging the resting (polarized) myocardial cells producing the P, P′, F, and f waves and causing the atria to contract.

ATRIAL DIASTOLE The interval or period during which the atria are relaxed and filling with blood. The period between atrial complexes.

ATRIAL DILATATION Distention of the atria because of increased pressure and/or volume within the atria; it may be acute or chronic.

ATRIAL DYSRHYTHMIA Dysrhythmia originating in the atria, such as wandering atrial pacemaker (WAP), premature atrial complexes (PACs), atrial tachycardia (ectopic atrial tachycardia, multifocal atrial tachycardia), atrial flutter, and atrial fibrillation.

ATRIAL ENLARGEMENT Includes atrial dilatation and hypertrophy. Common causes include heart failure, ventricular hypertrophy from whatever cause, pulmonary diseases, pulmonary or systemic hypertension, heart valve stenosis or insufficiency, and acute myocardial infarction. See *Left*

atrial enlargement (left atrial dilatation and hypertrophy) and *Right atrial enlargement (right atrial dilatation and hypertrophy).*

ATRIAL FIBRILLATION A dysrhythmia arising in numerous ectopic pacemakers in the atria characterized by very rapid atrial fibrillation (f) waves and an irregular, often rapid ventricular response. Atrial fibrillation is "fast" if the ventricular rate is greater than 100 per minute and "slow" if it is less than 60. When fast, atrial fibrillation is considered uncontrolled (untreated) atrial fibrillation; when slow, it is controlled (treated) atrial fibrillation.

ATRIAL FIB-FLUTTER Occurs when the rhythm may exhibit atrial fibrillation with an irregularly irregular rhythm.

ATRIAL FIBRILLATION (F) WAVES Irregularly shaped, rounded (or pointed), and dissimilar atrial waves originating in multiple ectopic pacemakers in the atria at a rate between 350 and 600 (average 400) beats per minute. May be "fine" (less than 1 mm in height) or "coarse" (1 mm or greater in height).

ATRIAL FLUTTER A dysrhythmia arising in an ectopic pacemaker in the atria, characterized by abnormal atrial flutter waves with a sawtooth appearance and usually a regular ventricular response after every other or every fourth F wave. If the QRS complexes occur irregularly at varying F wave-to-QRS complex ratios, a variable AV block is present. Atrial flutter may be transient (paroxysmal) or chronic (persistent). When fast, atrial flutter is considered uncontrolled (untreated) atrial flutter; when slow, it is controlled (treated) atrial flutter.

ATRIAL FLUTTER-FIBRILLATION A dysrhythmia arising in the atria alternating between atrial flutter and atrial fibrillation.

ATRIAL FLUTTER (F) WAVES Regularly shaped, usually pointed atrial waves with a sawtooth appearance originating in an ectopic pacemaker in the atria at a rate between 240 and 360 (average 300) beats per minute.

ATRIAL HYPERTROPHY Increase in the thickness of the atrial wall because of chronic increase in pressure and/or volume within the atria.

"ATRIAL KICK" Refers to the complete filling of the ventricles brought on by the contraction of the atria during the last part of ventricular diastole just before the ventricles contract.

ATRIAL OVERLOAD Refers to increased pressure and/or volume within the atria.

ATRIAL REPOLARIZATION The electrical process by which the depolarized atria return to their polarized, resting state. Atrial repolarization produces the atrial T (Ta) wave.

ATRIAL STANDSTILL Absence of electrical activity of the atria.

ATRIAL SYNCHRONOUS VENTRICULAR PACEMAKER (VDD) An artificial pacemaker that is synchronized with the patient's atrial rhythm and paces the ventricles when an AV block occurs.

ATRIAL SYSTOLE The interval or period during which the atria are contracting and emptying of blood.

ATRIAL TACHYCARDIA A dysrhythmia originating in an ectopic pacemaker in the atria with a rate between 160 and 240 beats per minute. It includes ectopic atrial tachycardia and multifocal atrial tachycardia (MAT). Atrial tachycardia may occur with or without an AV block, which may be constant or variable. It may occur with narrow QRS complexes or abnormally wide QRS complexes because of preexisting bundle branch block, aberrant ventricular conduction, or ventricular preexcitation. When abnormal QRS complexes occur with the tachycardia because of aberrant ventricular conduction, the tachycardia is called atrial tachycardia with aberrant ventricular conduction (aberrancy).

ATRIAL TACHYCARDIA WITH ABERRANCY A dysrhythmia with abnormal QRS complexes only during tachycardia. See *Aberrant ventricular conduction*.

ATRIAL TACHYCARDIA WITH BLOCK When the AV block occurs only during tachycardia.

ATRIAL T WAVE (Ta) Represents atrial repolarization; often buried in the following QRS complex.

ATRIO-HIS PREEXCITATION Abnormal conduction of the electrical impulses from the atria to the bundle of His via the atrio-His fibers (James fibers) bypassing the AV node, resulting in PR intervals that are usually shortened to less than 0.12 second and normal QRS complexes.

ATRIO-HIS FIBERS (JAMES FIBERS) Abnormal accessory conduction pathways connecting the atria with the lower part of the AV node at its junction with the bundle of His. See *Atrio-His preexcitation*.

ATRIOVENTRICULAR (AV) BLOCK See *AV block* and specific AV blocks.

ATRIOVENTRICULAR (AV) DISSOCIATION Occurs when the atria and ventricles beat independently.

ATRIOVENTRICULAR (AV) JUNCTION The part of the electrical conduction system that normally conducts the electrical impulse from the atria to the ventricles. It consists of the AV node and the bundle of His.

ATRIOVENTRICULAR (AV) NODE The part of the electrical conduction system, located in the posterior floor of the right atrium near the interatrial septum, through which the electrical impulses are normally conducted from the atria to the bundle of His.

ATRIOVENTRICULAR VALVES Tricuspid and mitral valves.

ATRIUM The thin-walled chamber into which venous blood flows before reaching the ventricle. The two atria, the right and left atria, form the upper part of the heart, or the base, and are separated from the ventricles by the mitral and tricuspid valves.

ATROPINE A drug that counteracts parasympathetic activity in the heart, thereby increasing the heart rate and enhancing the conduction of the electrical impulses through the AV node; used to treat sinus bradycardia, sinus arrest/sinoatrial exit block, and second- and third-degree AV blocks with narrow QRS complexes.

AUGMENTED (UNIPOLAR) LEADS Leads aVR, aVL, and aVF; each obtained using a positive electrode attached to one extremity and a negative electrode to a central terminal.

Lead aVR. The positive electrode attached to the right arm and the negative electrode to the central terminal.

Lead aVL. The positive electrode attached to the left arm and the negative electrode to the central terminal.

Lead aVF. The positive electrode attached to the left leg and the negative electrode to the central terminal.

AUTOMATICITY, PROPERTY OF The property of a cell to reach a threshold potential and generate electrical impulses spontaneously. Also referred to as the *property of self-excitation*.

AUTONOMIC NERVOUS SYSTEM Part of the nervous system that is involved in the constant control of involuntary bodily functions, including the control of cardiac output (by regulating the heart rate and stroke volume) and blood pressure (by regulating blood vessel activity). It includes the sympathetic (adrenergic) and parasympathetic (cholinergic or vagal) nervous systems, each producing opposite effects when stimulated.

AV Abbreviation for atrioventricular.

AV BLOCK Delay or failure of conduction of electrical impulses through the AV junction.

AV BLOCK, FIRST-DEGREE A dysrhythmia in which there is a constant delay in the conduction of electrical impulses through the AV node. It is characterized by abnormally prolonged PR intervals (greater than 0.20 second).

AV BLOCK, SECOND-DEGREE, TYPE I (WENCKEBACH) A dysrhythmia in which progressive prolongation of the conduction of electrical impulses through the AV node occurs until conduction is completely blocked. It is characterized by progressive lengthening of the PR interval until a QRS complex fails to appear after a P wave. This phenomenon is cyclical.

AV BLOCK, SECOND-DEGREE, TYPE II A dysrhythmia in which a complete block of conduction of the electrical impulses occurs in one bundle branch and an intermittent block in the other. It is characterized by regularly or irregularly absent QRS complexes (producing, commonly, an AV conduction ratio of 4:3 or 3:2) and a bundle branch block.

AV BLOCK, SECOND-DEGREE, 2:1 AND ADVANCED A dysrhythmia caused by defective conduction of electrical impulses through the AV node or bundle branches or both. It is characterized by regularly or irregularly absent QRS complexes (commonly producing an AV conduction ratio of 2:1 or greater) with or without a bundle branch block.

AV BLOCKS WITH WIDE QRS COMPLEXES Second-degree AV block, type II and 2:1 and advanced AV block, and third-degree AV block with wide QRS complexes require a temporary transcutaneous pacemaker immediately, regardless of whether not the bradycardia is symptomatic.

AV BLOCK, THIRD-DEGREE (COMPLETE AV BLOCK) A dysrhythmia in which there is a complete block of the conduction of electrical impulses through the AV node, bundle of His, or bundle branches. It is characterized by independent beating of the atria and ventricles. Third-degree AV block may be transient and reversible or permanent (chronic).

AV CONDUCTION RATIO The ratio of P, P′, F, or f waves to QRS complexes. For example, an AV conduction ratio of 4:3 indicates that for every four P waves, three are followed by QRS complexes.

AV DISSOCIATION Occurs when the atria and ventricles beat independently. Occurs when QRS complexes occur totally unrelated to the P, P′, or F waves.

AV JUNCTION See *Atrioventricular (AV) junction.*

AV NODE See *Atrioventricular (AV) node.*

AV REENTRY TACHYCARDIA (AVRT) A dysrhythmia when both the AV node and an accessory conduction pathway are involved in the reentry mechanism.

AV SEQUENTIAL PACEMAKER (DVI) An artificial pacemaker that paces either the atria or ventricles or both sequentially when spontaneous ventricular activity is absent.

AXIS Used alone, usually refers to the QRS axis—the single large vector representing the mean (or average) of all the ventricular vectors. It is usually graphically displayed as an arrow. See *P axis*, *ST axis*, and *T axis*.

AXIS OF A LEAD (LEAD AXIS) A hypothetical line joining the poles of a lead. A lead axis has a direction and a polarity.

B

β-BLOCKER, BETA-BLOCKER, BETA-ADRENERGIC BLOCKING AGENT, β-ADRENERGIC BLOCKING AGENT See *Beta-blockers.*

BACHMANN'S BUNDLE A branch of the internodal atrial conduction tracts that extends across the atria, conducting the electrical impulses from the SA node to the left atrium.

BALLOON ANGIOPLASTY The insertion of a balloon-tipped catheter into the occluded or narrowed coronary artery to reopen the artery by inflating the balloon, fracturing the atheromatous plaque, and dilating the arterial lumen. This procedure, also called *percutaneous transluminal coronary angioplasty* (PTCA), is often followed by insertion of a coronary artery stent.

BASELINE The part of the ECG during which electrical activity of the heart is absent. Commonly the interval between the end of the T wave and the onset of the P wave (the TP segment) is considered the baseline and is used as the reference for the measurement of the amplitude of the ECG waves and complexes.

BASE OF THE HEART The upper part of the heart formed by the right and left atria.

BETA-BLOCKERS A group of drugs that block sympathetic activity; used primarily to treat tachydysrhythmia, hypertension, angina, and acute MI. Atenolol, esmolol, and metoprolol.

BIDIRECTIONAL VENTRICULAR TACHYCARDIA Ventricular tachycardia characterized by two distinctly different forms of QRS complexes alternating with each other, indicating the presence of two ventricular ectopic pacemakers.

BIGEMINY A dysrhythmia in which every other beat is a premature complex. The premature beat may be atrial, junctional, or ventricular in origin (i.e., atrial bigeminy, junctional bigeminy, ventricular bigeminy).

BIOLOGICAL DEATH Present when irreversible brain damage has occurred, usually within 10 minutes after cardiac arrest, if untreated.

BIPHASIC DEFLECTION A deflection having both a positive and a negative component (e.g., a biphasic P wave, a biphasic T wave).

BIPOLAR LEAD A lead that has both a positive and negative electrode that measures the electrical potential between the electrodes.

BIPOLAR LIMB LEADS Leads I, II, and III.

BLEEDING DIATHESIS A tendency toward abnormally inadequate blood clotting and an increase in bleeding.

BLOCK Delay or failure of conduction of an electrical impulse through the electrical conduction system because of tissue damage or increased parasympathetic (vagal) tone.

BLOCKED PAC A P′ wave not followed by a QRS complex.

BLOOD THINNER A term used to indicate an anticoagulant, such as warfarin, used to reduce the prothrombin activity, thus inhibiting clot formation.

BOLUS A single large dose of a drug that provides an initial high therapeutic blood level of the drug.

BRADYCARDIA A dysrhythmia with rates of less than 60 beats per minute (e.g., sinus bradycardia; sinus arrest and sinoatrial [SA] exit block; junctional escape rhythm; ventricular escape rhythm; second-degree, type I AV block [Wenckebach]; second-degree, type II AV block; second-degree, 2:1, and advanced AV block; and third-degree AV block).

BRETYLIUM TOSYLATE An antiarrhythmic once used in the treatment of premature ventricular complexes (PVCs), ventricular fibrillation, and ventricular tachycardia.

BRUGADA SYNDROME Sudden cardiac arrest from ST-segment elevation in the right precordial leads, right bundle branch block, susceptibility to ventricular tachydysrhythmias, and structurally normal hearts.

BUNDLE BRANCH BLOCK (BBB) Defective conduction of electrical impulses through the right or left bundle branch from the bundle of His to the Purkinje network, causing a right or left bundle branch block. It may be complete or incomplete (partial) or permanent (chronic) or intermittent (transient). It may be present with or without an intact interventricular septum.

BUNDLE BRANCHES The part of the electrical conduction system in the ventricles consisting of the right and left bundle branches that conducts the electrical impulses from the bundle of His to the Purkinje network of the myocardium.

BUNDLE OF HIS The part of the electrical conduction system located in the upper part of the interventricular septum that conducts the electrical impulses from the AV node to the right and left bundle branches. The bundle of His and the AV node form the AV junction.

BUNDLES OF KENT See *Accessory atrioventricular (AV) pathways.*

BURIED P WAVE Refers to a P wave partially or completely hidden in a preceding T wave. This occurs when a sinus, atrial, or junctional P wave occurs during the repolarization of a previous beat as in a sinus, atrial, or junctional tachycardia or a premature atrial or junctional premature beat.

BURSTS (OR SALVOS) Refers to the occurrence of two or more consecutive premature atrial, junctional, or ventricular complexes.

C

CABG See *Coronary artery bypass grafting (CABG).*

CALCIUM CHANNEL BLOCKER A drug that blocks the entry of calcium ions (Ca^{++}) into cells, especially those of cardiac and vascular smooth muscle. Used as an antiarrhythmic, antihypertensive, and antianginal drug. Diltiazem.

CALCIUM CHLORIDE A calcium salt (electrolyte) used to replenish blood calcium levels after administration of excessive calcium channel blockers or to reverse the effects of hyperkalemia and hypermagnesemia on the heart.

CALIBRATION (OR STANDARDIZATION) Accomplished by inserting a standard 1-millivolt (mV) electrical signal to produce a 10-mm deflection (two large squares) on the ECG.

CAMEL'S HUMP Descriptive term referring to the distinctive narrow, positive wave—the Osborn wave—that occurs at the junction of the QRS complex and the ST segment in hypothermic patients with a core body temperature of 95°F. Also referred to as the "J wave" or the "J deflection."

CAPTURE Refers to the ability of a pacemaker's electrical impulse to depolarize the atria or ventricles or both.

CAPTURE BEAT A normally conducted QRS complex of the underlying rhythm occurring within a ventricular tachycardia.

CARDIAC ACTION POTENTIAL Refers to the membrane potential of a myocardial cell and the changes it undergoes during depolarization and repolarization. The phases of the cardiac action potential include the following:
Phase 0: depolarization phase
Phase 1: early rapid repolarization phase
Phase 2: plateau phase of slow repolarization
Phase 3: terminal phase of rapid repolarization
Phase 4: period between action potentials

CARDIAC ARREST The sudden and unexpected cessation of an adequate circulation to maintain life in a patient who was not expected to die.

CARDIAC CELLS Cells of the heart, consisting of the myocardial (or "working") cells and the specialized cells of the electrical conduction system of the heart.

CARDIAC CYCLE The interval from the beginning of one heart beat to the beginning of the next one. The cardiac cycle normally consists of a P wave, a QRS complex, and a T wave. It represents a sequence of atrial contraction and relaxation and ventricular contraction and relaxation, in that order.

CARDIAC OUTPUT The amount of blood circulated by the heart in 1 minute, in liters per minute. Obtained by multiplying the amount of blood expelled by the left ventricle with each contraction (stroke volume) by the heart rate per minute.

CARDIAC PACEMAKER An artificial pacemaker. See *Artificial pacemaker.*

CARDIAC STANDSTILL Absence of atrial and ventricular complexes. This term is used interchangeably with ventricular asystole.

CARDIAC TAMPONADE Acute compression of the heart because of effusion of fluid into the pericardial cavity (as occurs in pericarditis) or accumulation of blood in the pericardium from rupture of the heart or penetrating trauma.

CARDIAC VECTOR A graphic presentation, using an arrow, representing the moment-to-moment electric current generated by depolarization or repolarization of a small segment of the atrial or ventricular wall.

CARDIOACCELERATOR CENTER One of the nerve centers of the sympathetic nervous system located in the medulla oblongata, a part of the brainstem. Impulses from the cardioaccelerator center reach the electrical conduction system of the heart and the atria and ventricles by way of the sympathetic nerves.

CARDIOGENIC Originating in the heart.

CARDIOGENIC SHOCK A life-threatening complication of acute myocardial infarction caused by the inability of the damaged ventricles to maintain an adequate systemic circulation. One of the consequences of pump failure.

CARDIOINHIBITOR CENTER One of the nerve centers of the parasympathetic nervous system located in the medulla oblongata, a part of the brainstem. Impulses from the cardioinhibitor center by way of the right and left vagus nerves innervate the atria, SA node, and AV junction, and to a small extent the ventricles.

CARDIOMYOPATHY A primary disease of the myocardium affecting the bundle branches, causing bundle branch and fascicular blocks, often of unknown etiology.

CARDIOVERSION Application of a synchronized countershock to convert certain dysrhythmias—atrial flutter, atrial fibrillation, paroxysmal supraventricular tachycardia (PSVT), wide-QRS-complex tachycardia of unknown origin with pulse, and ventricular tachycardia with pulse—to an organized supraventricular rhythm.

CAROTID ARTERY DISEASE Primarily atherosclerotic in nature, with progressive formation of lumen-narrowing (stenotic) atheromatous plaques. A carotid occlusive disease.

CAROTID BRUIT An abnormal sound or murmur heard by auscultation over a stenotic (narrowed) carotid artery, usually a sign of an atheromatous plaque.

CAROTID SINUS A slightly dilated section of the common carotid artery at the point where it bifurcates, containing sensory nerve endings involved in the nervous reflexes regulating blood pressure and heart rate.

CAROTID SINUS MASSAGE Application of pressure to one of the carotid sinuses with the fingertips to convert paroxysmal supraventricular tachycardia (PSVT) and narrow-QRS-complex tachycardia of unknown origin (with pulse).

CATECHOLAMINES Hormone-like substances, such as epinephrine and norepinephrine, that have a strong sympathetic action on the heart and peripheral blood vessels, increasing the cardiac output and blood pressure.

CATION An ion with a positive charge (e.g., K$^+$, Na$^+$).

cc Abbreviation for cubic centimeter. It is often substituted for mL (milliliter).

CELL MEMBRANE POTENTIAL The difference in electrical potential across the cell membrane (i.e., the difference between the electrical potential within the cell and a reference potential in the extracellular fluid surrounding the cell).

CENTRAL TERMINAL The central terminal, in the case of the augmented ECG leads, consists of connecting together two of the three electrodes used (the right and left arm electrodes and the left leg electrode) other than the positive electrode. In the case of the precordial leads, the central terminal consists of connecting all three extremity electrodes—the right and left arm electrodes and the left leg electrode. The central terminal is considered to be an indifferent, zero reference point.

CEREBROVASCULAR ACCIDENT (CVA) Cerebral ischemia caused by a decrease in blood flow resulting from obstruction of a blood vessel by an embolus or a thrombus, or from cerebrovascular hemorrhage. Cerebral stroke.

CEREBROVASCULAR DISEASE General term for a brain dysfunction caused by an inadequacy of the cerebral blood supply.

CHAMBERS OF THE HEART Consists of the two thin-walled atria (the right and left atrium) and the two thick-walled ventricles (the right and left ventricle).

CHEST DISCOMFORT Described as a crushing, vice-like constriction, a feeling equivalent to an "elephant sitting on the chest," or heartburn.

CHIEF COMPLAINT Short statement of the patient's major symptoms requiring emergency medical care.

CHRONIC OBSTRUCTIVE PULMONARY DISEASE (COPD) A chronic disease of the lungs characterized by a chronic productive cough and dyspnea. Typical ECG pattern: poor R-wave progression in the precordial leads V_1-V_5 or V_1-V_6.

CIRCULATORY SYSTEM The blood vessels in the body, including the systemic and pulmonary circulatory systems.

CLINICAL DEATH Present the moment the patient's cardiac output ceases, as evidenced by the absence of a pulse and blood pressure; occurs immediately after the onset of cardiac arrest. Common causes are ventricular fibrillation, pulseless ventricular tachycardia, ventricular asystole, and pulseless electrical activity.

COAGULATION CLOTTING The process of changing from a liquid to a solid (i.e., changing from liquid blood to a solid blood clot or thrombus).

COARSE ATRIAL FIBRILLATION Atrial fibrillation with large fibrillatory waves—1 mm or greater in height.

COARSE VENTRICULAR FIBRILLATION Ventricular fibrillation with large fibrillatory waves—greater than 3 mm in height.

COLLAGEN FIBERS The white protein fibers present in the connective tissue within the intima of the arterial wall that, when exposed to blood after an injury, immediately bind to the platelets directly (via GP Ia receptors) and indirectly through vWF (via GP Ib and GP IIb/IIIa receptors). This action adheres the platelets to the arterial wall and activates them.

COMPENSATORY PAUSE The R-R interval following a premature complex. It may be full or incomplete, depending on whether the SA node, for example, is depolarized by the premature complex. If the SA node is not depolarized by the premature complex, the compensatory pause is called "full"; the sum of a "full" compensatory pause and the preceding R-R interval is equal to the sum of two R-R intervals of the underlying rhythm. If the SA node is depolarized by the premature complex, resetting the timing of the SA node, the compensatory pause is called "incomplete"; the sum of an "incomplete" compensatory pause and the preceding R-R interval is less than the sum of two R-R intervals of the underlying rhythm.

COMPLETE ATRIOVENTRICULAR (AV) BLOCK See *AV block, third-degree.*

COMPLETE BUNDLE BRANCH BLOCK (RIGHT, LEFT) Complete disruption of the conduction of electrical impulses through the right or left bundle branch. The duration of the QRS complex is 0.12 second or greater.

COMPONENTS OF THE ELECTROCARDIOGRAM Includes the P wave, PR interval, PR segment, QRS complex, ST segment, T wave, U wave, QT interval, TP segment, and R-R interval.

CONDUCTED PAC A positive P′ wave (in Lead II) followed by a QRS complex.

CONDUCTED PJC A negative P′ wave (in Lead II) followed by a QRS complex.

CONDUCTIVITY, PROPERTY OF The property of cardiac cells to conduct electrical impulses.

CONGESTIVE HEART FAILURE (CHF) Excessive blood or tissue fluid in the lungs or body or both caused by the inefficient pumping of the ventricles. One of the consequences of pump failure. May be of recent origin (acute) or of prolonged duration (chronic).

CONTRACTILE FILAMENT See *Myofibril.*

CONTRACTILITY, PROPERTY OF The property of cardiac cells to contract when they are depolarized by an electrical impulse.

CONTROLLED ATRIAL FIBRILLATION When less than 100 QRS complexes per minute are conducted.

CONTROLLED ATRIAL FLUTTER A "treated" atrial flutter with a slow ventricular rate of about 60 to 75 beats per minute.

COPD See *Chronic obstructive pulmonary disease (COPD).*

CORONARY ARTERY ANGIOPLASTY See *Percutaneous transluminal coronary angioplasty (PTCA).*

CORONARY ARTERY CIRCULATION The coronary artery circulation consists of the left coronary artery (LCA) and the right coronary artery (RCA). The left coronary artery has a short main stem, the left main coronary artery, which branches into the left anterior descending (LAD) coronary artery and the left circumflex coronary artery. The arteries that commonly arise from the LAD coronary artery, the left circumflex coronary artery, and the right coronary artery are listed below.

Left anterior descending coronary artery	Right coronary artery
Diagonal arteries	Conus artery
Septal perforator arteries	Sinoatrial node artery
Right ventricular arteries	Anterior right ventricular artery
Left circumflex coronary artery	Right atrial artery
Left atrial circumflex arteries	Acute marginal artery
Anterolateral marginal artery	Posterior descending coronary artery
Posterolateral marginal arteries	AV node artery
Distal left circumflex artery	Posterior left ventricular arteries

CORONARY ARTERY DISEASE Progressive narrowing and eventual obstruction of the coronary arteries by atherosclerosis.

CORONARY ARTERY BYPASS GRAFTING (CABG) The surgical procedure of bypassing a critically narrowed or obstructed coronary artery using an internal mammary (thoracic) artery or a saphenous vein. Other arteries used for grafting include the radial artery, the inferior gastroepiploic artery, and the inferior epigastric artery.

CORONARY ARTERY STENT A cylindrical coil or wire mesh. See *Coronary artery stenting.*

CORONARY ARTERY STENTING The procedure of inserting a cylindrical coil or wire mesh into an obstructed coronary artery and expanding it (usually by balloon inflation) to compress the surrounding atherosclerotic tissue and dilate the obstructed lumen.

CORONARY CIRCULATION Passage of blood through the coronary arteries and their branches and the capillaries in the heart and then back to the right atrium via the coronary venules and veins and the coronary sinus.

CORONARY OCCLUSION (OR OBSTRUCTION) Obstruction of a coronary artery, usually by a blood clot (coronary thrombus); the major cause of acute myocardial infarction.

CORONARY SINUS The outlet in the right atrium draining the coronary venous system.

CORONARY THROMBOSIS The formation of a blood clot (thrombus) within a coronary artery, resulting in coronary artery obstruction; the major cause of acute myocardial infarction.

CORONARY VASOSPASM Coronary artery spasm. One of the causes of coronary artery obstruction.

COR PULMONALE Right heart disease with right ventricular hypertrophy and right atrial dilatation caused by pulmonary hypertension secondary to chronic lung disease.

CORRECTED QT INTERVAL (QTc) The average duration of the QT interval normally expected at a given heart rate.

COUMADIN Trade name for warfarin, an anticoagulant.

COUNTERSHOCK See *Synchronized countershock.*

COUPLED BEATS Atrial or ventricular ectopic beats occurring in groups of two. Also called paired beats, couplet.

COUPLET Two consecutive premature complexes. Also referred to as coupled beats, paired beats.

COUPLING Ventricular bigeminy with the premature ventricular complexes following the QRS complexes of the underlying rhythm at equal coupling intervals.

COUPLING INTERVAL The R-R interval between a premature complex and the preceding QRS complex of the underlying rhythm.

COURSE FIBRILLATORY WAVES When the f waves are greater than 1 mm high.

C-REACTIVE PROTEIN A plasma protein that becomes abnormally elevated in many acute inflammatory conditions and in tissue necrosis as occurs in acute MI. It becomes elevated in about 24 hours after acute MI.

CURRENT OF INJURY The theoretical cause of ST-segment elevation in acute myocardial infarction; an electrical manifestation of the inability of cardiac cells "injured" by severe ischemia to maintain a normal resting membrane potential during diastole.

CVA See *Cerebrovascular accident (CVA).*

CYANOSIS Slightly bluish, grayish, slatelike, or purplish discoloration of the skin caused by the presence of unoxygenated blood.

D

DEFIBRILLATION SHOCK An unsynchronized direct current (DC) shock used to terminate pulseless ventricular tachycardia and ventricular fibrillation.

DEFLECTION Refers to the waves in the ECG. A deflection may be positive (upright), negative (inverted), biphasic (both positive and negative), or equiphasic (equally positive and negative). When a series of waves, such as a QRS complex, is composed of positive and negative deflections, it may be (1) predominantly positive (the sum total of the positive and negative deflections is positive, no matter by how much); (2) predominantly negative (the sum total of the positive and negative deflections is negative, no matter by how much); or (3) equiphasic (the positive deflections are equal to the negative deflections).

DELAYED AFTERDEPOLARIZATION See *Afterdepolarization.*

DELTA WAVE The slurring of the onset of the QRS complex—the fusion of the depolarization wave of a prematurely activated ventricle, the result of premature ventricular excitation, and the depolarization wave of the other, normally activated ventricle. Present in ventricular preexcitation and nodoventricular/fasciculoventricular preexcitation.

DEMAND PACEMAKERS Artificial pacemakers that have a sensing device that senses the heart's electrical activity and fires at a preset rate when the heart's electrical activity drops below a predetermined rate level.

DEMAND PACING Refers to a mode of pacing by an artificial pacemaker in which the pacemaker is turned on when an appropriate underlying spontaneous atrial or ventricular rhythm fails to occur.

DEPOLARIZATION The electrical process by which the resting potential of a polarized, resting cell of the atria, ventricles, or electrical conduction system is reduced to a less negative value.

DEPOLARIZATION WAVES The parts of the ECG representing the depolarization of the atria and ventricles—the P wave (atrial depolarization) and the QRS complex (ventricular depolarization).

DEPOLARIZED STATE The condition of the cell when it has been completely depolarized.

DIABETIC HEMORRHAGIC RETINOPATHY A disorder of the retinal blood vessels characterized by degeneration of the blood vessels and hemorrhage within the eye, the result of long-standing, poorly controlled diabetes.

DIAGONAL CORONARY ARTERY Arises from the left main coronary artery instead of from the left anterior descending coronary artery.

DIASTOLE (ELECTRICAL) Phase 4 of the action potential.

DIASTOLE (MECHANICAL) The period of atrial or ventricular relaxation.

DIAZEPAM An antianxiety agent used to produce amnesia in conscious patients before cardioversion of certain dysrhythmias. A drug that relieves apprehension and anxiety. Trade name: Valium.

DIGITALIS A cardiac glycoside obtained from the leaves of *Digitalis lanata*, used to decrease rapid ventricular rate in atrial flutter, atrial fibrillation, and paroxysmal supraventricular tachycardia (PSVT) and to improve ventricular contraction in congestive heart failure.

DIGITALIS EFFECT The changes in the ECG caused by the administration of digitalis. They include prolongation of the PR interval over 0.2 second; depression of the ST segment by 1 mm or more in many of the leads, with a characteristic "scooped-out" appearance; alteration of the T waves so that they appear flattened, inverted, or biphasic; and shortening of the QT interval to less than normal for the heart rate.

DIGITALIS OVERDOSE Excessive administration of digitalis, often accompanied by signs and symptoms of digitalis toxicity, which includes the appearance of dysrhythmias, such as sinus dysrhythmia and bradycardia; premature atrial, junctional, and ventricular complexes; atrial, junctional, and ventricular tachycardias; accelerated idioventricular rhythm (AIVR); ventricular fibrillation; and AV blocks. In fact, almost any dysrhythmia may be caused by excess digitalis.

DIGITALIS TOXICITY Digitalis overdose.

DIGITALIZATION The process of administering an adequate amount of digitalis over a period of time in the treatment of certain dysrhythmias. See *Digoxin*.

DIGOXIN A cardiac glycoside obtained from the leaves of *Digitalis lanata*, used in the treatment of atrial flutter, atrial fibrillation, and paroxysmal supraventricular tachycardia (PSVT) and to improve ventricular contraction in congestive heart failure.

DILATATION AND HYPERTROPHY Refers to the two kinds of enlargement of the atria and ventricles. Distention of an individual heart chamber; it may be acute or chronic.

DILTIAZEM HYDROCHLORIDE A calcium channel blocker drug used to treat atrial tachycardia without block, atrial flutter, atrial fibrillation, and paroxysmal supraventricular tachycardia (PSVT).

DIRECT CURRENT (DC) SHOCK Used as defibrillation shock, synchronized countershock, and unsynchronized shock to terminate various dysrhythmias. See *Defibrillation shock, Synchronized countershock*, and *Unsynchronized shock*.

DIRECTIONAL CORONARY ATHERECTOMY (DCA) The mechanical removal of a noncalcified thrombus through a catheter inserted in the occluded or narrowed coronary artery.

DIURETIC A drug used in congestive heart failure to decrease excess body fluid by increasing the secretion of urine by the kidney.

DIVING REFLEX The technique of immersing the patient's face in ice water to elicit the parasympathetic reflex in an attempt to terminate paroxysmal supraventricular tachycardia (PSVT) and narrow-QRS-complex tachycardia of unknown origin (with pulse). It should only be tried if other vagal maneuvers are not effective and ischemic heart disease is not present or suspected.

DOBUTAMINE (DOBUTREX) Adrenergic agent used to increase cardiac output and elevate the blood pressure.

DOMINANT CORONARY ARTERY (RIGHT, LEFT) Refers to the coronary artery, right or left, that gives rise to both the posterior left ventricular arteries and the posterior descending coronary artery.

DOMINANT (OR PRIMARY) PACEMAKER OF THE HEART The SA node.

DOPAMINE HYDROCHLORIDE A sympathomimetic that increases blood pressure; used in the treatment of hypotension and shock.

DOWNSLOPING ST-SEGMENT DEPRESSION A type of ST-segment depression that is most specific for myocardial ischemia, including that present in acute subendocardial non-Q-wave MI.

DROPPED BEATS Nonconducted P waves in AV blocks.

DROPPED P WAVES Absent P waves in sinus arrest and sinoatrial (SA) exit block.

DUAL-CHAMBER PACEMAKER An artificial pacemaker that paces the atria, ventricles, or both when appropriate.

DYING HEART A heart with feeble, ineffectual ventricular contractions and an ECG showing markedly abnormal QRS complexes, usually a ventricular escape rhythm.

DYSRHYTHMIA A rhythm other than a normal sinus rhythm when (1) the heart rate is less than 60 or greater than 100 beats per minute, (2) the rhythm is irregular, (3) premature complexes occur, or (4) the normal progression of the electrical impulse through the electrical conduction system is blocked. A term more correct than "arrhythmia" but used less frequently.

E

EARLY AFTERDEPOLARIZATION See *Afterdepolarization*.

EARLY REPOLARIZATION A normal variant of myocardial repolarization in which the ST segment is elevated or depressed 1 to 3 mm above or below the baseline, respectively. Most commonly elevated in leads I, II, and aVF and the precordial leads V_2-V_6.

ECG Abbreviation for electrocardiogram.

ECG ARTIFACTS See *Artifacts*.

ECG CALIPERS A device used to measure distances and intervals on an ECG tracing as an aid in determining the heart rate and rhythm.

ECG GRID The grid on the ECG paper is formed by dark and light horizontal and vertical lines. It is used to measure the time in seconds (sec) and distance in millimeters (mm) along the horizontal lines and voltage (amplitude) in millimeters (mm) along the vertical lines. The dark vertical lines are 0.20 second (5 mm) apart; the light vertical lines 0.04 second (1 mm) apart. The dark horizontal lines are 5 mm apart; the light horizontal lines 1 mm apart.

ECG LEAD An ECG lead measures the difference in electrical potential generated by the heart, obtained by using a positive and a negative electrode—the positive electrode attached to an extremity or the anterior chest wall and the negative electrode to an extremity or a central terminal. Includes leads I, II, III, aVR, aVL, aVF, and V_1-V_6.

ECG LEAD V_4 R A precordial lead obtained by placing the positive electrode in the right midclavicular line in the right fifth intercostal space. Used primarily to rule out a right ventricular myocardial infarction after the initial finding of an inferior myocardial infarction.

ECG MONITOR The screen of an oscilloscope used in viewing the ECG.

ECTOPIC ATRIAL TACHYCARDIA An atrial tachycardia that originates in a single atrial ectopic pacemaker site, characterized by P′ waves that are usually identical.

ECTOPIC BEATS Premature beats originating in ectopic pacemakers in the atria, AV junction, and ventricles (e.g., premature atrial complexes [PACs], premature junctional complexes [PJCs], and premature ventricular complexes [PVCs]).

ECTOPIC FOCUS A pacemaker other than the SA node.

ECTOPIC PACEMAKERS Abnormal pacemakers in the atria, AV junction, bundle branches, Purkinje network, and ventricular myocardium.

ECTOPIC P WAVE (P′ WAVE) A P wave produced by the depolarization of the atria in an abnormal direction, initiated by an electrical impulse arising in an ectopic pacemaker in the atria, AV junction, or ventricles. The ectopic P wave may be either positive (upright) or negative (inverted) in lead II and may precede or follow the QRS complex.

ECTOPIC RHYTHMS Dysrhythmias originating in ectopic pacemakers in the atria, AV junction, and ventricles.

Atrial. Wandering atrial pacemaker (WAP), premature atrial complexes (PACs), atrial tachycardia (ectopic atrial tachycardia, multifocal atrial tachycardia), atrial flutter, atrial fibrillation

Junctional. Premature junctional complexes (PJCs), nonparoxysmal junctional tachycardia (accelerated junctional rhythm, junctional tachycardia), paroxysmal supraventricular tachycardia (PSVT)

Ventricular. Accelerated idioventricular rhythm (AIVR), premature ventricular complexes (PVCs), ventricular tachycardia (VT), ventricular fibrillation (VF)

ECTOPIC TACHYCARDIAS Abnormal rhythms originating in ectopic pacemakers having a rate of over 100 beats per minute, such as atrial tachycardia (ectopic atrial tachycardia, multifocal atrial tachycardia), atrial flutter, atrial fibrillation, junctional tachycardia, paroxysmal supraventricular tachycardia (PSVT), and ventricular tachycardia (VT).

ECTOPIC VENTRICULAR DYSRHYTHMIAS Abnormal rhythms originating in ectopic pacemakers in the ventricles, such as accelerated idioventricular rhythm (AIVR), premature ventricular complexes (PVCs), ventricular tachycardia, and ventricular fibrillation.

ECTOPY A condition signifying the presence of ectopic beats and rhythms (e.g., ventricular ectopy).

EDEMA A condition in which the body tissues have accumulated excessive tissue fluid or exudate (as in congestive heart failure).

EINTHOVEN'S EQUILATERAL TRIANGLE An equilateral triangle depicted in the frontal plane using the lead axes of the three limb leads as the sides with the heart and its zero reference point in the center.

EINTHOVEN'S LAW The sum of the electrical currents recorded in leads I and III equals the sum of the electrical currents recorded in lead II.

ELECTRIC CURRENT The flow of electricity along a conductor in a closed circuit.

ELECTRICAL ACTIVITY OF THE HEART The electric current generated by the depolarization and repolarization of the atria and ventricles, which can be graphically displayed on the ECG.

ELECTRICAL ALTERNANS Periodic alternation in the size of the QRS complexes between normal and small, coincident with respiration; typically present in cardiac tamponade.

ELECTRICAL AXIS AND VECTOR A graphic presentation, using an arrow, of the electric current generated by the depolarization and repolarization of the atria and ventricles.

ELECTRICAL CONDUCTION SYSTEM OF THE HEART Includes the sinoatrial (SA) node, internodal atrial conduction tracts, interatrial conduction tract (Bachmann's bundle), atrioventricular (AV) node, bundle of His, right and left bundle branches, and Purkinje network.

ELECTRICAL CONDUCTION SYSTEM OF THE VENTRICLES The His-Purkinje system, which includes the bundle of His, the right and left bundle branches, and the Purkinje network.

ELECTRICAL IMPULSE The tiny electric current that normally originates in the SA node automatically and is conducted through the electrical conduction system to the atria and ventricles, causing them to depolarize and contract.

ELECTRICAL NONUNIFORMITY A condition of the ventricles during the vulnerable period of ventricular repolarization (i.e., the relative refractory period of the ventricles coincident with the peak of the T wave) when the ventricular muscle fibers may be completely repolarized, partially repolarized, or completely refractory. Stimulation of the ventricles at this point by an intrinsic electrical impulse, such as that generated by a PVC or by an extrinsic impulse from a cardiac pacemaker or an electrical countershock, may result in nonuniform conduction of the electrical impulse through the muscle fibers, setting up a reentry mechanism that may precipitate repetitive ventricular complexes and result in ventricular tachycardia or fibrillation. Responsible for the "R-on-T phenomenon."

ELECTRICAL POTENTIAL Refers to the amount of electric current generated by the depolarization and repolarization of the heart and expressed as millivolts (mV). It ranges between 0-620 mV or more.

ELECTROCARDIOGRAM (ECG) The graphic display of the electrical activity of the heart generated by the depolarization and repolarization of the atria and ventricles. The ECG includes the QRS complex; the P, T, and U waves; the PR, ST, and TP segments; and the PR, QT, and R-R intervals.

ELECTRODE A sensing device that detects electrical activity, such as that of the heart. May be positive or negative.

ELECTROLYTE A substance that when in solution dissociates into cations and anions, thus becoming capable of conducting electricity.

ELECTROLYTE IMBALANCE Abnormal concentrations of serum electrolytes within the body caused by excessive intake or loss of such electrolytes as calcium, chloride, potassium, and sodium.

ELECTROMECHANICAL DISSOCIATION (EMD) A term no longer used that referred to a condition in which the electrical activity of the heart is present and can be recorded on the ECG, but effective ventricular contractions, blood pressure, and pulse are absent. See *Pulseless electrical activity*.

EMBOLISM Obstruction of a blood vessel by an embolus that reduces or stops blood flow, resulting in ischemia or necrosis of the tissue supplied by the blood vessel.

EMBOLUS A mass of solid, liquid, or gaseous material carried from one part of the circulatory system to another.

ENDOCARDIUM The thin membrane lining the inside of the heart.

ENHANCED AUTOMATICITY An abnormal condition of latent pacemaker cells in which their firing rate is increased beyond their inherent rate because of a spontaneous increase in the slope of phase-4 depolarization. See *Slope of phase-4 depolarization*.

ENOXAPARIN A low-molecular-weight (LMW) heparin used as an anticoagulant. See *Anticoagulant*.

EPICARDIAL SURFACE The outside surface of the heart.

EPICARDIUM The thin connective tissue lining the outside of the heart.

EPINEPHRINE (ADRENALIN) A hormone produced by the adrenal gland and other tissues of the body. It is an alpha- and beta-stimulator causing an increase in blood pressure by means of peripheral artery vasoconstriction and an increase in cardiac output by increasing heart rate and force of ventricular contraction. Used in the treatment of bronchial asthma, acute allergic disorders, bradycardia from whatever cause, ventricular fibrillation/pulseless ventricular tachycardia, ventricular asystole, and pulseless electrical activity.

EPTIFIBATIDE A platelet GP IIb/IIIa receptor inhibitor that blocks the GP IIb/IIIa receptors on activated platelets from binding to vWF and fibrinogen, thus inhibiting platelet adhesion and aggregation and further thrombus formation.

EQUIPHASIC DEFLECTION A biphasic deflection in which the sum of the positive (upright) deflection or deflections in an ECG are equal to that of the negative (inverted) deflection or deflections.

EROSION Occurs when the endothelial cover of the plaque is torn away, exposing the plaque itself.

ESCAPE BEAT OR COMPLEX A QRS complex arising in an escape (or secondary pacemaker) in the AV junction or ventricles when the underlying rhythm slows to less than the escape or secondary pacemaker's inherent firing rate. Such rhythms are called junctional or ventricular escape beats or complexes.

ESCAPE (OR SECONDARY) PACEMAKER A latent pacemaker in the AV junction or ventricles that takes over pacing the heart when the pacemaker of the underlying rhythm slows to less than the latent pacemaker's inherent firing rate or stops functioning altogether.

ESCAPE PACEMAKER CELLS The pacemaker cells in the rest of the electrical conduction system that hold the property of automaticity in reserve should the SA node fail to function properly or electrical impulses fail to reach them for any reason, such as disruption in the electrical conduction system.

ESCAPE RHYTHM Three or more consecutive QRS complexes that result when the underlying rhythm slows to less than the escape or secondary pacemaker's inherent firing rate, or stops altogether and the escape pacemaker takes over. Examples of escape rhythms are junctional escape rhythm and ventricular escape rhythm.

ESMOLOL A beta-adrenergic blocking agent used primarily in the treatment of tachydysrhythmias, hypertension, angina pectoris, and acute MI.

ESSENTIALLY REGULAR RHYTHM A rhythm in which the shortest and longest R-R interval varies by less than 0.08 second (two small squares) in an ECG tracing.

EVOLVING MI Necrosis progresses from the endocardium to the epicardium.

EXCITABILITY, PROPERTY OF The ability of a cell to respond to stimulation.

EXTENSIVE ANTERIOR MI A myocardial infarction commonly caused by occlusion of the left anterior descending (LAD) coronary artery alone or in conjunction with the anterolateral marginal artery of the left circumflex coronary artery and characterized by early changes in the ST segments and T waves (i.e., ST elevation and tall, peaked T waves) in leads I, aVL, and V_1-V_6. and the appearance early of abnormal Q waves in leads V_1-V_2 and then later in leads I, aVL, and V_3-V_6.

EXTERNAL CARDIAC PACING Transcutaneous pacing (TCP, TC pacing). A technique to treat bradycardias from whatever cause, ventricular asystole, and pulseless electrical activity using an external artificial pacemaker.

EXTRASYSTOLE A premature beat or complex independent of the underlying rhythm caused by an electrical impulse originating in an ectopic focus in the atria, AV junction, or ventricles. Examples of extrasystoles are premature atrial complexes (PACs), premature junctional complexes (PJCs), and premature ventricular complexes (PVCs).

EXTREME RAD When a QRS axis falls between −90° and ±180°. Also called an indeterminate axis (IND).

F

FACING ECG LEADS Leads that view specific surfaces of the heart (e.g., leads V_1-V_4 are facing leads viewing the anterior of the heart).

FASCICLE A band or bundle of muscle or nerve fibers. The left anterior fascicle and the left posterior fascicle form the two major divisions of the left bundle branch before it divides into the Purkinje fibers, forming the Purkinje network. See *Left bundle branch (LBB).*

FASCICULAR BLOCK Absent conduction of electrical impulses through one of the fascicles of the left bundle branch (i.e., left anterior fascicular block, left posterior fascicular block).

FASCICULOVENTRICULAR FIBERS (MAHAIM FIBERS) An accessory conduction pathway located between the bundle of His and the ventricles, resulting in fasciculoventricular preexcitation.

FASCICULOVENTRICULAR PREEXCITATION Abnormal conduction of the electrical impulses through the fasciculoventricular fibers, resulting in abnormally wide QRS complexes of greater than 0.10 second in duration and of abnormal shape, with a delta wave. PR intervals are normal.

FAST SODIUM CHANNELS Structures in the cell membrane called "pores" that facilitate the rapid flow of sodium ions into the cell during depolarization, rapidly changing the electrical potential within the cell from negative to positive. Fast sodium channels are typically found in the myocardial cells and the cells of the electrical conduction system other than those of the SA and AV nodes.

FIBRILLATION Chaotic, disorganized beating of the myocardium in which each myofibril contracts and relaxes independently, producing rapid, tremulous, and ineffectual contractions. Fibrillation may occur in both the atria and ventricles.

FIBRILLATION (F) WAVES On the ECG, these waves appear as numerous irregularly shaped, rounded (or pointed), and dissimilar waves originating in multiple ectopic foci in the atria or ventricles.

FIBRIN An elastic threadlike filament that binds the platelets firmly together to form the thrombus after being converted from fibrinogen.

FIBRINOGEN A plasma protein that converts to fibrin, an elastic threadlike filament, when exposed to thrombin.

FIBRINOLYSIS The process of dissolving the fibrin strands binding the platelets together within a thrombus, initiating the breakup of the thrombus (thrombolysis).

FIBROUS PERICARDIUM The outer tough layer of the pericardium that comes in contact with the lung.

FINE ATRIAL FIBRILLATION Atrial fibrillation with fine fibrillatory waves—less than 1 mm in height.

FINE FIBRILLATORY WAVES When the f waves are less than 1 mm high.

FINE VENTRICULAR FIBRILLATION Ventricular fibrillation with small fibrillatory waves—less than 3 mm in height.

FIRING RATE The rate at which electrical impulses are generated in a pacemaker, whether it is the SA node or an ectopic or escape pacemaker.

FIRST-DEGREE AV BLOCK A dysrhythmia in which there is a constant delay in the conduction of electrical impulses through the AV node. It is characterized by abnormally prolonged PR intervals (greater than 0.20 second).

FIXED COUPLING Equal intervals of time between each premature beat and the preceding QRS complex of the underlying rhythm (i.e., equal [constant] coupling intervals).

FIXED-RATE PACEMAKERS Artificial pacemakers designed to fire constantly at a preset rate without regard to the patient's own heart's electrical activity.

FLUID BOLUS A rapidly administered predetermined volume of IV fluid, such as 0.9% saline or Ringer's lactate solution, to reverse hypotension and shock.

FLUTTER Rapid, regular, repetitive beating of the atria or ventricles.

FLUTTER-FIBRILLATION Refers to the simultaneous occurrence of flutter and fibrillation as in atrial flutter-fibrillation.

FLUTTER (F) WAVES On the ECG, these waves appear as numerous repetitive, similar, usually pointed waves originating in an ectopic pacemaker in the atria or ventricles.

FREQUENT PVCs Five or more PVCs per minute.

FRONTAL PLANE A flat surface passing through the body at right angles to a plane passing through the body from front to back in the midline (sagittal plane), as viewed from the front of the body.

FULL (FULLY) COMPENSATORY PAUSE See *Compensatory pause.*

FUROSEMIDE A rapid-acting diuretic used to treat congestive heart failure by promoting the excretion of urine to reduce pulmonary congestion and edema. Trade name: Lasix.

FUSION BEAT, VENTRICULAR A ventricular complex unlike the QRS complexes of the underlying rhythm and those of the ventricular dysrhythmia in a given ECG lead, having features of both. This results from the stimulation of the ventricles by two electrical impulses, one originating in the SA node or an ectopic focus in the atria or AV junction and the other in an ectopic focus in the ventricles. A fusion beat can occur in accelerated idioventricular rhythm (AIVR), pacemaker rhythm, premature ventricular complexes (PVCs), and ventricular tachycardia.

f WAVES See *Atrial fibrillation (f) waves.*

F WAVES See *Atrial flutter (F) waves.*

G

GAP JUNCTION A structure within the intercalated disks located at the junctions of the branches of myocardial cells, permitting very rapid conduction of electrical impulses from one cell to another.

GLYCOPROTEIN (GP) RECEPTORS Adhesive glycoproteins located on platelet surface that bind with various components of connective tissue and blood to form thrombi. The major receptors and their function include the following:
GP Ia binds the platelets directly to collagen fibers present in connective tissue.
GP Ib binds the platelets to von Willebrand factor (vWF).
GP IIb/IIIa binds the platelets to vWF and, after the platelets are activated, to fibrinogen.

GOALS IN THE MANAGEMENT OF AN ACUTE MI The three major goals in the management of acute MI are:
- Prevent the further expansion of the original thrombus and/or prevent the formation of a new thrombus

- Dissolve or lyse the existing thrombus (thrombolysis)
- Enlarge the lumen of the occluded section of the affected coronary artery

GP Ia RECEPTOR The platelet receptor that binds the platelets directly to collagen fibers present in connective tissue.

GP Ib RECEPTOR The platelet receptor that binds the platelets to von Willebrand factor (vWF).

GP IIb/IIIa RECEPTOR The platelet receptor that binds the platelets to vWF and, after the platelets are activated, to fibrinogen.

GP IIb/IIIa RECEPTOR INHIBITOR Inhibits platelet adhesion and aggregation by blocking the platelets' GP IIb/IIIa receptors. Abciximab, eptifibatide.

GRAM (g) Measurement of metric weight equal to about 1 cubic centimeter (cc) or 1 milliliter (mL) of water. 1000 g is equal to 1 kilogram (kg).

GRID, ECG See *ECG grid*.

GROSSLY IRREGULAR RHYTHM When there appears to be no fixed pattern or ratio of the R-R intervals on an ECG.

GROUND ELECTRODE The ECG lead other than the positive and negative leads that grounds the input to prevent extraneous noise from entering the amplifier circuit.

GROUP BEATING Repetitive sequence of two or more consecutive beats followed by a dropped beat as seen in second-degree AV block.

GROUP BEATS Occurrence of two or more consecutive atrial, junctional, or ventricular premature complexes preceded and followed by the underlying rhythm.

GRUEL The semiliquid, lipid-rich mixture often seen within the atherosclerotic plaque.

H

HEART RATE The number of heart beats, QRS complexes, or R-R intervals per minute.

HEART RATE CALCULATOR RULER A rulerlike device used to calculate the heart rate.

HEMIBLOCK Blockage to the conduction of electrical impulses in one of the fascicles (anterior or posterior) of the left bundle branch. See *Left anterior fascicular block (LAFB), Left posterior fascicular block (LPFB)*.

HEMODYNAMICALLY STABLE (OR UNSTABLE) Refers to a patient who is normotensive, without chest pain or congestive heart failure, and not having an acute myocardial infarction or ischemic episode. A patient who is hemodynamically unstable, on the other hand, is hypotensive with evidence of poor peripheral perfusion, has chest pain or congestive heart failure, or is having an acute myocardial infarction or ischemic episode.

HEMORRHAGIC DIATHESIS Any tendency to spontaneous bleeding or bleeding from minor trauma caused by a defect in clotting or a defect in the structure of blood vessels.

HEMOSTATIC DEFECTS Abnormal conditions that stop the flow of blood within the vessels.

HEPARIN An anticoagulant. Types of heparin include low-molecular-weight (LMW) heparin and unfractionated heparin. See *Anticoagulant*.

HEXAXIAL REFERENCE FIGURE A guide for determining the direction of the QRS axis in the frontal plane, formed by the lead axes of the three limb leads and three augmented leads, spaced 30° apart around a zero reference point.

HIS-PURKINJE SYSTEM (OF THE VENTRICLES) The part of the electrical system consisting of the bundle of His, bundle branches, and Purkinje network.

"HOCKEY STICK" PATTERN The ventricular "strain" pattern in the QRS-ST-T complex produced by a downsloping ST-segment depression and T wave inversion; characteristic of long-standing right or left ventricular hypertrophy. Synonymous with left or right ventricular strain pattern.

HORIZONTAL PLANE A flat surface passing through the body at right angles to the sagittal and frontal planes and, in the case of electrocardiography, dividing the chest into an upper and a lower half at the level of the heart.

HYPERCALCEMIA Elevated levels of serum calcium in the blood.

HYPERCAPNIA Excessive amount of carbon dioxide in the blood defined as a blood gas carbon dioxide level over 45 mm Hg.

HYPERCARBIA Hypercapnia.

HYPERKALEMIA Excessive amount of serum potassium in the blood. Normal is 3.5 to 5.0 mEq/L.

HYPERTENSION Blood pressure over 140/90 mm Hg.

HYPERTROPHY Chronic condition of the heart characterized by an increase in the thickness of a chamber's myocardial wall secondary to the increase in the size of the muscle fibers.

HYPERVENTILATION Increased ventilation of the alveoli caused by abnormally rapid, deep, and prolonged respirations; the result is a loss of carbon dioxide from the body and eventually alkalosis.

HYPOCALCEMIA Low amount of serum calcium in the blood.

HYPOCAPNIA Low amount of carbon dioxide in the blood.

HYPOCARBIA Hypocapnia. Low amount of carbon dioxide in the blood.

HYPOKALEMIA Low amount of serum potassium in the blood.

HYPOTENSION Low blood pressure; generally considered to be a systolic blood pressure of 80 to 90 mm Hg or less.

HYPOTHERMIA A state of low body temperature. When the core body temperature drops to 95°F, a distinctive narrow, positive wave—the Osborn wave—appears in the ECG. See *Osborn wave*.

HYPOVENTILATION Decreased ventilation of the alveoli.

HYPOVOLEMIA Decreased amount of blood in the body's cardiovascular system.

HYPOXEMIA Reduced oxygenation of the blood.

HYPOXIA Reduced amount of oxygen.

I

ICHD CODE See *Intersociety Commission for Heart Disease Resources (ICHD) Code*.

IDIOVENTRICULAR Pertaining to the ventricles.

IDIOVENTRICULAR RHYTHM See *Ventricular escape rhythm*.

IDIOVENTRICULAR TACHYCARDIA See *Accelerated idioventricular rhythm (AIVR)*.

IM Abbreviation for intramuscular.

IMPLANTABLE CARDIOVERTER-DEFIBRILLATOR (ICD) Internal placement of a device capable of delivering electrical shocks to the heart to interrupt a life-threatening run of ventricular tachycardia or ventricular fibrillation. Prevents syncope or sudden death.

IMPLANTED CARDIAC PACEMAKER-INDUCED QRS COMPLEX Generally 0.12 second or greater in width and appear bizarre.

INCOMPLETE AV BLOCK (SECOND-DEGREE AV BLOCK) A dysrhythmia in which one or more P waves are not conducted to the ventricles. See *Second-degree, type I AV block (Wenckebach); Second-degree, type II AV block; Second-degree, 2:1,* and *advanced AV block.*

INCOMPLETE BUNDLE BRANCH BLOCK (RIGHT, LEFT) Defective conduction of electrical impulses through the right or left bundle branch from the bundle of His to the Purkinje network in the myocardium, resulting in a slightly widened QRS complex (i.e., greater than 0.10 second but less than 0.12 second).

INCOMPLETE COMPENSATORY PAUSE The R-R interval following a premature complex that if added to the R-R interval preceding the premature complex would result in a sum less than the sum of two R-R intervals of the underlying rhythm. See *Compensatory pause.*

INDETERMINATE AXIS A QRS axis between 90° and 180° (i.e., extreme right axis deviation).

INDIFFERENT, ZERO REFERENCE POINT See *Central terminal.*

INFARCTION Death (necrosis) of tissue caused by interruption of the blood supply to the affected tissue.

INFERIOR (DIAPHRAGMATIC) MI A myocardial infarction commonly caused by occlusion of the posterior left ventricular arteries of the right coronary artery or, less commonly, of the left circumflex coronary artery of the left coronary artery and characterized by early changes in the ST segments and T waves (i.e., ST elevation and tall, peaked T waves) and the appearance later of abnormal Q waves in leads II, III, and aVF.

INFERIOR VENA CAVA One of the two largest veins in the body that empty venous blood into the right atrium.

INFEROLATERAL MI A myocardial infarction that may be caused by (1) occlusion of (a) the laterally located diagonal arteries of the left anterior descending (LAD) coronary artery and/or the anterolateral marginal artery of the left circumflex coronary artery, and (b) the posterior left ventricular arteries of the right coronary artery, or, less commonly, of the left circumflex coronary artery of the left coronary artery; or (2) occlusion of the left circumflex artery of a dominant left coronary artery. The infarct is characterized by early changes in the ST segments and T waves (i.e., ST elevation and tall, peaked T waves) and the appearance later of abnormal Q waves in leads I, II, III, aVL, aVF, and V_5 or V_6.

INFRANODAL Below the AV node.

INFREQUENT PVCs Less than five PVCs per minute.

INFUSION Administration of a fluid into a vein.

INHERENT FIRING RATE The rate at which a given pacemaker of the heart normally generates electrical impulses.

INR International Normalized Ratio, the standard measure of the degree of anticoagulation attained by the administration of an anticoagulant such as warfarin. Based on the prothrombin time (PT), the optimal degree of anticoagulation is present when the INR is within the range of 2.0 to 3.0.

INSTANTANEOUS ELECTRICAL OR CARDIAC AXIS OR VECTOR A graphic presentation, using an arrow, of the electric current generated by the depolarization or repolarization of the atria and ventricles at any given moment.

INTEGRILIN Trade name for eptifibatide, a GP IIb/IIIa receptor inhibitor.

INTERATRIAL CONDUCTION TRACT See *Bachmann's bundle.*

INTERATRIAL SEPTUM The membranous wall separating the right and left atria.

INTERCALATED DISKS Specialized structures located at the junctions of the branches of myocardial cells that permit very rapid conduction of electrical impulses from one cell to another.

INTERNODAL ATRIAL CONDUCTION TRACTS Part of the electrical conduction system of the heart consisting of three pathways of specialized conducting tissue located in the walls of the right atrium between the SA node and AV node.

INTERPOLATED PVC A PVC that occurs between two normally conducted QRS complexes without greatly disturbing the underlying rhythm. A full compensatory pause, commonly present with PVCs, is absent.

INTERSOCIETY COMMISSION FOR HEART DISEASE RESOURCES (ICHD) CODE A five-letter code specifying the capabilities of an artificial pacemaker. The first letter of the code indicates which chamber is paced (A, atria; V, ventricles; D, both atria and ventricles); the second letter indicates which chamber is sensed (A, atria; V, ventricles; D, both atria and ventricles); the third letter indicates the response of the pacemaker to a P wave or QRS complex (I, pacemaker output inhibited by a P wave or QRS complex; D, pacemaker output inhibited by a QRS complex and triggered by a P wave). The fourth letter indicates the programmability of the device. The fifth letter indicates whether the device is a combined pacemaker/defibrillator.

INTERVALS The sections of the ECG between waves and complexes. Includes waves, complexes, and segments. See *P-P interval, PR interval, QT interval, and R-R interval.*

INTERVENTRICULAR SEPTUM The membranous, muscular wall separating the right and left ventricles. The anterior portion of the interventricular septum is supplied by the left anterior descending (LAD) coronary artery; the posterior portion is supplied by the posterior descending coronary artery.

INTIMA The innermost layer lining a blood vessel.

INTRACARDIAC Within the heart.

INTRAVENOUS (IV) DRIP The very slow administration of fluid into a vein.

INTRAVENTRICULAR CONDUCTION DISTURBANCE Defective conduction of electrical impulses from the AV junction to the myocardium via the bundle branches and Purkinje fibers, resulting in an abnormally wide QRS complex. It occurs most commonly as a right or left bundle branch block and to a lesser extent as a nonspecific, diffuse intraventricular conduction defect (IVCD) seen in myocardial infarction, fibrosis, and hypertrophy; electrolyte imbalance; and excessive administration of certain cardiac drugs.

INTRINSICOID DEFLECTION The downstroke of the R wave; the part of the QRS complex that begins at the peak of the last R wave and ends at the J point or tip of the following S wave. Follows the ventricular activation time (VAT) (or preintrinsicoid deflection).

INTRINSICOID DEFLECTION TIME (IDT) The downstroke of the R wave, which begins at the peak of the R wave and ends at the J point or tip of the following S wave.

ION An atom or group of atoms having a positive charge (cation) or a negative one (anion).

IRREGULARLY IRREGULAR RHYTHM See *Grossly irregular rhythm.*

ISCHEMIA Reduced blood flow to tissue caused by narrowing or occlusion of the artery supplying blood to it. Ischemia results in tissue anoxia. Ischemia may be localized under the endocardium (subendocardial ischemia) or under the epicardium (subepicardial ischemia).

ISCHEMIC HEART DISEASE Heart disease caused by a deficiency of the blood supply to the heart (the myocardium, the electrical conduction system, and other structures), caused by obstruction or constriction of the coronary arteries. Manifestations of ischemic heart disease include acute MI, angina pectoris, bundle branch and fascicular blocks, right and left heart failure, and arrhythmias.

ISCHEMIC T WAVES Symmetrically positive and abnormally tall, peaked T waves, or symmetrically and deeply inverted T waves that appear over an ischemic myocardium. Generally, the ischemic T waves are upright over subendocardial ischemia and inverted over subepicardial ischemia.

ISOELECTRIC LINE The flat (sometimes wavy) line in an ECG during which electrical activity is absent. Synonymous with baseline.

ISOLATED BEAT A premature complex occurring singly.

IV Abbreviation for intravenous.

IV BOLUS A single, relatively large dose of a drug given intravenously.

IV FLUIDS Sterile fluids such as 0.9% saline or Ringer's lactate solution administered intravenously.

IV LINE A catheter or needle, a solution administration set, and an intravenous solution used to administer drugs and fluids intravenously.

J

JAMES FIBERS The other name for atrio-His fibers, the abnormal accessory conduction pathway connecting the atria with the lower part of the AV node at its junction with the bundle of His.

J DEFLECTION See *Osborn wave.*

JOULES Unit of electrical energy delivered for 1 second by an electrical source, such as a defibrillator. Used interchangeably with the term Watt-seconds.

J POINT See *Junction (or "J") point.*

JUNCTION Between the QRS complex and the ST segment.

JUNCTION (OR "J") POINT The point where the QRS complex becomes the ST segment or the ST-T wave.

JUNCTION (AV) See *Atrioventricular (AV) junction.*

JUNCTIONAL DYSRHYTHMIA A dysrhythmia arising in an ectopic or escape pacemaker in the AV junction, such as premature junctional complexes, junctional escape rhythm, nonparoxysmal junctional tachycardia (accelerated junctional rhythm, junctional tachycardia), and paroxysmal supraventricular tachycardia (PSVT).

JUNCTIONAL ESCAPE BEATS (COMPLEXES) AND RHYTHMS Beats (or complexes) and rhythms originating in an escape pacemaker in the AV junction that occur when the rate of the underlying supraventricular rhythm drops to less than 40 to 60 beats per minute.

JUNCTIONAL ESCAPE RHYTHM A dysrhythmia originating in an escape pacemaker in the AV junction with a rate of 40 to 60 beats per minute.

JUNCTIONAL TACHYCARDIA A dysrhythmia originating in an ectopic pacemaker in the AV junction with a rate greater than 100 beats per minute. When abnormal QRS complexes occur with tachycardia because of aberrant ventricular conduction, the tachycardia is called *junctional tachycardia with aberrant ventricular conduction (aberrancy).*

JUNCTIONAL TACHYCARDIA WITH ABERRANCY See *Aberrant ventricular conduction.*

J WAVE See *Osborn wave.*

K

K+ Symbol for potassium.

kg Abbreviation for kilogram.

KILOGRAM A unit of metric weight measurement. One kilogram (kg) is equal to 1000 grams, or 2.2 pounds.

KVO Abbreviation for "keep the vein open."

L

L Abbreviation for liter.

LAD Left anterior descending coronary artery. See *Coronary circulation.*

LARGE SQUARES The areas on ECG paper enclosed by the dark horizontal and vertical lines of the grid.

LATENT (OR SUBSIDIARY) PACEMAKER CELLS Cells in the electrical conduction system with the property of automaticity, located below the SA node. These cells hold the property of automaticity in reserve should the SA node fail to function properly or electrical impulses fail to reach them for any reason, such as a disruption in the electrical conduction system.

LATERAL LEADS Leads V_5 and V_6. The left precordial leads.

LATERAL MI A myocardial infarction commonly caused by occlusion of the laterally located diagonal arteries of the left anterior descending (LAD) coronary artery and/or the anterolateral marginal artery of the left circumflex coronary artery and characterized by early changes in the ST segments and T waves (i.e., ST elevation and tall, peaked T waves) and the appearance later of abnormal Q waves in leads I, aVL, and V₅ or V₆.

LBB See *Left bundle branch (LBB)*.

LBBB See *Left bundle branch block (LBBB)*.

LEAD A lead of the ECG. See *ECG lead*.

LEAD AXIS See *Axis of a lead (lead axis)*.

LEAD I, MONITORING LEAD See *Monitoring lead I*.

LEAD II, MONITORING LEAD See *Monitoring lead II*.

LEAD III, MONITORING LEAD See *Monitoring lead III*.

LEAD MCL1, MONITORING LEAD See *Monitoring lead MCL1*.

LEAD MCL6, MONITORING LEAD See *Monitoring lead MCL6*.

LEFT ANTERIOR DESCENDING CORONARY ARTERY Travels anteriorly and downward within the interventricular groove over the interventricular septum and circles the apex of the heart to end behind it.

LEFT ANTERIOR FASCICULAR BLOCK (LAFB) Absent conduction of electrical impulses through the left anterior fascicle of the left bundle branch. Typical ECG pattern: q1r3 pattern. Also referred to as *left anterior hemiblock*.

LEFT ATRIAL ENLARGEMENT (LEFT ATRIAL DILATATION AND HYPERTROPHY) Usually caused by increased pressure and/or volume in the left atrium. It is found in mitral valve stenosis and insufficiency, acute myocardial infarction, left heart failure, and left ventricular hypertrophy from various causes such as aortic stenosis or insufficiency, systemic hypertension, and hypertrophic cardiomyopathy.

LEFT AXIS DEVIATION (LAD) A QRS axis greater than 230° (230° to 290°).

LEFT BUNDLE BRANCH (LBB) Part of the electrical conduction system of the heart that conducts electrical impulses into the left ventricle. It consists of the left common bundle branch (or main stem), which divides into two bundles of fibers, the left anterior fascicle (LAF) and the left posterior fascicle (LPF).

LEFT BUNDLE BRANCH BLOCK (LBBB) Defective conduction of electrical impulses through the left bundle branch. Left bundle branch block may be complete or incomplete and be present with or without an intact interventricular septum.

LEFT CIRCUMFLEX CORONARY ARTERY Courses over the anterior and lateral surface of the left ventricle between the left anterior descending coronary artery and the anterolateral marginal branch of the left circumflex coronary artery.

LEFT CORONARY ARTERY Arises from the base of the aorta just above the left coronary cusp of the aortic valve.

LEFT HEART Left side of the heart consisting of the left atrium and left ventricle.

LEFT MAIN CORONARY ARTERY Short main stem of about 2 to 10 mm in length that divides into two equal major branches, the left anterior descending coronary artery (LAD) and the left circumflex coronary artery (LCx).

LEFT POSTERIOR FASCICULAR BLOCK (LPFB) Absent conduction of electrical impulses through the left posterior fascicle of the left bundle branch. Typical ECG pattern: q3r1 pattern. Also referred to as *left posterior hemiblock*.

LEFT PRECORDIAL (OR LATERAL) LEADS Leads V₅ and V₆.

LEFT VENTRICULAR FAILURE Inadequacy of the left ventricle to maintain normal circulation of blood. This results in pulmonary congestion and edema.

LEFT VENTRICULAR HYPERTROPHY (LVH) Increase in the thickness of the left ventricular wall because of chronic increase in pressure and/or volume within the ventricle. Common causes include mitral insufficiency, aortic stenosis or insufficiency, and systemic hypertension.

LENEGRE'S DISEASE/LEV'S DISEASE Idiopathic degenerative disease of the electrical conduction system with fibrosis and/or sclerosis and disruption of the conduction fibers. A cause of bundle branch and fascicular blocks.

LEUKOCYTES White blood cells.

LIDOCAINE An antiarrhythmic used to treat premature ventricular complexes (PVCs) and monomorphic and polymorphic ventricular tachycardia with a pulse.

LIFE-THREATENING DYSRHYTHMIAS Include ventricular fibrillation, pulseless ventricular tachycardia, ventricular asystole, and pulseless electrical activity.

LIMB OR EXTREMITY LEADS The three standard (bipolar) limb leads (leads I, II, and III) and the three augmented (unipolar) leads (leads aVR, aVL, and aVF).

LINGUAL AEROSOL Pertains to a method of delivering a drug by spraying it under the tongue.

LITER (L) A metric measurement of volume. One liter is equal to 1000 milliliters (mL), or 1.1 quarts.

LOADING DOSE A single large dose of a drug that produces an initial high therapeutic blood level necessary to treat certain conditions.

LOVENOX Trade name for enoxaparin, a low-molecular-weight (LMW) heparin used as an anticoagulant. See *Anticoagulant*.

LOW-MOLECULAR-WEIGHT (LMW) HEPARIN An anticoagulant.

LOWER CASE LETTERS Lower case letters, such as q, r, s, are used to designate small deflections of the ECG.

LOWN-GANONG-LEVINE (LGL) SYNDROME Atrio-His preexcitation typified by an abnormally short PR interval.

LPFB See *Left posterior fascicular black (LPFB)*.

LVH See *Left ventricular hypertrophy (LVH)*.

LYSE To break up, to disintegrate (e.g., to lyse a thrombus).

LYSIS The process of breaking up or disintegrating (e.g., thrombolysis).

M

MAGNESIUM SULFATE An electrolyte solution used to treat polymorphic ventricular tachycardia (with pulse), Torsades de pointes (with pulse), and ventricular fibrillation/pulseless ventricular tachycardia if indicated.

MAHAIM FIBERS See *Nodoventricular fibers and Fasciculoventricular fibers*.

MARKED BRADYCARDIA A bradycardia with a heart rate between 30 and 45 beats per minute or less accompanied by hypotension and signs and symptoms of decreased perfusion of the brain and other organs.

MARKED SINUS BRADYCARDIA See *Marked bradycardia*.

MAT See *Multifocal atrial tachycardia (MAT)*.

MCL1 See *Monitoring lead MCL1.*

MEAN QRS AXIS The average of all the ventricular vectors; the QRS axis, or simply, the axis.

MEAN VECTOR An average of one or more vectors.

MEDULLA OBLONGATA Part of the brainstem connecting the cerebral hemispheres with the spinal cord; it contains specialized nerve centers for special senses, respiration, and circulation, including the sympathetic and parasympathetic nervous systems with their respective cardioaccelerator and cardioinhibitor centers.

MEMBRANE POTENTIAL The electrical potential measuring the difference between the interior of a cell and the surrounding extracellular fluid.

mEq Abbreviation for milliequivalents.

METER A metric unit of linear measurement. One meter is equal to 1000 millimeters, or 39.37 inches.

METOPROLOL A BETA BLOCKER See *Beta blockers.*

mg Abbreviation for milligrams.

µg Abbreviation for microgram.

MICROGRAM (µg) A metric unit of measurement of weight. One thousand micrograms are equal to 1 milligram.

MIDCLAVICULAR LINE An imaginary line beginning in the middle of the left clavicle and running parallel to the sternum slightly inside the left nipple.

MIDPRECORDIAL (OR ANTERIOR) LEADS Leads V_3 and V_4.

MILD BRADYCARDIA A bradycardia with a heart rate between 50 and 59 beats per minute and absence of hypotension and signs and symptoms of decreased perfusion of the brain or other organs.

MILD SINUS BRADYCARDIA See *Mild bradycardia.*

MILLIEQUIVALENTS (mEq) The weight of a substance dissolved in 1 milliliter of solution.

MILLIGRAM (mg) A metric unit of weight. One thousand milligrams are equal to 1 kilogram, or 2.2 pounds.

MILLILITER (mL) A metric unit of measurement of volume. One thousand milliliters are equal to 1 liter, or 1.1 quarts.

MILLIMETER (mm) A metric unit of linear measurement. One thousand millimeters are equal to 1 meter, or 39.37 inches.

MILLIMETER OF MERCURY (mm Hg) A metric unit of weight used in the determination of blood pressure.

MILLIVOLT (mV) A unit of electrical energy. One thousand millivolts are equal to 1 volt.

MITRAL STENOSIS Pathologic narrowing of the orifice of the mitral valve, commonly the result of rheumatic fever or age-related calcification of the valve leaflets. One of the causes of left atrial enlargement.

MITRAL VALVE The one-way valve located between the left atrium and the left ventricle.

mL Abbreviation for milliliter.

mm Abbreviation for millimeter.

mm Hg Abbreviation for millimeters of mercury.

MOBITZ TYPE I AV BLOCK Type I AV block. A form of second-degree atrioventricular heart block characterized by progressively lengthening PR intervals until a QRS complex fails to occur.

MOBITZ TYPE II AV BLOCK Type II AV block. A form of 2nd degree atrioventricular heart block characterized by constant PR intervals. There are more P waves than QRS complexes, usually in a fixed ratio (2:1, 3:2, etc.).

MONITORED CARDIAC ARREST Cardiac arrest in a patient who is being monitored.

MONITORING LEAD I The single ECG lead used for monitoring the heart for dysrhythmias. Lead I is obtained by attaching the negative electrode to the right arm or the upper right anterior chest wall and the positive electrode to the left arm or the upper left anterior chest wall.

MONITORING LEAD II The single ECG lead commonly used for monitoring the heart solely for dysrhythmias. Lead II is obtained by attaching the negative electrode to the right arm or the upper right anterior chest wall and the positive electrode to the left leg or the lower left anterior chest wall at the intersection of the left fifth intercostal space and the midclavicular line.

MONITORING LEAD III The single ECG lead used for monitoring the heart for dysrhythmias. Lead III is obtained by attaching the negative electrode to the left arm or the upper left anterior chest wall and the positive electrode to the left leg or the lower left anterior chest wall at the intersection of the fifth intercostal space and the midclavicular line.

MONITORING LEAD MCL1 An ECG lead commonly used in the monitoring of dysrhythmias in the hospital, particularly in differentiating supraventricular dysrhythmias with aberrant ventricular conduction (aberrancy) from ventricular dysrhythmias. Lead MCL1 is obtained by attaching the positive electrode to the right side of the anterior chest in the fourth intercostal space just right of the sternum. The negative electrode is attached to the left chest in the midclavicular line below the clavicle.

MONITORING LEAD MCL6 The single ECG lead commonly used for monitoring the heart solely for dysrhythmias. Lead MCL6 is obtained by attaching the negative electrode to the upper left anterior chest wall and the positive electrode to the lower left anterior chest wall at the intersection of the sixth intercostal space and the midaxillary line.

MONOMORPHIC V-TACH V-Tach with QRS complexes that are of the same or almost the same shape, size, and direction.

MORPHINE SULFATE A narcotic analgesic and sedative used to produce amnesia in conscious patients before cardioversion of certain dysrhythmias. Also used as a vasodilator to relieve congestive heart failure secondary to left heart failure.

"M" (OR RABBIT EARS) PATTERN Refers to the rSR′ pattern of the QRS complex in V_1, representative of a right bundle branch block.

MULTIFOCAL Indicates a dysrhythmia originating in different pacemaker sites (e.g., a ventricular dysrhythmia with QRS complexes that differ in size, shape, and direction).

MULTIFOCAL ATRIAL TACHYCARDIA (MAT) An atrial tachycardia that originates in three or more different ectopic pacemaker sites, characterized by P′ waves that usually vary in size, shape, and direction in each given lead.

MULTIFOCAL PREMATURE VENTRICULAR COMPLEXES (PVCs) Different-appearing premature ventricular complexes (PVCs) in the same tracing that originate from different ectopic pacemaker sites in the ventricles.

MULTIFORM Applies to a ventricular dysrhythmia with QRS complexes that differ in size, shape, and direction, originating in single or multiple pacemaker sites.

MULTIFORM PREMATURE VENTRICULAR COMPLEXES (PVCs) Different-appearing premature ventricular complexes (PVCs) in the same tracing that originate in one or more ectopic pacemaker sites in the ventricles.

MULTIFORM VENTRICULAR TACHYCARDIA Ventricular tachycardia with QRS complexes that differ markedly from beat to beat.

MUSCLE TREMOR The cause of extraneous spikes and waves in the ECG brought on by voluntary or involuntary muscle movement or shivering; often seen in elderly persons or in a cold environment.

mV Abbreviation for millivolt.

MYOCARDIAL Pertaining to the muscular part of the heart.

MYOCARDIAL INFARCTION (MI) See *Acute myocardial infarction (acute MI, AMI)*.

MYOCARDIAL INJURY Reversible changes in the myocardial cells from prolonged lack of oxygen. ECG manifestations include ST elevation or depression over injured myocardial cells.

MYOCARDIAL ISCHEMIA Reversible changes in myocardial cells from a temporary lack of oxygen. ECG manifestations include symmetrical T wave elevation or inversion over ischemic myocardial cells.

MYOCARDIAL NECROSIS (INFARCTION) Irreversible damage to myocardial cells causing their death, the result of prolonged lack of oxygen. ECG manifestations include abnormal Q waves over necrotic myocardial cells.

MYOCARDIAL (OR "WORKING") CELLS Myocardial cells other than those in the electrical conduction system of the ventricles.

MYOCARDIAL RUPTURE Rupture of the myocardial wall, usually occurring in the left ventricle in the area of necrosis following an acute transmural myocardial infarction.

MYOCARDIUM Middle layer of heart tissue that contains the muscle cells.

MYOFIBRIL Tiny structure within a muscle cell that contracts when stimulated. Contains the contractile protein filaments actin and myosin.

MYOSIN One of the contractile protein filaments in myofibrils that give the myocardial cells the property of contractility. The other is actin.

N

Na⁺ Symbol for sodium ion.

NECROSIS Death of tissue.

NEGATIVE DEFLECTION Occurs when an electric current flows away from the positive electrode.

NERVOUS CONTROL OF THE HEART Emanates from the autonomic nervous system, which includes the sympathetic (adrenergic) and parasympathetic (cholinergic or vagal) nervous systems, each producing opposite effects when stimulated.

NITROGLYCERIN A drug used as a vasodilator to relieve angina pectoris and to relieve severe pulmonary congestion and edema (congestive heart failure) secondary to left heart failure. Also used in acute coronary syndromes to enhance coronary blood flow and to reduce ventricular preload by decreasing venous return through venous dilation.

NODAL REENTRY TACHYCARDIA (AVNRT) A dysrhythmia when the reentry mechanism involved only the AV node.

NODOVENTRICULAR FIBERS (MAHAIM FIBERS) An accessory conduction pathway located between the lower part of the AV node and the ventricles, resulting in nodoventricular preexcitation.

NODOVENTRICULAR PREEXCITATION Abnormal conduction of the electrical impulses through the nodoventricular fibers, resulting in abnormally wide QRS complexes of greater than 0.10 second in duration and of abnormal shape, with a delta wave. PR intervals are normal.

NOISE Extraneous spikes, waves, and complexes in the ECG signal caused by muscle tremor, 60-cycle AC interference, improperly attached electrodes, and biomedical telemetry-related events, such as out-of-range ECG transmission and weak transmitter batteries. See *Artifact*.

NONCOMPENSATORY PAUSE The R-R interval following a premature complex that, if added to the R-R interval preceding the premature complex, would result in a sum less than the sum of two R-R intervals of the underlying rhythm. Synonymous with incomplete compensatory pause. See *Compensatory pause*.

NONCONDUCTED PAC A positive P′ wave (in Lead II) not followed by a QRS complex. A blocked PAC.

NONCONDUCTED PJC A negative P′ wave (in Lead II) not followed by a QRS complex. A blocked PJC.

NONCONDUCTED P WAVE A P wave not followed by a QRS complex. A dropped beat.

NONPACEMAKER CELL A cardiac cell without the property of automaticity.

NONPAROXSYMAL ATRIAL TACHYCARDIA When atrial tachycardia starts and ends gradually.

NONPAROXYSMAL JUNCTIONAL TACHYCARDIA A dysrhythmia originating in an ectopic pacemaker in the AV junction with a rate between 60 and 150 beats per minute. It includes accelerated junctional rhythm (60 to 100 beats per minute) and junctional tachycardia (100 to 150 beats per minute). It may occur with narrow QRS complexes or abnormally wide QRS complexes because of preexisting bundle branch block or aberrant ventricular conduction. When abnormal QRS complexes occur with the tachycardia because of aberrant ventricular conduction, the tachycardia is called *junctional tachycardia with aberrant ventricular conduction (aberrancy)*.

NONPITTING EDEMA Results from swelling caused by trauma or inflammation.

NON–Q WAVE MI A myocardial infarction where abnormal Q waves are absent in the ECG. In the majority of such MIs, a nontransmural MI is present; in the rest, it is transmural.

NONSUSTAINED VENTRICULAR TACHYCARDIA Paroxysms of three or more PVCs separated by the underlying rhythm. Paroxysmal ventricular tachycardia.

NONTRANSMURAL Not extending from the endocardium to the epicardium (i.e., partial involvement of the myocardial wall, either in the subendocardial area or the midportion of the myocardium).

NONTRANSMURAL MYOCARDIAL INFARCTION A myocardial infarction in which the ventricular wall is only partially involved by the infarction.

NOREPINEPHRINE (LEVARTERENOL) Adrenergic agent used in the treatment of hypotension and shock. Levophed.

NORMAL QRS AXIS A QRS axis between −30° and 190°.

NORMAL SALINE Incorrect term for the intravenous saline solution containing 0.9% sodium chloride (0.9% saline).

NORMAL SINUS RHYTHM (NSR) Normal rhythm of the heart, originating in the SA node with a rate of 60 to 100 beats per minute.

NOTCH A sharply pointed upright or downward wave in the QRS complex or T wave that does not go below or above the baseline, respectively.

O

OCCASIONALLY IRREGULAR RHYTHM Occurs when premature complexes occur in an otherwise regular rhythm. Seen in premature atrial complexes and premature ventricular complexes.

OPPOSITE (OR RECIPROCAL) ECG LEADS See *"Reciprocal" ECG changes*.

OPTIMAL SEQUENTIAL PACEMAKER (DDD) An artificial pacemaker that paces the atria or ventricles or both when spontaneous atrial or ventricular activity is absent.

ORTHOPNEA Severe dyspnea that is relieved only by the patient assuming a sitting or semi-reclining position of standing up.

OSBORN WAVE The distinctive narrow, positive wave that occurs at the junction of the QRS complex and the ST segment—the QRS-ST junction—in hypothermic patients with a core body temperature of 95°F. Also referred to as the "J wave," the "J deflection," or the "camel's hump." Associated ECG changes include prolonged PR and QT intervals and widening of the QRS complex.

OVERDRIVE SUPPRESSION The suppression of spontaneous depolarization of the SA node or an escape or ectopic pacemaker by a series of electrical impulses (from whatever source) that depolarize the pacemaker cells prematurely. Following termination of the electrical impulses, there may be a slight delay in the appearance of the next expected spontaneous depolarization of the affected pacemaker cells because of a depressing effect that premature depolarization has on their automaticity.

OVERLOAD Refers to increased pressure, volume, or both within a chamber of the heart from various causes, resulting in chamber enlargement from dilatation, hypertrophy, or both. Examples are right atrial enlargement, left atrial enlargement, right ventricular hypertrophy, and left ventricular hypertrophy.

P

PAC Abbreviation for premature atrial complex.

PACEMAKER, ARTIFICIAL An electronic device used to stimulate the heart to beat when the electrical conduction system of the heart malfunctions, causing bradycardia or ventricular asystole. An artificial pacemaker consists of an electronic pulse generator, a battery, and a wire lead that senses the electrical activity of the heart and delivers electrical impulses to the atria or ventricles or both when the pacemaker senses an absence of electrical activity.

PACEMAKER CELL A myocardial cell with the property of automaticity.

PACEMAKER OF THE HEART The SA node or an escape or ectopic pacemaker in the electrical system of the heart or in the myocardium. May be sinus nodal, atrial, AV junctional, or ventricular.

PACEMAKER RHYTHM A cardiac rhythm produced by an artificial pacemaker.

PACEMAKER SITE The site of the origin of an electrical impulse. It can be the SA node or an escape or ectopic pacemaker in any part of the electrical system of the heart or in the myocardium.

PACEMAKER SPIKE The narrow sharp deflection in the ECG caused by the electrical impulse generated by an artificial pacemaker.

PACEMAKER'S INHERENT FIRING RATE The rate at which the SA node or an escape pacemaker normally generates electrical impulses.

PAIRED BEATS Atrial or ventricular ectopic beats occurring in groups of two. Also called *coupled beats*, *couplet*.

PAIRED PVCs Two consecutive PVCs.

PARASYMPATHETIC (CHOLINERGIC OR VAGAL) ACTIVITY The inhibitory action on the heart, blood vessels, and other organs brought on by the stimulation of the parasympathetic nervous system. The effect on the heart and blood vessels results in a decrease in heart rate, cardiac output, and blood pressure and, sometimes, an AV block.

PARASYMPATHETIC (CHOLINERGIC OR VAGAL) NERVOUS SYSTEM Part of the autonomic nervous system involved in the control of involuntary bodily functions, including the control of cardiac and blood vessel activity. Activation of this system depresses cardiac activity and produces effects opposite those of the sympathetic nervous system. Some effects of parasympathetic stimulation are slowing of the heart rate, decreased cardiac output, drop in blood pressure, nausea, vomiting, bronchial spasm, sweating, faintness, and hypersalivation.

PARASYMPATHETIC (CHOLINERGIC OR VAGAL) TONE Pertains to the degree of parasympathetic activity.

PAROXYSM Sudden unexpected occurrence.

PAROXYSMAL NOCTURNAL DYSPNEA (PND) Sudden attacks of dyspnea, occurring at night, in a patient who may be asymptomatic during the day.

PAROXYSMAL SUPRAVENTRICULAR TACHYCARDIA (PSVT) A dysrhythmia with a rate between 160 and 240 beats per minute and usually an abrupt onset and termination. It originates in the AV junction as a reentry mechanism involving the AV node alone (AV nodal reentry tachycardia—AVNRT) or the AV node and an accessory conduction pathway (AV reentry tachycardia—AVRT). It may occur with narrow QRS complexes or abnormally wide QRS complexes because of preexisting bundle branch block or aberrant ventricular conduction. When abnormal QRS complexes occur only with the paroxysmal supraventricular tachycardia because of aberrant ventricular conduction, the tachycardia is called *paroxysmal supraventricular tachycardia (PSVT) with aberrant ventricular conduction (aberrancy).*

PAROXYSMAL SUPRAVENTRICULAR TACHYCARDIA WITH ABERRANCY See *Aberrant ventricular conduction.*

PAROXYSMAL VENTRICULAR TACHYCARDIA A short burst of ventricular tachycardia consisting of three or more QRS complexes.

PAROXYSMS OF BEATS Bursts of three or more beats. Three or more beats are considered to be a tachycardia.

PAST CARDIAC HISTORY Brief review of previous cardiovascular disease and their treatment.

PATTERNED IRREGULARITY Occurs when there is an ECG pattern seen between the measured R-R intervals.

P AXIS The mean of all the vectors generated during the depolarization of the atria.

PEA See *Pulseless electrical activity.*

PCI See *Percutaneous coronary interventions (PCI).*

PEAK OF THE T WAVE Coincident with the vulnerable period of ventricular repolarization, during which a premature ventricular complex (PVC) can initiate ventricular tachycardia or ventricular fibrillation.

PERCUTANEOUS CORONARY INTERVENTIONS (PCI) Catheter-based techniques to enlarge the lumen of the occluded section of the affected coronary artery mechanically by means of one or more of the following:
- Percutaneous transluminal coronary angioplasty (PTCA)
- Coronary artery stenting
- Directional coronary atherectomy (DCA)
- Rotational atherectomy

PERCUTANEOUS TRANSLUMINAL CORONARY ANGIOPLASTY (PTCA) Inserting a balloon-tipped catheter into the occluded or narrowed coronary artery and then inflating the balloon, thus fracturing the atheromatous plaque and dilating the arterial lumen. This procedure, also referred to as balloon angioplasty, is the most commonly performed invasive treatment for coronary artery occlusion. It is often followed by insertion of a coronary artery stent.

PERFUSION Passage of a fluid such as blood through the vessels of a tissue or organ.

PERICARDIAL EFFUSION Fluid within the pericardial cavity or sac.

PERICARDIAL FLUID Helps lubricate the movements of the heart within the pericardium.

PERICARDIAL SPACE OR CAVITY Located between the visceral pericardium and the pericardial sac. It contains up to 50 mL of pericardial fluid.

PERICARDIAL TAMPONADE Accumulation of fluid under pressure within the pericardial cavity.

PERICARDITIS Inflammation of the pericardium accompanied by chest pain somewhat resembling that of acute myocardial infarction. The ECG in acute pericarditis mimics that of acute myocardial infarction because of marked ST-segment elevation.

PERICARDIUM The tough fibrous sac containing the heart and origins of the superior vena cava, inferior vena cava, aorta, and pulmonary artery. The pericardium consists of an inner, two-layered, fluid-secreting membrane (serous pericardium) and an outer, tough, fibrous sac (fibrous pericardium). The inner layer of the serous pericardium, the visceral pericardium, or as it is more commonly known, the epicardium, covers the heart itself; the outer layer, the parietal pericardium, lines the fibrous pericardium. Between the two layers of the serous pericardium is the pericardial space or cavity (or sac), which contains the pericardial fluid.

PERIPHERAL VASCULAR RESISTANCE The resistance to blood flow in the systemic circulation that depends on the degree of constriction or dilation of the small arteries, arterioles, venules, and small veins making up the peripheral vascular system.

PERIPHERAL VASOCONSTRICTION Constriction of blood vessels, especially the small arteries, arterioles, venules, and small veins, causing an increase in blood pressure and a decrease in the circulation of blood beyond the point of vasoconstriction.

PERIPHERAL VASODILATATION Dilation of blood vessels, especially the small arteries, arterioles, venules, and small veins, causing a decrease in blood pressure.

PERPENDICULAR OF A LEAD AXIS (PERPENDICULAR AXIS) A line intersecting or connecting with the lead axis at 90° (or a right angle), at its electrically "zero" point. Also referred to simply as "the perpendicular."

pH Symbol for the concentration of hydrogen ions (H^+) in a solution.

PHASES OF ACUTE MI
Phase 1: (0 to 2 hours)
Phase 2: (2 to 24 hours)
Phase 3: (24 to 72 hours)
Phase 4: (2 to 8 weeks)

PHASES OF DEPOLARIZATION AND REPOLARIZATION See *Cardiac action potential.*

PHASES OF THROMBOLYSIS (1) Release of tPA from the endothelium of the blood vessel wall into the plasma; (2) plasmin formation by conversion of plasminogen attached to the fibrin strands within the thrombus through the action of tPA; (3) fibrinolysis by the breakdown of fibrin through the action of plasmin, causing the platelets to separate from each other and the thrombus to break apart.

PHYSIOLOGICAL AV BLOCK An AV block that occurs only when a rapid atrial dysrhythmia, such as atrial fibrillation, atrial flutter, and atrial tachycardia, is present.

PITTING EDEMA When pressure is applied with a finger, a dent appears in the edematous tissue that does not disappear immediately upon withdrawal of pressure. Sign of peripheral edema.

PJC Abbreviation for premature junctional complex.

PLASMIN An enzyme that dissolves fibrin within the thrombus, helping to break the thrombus apart (thrombolysis). See *Plasminogen.*

PLASMINOGEN A plasma glycoprotein that converts to an enzyme, plasmin, when activated by tissue-type plasminogen activator (tPA). Plasmin, in turn, dissolves the fibrin strands (fibrinolysis) binding the platelets together within a thrombus, initiating thrombolysis.

PLATELET ACTIVATION The second phase of thrombus formation that occurs after the platelets become bound to the collagen fibers. The platelets become activated and change their shape from smooth ovals to tiny spheres while releasing adenosine diphosphate (ADP), serotonin, and thromboxane A2 (TxA2), substances that stimulate platelet aggregation. Platelet activation is also stimulated by the lipid-rich gruel within the atherosclerotic plaque. At the same time, the GP IIb/IIIa receptor is turned on to bind with fibrinogen. While this is happening, tissue factor is being released from the tissue and platelets.

PLATELET ADHESION The first phase of thrombus formation. After the denudation or rupture of an atherosclerotic plaque, the platelets are exposed to collagen fibers and von Willebrand factor (vWF). The platelets' receptors GP Ia binds with the collagen fibers and GP Ib and GP IIb/IIIa with vWF, which in turn also binds with collagen fibers. The result is the adhesion of platelets to the collagen fibers within the plaque, forming a layer of platelets overlying the damaged plaque.

PLATELET AGGREGATION The third phase of thrombus formation. Once activated, the platelets bind to each other by means of fibrinogen, which binds to the platelets' GP IIb/IIIa receptors. Stimulated by ADP and TxA2, the binding of fibrinogen to the GP IIb/IIIa receptors is greatly enhanced, resulting in a rapid growth of the platelet plug. By this time, the prothrombin has been converted to thrombin by the tissue factor.

PLATELET GP IIb/IIIa RECEPTOR INHIBITOR A compound that blocks the GP IIb/IIIa receptors on activated platelets from binding to fibrinogen, thus inhibiting platelet adhesion and aggregation and further thrombus formation. GP IIb/IIIa receptor inhibitors include abciximab and eptifibatide.

PLATELETS Small cells present in the blood that are necessary for coagulation of blood and maintenance of hemostasis. Contain adhesive glycoprotein (GP) receptors that bind with various components of connective tissue and blood to form thrombi. The major receptors are GP Ia, GP Ib, and GP IIb/IIIa. Platelets also contain several substances that, when released upon platelet activation, promote thrombus formation by stimulating platelet aggregation. These include adenosine diphosphate (ADP), serotonin, and thromboxane A2 (TxA2).

PLEURA The serous membrane enveloping the lungs and lining the thoracic cavity, completely enclosing a space filled with fluid, the pleural cavity.

P MITRALE A wide, notched P wave occurring in the presence of left atrial dilatation and hypertrophy. Typically associated with severe mitral stenosis.

PNEUMOTHORAX, TENSION Accumulation of air under positive pressure within the pleural cavity.

POLARITY The condition of being positive or negative.

POLARIZED (OR RESTING) STATE OF THE CELL The condition of the cell after repolarization, when the interior of the cell is negative and the outside is positive.

POLYMORPHIC V-TACH V-Tach in which the QRS complexes differ markedly in shape, size, and direction from beat to beat.

POOR R-WAVE PROGRESSION Refers to the presence of small R waves in the precordial leads V_1-V_5 V_1-V_6, characteristic of chronic obstructive pulmonary disease (COPD). Also seen after an anterior myocardial infarction.

POSITIVE DEFLECTION Occurs when an electric current flows toward the positive electrode of a lead.

POSTDEFIBRILLATION DYSRHYTHMIA A dysrhythmia occurring after defibrillatory shocks (e.g., premature beats, bradycardias, and tachycardias).

POSTERIOR MI A myocardial infarction commonly caused by occlusion of the distal left circumflex artery and/or posterolateral marginal artery of the left circumflex artery and characterized by early changes in the ST segments and T waves (i.e., ST depression in V_1-V_4, inverted T waves in V_1-V_2).

POTENTIAL (ELECTRICAL) The difference in the concentration of ions across a cell membrane, for instance, measured in millivolts.

P-P INTERVAL The section of the ECG between the onset of one P wave and the onset of the following P wave.

P PRIME (P') WAVE An abnormal P wave originating in an ectopic pacemaker in the atria or AV junction or, rarely, in the ventricles. Usually negative in lead II.

P PULMONALE A wide, tall P wave (greater than 2.5 mm in height) occurring in the presence of right atrial dilatation and hypertrophy. Typically associated with pulmonary disease such as COPD, pulmonary embolism, and cor pulmonale.

PRECORDIAL Pertaining to the precordium.

PRECORDIAL REFERENCE FIGURE An outline of the chest wall in the horizontal plane superimposed by the six precordial lead axes and their angles of reference in degrees, radiating out from the heart's zero reference point.

PRECORDIAL THUMP A sharp, brisk blow delivered to the midportion of the sternum with a clenched fist in an initial attempt to terminate ventricular fibrillation or pulseless ventricular tachycardia.

PRECORDIAL (UNIPOLAR) LEADS Leads V_1, V_2, V_3, V_4, V_5, and V_6; each obtained using a positive electrode attached to a specific area of the anterior chest wall and a central terminal. The positive electrode for each precordial lead is attached as follows:

V_1: Right side of the sternum in the fourth intercostal space.

V_2: Left side of the sternum in the fourth intercostal space.

V_3: Midway between V_2 and V_4.

V_4: Left midclavicular line in the fifth intercostal space.

V_5: Left anterior axillary line at the same level as V_4.

V_6: Left midaxillary line at the same level as V_4.

V_1 and V_2: The right precordial (or septal) leads overlie the right ventricle.

V_3 and V_4: The midprecordial (or anterior) leads overlie the interventricular septum and part of the left ventricle.

V_5 and V_6: The left precordial (or lateral) leads overlie the left ventricle.

PRECORDIUM The region of the thorax over the heart, the midportion of the sternum.

PREEXCITATION SYNDROME An abnormal ECG pattern consisting of an abnormally short PR interval or an abnormally wide QRS complex with a delta wave, or both, that results when electrical impulses travel from the atria or AV junction into the ventricles through accessory conduction pathways, causing the ventricles to depolarize earlier than they normally would. Accessory conduction pathways are abnormal strands of myocardial fibers that conduct electrical impulses (1) from the atria to the ventricles (accessory AV pathways); (2) from the atria to the AV junction (atrio-His fibers); or (3) from the AV junction to the ventricles (nodoventricular/fasciculoventricular fibers), bypassing various parts of the normal electrical conduction system. Preexcitation syndromes include ventricular preexcitation, atrio-His preexcitation, and nodoventricular/fasciculoventricular preexcitation.

PREINTRINSICOID DEFLECTION The part of the QRS complex measured from its onset to the peak of the R wave, or, if there is more than one R wave, to the peak of the last R wave. See *Ventricular activation time (VAT)*.

PREMATURE ATRIAL COMPLEX (PAC) An extra beat consisting of an abnormal P wave originating in an ectopic pacemaker in the atria followed by a normal or abnormal QRS complex. PACs with abnormal QRS complexes that occur only with the PACs are called *PACs with aberrancy*; such PACs resemble PVCs. Also called *premature atrial beats (PABs)* or *complexes*.

PREMATURE ATRIAL COMPLEX WITH ABERRANCY See *Aberrant ventricular conduction*.

PREMATURE COMPLEX QRS complex that occurs unexpectedly at some point in the P-QRS-T cycle or between cycles.

PREMATURE ECTOPIC BEAT (COMPLEX) An extra beat or complex originating in the atria, AV junction, or ventricles, such as premature atrial complex (PAC), premature junctional complex (PJC), and premature ventricular complex (PVC).

PREMATURE JUNCTIONAL COMPLEX WITH ABERRANCY See *Aberrant ventricular conduction*.

PREMATURE JUNCTIONAL COMPLEX (PJC) An extra beat that originates in an ectopic pacemaker in the AV junction, consisting of a normal or abnormal QRS complex with or without an abnormal P wave. If a P wave is present, the PR interval is shorter than normal. PJCs with abnormal QRS complexes that occur only with the PJCs are called *PJCs with aberrancy*. Such PJCs resemble PVCs.

PREMATURE VENTRICULAR COMPLEX (PVC) An extra beat consisting of an abnormally wide and bizarre QRS complex originating in an ectopic pacemaker in the ventricles.

PRINZMETAL'S ANGINA A severe form of angina pectoris occurring at rest, caused by coronary artery spasm.

PROCAINAMIDE HYDROCHLORIDE An antiarrhythmic used to treat premature ventricular complexes and ventricular tachycardia.

PROCAINAMIDE TOXICITY Excessive administration of procainamide, manifested by wide QRS complexes, low and wide T waves, U waves, prolonged PR intervals, depressed ST segments, and prolonged QT intervals.

PRODUCTIVE COUGH Cough accompanied by sputum.

PROMETHAZINE HYDROCHLORIDE A drug used primarily for the prevention and control of nausea and vomiting.

PROPERTY OF AUTOMATICITY When pacemaker cells are capable of generating electrical impulses simultaneously.

PROPERTY OF CONDUCTIVITY The ability of cardiac cells to conduct electrical impulses.

PROPERTY OF CONTRACTILITY The ability of myocardial cells to shorten and return to their original length when stimulated by an electrical impulse.

PROPHYLAXIS Preventive treatment.

PROTHROMBIN A plasma protein that, when activated by exposure of the blood-to-tissue factor released from damaged arterial wall tissue, converts to thrombin. Thrombin in turn converts fibrinogen to fibrin.

PR (P'R) INTERVAL The section of the ECG between the onset of the P (or P') wave and the onset of the QRS complex. Normal PR interval is 0.12 to 2.0 second.

PR SEGMENT The section of the ECG between the end of the P wave and the onset of the QRS complex.

PSEUDOELECTROMECHANICAL DISSOCIATION A life-threatening condition in which the ventricular contractions are too weak to produce a detectable pulse and blood pressure because of the failure of the myocardium or electrical conduction system or both from a variety of causes. A form of pulseless electrical activity.

PTCA Percutaneous transluminal coronary angioplasty (PTCA).

PULMONARY CIRCULATION Passage of blood from the right ventricle through the pulmonary artery, all of its branches, and capillaries in the lungs and then to the left atrium through the pulmonary venules and veins. The blood vessels within the lungs and those carrying blood to and from the lungs.

PULMONARY EMBOLISM Obstruction (occlusion) of pulmonary arteries by small amounts of solid, liquid, or gaseous material carried to the lungs through the veins. Typical ECG pattern: S1Q3T3 pattern.

PULMONARY INFARCTION Localized necrosis of lung tissue caused by obstruction of the arterial blood supply, commonly caused by pulmonary embolism.

PULMONIC VALVE The one-way valve located between the right ventricle and the pulmonary artery.

PULSE DEFICIT Occurs when some cardiac contractions are weak and cannot produce a strong enough pulse wave to reach the radial artery.

PULSE OXIMETRY The continuous measurement of the oxygen saturation of hemoglobin and the pulse.

PULSELESS ELECTRICAL ACTIVITY The absence of a detectable pulse and blood pressure in the presence of electrical activity of the heart as evidenced by some type of an ECG rhythm other than ventricular fibrillation or ventricular tachycardia.

PULSELESS VENTRICULAR TACHYCARDIA A life-threatening dysrhythmia equivalent to ventricular fibrillation and treated the same way, by immediate defibrillation.

PUMP FAILURE Partial or total failure of the heart to pump blood forward effectively, causing congestive heart failure and cardiogenic shock. It is a complication of acute myocardial infarction, occurring more frequently in the presence of a bundle branch block.

PURKINJE FIBERS Tiny, immature muscle fibers forming an intricate web, the Purkinje network, spread widely throughout the subendocardial tissue of the ventricles, whose ends finally terminate at the myocardial cells.

PURKINJE NETWORK OF THE VENTRICLES The part of the electrical conduction system between the bundle branches and the ventricular myocardium consisting of the Purkinje fibers and their terminal branches.

PVC Abbreviation for premature ventricular complex.

P WAVE Normally, the first wave of the P-QRS-T complex representing the depolarization of the atria. The P wave may be positive (upright), symmetrically tall and peaked, or wide and notched; negative (inverted); biphasic (partially upright, partially inverted); or flat.

Q

q1r3 PATTERN Typical ECG pattern of an initial small q wave in lead I and an initial small r wave in lead III indicative of a left anterior fascicular block.

q3r1 PATTERN Typical ECG pattern of an initial small q wave in lead III and an initial small r wave in lead I indicative of a left posterior fascicular block.

QRS AXIS The single large vector representing the mean (or average) of all the ventricular vectors.

QRS COMPLEX Normally, the wave following the P wave, consisting of the Q, R, and S waves, and representing ventricular depolarization. May be normal (narrow), 0.10 second or less, or abnormal (wide), greater than 0.10 second.

QRS PATTERN The QRS pattern present in leads V_5-V_6 typical of right bundle branch block with an intact interventricular septum. An example of a QRS complex with a "terminal S" wave.

QRS-ST-T PATTERN Refers to the abnormally wide "sine-wave"–appearing QRS-ST-T complex that occurs in hyperkalemia.

qSR PATTERN The QRS pattern present in leads V_1-V_2 typical of right bundle branch block with a damaged interventricular septum.

QS WAVE A QRS complex that consists entirely of a single, large negative deflection.

QTc See *Corrected QT interval (QTc)*.

QT INTERVAL The section of the ECG between the onset of the QRS complex and the end of the T wave, representing ventricular depolarization and repolarization.

QUADRANTS Refers to the four quadrants of the hexaxial reference figure—quadrants I, II, III, and IV.

QUADRIGEMINY A series of groups of four beats, usually consisting of three normally conducted QRS complexes followed by a premature complex that may be atrial, junctional, or ventricular in origin (i.e., atrial quadrigeminy, junctional quadrigeminy, ventricular quadrigeminy).

QUINIDINE SULFATE An antiarrhythmic used to treat premature atrial and junctional complexes.

QUINIDINE TOXICITY Excessive administration of quinidine, manifested electrocardiographically by wide, often notched, P waves; wide QRS complexes; low, wide T waves; U waves; prolonged PR intervals; depressed ST segments; and prolonged QT intervals.

Q WAVE The first negative deflection of the QRS complex not preceded by an R wave.

Q WAVE MYOCARDIAL INFARCTION (MI) A myocardial infarction in which abnormal Q waves are present in the ECG. In the majority of the Q wave MIs, a transmural myocardial infarction is present; in the rest, the infarction involves only the subendocardium or midportion of the myocardium.

R

RABBIT EARS PATTERN See *rSR' pattern*.

RATE CONVERSION TABLE A table converting the number of small squares between two adjacent R waves into the heart rate per minute.

RATE OF IMPULSE FORMATION (THE FIRING RATE) See *Slope of phase-4 depolarization*.

R DOUBLE PRIME (R″) The third R wave in a QRS complex.

"RECIPROCAL" ECG CHANGES ECG changes of evolving acute myocardial infarction present in opposite ECG leads, being, for the most part, opposite in direction to those in the facing ECG leads (i.e., a mirror image). For example, an elevated ST segment and a symmetrically tall, peaked T wave in a facing ECG lead is mirrored as a depressed ST segment and a deeply inverted T wave in an opposite ECG lead.

REENTRY A condition in which the progression of an electrical impulse is delayed or blocked in one or more segments of the electrical conduction system while being conducted normally through the rest of the conduction system.

REENTRY MECHANISM A mechanism by which an electrical impulse repeatedly exits and reenters an area of the heart causing one or more ectopic beats.

REFRACTORY Inability to respond to a stimulus.

REFRACTORY PERIOD The time during which a cell or fiber may or may not be depolarized by an electrical stimulus depending on the strength of the electrical impulse. It extends from phase 0 to the end of phase 3 and is divided into the absolute refractory period (ARP) and relative refractory period (RRP). The absolute refractory period extends from phase 0 to about midway through phase 3. The relative refractory period extends from about midway through phase 3 to the end of phase 3.

REGULARLY IRREGULAR RHYTHM See *Patterned irregularity.*

RELATIVE BRADYCARDIA The heart rate is too slow relative to the existing metabolic needs.

RELATIVE REFRACTORY PERIOD (RRP) OF THE VENTRICLES The period of ventricular repolarization during which the ventricles can be stimulated to depolarize by an electrical impulse stronger than usual. It begins at about the peak of the T wave and ends with the end of the T wave.

ReoPro Trade name for abciximab.

REPERFUSION THERAPY Treatment to reopen an occluded atherosclerotic coronary artery using a thrombolytic agent or a mechanical means such as percutaneous coronary interventions that include percutaneous transluminal coronary angioplasty (PTCA), coronary artery stenting, directional coronary atherectomy (DCA), and rotational atherectomy.

REPOLARIZATION The electrical process by which a depolarized cell returns to its polarized, resting state.

REPOLARIZATION WAVE The progression of the repolarization process through the atria and ventricles that appears on the ECG as the atrial and ventricular T waves.

REPOLARIZED STATE The condition of the cell when it has been completely repolarized.

RESTING MEMBRANE POTENTIAL Electrical measurement of the difference between the electrical potential of the interior of a fully repolarized, resting cell and that of the extracellular fluid surrounding it.

RESTING STATE OF A CELL The condition of a cell when a layer of positive ions surrounds the cell membrane and an equal number of negative ions lines the inside of the cell membrane directly opposite each positive ion. A cell in such a condition is called a polarized cell.

RESUSCITATION The restoration of life by artificial respiration and external chest compression.

RETAVASE Trade name for reteplase (r-PA), a thrombolytic agent.

RETEPLASE (r-PA) A thrombolytic agent that converts plasminogen, a plasma protein, to plasmin, which in turn dissolves the fibrin binding the platelets together within a thrombus (fibrinolysis), causing the thrombus to break apart (thrombolysis). Trade name: Retavase.

RETROGRADE The movement in the opposite direction compared with normal.

RETROGRADE ATRIAL DEPOLARIZATION Abnormal depolarization of the atria that begins near the AV junction, producing a negative P′ wave in Lead II; typically associated with junctional dysrhythmias.

RETROGRADE AV BLOCK Delay or failure of backward conduction through the AV junction into the atria of electrical impulses originating in the bundle of His or ventricles.

RETROGRADE CONDUCTION Conduction of an electrical impulse in a direction opposite to normal (i.e., from the AV junction or ventricles [through the AV junction] to the atria or SA node). Same as retrograde AV conduction.

RIGHT AND LEFT ATRIA Two upper chambers of the heart; are thin-walled.

RIGHT AND LEFT VENTRICLES The lower two chambers of the heart; are thick-walled and muscular.

RIGHT ATRIAL ENLARGEMENT (RIGHT ATRIAL DILATATION AND HYPERTROPHY) Usually caused by increased pressure and/or volume in the right atrium. It is found in pulmonary valve stenosis, tricuspid valve stenosis and insufficiency (relatively rare), and pulmonary hypertension and right ventricular hypertrophy from various causes. These include chronic obstructive pulmonary disease (COPD), cor pulmonale, status asthmaticus, pulmonary embolism, pulmonary edema, mitral valve stenosis or insufficiency, and congenital heart disease.

RIGHT ATRIAL OVERLOAD Increased pressure and/or volume in the right atrium.

RIGHT AXIS DEVIATION (RAD) A QRS axis greater than 190°. Extreme right axis deviation—a QRS axis between 290° and 6180° (indeterminate axis).

RIGHT BUNDLE BRANCH (RBB) Part of the electrical conduction system of the heart that conducts electrical impulses into the right ventricle.

RIGHT BUNDLE BRANCH BLOCK (RBBB) Defective conduction of electrical impulses through the right bundle branch. It may be complete or incomplete and be present with or without an intact interventricular septum. Typical ECG patterns:

- rSR′ pattern in lead V_1, the so-called "M" (or rabbit ears) pattern
- Tall "terminal" R waves in leads aVR and V_1-V_2
- Deep and slurred "terminal" S waves in leads I, aVL, and V_5-V_6
- qRS pattern in leads V_5-V_6—typical of right bundle branch block with an intact interventricular septum
- QSR pattern in leads V_1-V_2—typical of right bundle branch block without an intact interventricular septum.

RIGHT CORONARY ARTERY Arises from the aorta just above the right aortic coronary cusp.

RIGHT HEART The right half of the heart consisting of the right atrium and right ventricle.

RIGHT HEART FAILURE Inadequacy of the right ventricle to maintain the normal circulation of blood. This results in distended veins of the body, especially the jugular veins; body tissue edema; and congestion and distension of the liver and spleen. The lungs are typically clear.

RIGHT PRECORDIAL (OR SEPTAL) LEADS Leads V_1-V_2.

RIGHT PRECORDIAL (UNIPOLAR) LEADS Leads V_2 R, V_3 R, V_4 R, V_5 R, and V_6 R; each obtained using a positive electrode attached to a specific area of the right anterior chest wall and a central terminal. The right precordial leads overlie the right ventricle. The positive electrode for each right precordial lead is attached as follows:

V_2 R: Right side of the sternum in the fourth intercostal space

V_3 R: Midway between V_2 R and V_4 R

V_4 R: Right midclavicular line in the right fifth intercostal space

V_5 R: Right anterior axillary line at the same level as V_4 R

V_6 R: Right midaxillary line at the same level as V_4 R

RIGHT VENTRICULAR HYPERTROPHY (RVH) Increase in the thickness of the right ventricular wall because of chronic increase in pressure and/or volume within the ventricle. It is found in pulmonary valve stenosis and other congenital heart defects (e.g., atrial and ventricular septal defects), tricuspid valve insufficiency (relatively rare), and pulmonary hypertension from various causes. These include chronic obstructive pulmonary disease (COPD), status asthmaticus, pulmonary embolism, pulmonary edema, and mitral valve stenosis or insufficiency.

RIGHT VENTRICULAR MI A myocardial infarction caused by the occlusion of the right coronary artery and characterized by early changes in the ST segments and T waves (i.e., ST elevation and tall, peaked T waves) and taller than normal R waves in leads II, III, and aVF, and ST-segment elevation in V4 R and the appearance later of abnormal QS waves or complexes with T wave inversion in leads II, III, and aVF and T wave inversion in V4 R.

RIGHT VENTRICULAR OVERLOAD Increased pressure and/or volume in the right ventricle.

RINGER'S LACTATE SOLUTION Frequently used sterile IV solution containing sodium, potassium, calcium, and chloride ions in about the same concentrations as present in blood, in addition to lactate ions.

R-ON-T PHENOMENON An ominous type of premature ventricular complex (PVC) that falls on the T wave of the preceding QRS-T complex. This can cause ventricular tachycardia or ventricular fibrillation.

ROTATIONAL ATHERECTOMY The use of a rotational, drill-like device to remove a calcified thrombus.

r-PA See *Reteplase (r-PA)*.

RP' INTERVAL The section of the ECG between the onset of the QRS complex and the onset of the P' wave following it. This is present in junctional dysrhythmias and occasionally in ventricular dysrhythmias.

R PRIME (R') The second R wave in a QRS complex.

R-R INTERVAL The section of the ECG between the onset of one QRS complex and the onset of an adjacent QRS complex or between the peaks of two adjacent R waves.

RS PATTERN Refers to the appearance of a QRS complex in which there is an initial tall R wave followed by a deep S wave.

rSR' PATTERN A typical QRS complex pattern in V_1 present in right bundle branch block. Also referred to as the "M" or "rabbit ears" pattern.

RUPTURE (DISRUPTION) OF THE FIBROUS CAP An abrupt tear in the leading edge of atheromatous plaque. Most likely to occur at its leading edge, the area of the cap where it connects with the normal arterial wall.

R WAVE The positive wave or deflection in the QRS complex. An upper case "R" indicates a large R wave; a lower case "r," a small R wave. May be tall or small; narrow or wide, slurred, or notched.

S

SALVOS Refers to two or more consecutive premature complexes. Bursts.

SA NODE The dominant pacemaker of the heart located in the wall of the right atrium near the inlet of the superior vena cava.

SAWTOOTH APPEARANCE Description given to atrial flutter waves.

SCOOPED-OUT APPEARANCE Description given to the depression of the ST segment caused by digitalis. Also referred to as the "digitalis effect."

S DOUBLE PRIME (S") The third S wave in the QRS complex.

SECONDARY PACEMAKER OF THE HEART A pacemaker in the electrical system of the heart other than the SA node; an escape or ectopic pacemaker.

SECOND-DEGREE AV BLOCK A dysrhythmia in which one or more P waves are not conducted to the ventricles. Incomplete AV block. See *AV block, second-degree, type I (Wenckebach)*; *AV block, second-degree, type II*; and *AV block, second-degree, 2:1, and advanced*.

SECOND-DEGREE, TYPE I AV BLOCK (WENCKEBACH) A dysrhythmia in which progressive prolongation of the conduction of electrical impulses through the AV node occurs until conduction is completely blocked. It is characterized by progressive lengthening of the PR interval until a QRS complex fails to appear after a P wave. This phenomenon is cyclical. See *Mobitz I AVB*.

SECOND-DEGREE, TYPE II AV BLOCK A dysrhythmia in which a complete block of conduction of the electrical impulses occurs in one bundle branch and an intermittent block in the other. It is characterized by regularly or irregularly absent QRS complexes (producing, commonly, an AV conduction ratio of 4:3 or 3:2). The QRS complexes, typically, are abnormally wide (greater than 0.12 second in duration). See *Mobitz II AVB*.

SECOND-DEGREE, 2:1, AND ADVANCED AV BLOCK A dysrhythmia caused by defective conduction of the electrical impulses through the AV node or the bundle branches or both. It is characterized by regularly or irregularly absent QRS complexes (producing, commonly, an AV conduction ratio of 2:1 or greater). The QRS complexes may be narrow (0.10 second or less) or abnormally wide (greater than 0.12 second in duration).

SEGMENT A section of the ECG between two waves (e.g., PR segment, ST segment, and TP segment). A segment does not include waves or intervals.

SELF-EXCITATION, PROPERTY OF The property of a cell to reach a threshold potential and generate electrical impulses spontaneously without being externally stimulated. Also referred to as the "property of automaticity."

SEPTAL DEPOLARIZATION Refers to the depolarization of the interventricular septum early in ventricular depolarization, producing the septal q and r waves.

SEPTAL LEADS Leads V_1-V_2. The right precordial leads.

SEPTAL MI A myocardial infarction commonly caused by occlusion of the left anterior descending (LAD) coronary artery beyond the first diagonal branch, involving the septal perforator arteries and characterized by early changes in the ST segments and T waves (i.e., ST elevation and tall, peaked T waves) and the early appearance of abnormal Q waves in leads V_1-V_2.

SEPTAL q WAVES The small q waves produced by the normal left-to-right depolarization of the interventricular septum early in ventricular depolarization. Present in one or more of leads I, II, III, aVL, aVF, and V_5-V_6.

SEPTAL r WAVES The small r waves produced by the normal left-to-right depolarization of the interventricular septum early in ventricular depolarization. Present in the right precordial leads V_1 and V_2.

SEPTUM A wall separating two cavities.

SEROTONIN A substance released from platelets after the platelets are activated after damage to the blood vessel walls. Serotonin is a potent vasoconstrictor and promotes thrombus formation by stimulating platelet aggregation. Other substances released on platelet activation are adenosine diphosphate (ADP) and thromboxane A2 (TxA2).

SEROUS PERICARDIUM The inner layer of the pericardium.

SERUM CARDIAC MARKERS Proteins and enzymes released from damaged or necrotic myocardial tissue into the blood. These serum markers include myoglobin, CK-MB (creatinine kinase MB isoenzyme), and troponin T and I (cTnT, cTnI).

SHOCK A state of cardiovascular collapse caused by numerous factors such as severe AMI, hemorrhage, anaphylactic reaction, severe trauma, pain, strong emotions, drug toxicity, or other causes. A patient in decompensated shock typically has dulled senses and staring eyes, a pale and cyanotic color, cold and clammy skin, systolic blood pressure of 80 to 90 mm Hg or less, a feeble rapid pulse (over 110 beats per minute), and a urinary output of less than 20 mL per hour.

SHORT VERTICAL LINES The vertical lines inscribed at every 3-second interval along the top of the ECG paper.

SICK SINUS SYNDROME A clinical entity manifested by syncope or near-syncope, dizziness, increased congestive heart failure, angina, and/or palpitations as a result of a dysfunctioning sinus node, especially in the elderly. The ECG may show marked sinus bradycardia, sinus arrest, sinoatrial (SA) block, chronic atrial fibrillation or flutter, AV junctional escape rhythm, or tachydysrhythmias interspersing with the bradycardias (sinus-tachydysrhythmia syndrome).

SIGNS Physical findings seen on the patient's body structure and function that are detected by initial inspection of the patient and by the physical examination.

SINGLE-CHAMBER PACEMAKER Artificial pacemaker that paces either the atria or the ventricles when appropriate.

SINOATRIAL (SA) EXIT BLOCK A dysrhythmia caused by a block in the conduction of the electrical impulse from the SA node to the atria, resulting in bradycardia, episodes of asystole, or both.

SINOATRIAL (SA) NODE See *SA node*.

SINUS ARREST A dysrhythmia caused by a decrease in the automaticity of the SA node, resulting in bradycardia, episodes of asystole, or both.

SINUS ARRHYTHMIA Irregularity of the heart rate caused by fluctuations of parasympathetic activity on the SA node during breathing.

SINUS BRADYCARDIA A dysrhythmia originating in the SA node with a rate of less than 60 beats per minute.

SINUS NODE DYSRHYTHMIAS Dysrhythmias arising in the sinus (SA) node include sinus dysrhythmia, sinus bradycardia, sinus arrest and sinoatrial (SA) exit block, and sinus tachycardia.

SINUS P WAVE A P wave produced by the depolarization of the atria initiated by an electrical impulse arising in the SA node.

SINUS TACHYCARDIA A dysrhythmia originating in the SA node with a rate of over 100 beats per minute.

SITE OF ORIGIN Pacemaker site.

6-SECOND COUNT METHOD A method of determining the heart rate by counting the number of QRS complexes within a 6-second interval and multiplying this number by 10 to get the heart rate per minute.

6-SECOND INTERVALS The period between every third 3-second interval mark.

SLIGHTLY IRREGULAR RHYTHM Over the length of the ECG the amount of R-R interval variation is rarely more than 0.08 seconds.

SLOPE OF PHASE-4 DEPOLARIZATION Refers to the rate at which a cell membrane depolarizes spontaneously, becoming progressively less negative, during phase 4—the period between action potentials. As soon as the threshold potential is reached, rapid depolarization of the cell (phase 0) occurs. The rate of spontaneous depolarization is dependent on the degree of sloping of phase-4 depolarization. The steeper the slope of phase-4 depolarization, the faster the rate of spontaneous depolarization and the rate of impulse formation (the firing rate). The flatter the slope, the slower the firing rate.

SLOW CALCIUM-SODIUM CHANNELS A mechanism in the membrane of certain cardiac cells, predominantly those of the SA and AV nodes, by which positively charged calcium and sodium ions enter the cells slowly during depolarization, changing the potential within these cells from negative to positive. The result is a slower rate of depolarization compared with the depolarization of cardiac cells with fast sodium channels.

SLOW VENTRICULAR TACHYCARDIA See *Accelerated idioventricular rhythm (AIVR)*.

SLURRING OF THE QRS COMPLEX The delta wave.

SMALL SQUARES The areas on ECG paper enclosed by the light horizontal and vertical lines of the grid.

SODIUM BICARBONATE Chemical substance with alkaline properties used to increase the pH or alkalinity of the body when acidosis is present; considered in the treatment of ventricular fibrillation, pulseless ventricular tachycardia, ventricular asystole, and pulseless electrical activity if indicated.

SODIUM-POTASSIUM PUMP A mechanism in the cell membrane, activated during phase 4—the period between action potentials—that transports excess sodium out of the cell and potassium back in to help maintain a stable membrane potential between action potentials.

SPECIALIZED CELLS OF THE ELECTRICAL CONDUCTION SYSTEM OF THE HEART One of two kinds of cardiac cells in the heart, the other being the myocardial (or "working") cells. The specialized cells conduct electrical impulses extremely rapidly (six times faster than do the myocardial cells), but do not contract. Some of these cells, the pacemaker cells, are also capable of generating electrical impulses spontaneously, having the property of automaticity.

SPIKES Artifacts in the ECG. If numerous and occurring randomly, they are most likely caused by muscle tremor, AC interference, loose electrodes, or biotelemetry-related interference. If they are regular, occurring at a rate of about 60 to 80/minute, they are most likely caused by an artificial pacemaker.

SPONTANEOUS DEPOLARIZATION Property possessed by pacemaker cells allowing them to achieve threshold potential and depolarize without external stimulation.

S PRIME (S′) The second S wave in the QRS complex.

S1Q3T3 PATTERN Typical ECG changes in lead I and lead III that occur in acute pulmonary embolism (i.e., large S wave in lead I and a Q wave and inverted T wave in lead III).

STANDARD (BIPOLAR) LIMB LEADS Standard limb leads I, II, and III; each obtained using a positive electrode attached to one extremity and a negative electrode to another extremity as follows:

Lead I: The positive electrode attached to the left arm and the negative electrode to the right arm.

Lead II: The positive electrode attached to the left leg and the negative electrode to the right arm. Commonly used as a monitoring lead in prehospital emergency cardiac care.

Lead III: The positive electrode attached to the left leg and the negative electrode to the left arm.

STANDARD LEADS Usually refers to the 12 ECG leads—leads I, II, III, aVR, aVL, aVF, and V_1-V_6.

STANDARD LIMB LEADS Leads I, II, and III.

STANDARD PAPER SPEED A rate of 25 mm per second.

STANDARDIZATION OF THE ECG TRACING A means of standardizing the amplitude of the waves and complexes of the ECG using a 1 mV/10 mm standardization impulse.

ST AXIS The mean of all the vectors generated during the ST-segment.

STENT A cylindrical coil or wire mesh. See *Coronary artery stenting.*

STRAIN PATTERN Refers to the combination of a downsloping ST-segment depression and a T wave inversion, characteristic of long-standing right or left ventricular hypertrophy. Along with the R wave, gives the so-called "hockey stick" appearance to the QRS-ST-T complex.

ST SEGMENT The section of the ECG between the end of the QRS complex, the "J" point, and onset of the T wave. May be flat (horizontal), downsloping, or upsloping.

ST-SEGMENT DEPRESSION An ECG sign of severe myocardial ischemia, appearing in the leads facing the ischemia. An ST segment is considered to be depressed when it is 1 mm (0.1 mV) below the baseline, measured 0.04 second (1 small square) after the J point of the QRS complex. It may be flat, upsloping, or downsloping. ST depression is also seen in the leads opposite those with ST elevation.

ST-SEGMENT ELEVATION An ECG sign of severe, extensive, myocardial ischemia and injury in the evolution of an acute Q-wave MI, usually indicating a transmural involvement. Less frequently, it may be seen in an acute non–Q-wave MI. An ST segment is considered to be elevated when it is 1 mm (0.1 mV) above the baseline, measured 0.04 second (1 small square) after the J point of the QRS complex. ST elevation usually occurs in the leads facing the myocardial ischemia and injury. ST elevation is also present in pericarditis and early repolarization.

ST-T WAVE The section of the ECG between the end of the QRS complex and the end of the T wave that includes the ST-segment and T wave.

SUBENDOCARDIAL Located under the endocardium.

SUBENDOCARDIAL AREA The inner half of the myocardium.

SUBENDOCARDIAL, NON–Q-WAVE MI A myocardial infarction localized in the subendocardial area of the myocardium with absent Q waves in the ECG most of the time. See *Non–Q wave myocardial infarction.*

SUBEPICARDIAL Located under the epicardium.

SUBEPICARDIAL AREA The outer half of the myocardium.

SUBLINGUAL Under the tongue. Subglossal.

SUBSTERNAL Under the sternum (retrosternal).

SUDDEN CARDIAC DEATH Sudden and unexpected death usually from coronary heart disease in patients with relatively minor or vague premonitory symptoms who appear well. Usual cause: a life-threatening dysrhythmia.

SUPERIOR VENA CAVA One of the two largest veins in the body that empty venous blood into the right atrium.

SUPERNORMAL PERIOD The short terminal phase of repolarization (phase 3) of cardiac cells near the end of the T wave, just before the cells return to their resting potential, during which a stimulus weaker than is normally required can depolarize the cardiac cells.

SUPERNORMAL PERIOD OF VENTRICULAR REPOLARIZATION The last phase of repolarization during which the cell can be stimulated to depolarize by an electrical stimulus weaker than usual (i.e., a subthreshold stimulus).

SUPERVENTRICULAR DYSRHYTHMIA Dysrhythmias originating in the SA node, atria or AV junction with bundle branch block, intraventricular conduction defect, aberrant ventricular conduction, or ventricular preexcitation.

SUPRAVENTRICULAR Refers to the part of the heart above the bundle branches; includes the SA node, atria, and AV junction.

SUPRAVENTRICULAR DYSRHYTHMIA A dysrhythmia originating above the bifurcation of the bundle of His.

SUPRAVENTRICULAR TACHYCARDIA A dysrhythmia originating above the bifurcation of the bundle of His in the SA node, atria, or AV junction, with a rate of over 100 beats per minute.

SUSTAINED VENTRICULAR TACHYCARDIA Prolonged ventricular tachycardia.

S WAVE The first negative or downward wave of deflection of the QRS complex that is preceded by an R wave. An upper case "S" indicates a large S wave; a lower case "s" indicates a small S wave. May be deep and narrow or wide and slurred.

SYMPATHETIC (ADRENERGIC) ACTIVITY The excitatory action on the heart, blood vessels, and other organs brought on by the stimulation of the sympathetic nervous system. The effect on the heart and blood vessels results in an increase in heart rate, cardiac output, and blood pressure.

SYMPATHETIC (ADRENERGIC) NERVOUS SYSTEM Part of the autonomic nervous system involved in the control of involuntary bodily functions, including the control of cardiac and blood vessel activity. This system stimulates cardiac activity and produces effects opposite those of the parasympathetic nervous system, which depresses cardiac activity. Some effects of sympathetic stimulation are an increase in heart rate, cardiac output, and blood pressure.

SYMPATHETIC TONE Pertains to the degree of sympathetic activity.

SYMPATHOMIMETIC DRUGS Drugs that mimic the effects of stimulation of the sympathetic nervous system (e.g., epinephrine and norepinephrine).

SYMPTOM An abnormal feeling of distress or an awareness of disturbances in bodily function experienced by the patient.

SYMPTOMATIC BRADYCARDIA A bradycardia with one or more of the following signs or symptoms: (1) hypotension (systolic blood pressure less than 90 mm Hg); (2) congestive heart failure; (3) chest pain; (4) dyspnea; (5) signs and symptoms of decreased cardiac output; or (6) premature ventricular complexes. Requires treatment immediately.

SYMPTOMATIC "RELATIVE" BRADYCARDIA Normal sinus rhythm or a dysrhythmia with a heart rate somewhat above 60 beats per minute with signs or symptoms associated with a symptomatic bradycardia because of the heart rate being too slow relative to the existing metabolic needs. Requires treatment immediately.

SYNCHRONIZED COUNTERSHOCK A direct current (DC) shock synchronized with the QRS complex used to terminate the following:

- Atrial flutter/Atrial fibrillation
- Paroxysmal supraventricular tachycardia (PSVT) with narrow QRS complexes
- Wide-QRS-complex tachycardia of unknown origin (with pulse)
- Ventricular tachycardia, monomorphic (with pulse)
- Ventricular tachycardia, polymorphic, with normal QT interval (with pulse)

SYNCYTIUM A branching and anastomosing network of cells, such as that formed by the interconnection of the cardiac cells to form the myocardium.

SYSTEMIC CIRCULATION Passage of blood from the left ventricle through the aorta, all its branches, and capillaries in the tissue of the body and then to the right atrium through the venules, veins, and vena cavae. The blood vessels in the body (except those in the lungs) and those carrying blood to and from the body.

SYSTOLE (ELECTRICAL) The period of time from phase 0 to the end of phase 3 of the cardiac action potential.

SYSTOLE (MECHANICAL) The period of atrial or ventricular contraction.

T

TACHYCARDIA Considered to be three or more beats occurring at a rate exceeding 100 beats per minute.

TA WAVE Atrial T wave; usually buried in the following QRS complex.

T AXIS The mean of all the vectors generated during the repolarization of the ventricles (i.e., during the T wave).

TEMPORARY TRANSVENOUS PACEMAKER Delivery of electrical impulses generated by an external artificial pacemaker through a catheter threaded through a vein and positioned in the right ventricle.

TENECTEPLASE (TNK-tPA) A thrombolytic agent that converts plasminogen, a plasma protein, to plasmin, which in turn dissolves the fibrin binding the platelets together within a thrombus (fibrinolysis), causing the thrombus to break apart (thrombolysis). Trade name: TNKase.

TERMINAL The final wave of the QRS complex.

TERMINAL R AND S WAVES Typical ECG findings in right bundle branch block—tall "terminal" R waves in leads aVR and V_1-V_2; deep and slurred "terminal" S waves in leads I, aVL, and V_5-V_6.

THIRD-DEGREE AV BLOCK (COMPLETE AV BLOCK) Complete absence of conduction of electrical impulses from the atria to the ventricles through the AV junction. May be transient and reversible or permanent (chronic). Usually associated with abnormally wide QRS complexes, but the QRS complexes may be narrow. See *AV block, third-degree.*

3-SECOND INTERVAL The period between two adjacent 3-second interval lines.

THRESHOLD POTENTIAL The value of intracellular negativity at which point a cardiac cell must reach before the cell will depolarize.

THROMBIN An enzyme formed from prothrombin when prothrombin is exposed to tissue factor released from damaged arterial wall tissue. Thrombin in turn converts fibrinogen to fibrin.

THROMBOLYSIS The breakdown (lysis) of a thrombus (blood clot) by thrombolytic agents such as the normally occurring tissue plasminogen activator (tPA), which converts plasminogen attached to the fibrin strands within the thrombus to plasmin (an enzyme). Plasmin in turn breaks down the fibrin into soluble fragments (fibrinolysis) causing the platelets to separate from each other and the thrombus to break apart. Drugs used for thrombolysis include: alteplase (t-PA) (Activase), reteplase (r-PA) (Retavase), and tenecteplase (TNK-tPA) (TNKase).

THROMBOLYTIC AGENTS A tissue plasminogen activator that converts plasminogen, normally present in the blood, to plasmin, an enzyme that dissolves fibrin (fibrinolysis) within the thrombus, helping to break the thrombus apart (thrombolysis). The following are thrombolytic agents: alteplase (t-PA), reteplase (r-PA), and tenecteplase (TNK-tPA).

THROMBOXANE A2 (TxA2) A substance released from platelets after the platelets are activated following damage to the blood vessel walls. Thromboxane A2 promotes thrombus formation by stimulating platelet aggregation. Other substances released on platelet activation are adenosine diphosphate (ADP) and serotonin. Aspirin inhibits thromboxane A2 (TxA2) formation and its release from the platelets, thus partially impeding platelet aggregation.

THROMBUS (BLOOD CLOT) An aggregation of platelets, fibrin, clotting agents, and red and white blood cells attached to a blood vessel wall.

TISSUE FACTOR A substance present in tissue, platelets, and leukocytes that, when released after injury, initiates the conversion of prothrombin to thrombin.

THROMBUS FORMATION The formation of a blood clot (coagulation) involving a complex interaction between certain blood components (i.e., platelets, prothrombin, and fibrinogen) and von Willebrand factor (vWF), collagen fibers, and tissue factor present in the endothelium and intima lining the blood vessel walls. The four phases of thrombus formation are as follows:

Phase I: Platelet adhesion. See *Platelet adhesion*.

Phase II: Platelet activation. See *Platelet activation*.

Phase III: Platelet aggregation. See *Platelet aggregation*.

Phase IV: Thrombus formation.

Also refers to the fourth phase of thrombus formation when the fibrinogen between the platelets is converted into stronger strands of fibrin by the action of thrombin, itself converted from prothrombin by tissue factor. Plasminogen usually becomes attached to the fibrin during its formation. As the thrombus grows, red cells and leukocytes (white cells) become entrapped in the platelet-fibrin mesh.

TISSUE PLASMINOGEN ACTIVATOR (tPA) A clot-dissolving enzyme normally present in the endothelium of the blood vessel wall that activates plasminogen to convert to plasmin, which, in turn, dissolves the fibrin (fibrinolysis), causing the thrombus to break apart (thrombolysis).

TNK-tPA Tenecteplase (TNK-tPA), a thrombolytic agent.

TNKase Trade name for tenecteplase (TNK-tPA), a thrombolytic agent.

TORSADES DE POINTES A form of ventricular tachycardia characterized by QRS complexes that gradually change back and forth from one shape and direction to another over a series of beats. A French expression meaning "twisting around a point."

TOTALLY IRREGULAR RHYTHM See *Grossly irregular rhythm*.

tPA TISSUE PLASMINOGEN ACTIVATOR (tPA) See *Alteplase (t-PA)*.

TP-SEGMENT The section of the ECG between the end of the T wave and the onset of the P wave. Used as the baseline reference for the measurement of the amplitude of the ECG waves and complexes.

TRANSCUTANEOUS OVERDRIVE PACING The use of a transcutaneous pacemaker to terminate certain dysrhythmias such as polymorphic ventricular tachycardia with a prolonged QT interval (with pulse) and torsades de pointes (with pulse). This is done by adjusting the pacemaker's rate to one that is greater than that of the dysrhythmia.

TRANSCUTANEOUS PACING (TCP, TC PACING) The delivery of electrical impulses through the skin to treat bradycardia from whatever cause, ventricular asystole, and pulseless electrical activity using an external artificial pacemaker. External cardiac pacing.

TRANSMURAL Extending from the endocardium to the epicardium.

TRANSMURAL INFARCTION When the zone of infarction involves the entire or almost entire thickness of the ventricular wall, including both the subendocardial and subepicardial areas of the myocardium.

TRANSMURAL, Q WAVE MI An infarction in which the zone of infarction involves the entire full thickness of the ventricular wall, from the endocardium to the epicardial surface. Abnormal Q waves are usually present.

TRENDELENBURG POSITION One in which the patient is supine on the backboard, the head of which is tilted downward 30 to 40 degrees, and the patient's knees are bent.

TRIAXIAL REFERENCE FIGURE A guide for determining the direction of the QRS axis in the frontal plane, formed by the lead axes of the three limb leads or the three augmented leads, spaced 60° apart around a zero reference point. The two triaxial reference figures, one formed by the standard limb leads and the other by the augmented leads, superimposed, form the hexaxial reference figure.

TRICUSPID VALVE The one-way valve located between the right atrium and the right ventricle.

TRIGEMINY A series of groups of three beats, usually consisting of two normally conducted QRS complexes followed by a premature complex. The premature complex may be atrial, junctional, or ventricular in origin (i.e., atrial trigeminy, junctional trigeminy, ventricular trigeminy).

TRIGGERED ACTIVITY See *Afterdepolarization*.

TRIPHASIC rSR′ PATTERN OF RBBB See *"M" (or rabbit ears) pattern*.

TRIPLICATE METHOD A method used to determine the heart rate.

T WAVE The part of the ECG representing repolarization of the ventricles that follows the QRS complex from which it is separated by the ST-segment if it is present. It may be positive (symmetrically tall and peaked) or negative (deeply inverted).

T WAVE ELEVATION/INVERSION See *Ischemic T waves*.

TxA2 Thromboxane A2 (TxA2).

12-LEAD ELECTROCARDIOGRAM (ECG) The routine (or conventional) ECG consisting of three standard (bipolar) limb leads (leads I, II, and III), three augmented (unipolar) leads (leads aVR, aVL, and aVF), and six precordial (unipolar) leads (leads V_1, V_2, V_3, V_4, V_5, and V_6).

2:1 AV BLOCK An AV block with a 2:1 AV conduction ratio. Also referred to as an *Advanced AV block*.

U

UNCONTROLLED Refers to dysrhythmias such as atrial flutter and atrial fibrillation that are untreated and, consequently, have rapid ventricular rates.

UNCONTROLLED ATRIAL FIBRILLATION When greater than 100 QRS complexes per minute are conducted in the presence of atrial fibrillation.

UNDERLYING RHYTHM The basic rhythm upon which certain dysrhythmias are superimposed, such as sinus arrest and sinoatrial (SA) exit block; AV blocks; pacemaker rhythm; and premature atrial, junctional, and ventricular complexes.

UNFRACTIONATED HEPARIN An anticoagulant.

UNIFOCAL Pertains to a single ectopic pacemaker.

UNIFOCAL PVCs PVCs that originate in the same ventricular ectopic pacemaker site, usually appearing identical (i.e., uniform).

UNIFORM PVCs PVCs having the same appearance and configuration, presumably arising from the same ventricular ectopic pacemaker site (i.e., unifocal).

UNIPOLAR CHEST ("V") LEADS Leads V_1 to V_6.

UNIPOLAR LEADS A lead that has only one electrode, which is positive.

UNIPOLAR LIMB LEADS Leads aVR, aVL, and aVF.

UNMONITORED CARDIAC ARREST Cardiac arrest that is witnessed by the resuscitation team or that has occurred before the arrival of the team and the patient is not being monitored.

UNSYNCHRONIZED SHOCK A direct current (DC) shock not synchronized with the QRS complex, used to treat the following:
- Ventricular tachycardia, polymorphic, with prolonged QT interval (with pulse)
- Torsades de pointes (with pulse)
- Pulseless ventricular tachycardia
- Ventricular fibrillation

UPPERCASE LETTERS Uppercase letters, such as Q, R, S, are used to designate large deflections of the ECG.

U WAVE The positive wave superimposed on or following the T wave. Possibly represents the final phase of repolarization of the ventricles.

V

VAGAL MANEUVERS Methods to increase the vagal (parasympathetic) tone to convert paroxysmal supraventricular tachycardia. See *Valsalva maneuver*.

VAGAL (PARASYMPATHETIC) TONE See *Parasympathetic (vagal) tone*.

VAGUS NERVE The parasympathetic nerve. Consists of the right and left vagus nerves.

VALSALVA MANEUVER Forceful act of expiration against a closed glottis (nose and mouth), producing a bearing down and subsequent rise in intrathoracic pressure. Also accomplished by gentle massage of the carotid bodies on the side of the neck. Used to increase the parasympathetic tone to convert paroxysmal supraventricular tachycardia.

VARIABLE AV BLOCK Refers to an AV block with varying AV conduction ratios (i.e., the ratio of P, P′, F, or f waves to QRS complexes varies).

VASOCONSTRICTION Narrowing the lumen of blood vessels.

VASOCONSTRICTOR A drug, hormone, or substance that constricts the lumen of blood vessels.

VASODILATATION Widening the lumen of blood vessels.

VASODILATOR A drug, hormone, or substance that dilates or widens the lumen of blood vessels.

VASOPRESSOR A drug that causes vasoconstriction.

VASOVAGAL Pertaining to a vascular and neurogenic cause.

VAT See *Ventricular activation time (VAT)*.

VECTOR A graphic presentation, using an arrow, of the electric current generated by the depolarization or repolarization of the atria and ventricles at any one moment of time.

VENTRICLE The thick-walled muscular chamber that receives blood from the atrium and pumps it into the pulmonary or systemic circulation. The two ventricles form the larger lower part of the heart and the apex. They are separated from the atria by the mitral and tricuspid valves.

VENTRICULAR ACTIVATION TIME (VAT) The time it takes for depolarization of the interventricular septum, the right ventricle, and most of the left ventricle, up to and including the endocardial to epicardial depolarization of the left ventricular wall under the facing lead. Also called the "preintrinsicoid deflection or intrinsicoid deflection time (IDT)".

VENTRICULAR ASYSTOLE (CARDIAC STANDSTILL) Cessation of ventricular complexes. See *Asystole*

VENTRICULAR BIGEMINY When PVCs alternate with the QRS complexes of the underlying rhythm.

VENTRICULAR DEMAND PACEMAKER (VVI) A pacemaker that senses spontaneously occurring QRS complexes and paces the ventricles when they do not appear.

VENTRICULAR DIASTOLE The interval or period during which the ventricles are relaxed and filling with blood. The period between ventricular contractions.

VENTRICULAR DILATATION Distention of the ventricle because of increased pressure and/or volume within the ventricle; it may be acute or chronic.

VENTRICULAR DYSRHYTHMIA A dysrhythmia originating in an ectopic pacemaker in the ventricles. Also referred to as "ventricular ectopy".

VENTRICULAR ECTOPY Occurrence of ventricular ectopic beats or rhythms.

VENTRICULAR ENLARGEMENT Ventricular enlargement includes ventricular dilatation and hypertrophy. Common causes include heart failure, pulmonary diseases, pulmonary or systemic hypertension, heart valve stenosis or insufficiency, congenital heart defects, and acute myocardial infarction. See *Left ventricular hypertrophy (LVH)*, *Right ventricular hypertrophy (RVH)*.

VENTRICULAR ESCAPE RHYTHM A dysrhythmia arising in an escape pacemaker in the ventricles with a rate of less than 40 beats per minute.

VENTRICULAR FIBRILLATION/PULSELESS VENTRICULAR TACHYCARDIA Two life-threatening ventricular dysrhythmias that result in cardiac arrest. Treatment is immediate defibrillation.

VENTRICULAR FIBRILLATION (VF, V-FIB) A dysrhythmia originating in multiple ectopic pacemakers in the ventricles characterized by numerous ventricular fibrillatory waves and no QRS complexes.

VENTRICULAR FIBRILLATION (VF) WAVES Bizarre, irregularly shaped, rounded or pointed, and markedly dissimilar waves originating in multiple ectopic pacemakers in the ventricles.

VENTRICULAR FUSION BEAT See *Fusion beat, ventricular.*

VENTRICULAR HYPERTROPHY Enlargement of the ventricular myocardium, the result of an increase in the size of the muscle fibers because of chronic increase in pressure and/or volume within the ventricle. Common causes include heart failure, pulmonary diseases, pulmonary or systemic hypertension, heart valve stenosis or insufficiency, and congenital heart defects. See *Left ventricular hypertrophy (LVH)*, *Right ventricular hypertrophy (RVH)*.

VENTRICULAR OVERLOAD Refers to increased pressure and/or volume within the ventricles.

VENTRICULAR PREEXCITATION The premature depolarization of the ventricles associated with an abnormal accessory conduction pathway, such as the accessory AV pathways or nodoventricular/fasciculoventricular fibers that bypass the AV junction or bundle of His, respectively, allowing the electrical impulses to initiate depolarization of the ventricles earlier than usual. This results in an abnormally wide QRS complex of greater than 0.10 second that characteristically has an abnormal slurring and sometimes notching at its onset—the delta wave. The PR interval is usually less than 0.10 second when ventricular preexcitation is the result of an accessory AV pathway and usually normal when nodoventricular/fasciculoventricular fibers are the cause. The term *ventricular preexcitation* is most commonly used to indicate ventricular preexcitation associated with accessory AV pathway conduction.

VENTRICULAR REPOLARIZATION The electrical process by which the depolarized ventricles return to their polarized, resting state. Ventricular depolarization is represented by the T wave on the ECG.

VENTRICULAR "STRAIN" PATTERN The changes in the QRS-ST-T complex produced by a downsloping ST-segment depression and T wave inversion, characteristic of longstanding right or left ventricular hypertrophy. Also known as the "hockey stick" pattern.

VENTRICULAR SYSTOLE The interval or period during which the ventricles are contracting and emptying of blood.

VENTRICULAR TACHYCARDIA (VT, V-TACH) A dysrhythmia originating in an ectopic pacemaker in the ventricles with a rate between 100 and 250 beats per minute.

VENTRICULAR TRIGEMINY Occurs when there is one PVC for every two QRS complexes of the underlying rhythm, or one QRS complex of the underlying rhythm for every two PVCs.

VENTRICULAR T WAVE (T WAVE) Represents ventricular repolarization.

VERAPAMIL An antiarrhythmic used to treat paroxysmal atrial and junctional tachycardias.

VISCERAL PERICARDIUM See *Epicardium.*

V LEADS Leads V_1, V_2, V_3, V_4, V_5, and V_6. See *Precordial (unipolar) leads.*

VOLTAGE (AMPLITUDE) See *Amplitude (voltage).*

VON WILLEBRAND FACTOR (vWF) A protein stored in the endothelium of blood vessels that, when exposed to blood, binds to the platelets' GP Ib and GP IIb/GP IIIa receptors, adhering the platelets to the collagen fibers in the blood vessel wall.

VULNERABLE PERIOD OF VENTRICULAR REPOLARIZATION The part of the last phase of repolarization during which the ventricles can be stimulated to depolarize prematurely by a greater-than-normal electrical stimulus. This corresponds to the downslope of the T wave.

vWF See *von Willebrand factor (vWF).*

W

WANDERING ATRIAL PACEMAKER (WAP) A dysrhythmia originating in pacemakers that shifts back and forth between the SA node and an ectopic pacemaker in the atria or AV junction. It is characterized by P waves varying in size, shape, and direction in any given lead.

WARNING DYSRHYTHMIAS PVCs that are more prone than others to initiate life-threatening dysrhythmias, particularly after an acute myocardial infarction or ischemic episode:
- PVCs falling on the T wave (the R-on-T phenomenon)
- Multiform and multifocal PVCs
- Frequent PVCs of more than five or six per minute
- Ventricular group beats with bursts or salvos of two, three, or more

WATT/SECONDS Units of electrical energy delivered by a source of energy, such as a defibrillator. One watt/second equals 1 joule.

WAVES Refers to various components of the ECG—the P, Q, R, S, T, and U waves. Waves may be large or small.

WENCKEBACH BLOCK See *Second-degree AV block type I AV block (Wenckebach)*.

WENCKEBACH PHENOMENON A progressive prolongation of the conduction of electrical impulses through the AV node, most commonly until conduction is completely blocked, occurring in cycles. Conduction block may also occur infranodally.

WIDE-QRS-COMPLEX TACHYCARDIA A tachycardia with abnormally wide QRS complexes (greater than 0.12 second) that may be ventricular tachycardia or a supraventricular tachycardia with wide QRS complexes resulting from a preexisting bundle branch block, aberrant ventricular conduction, or ventricular preexcitation.

"WINDOW" THEORY Refers to the popular theory of why Q waves occur over infarcted myocardium. According to this theory, the facing leads over electrically inert infarcted myocardium (or "window") view the endocardium of the opposite noninfarcted ventricular wall, and detect the R waves generated by the opposite wall as large Q waves.

WOLFF-PARKINSON-WHITE (WPW) CONDUCTION Accessory AV pathway conduction, resulting in abnormally wide QRS complexes.

WOLFF-PARKINSON-WHITE SYNDROME When Wolff-Parkinson-White conduction is associated with paroxysmal supraventricular tachycardia with normal QRS complexes.

Z

"ZERO" CENTER OF THE HEART Refers to the hypothetical reference point with an electrical potential of zero, located in the electrical center of the heart—left of the interventricular septum and below the AV junction. Formed by connecting the extremity electrodes together, the "indifferent" zero reference point is used as the central terminal for the unipolar leads. It also represents the central point for the hexaxial reference figure.

ZONES OF INFARCTION (NECROSIS), INJURY, AND ISCHEMIA A myocardial infarction at its height typically consists of a central area of dead, necrotic tissue—the zone of infarction (or necrosis), surrounded immediately by a layer of injured myocardial tissue—the zone of injury, and, lastly, by an outer layer of ischemic tissue—the zone of ischemia.

ZONE OF INJURY Layer of injured myocardial tissue.

ZONE OF ISCHEMIA Outer layer of ischemic tissue.

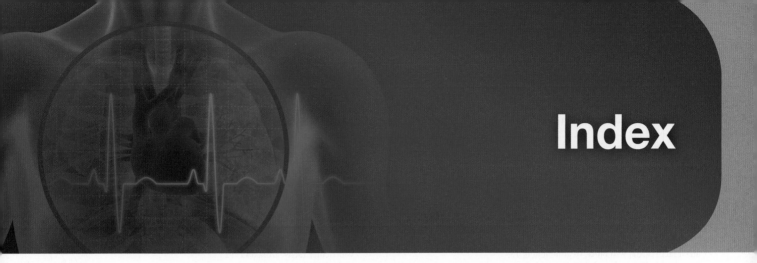

Index

R